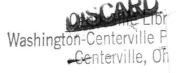

OXFORD MEDICAL PUBLICATIONS

nutrition
a reference handbook

nutrition
a reference handbook

David A. Bender
*Senior Lecturer, Department of Biochemistry and Molecular Biology,
University College London*

and

Arnold E. Bender
*Emeritus Professor of Nutrition,
University of London*

Oxford   New York   Melbourne   Toronto
OXFORD UNIVERSITY PRESS
1997

Oxford University Press, Walton Street, Oxford OX2 6DP
Oxford   New York
Athens   Auckland   Bangkok   Bombay
Calcutta   Cape Town   Dar es Salaam   Delhi
Florence   Hong Kong   Istanbul   Karachi
Kuala Lumpur   Madras   Madrid   Melbourne
Mexico City   Nairobi   Paris   Singapore
Taipei   Tokyo   Toronto

and associated companies in
Berlin   Ibadan

Oxford is a trade mark of Oxford University Press

Published in the United States
by Oxford University Press Inc., New York
© David A. Bender & Arnold E. Bender, 1997

A catalogue record for this book is available from the British
Library.

Library of Congress Cataloging in Publication Data
Bender, David A.
    Nutrition : a reference handbook / David A. Bender and Arnold E.
Bender. — [1st ed.]
       p.   cm. — (Oxford medical publications)
    1. Nutrition–Handbooks, manuals, etc.   2. Food—Handbooks,
manuals, etc.   3. Diet—Handbooks, manuals, etc.   I. Bender Arnold
E. (Arnold Eric)   II. title.   III. Series.
TX353.B45   1997
613.2—dc20   96-13459
                                                     CIP

ISBN 0-19-262368-0

Typeset by Keyword Typesetting Services Ltd
Printed in Great Britain by Biddles Short Run Books, King's Lynn

Preface

Our intention in preparing this reference handbook is to provide, in a single volume, as much as possible of the information about nutrition that is required by anyone working in the broad fields of diet and health, food and nutrition. Not all of the information will be relevant, or perhaps even of interest, to all specialists in all fields, but we hope that we have managed to include the information to answer any nutrition-related questions that any reader may ask.

At the end of each chapter we have included a list of further reading-books and review articles that we have found especially useful, and which we think would be helpful to those who want to delve further into specific topics. Specific references cited in the text, and as sources for the tables, are listed in the bibliography.

Where a single reference is cited as the source of a table, we are grateful to the copyright holder for permission to reproduce the table.

David A. Bender
Arnold E. Bender
March 1996

Acknowledgements

Permission to reproduce copyright material in the following tables is gratefully acknowledged.

2.4, 2.7, 2.10, 2.12, 2.14, 2.16, 2.18, 2.19, 2.20, 2.22, 3.3, 6.3, 6.4, 6.5, 6.7, 6.9, 6.10, 6.11, 8.9, 14.14. Snyder, W.S., Cook, M.J., Nassett, E.S., Karkhausen, L.R., Parry-Howells, G., and Tipton, I.H. (1975). International Commission on Radiological Protection, *Report of the Task Force on Reference Man*, Pergamon Press, Oxford. By permission of the International Commission on Radiological Protection.

2.8. Widdowson, E.M., McCance, R.A. and Spray, C.M. (1951). The chemical composition of the human body. *Clinical Science* 10, 113–25. By permission of the Biochemical Society and Portland Press Ltd.

2.9 Clarys, J.P., Martin, A.D., and Drinkwater, D.T. (1984). Gross tissue weights in the human body by cadaver dissection. *Human Biology* 56, 459–73. By permission of Wayne State University Press.

2.21 Frisancho, A.R. (1974). Triceps skin fold and upper arm muscle size norms for assessment of nutritional status. *American Journal of Clinical Nutrition* 27, 1052–8. By permission of the American Society for Clinical Nutrition.

2.26 Brozek, J. and Keys, A. (1951). The evaluation of leanness-fatness in man, norms and interrelationships. *British Journal of Nutrition* 5, 194–206. By permission of Cambridge University Press.

2.27 and 2.28. Durnin, J.V.G.A. and Womersley, J. (1974). Body fatness assessed from total body density and its estimation from skinfold thickness, measurements on 481 men and women aged from 16 to 72 years. *British Journal of Nutrition* 23, 77–97. By permission of Cambridge University Press.

2.30 Slaughter, M.H., Lohman, T.G., Boileau, R.A., Horswill, C.A., Stillman, R.J., van Loan, M.D., and Bemben, D. (1988). Skinfold equations for estimation of body fatness in children and youth. *Human Biology* 60, 709–23. By permission of Wayne State University Press.

3.11. Fomon, S.J., Haschke, F., Ziegler, E.E., and Nelson, S.E. (1982). Body composition of reference children from birth to age 10 years. *American Journal of Clinical Nutrition* 35, 1169–75. By permission of the American Society for Clinical Nutrition.

3.13, 3.15 and 3.17. Tanner, J.M., Whitehouse, R.H., and Takaishi, M. (1966). Standards from birth to maturity for height, weight, height velocity and weight velocity, British children, 1965, part 1. *Archives of Disease in Childhood* 41, 454–71. By permission of British Medical Journal Publishing Group.

3.14, 3.16, 3.18, 3.21, 3.22 and 3.24. Hamill, P.V., Drizd, T.A., Johnson, C.L., Reed, R.B., Roche, A.F., and Moore, W.M. (1979). Physical growth, National Center for Health Statistics percentiles. *American Journal of Clinical Nutrition* 32, 607–29. By permission of the American Society for Clinical Nutrition.

3.19, 3.20 and 3.23. Jelliffe, D.B., and Jelliffe, E.F.P. (1989). *Community Nutritional Assessment*, Oxford University Press. By permission of Oxford University Press.

3.25. Nellhaus, G. (1968). Head circumference from birth to eighteen years, practical composite international and interracial groups. *Pediatrics* 41, 106–14. By permission of *Pediatrics*.

3.26, 3.27, 3.28 and 3.29. Frisancho, A.R. (1981). New norms of upper limb fat and muscle areas for assessment of nutritional status. *American Journal of Clinical Nutrition* 34, 2540–5. By permission of the the American Society for Clinical Nutrition.

3.30. Frisancho, A.R. (1974). Triceps skin fold and upper arm muscle size norms for assessment of nutritional status. *American Journal of Clinical Nutrition* 27, 1052–8. By permission of the American Society of Clinical Nutrition.

6.16. McConalogue, K. and Furness, J.B. (1994). Gastrointestinal neurotransmitters. *Baillière's Clinical Endocrinology and Metabolism* 8, 1–6. By permission of Baillière-Tindall Ltd.

6.6 MacFarlane, T.W. and Samaranayake, L.P. (1989). *Clinical Oral Microbiology*. Wright, London. By permission of Butterworth-Heinemann Ltd.

7.6 Cummings, J.H. and Englyst, H.N. (1995). Gastrointestinal effects of food carbohydrates. *American Journal of Clinical Nutrition* 61, (suppl). 938–45s. By permission of the American Society for Clinical Nutrition.

7.9, 7.10 and 7.11. Livesey, G. (1992). The energy values of dietary fibre and sugar alcohols for man. *Nutrition Research Reviews* 5, 61–84. By permission of the editor and author.

8.6. British Nutrition Foundation (1995). *Trans fatty acids, Report of the British Nutrition Foundation Task Force*, British Nutrition Foundation, London. By permission of the British Nutrition Foundation.

10.38. Scriver, C.R., Gregory, D.M., Sovetts, D., and Tissenbaum, G. (1985). Normal plasma free amino acids in adults, the influence of some common physiological variables. *Metabolism* 34, 863–73. By permission of W B Saunders Company.

13.6 and 13.8. Xerophthalmia Club (1990). *Xerophthalmia Club Bulletin* no. 45. International Centre for Eye Health, 27 Cayton Street, London EC1V 9EJ. By permission of the Editor, Xerophthalmia Club Bulletin.

21.7 and 21.8. Herbert, V. (1987). The 1986 Herman Award Lecture, nutrition science as a continually unfolding story, the folate and vitamin B_{12} paradigm. *American Journal of Clinical Nutrition* 46, 387–402. By permission of Dr V Herbert.

24.14. Herbert, V. (1987). The 1986 Herman Award Lecture, nutrition science as a continually unfolding story, the folate and vitamin B_{12} paradigm. *American Journal of Clinical Nutrition* 46, 387–402. By permission of the American Society for Clinical Nutrition.

25.13. Milne, D.B. and Johnson, P.E. (1993). Assessment of copper status, effect of age and gender on reference ranges in healthy adults. *Clinical Chemistry* 39, 883–77. By permission of the American Association for Clinical Chemistry.

Contents

List of tables

List of figures

The historical development of nutritional concepts

If one distinguishes between nutrition—the study of foods in relation to the living organism—and dietetics—recommendations for treatment of disorders by dietary change—then dietetics has the longer history. Among the writings of Hippocrates (460–360 BC) is the injunction 'Let your food be your medicine, and your only medicine be your food.'

The ancient Egyptian medical text, Eber's Papyrus (1550–1570 BC) prescribed squeezing roasted beef liver against the eye for diseases of the eye, ancient Chinese writings (1600 BC) prescribed liver (dipped in honey), and Galen (AD 129–199) recommended regular consumption of goat liver for night blindness. Scurvy was described in Eber's Papyrus and Hippocrates (460–360 BC) listed the symptoms. Goitre is mentioned in ancient Chinese medical writings and the physician, Souen-Sse-mo (AD 581–682), recommended seaweed (a source of iodine) as a remedy. The description of rickets was more recent (Daniel Whistler in 1645), but cod-liver oil was a traditional remedy, first formally introduced into medical practice in the late eighteenth century.

Nutritional science was effectively founded by Lavoisier in the eighteenth century but had its roots in observations (rather than experimentation) made by the ancient Greeks. Some of the principles enunciated at that time were incorrect, while others waited two millennia for verification (Guggenheim 1981). Current science at that time, and for many centuries after, included the belief that exercise 'consumes the body', while food replenishes what exercise has consumed, that food supplies both building material and energy. A distinction was made between requirements for growth and maintenance, and for rest and muscular activity.

Aristotle (384–322 BC) stated that food is broken up mechanically in the mouth, undergoes a first 'concoction' in the stomach (pepsis), that the fluid portion is of use in nutrition and absorbed by the blood vessels of the stomach and intestine while the solid and indigestible portions are excreted in the faeces. 'When nourishment is abundant flesh is formed, whereas excess is converted into fat–too much fat is harmful'.

Most conclusions were reached from observation and direct experimentation was rare; the writings of Galen (AD 129–199) carried such authority that they formed the basis of medical science for the next 1500 years. He wrote that 'nutrition is a metabolic process occurring in the tissues–food must be prepared or altered by the action of saliva and further changed in the stomach'; the process was regarded as one of change of quality. He stated that any disturbance in the integrated process of absorption, distribution, metabolism, assimilation and excretion would upset the delicate balance of the body and lead to emaciation or obesity. He even advocated 'swift exercise' such as running as a means of reducing obesity—a concept only recently rediscovered.

Long before the time of Lavoisier, Galen compared the production of heat from food with the process of combustion as it occurs outside the body, a concept that waited 1500 years for evidence. Centuries later Avicenna (908–1037) codified ancient and Muslim medical knowledge along the lines of Galen.

Advances in knowledge came with the work of the Flemish anatomist Andreas Vesalius (1514–1564) who wrote 'On the fabric of the human body' in 1543, for teaching purposes and discussed nutrition in relation to the abdominal cavity, but still followed traditional Galenic physiology.

The venous system was centred on the liver until William Harvey (1578–1657) wrote his essay 'The circulation of the blood' in 1628, and centred the venous system on the heart; the liver lost its paramount place in nutritional physiology (Guggenheim, 1981).

Paracelsus (1493–1547) gathered together the agglomeration of primitive ideas into a more coherent form and challenged some of the ideas of classical medical science. He did, however, pass on the Doctrine of Signatures which stated that 'like cures like'—because beetroot is red it cures anaemia, herbs with yellow sap cure jaundice. However, more correctly, he introduced the concept that the properties of food could be measured in terms of its chemical composition, a concept that was not verified for several hundred years.

1.1   The development of modern concepts

While today we describe nutrition as an integrated science, including basic sciences such as chemistry and physics, allied sciences such as medicine, physiology, biochemistry, and microbiology, as well as the social sciences, over the centuries contributions were made by physicians, chemists, pharmacists, and physiologists in particular, with additional inputs from engineers and physicists, as well as scientists who developed appropriate techniques in their own specialities.

The development of current nutritional concepts can be divided into five overlapping phases.

1. Late eighteenth through nineteenth centuries. Energy balance, the concepts of utilization of foods as the source of energy for physical work, measurement of carbon balance. There are still outstanding problems of the metabolic energy yields of complex carbohydrates (see section 7.4) and alcohol (see section 9.1), and it was only with the development of dual-isotopically labelled water methods in the 1980s (see section 5.2.2.3) that it became possible to estimate energy expenditure over a period of more than a few hours.

2. Nineteenth century through the first half of the twentieth century. Recognition of the special importance of nitrogenous compounds (proteins), and the definition of essential amino acids. As recently as 1989 the established requirements for essential amino acids, based on studies of nitrogen balance, were challenged on the basis of studies of the rate of oxidation of isotopically labelled amino acids.

3. First half of the twentieth century. Discovery and elucidation of the structures and functions of the vitamins (see section 1.3). Vitamin deficiencies were common in industrialized countries during this period, as was simple hunger. New physiological functions of vitamins continue to be reported.

4. Second half of the twentieth century. A shift in emphasis in industrialized countries away from problems of deficiency and towards the role of diet in the aetiology of diseases of affluence; the problems of obesity rather than hunger. In less developed countries, problems of deficiency continue to be important, but the challenge is the practical one of how to alleviate hunger rather than the physiological one of explaining the role of nutrient deficiency in the aetiology of disease.

5. Last quarter of the twentieth century. Appreciation of the importance of free radicals in disease processes, and the protective roles of antioxidant nutrients (see sections 13.6, 15.5.1 and 22.4.4.4) and non-nutrient compounds in plant foods (see sections 7.6 and 23.3). A shift in the philosophy underlying determination of reference intakes away from prevention of deficiency and towards levels of intake that may be associated with optimum health.

Major scientific advances based on experiment as well as observation started in the seventeenth century and continued at an increasing pace after that. The Italian physician Santorio Sanctorius (1561–1636) published in 1614 the results of experiments in which he weighed his food, drink and excretions. Of a daily intake totalling 8 lb, 3 lb were excreted and 5 lb lost through 'insensible perspiration'. These findings, however, were largely ignored until the discovery of the various gases in air in the eighteenth century.

Thus the Irish scientist, Robert Boyle (1627–1691), showed in 1660 that air was necessary for the life of experimental animals; the English scientist John Mayow (1640–1679) demonstrated in 1674 the relation between combustion and respiration. Oxygen was discovered in 1771, 'fire air', by the Swedish pharmacist, Karl Wilhelm Scheele (1742–1786). The major advances were made by the French chemist Antoine-Laurent Lavoisier (1743–1794) starting with the demonstration of the conversion of oxygen, which he named, into carbon dioxide, both in respiration in the body and combustion outside the body. He quantified the heat generated by the amount of ice melted in an ice calorimeter. Together with the French mathematician Pierre-Simon Laplace (1749–1827) he calculated the relation between the amount of heat produced and the amount of carbon dioxide formed–the birth of calorimetry.

This was the first demonstration that respiration is a chemical, and not merely a mechanical, process. Lavoisier also showed that oxygen consumption increases during physical work and exposure to cold, that it is lower in the fasting state (later termed basal metabolism) and increases during digestion (later called specific dynamic action, then thermogenesis).

Lavoisier is thus designated the father of nutrition. He was also involved in public health nutrition through examining the food supply in prisons, the spoilage of meat and grain, improvements in agriculture and associated problems of sanitation and sewage disposal.

This knowledge was built on by the Italian physiologist and naturalist Lazzaro Spallanzani (1729–1799), whose findings, published posthumously in 1807, showed that all organs of the body take up oxygen and produce carbon dioxide. This finding did not make an impact until the German scientist Theodor Schwann (1810–1882) described, in 1829, tissue respiration and heat production. Lavoisier and the French Academicians in 1787 had given the name 'calorie' to the heat produced in the body, but at that time heat was regarded as an elastic fluid. It was not until 1824 that the French engineer Nicolas Leonard Sadi Carnot (1796–1832) showed in his heat engines that heat was transferred from high to low temperature regions, described heat as the motion of molecules, and showed that heat and mechanical energy are interconvertible .

The next major step forward was the work of 'the father of organic chemistry' Justus von Liebig (1803–1873) with his book 'Animal Chemistry or Organic Chemistry in its application to Physiology and Pathology' in 1834. He concluded that the heat involved in the combustion of food in the body explains the constant temperature of the body, that combustion can take place rapidly or slowly, at high or low temperature, and that the amount of heat liberated is constant. The law of conservation of energy was discovered independently by the German physician Julius Robert Mayer (1814–1878), who defined the calorie, the English physicist James Prescott Joule (1818–1889) and the German physiologist Hermann-Ludwig Fredinand Helmholz (1821–1894), in the same decade as Liebig's publication.

Liebig divided foods into nitrogenous and non-nitrogenous, and considered that the former were converted into blood and muscles, while the latter generated heat, and were therefore termed the respiratory foodstuffs. He believed that muscular work caused the breakdown of muscle and excretion of nitrogen in the urine, and that protein was the fuel for muscle work. Liebig's theory was proved wrong by two Swiss scientists, the physiologist Adolf Fick (1829–1901) and the chemist Johannes Adolf Wislicenus (1835–1902), in a 13 hour mountain climb up the Faulhorn in 1866. They took with them only fat and carbohydrate foods, having abstained from protein foods in the preceding 17 hours. During the climb they each lost less than 6 g of nitrogen in their urine, so demonstrating that muscle power cannot come from oxidation of protein. This was verified by the English chemist Edward Frankland (1825–1899) who measured the heat of combustion of a number of common foods (allowing for the heat of combustion of the excreted urea) and showed that less than half of the energy spent could be accounted for by the nitrogen excreted. (In keeping with modern nomenclature he used the Joule equivalent of mechanical energy for his calculations.)

The balance method of studying nutrition was replaced by a study of intermediary metabolism, stimulated by the French physiologist Claude Bernard (1813–1878). He showed that all animal blood contains sugar 'even when they do not eat it' and that it is especially rich in the blood leaving the liver. He made use of the liver perfusion technique and showed that the liver contains a special glycogenic animal substance (glycogen). Previously nutrition had been regarded as the replacement of worn out body substances; Bernard changed this to a much more complex series of transformations–'indirect nutrition'.

It was about a century later that Rudolf Schoenheimer and his coworkers in the USA labelled organic compounds with deuterium and the stable isotopes of nitrogen and carbon, and demonstrated the continuous process operating in the body–'dynamic equilibrium'.

From then on contributions were made by many scientists to the composition of foods, their energy potential, and the value of fat, carbohydrate and protein as sources of energy. Accurate measurements of energy and oxygen usage and carbon dioxide excretion were made on human beings in greatly improved respiratory chambers (Voit, Pettenkofer, Rubner, Atwater, Rosa, Benedict).

1.2 Proteins

Hippocrates' view that there was only one kind of universal nutrient present in all food was generally accepted until the beginning of the nineteenth century (Guggenheim, 1981). The first challenge came from the French physician François Magendie (1783–1855) in 1816, when he showed that nitrogenous foods were essential to the survival of dogs, and the English chemist and physician William Prout (1785–1850), who in 1834 distinguished between saccharine, oleaginous, and albumin groups of nutrients (and water).

Lavoisier had shown that living things, both vegetable and animal, were composed mainly of carbon, hydrogen, oxygen and nitrogen, but there was a long-standing puzzle as to how food could be converted into flesh and blood–'animalization' theories abounded. There was also the question how herbivorous animals could maintain the same body composition as carnivores when their foods were so low in nitrogen.

Most of the protein problems were solved in the nineteenth century (see Table 1.1). Wet weather early in that century led to the spoilage of cereals and a scarcity of food in parts of Europe. The Academy of Paris appointed a Gelatine Commission in 1815 to enquire whether gelatinous extract of bones could properly replace meat in the diet. In 1817 the Society for Promotion of Arts in Geneva investigated the practicability of utilizing the nutrient contained in bones. (It is interesting to note that a similar flurry of protein research took place about 150 years later when the rapid growth of populations and postulation of 'the protein gap' stimulated a vast amount of research into novel sources of protein ranging from oilseed residues and single-cell protein to vegetable protein texturized to resemble meat.)

Magendie reported on behalf of the Gelatine Commission in 1841 that dogs could not be maintained on gelatine alone, or bread alone, or bread and gelatine, indicating that proteins differ in their nutritional value. Muscle flesh together with fats and mineral salts was adequate, as was wheat gluten, but the Commission was unable to decide whether the results of animal experiments could be applied to man. The Society for the Promotion of Arts reported that 2 kg of bones yielded 500 g of gelatine, and that soup made from it was as nutritious as soup made from 3 kg of meat.

The Dutch chemist and physician Gerard Johann Mulder (1802–1880), at the suggestion of the Swedish chemist Jöns Jakob Berzelius (1779–1848), introduced the term 'protein' in 1839, from the Greek προτειοσ for primary or πρστοσ meaning first, since protein was believed to be the most important of the nutrients.

It had been thought for many years that all 'albuminous' substances were the same since they had the same basic analysis, but these observations and other experiments on animals indicated that this was not so.

The French chemist Jean Baptiste Boussingault (1802–1887), applied chemistry to the study of agriculture–and so is referred to as the founder of scientific agriculture–as well as the utilization of food by animals. He carried out balance experiments in which he analysed intake of food and output of urine, faeces and milk of cows–and showed that herbivorous animals can obtain all the nitrogen they need from fodder.

During the nineteenth century most of the amino acids were isolated from proteins and their structures determined. The British biochemists E.G. Willcock and Frederick Gowland Hopkins (1861–1947) showed in 1906 that maize as a source of protein could not maintain life unless supplemented with the amino acid tryptophan. This indicated the essential nature of this amino acid, a concept explained more fully by the Americans T.B. Osborne and L.B. Mendel in 1914, when they showed that the qualities of different proteins depended on their content of the essential amino acids. Considerable effort was devoted to biological evaluation of protein foodstuffs between 1890 and 1924 (K. Thomas 1909; Osborne *et al.* 1919; Mitchell 1924).

After the last two amino acids were identified, methionine in 1922 and threonine in 1935, it became possible to correlate protein quality with essential amino acid composition. It also became possible to quantify the amino acid requirements for growth and maintenance, first on experimental animals, as a basis for subsequent measurements on human beings (W.C. Rose 1957).

Measurements of the biological value of protein foods led to a misleading concept of first and second class proteins, misleading because diets are not composed of single sources of protein but of multiple mixtures in which many individual proteins complement one another. In the 1960s and 1970s work on proteins was mainly devoted to establishing safe intakes, first on the basis of quality and then on digestibility, as it was realized that the overall protein qualities of diets world-wide were very similar. At the same time it was becoming accepted that there was a 'food gap' rather than a 'protein gap' since, for adults at least, an adequate intake of energy invariably included an adequate intake of protein–even a diet based largely on cereals would supply enough protein for an adult–the end of the 'animalization puzzle' of the nineteenth century.

1.3   Accessory food factors

At the end of the nineteenth century it was generally accepted that adequate nutrition could be maintained by carbohydrates, fats, proteins and mineral salts, despite the expression of opinions and the results of direct experimentation indicating that other (essential) nutrients were present in foods in small amounts. For example, the English pharmacist J. Pereira had published a treatise on Food and Diet in 1843 drawing attention to the fact that the anti-scorbutic properties of lemon juice did not fall into any of the three nutrient categories, to the need for salt in the diet, to the value of fruits and vegetables in maintaining health, and to the need for superphosphate of lime and magnesia for bone formation. He listed 13 elements as dietary essentials—carbon, hydrogen, oxygen, nitrogen, sulphur, phosphorus, chlorine, calcium, sodium, potassium, magnesium, iron and fluorine.

G. Budd, Professor of Medicine at King's College, London, in his only foray into the field of nutrition, published articles in 1842 suggesting that the absence of 'accessory food factors' gave rise to disease–notably scurvy, ulceration of the cornea and imperfect bone formation–i.e. vitamins C, A and D, thus predicting the experimental findings of Lunin, Pekelharing and Hopkins.

On the experimental side, the Russian physician N. Lunin attempted in 1881 to keep mice alive on a purified diet of cane sugar, washed milk curd (casein), fat and a salt mixture resembling the ash from milk. They died in less than a month, whereas those fed solely on milk survived. This was confirmed, again in a single foray into the field, by C.A. Socin (1891) a student of von Bunge.

However, it was not until 1912, when the British biochemist F.G. Hopkins carried out a convincing controlled cross-over experiment, that the existence of 'accessory food factors' was accepted. Hopkins fed rats a diet of casein, lard, sugar, starch, and inorganic salts; they ceased to grow and began to lose weight. The addition of a small amount of milk rectified the situation. In a cross-over trial he fed the supplemented diet and showed that when the milk was withdrawn the animals failed to grow.

In fact the same results had been obtained earlier (in 1906) with mice, by the Dutch physiological chemist C.A. Pekelharing, who concluded that there was an unknown substance in milk which, even in small amounts, is of paramount importance in nutrition. However, his report was published in a Dutch journal and was not known to most investigators until a summary was published in English in 1926.

Until the experiments of Hopkins the germ theory of disease so dominated scientific thinking, following Pasteur's discovery of micro-organisms, that it was not feasible to consider the absence of a substance as the cause of a disease.

The laboratory findings were linked with the recognition of deficiency diseases–beriberi, scurvy and rickets–and gave rise to the concept of vitamins. These were defined as substances present in foods in very small amounts (relative to the three macronutrients) which are essential to life. They were later specified as organic substances, to distinguish them from mineral salts, also needed in small amounts, and it has been more recently shown that two vitamins, niacin (see Chapter 19) and vitamin D (see Chapter 14), can be made in the body from the essential amino acid tryptophan, and through the action of sunshine on the skin respectively, so they are not strictly essential in the diet.

Epidemiological observations and experimental evidence came from the Dutch military surgeon Christiaan Eijkman (1858–1930), investigating the disease beriberi in Batavia (in the Netherlands East Indies, now Indonesia). He showed in 1897 that chickens fed on polished rice developed a paralytic polyneuritis, analogous to human beriberi; it could be cured or prevented with brown rice. At first Eijkman postulated the presence of a toxin in the white rice that was neutralized by a substance in the outer layers of whole rice. His successor, G. Grijns concluded in 1901 that it was the absence of a 'protective factor' in the white rice that was the cause of the disease–thiamin (see Chapter 17) was isolated by Casimir Funk in 1911.

The experiments of Hopkins marked the turning point in acceptance of what was termed the vitamin theory. The name *vitamine* was coined by the Polish chemist Casimir Funk in 1912, working in London, but as more vitamins were identified and found not to be chemically amines, the English biochemist, J.C. Drummond suggested in 1920 that the final 'e' be dropped.

In 1915, Elmer Verner McCollum identified 'fat soluble factor' (vitamin A) and McCollum and Davis identified 'water-soluble B', later subdivided. During the twentieth century many laboratories turned their attention to accessory food factors and identified, isolated, elucidated the structures and finally synthesized, the thirteen vitamins. They can be classed in three groups:

(1) those which are important in public health, as a result of problems due to deficiency (A, B_1, B_2, niacin, C, D and folate);

(2) those rarely, if ever, involved in clinical problems, which were discovered through laboratory investigations (biotin, pantothenate, vitamin E);

(3) those that are occasionally of clinical importance (B_6, K and B_{12}).

During the course of identification of the vitamins, different laboratories found deficiency signs in their experimental organisms and curative effects to which they gave names such as anti-anaemic factor, bios, Wills factor, vitamin M, B_c, factor U, etc. Many of these were found to be the same compound or identical with known substances so the original names were discarded (see Table 23.1).

The original investigations gave rise to names and numbers such as fat-soluble A, B_1, B_2, E, K etc., but when the vitamins were identified chemically they were given their chemical names. However, the term vitamin is used as the generic descriptor of the chemical substances with the same or similar biological effect. Thus vitamin A is used to include both the carotenoids (previously called precursors of vitamin A) and retinol (preformed vitamin A); vitamin B_1 is specifically thiamin; B_6 includes all three forms of the vitamin; K includes the two naturally occurring forms and a range of synthetic variants; E includes four tocopherols and four tocotrienols. The history of the identification of the vitamins is summarized in Table 1.2.

Other substances have been found to be dietary essentials for certain organisms but not essential for man, although some may have a role in the diet in supplementing what is synthesized in the body. Thus inositol, choline, *p*-amino benzoic acid, and vitamin T (carnitine) are of nutritional interest (see Chapter 23).

1.3.1 International Units

When a substance with biological properties has been recognized, the next step is to purify and isolate it. Isolation is tracked by comparison of the extracts and concentrates with some standard material, such as a specific yeast extract or a vegetable or animal concentrate, that has the same biological effect. When comparisons are needed between laboratories, each having its own internal standard, it becomes necessary to establish a standard that can be used in all the laboratories involved, an international standard. An example is the early standard for vitamin A; at that time vitamin A itself, retinol, had not been isolated but there was available 'pure' crystalline carotene which had the biological activity of vitamin A. The international unit of vitamin A was established as 1 μg of a mixed sample of crystalline carotene supplied by the scientists involved. However, almost immediately the standard had been established it was found that the so-called pure carotene was a mixture of isomers and that 1 μg of the mixture was equivalent in potency to 0.6 μg of β-carotene. This then became the international unit for vitamin A, until the pure vitamin (retinol) had been isolated, when it became possible to measure potencies as micrograms of the pure substance.

1.4 Social nutrition

Edward Smith, an English physiologist, nutritionist and social reformer was the first to conduct a dietary survey (1862–3) in an investigation of the medical and nutritional effects of the cotton famine and to compile a 'least cost diet'. He measured protein and calorie intakes–subsequent examination of his data (Barker *et al.* 1970) in the light of modern knowledge could not assess the vitamin intake because of the enormous variability of the vitamin content of foods and the effects of storage and cooking.

Many surveys in developed and developing regions have been carried out in the twentieth century to monitor the health of the populations and assess the availability of food and the possible relations between diet and health.

Allied to that has been the development of social nutrition aimed at ascertaining the effect on nutrient intake of the vast array of factors that influence food choice. With the growing knowledge of the effect of diet on health and various disorders this has become a matter of prime importance. At the same time evidence has come to light of the potentially beneficial effects of some nutrients and other substances present in foods in amounts greater than required to maintain growth and development and the possible treatment of some genetic problems by dietary control.

Further reading

Guggenheim, K.Y. (1981). *Nutrition and Nutritional Diseases, the Evolution of Concepts*. The Collamore Press, D.C. Heath & Co. Lexington, Massachusetts, Toronto.

Munro, H.N. (1964). Historical introduction: the origin and growth of our present concepts of protein nutrition. In *Mammalian Protein Metabolism* (ed. H. N. Munro and J. B. Allison) Chapter 1, pp. 1–26. Academic Press, London.

Table 1.1: Chronology of protein nutrition (see Chapter 10)

1773	Discovery of urea as a major compound in urine
1787	Lavoisier discovered nitrogen (*azote* = without life)
1810	Wolaston isolated cystine from renal calculi
1816	Magendie fed animals a N-free diet; they did not survive, hence N is essential
1820	Discovery of leucine by hydrolysis of meat and wool
1828	Synthesis of urea (an organic compound) from ammonium carbamate (an inorganic compound) (Wöhler)
1839	Mulder coined the name protein for the basic nitrogenous substance present in all N-rich organic compounds
1840	Liebig fed animals on gelatine as sole protein source; showed they were unable to survive
1842	Liebig fed animals fed animals on sugar alone, showed urea continued to be excreted, increasing with exercise. Suggested that protein is the fuel for muscle work
1860	Voit measured difference between intake and excretion of nitrogenous compounds—established the technique of N balance; demonstrated that gelatine alone unable to support N balance
1865	Fick and Wislicenius climbed Faulhorn; showed that urea excreted would not account for protein being energy source for the work done
1901	Hopkins and Cole discovered tryptophan; first chemical reaction for detection and determination of a specific amino acid in proteins
1906	Willcock and Hopkins demonstrated improvement in nutritional value of protein by addition of tryptophan and lysine
1909	Development of biological assay of protein quality (Thomas)
1920-1950	Rose studied N balance with amino acid mixtures; defined essential amino acid requirements
1932	First description of kwashiorkor (Williams)—attributed to protein deficiency with adequate carbohydrate intake
1935	Discovery of threonine from N balance studies with amino acid mixtures
1940s	Schoenheimer *et al.* studied metabolism of [^{15}N]amino acids—concept of dynamic equilibrium
1950s	Perception that problems in developing countries were due specifically to lack of protein
1967	Development of constant infusion techniques with labelled amino acids for measurement of whole body protein turnover (Waterlow and Stephen)
1970s	Appreciation that protein quality of mixed diets varies little; major problem of developing countries is lack of total food (energy) rather than specifically of protein
1973	WHO/FAO estimates of protein requirements based on factorial calculation
1975	Discovery of essentiality of histidine for adults (Kopple and Swendseid)
1985	FAO/WHO/UNU lower estimates of protein requirements based on N balance studies
1988	Catabolic drive proposed to explain the need for protein in an adult (Millward and Rivers)
1989	Young *et al.* challenged essential amino acid requirements based on N balance studies; proposed higher requirements based on amino acid oxidation

Table 1.2: Chronology of the discovery of the vitamins

Vitamin A (see Chapter 13)

1600 BC	Night blindness described in Eber's Papyrus and liver recommended
1500 BC	Chinese prescribed liver and honey as treatment
1915	McCollum and Simmonds named fat-soluble A for the factor in some fats that cured eye disorders
1926	Carr-Price colour reaction for vitamin A developed, permitting chemical measurement
1928	Role in resistance to infection recognized—called 'anti-infective vitamin' (Green and Mellanby)
1930	Carotene from plant sources shown to be converted into vitamin A in the body (Moore; Capper)
1930	Structure of β-carotene and vitamin A (retinol) determined and certain derivatives (e.g. retinaldehyde) synthesized
1932	Retinol isolated (Heilbron) (carotene was isolated in 1831 by Wackenroder)
1947	Retinol synthesized (Isler)
1950	β-Carotene synthesized (Karrer and Inhoffen)
1958	Elucidation of isomerization of retinaldehyde in visual process (Wald)
1969	Role proposed in membrane mucopolysaccharide synthesis (Morton)
1979	Discovery of cellular retinol-binding proteins
1984	Antioxidant role of β-carotene proposed (Burton and Ingold)
1980s	Elucidation of role in controlling gene expression and tissue differentiation
1990s	Recognition of separate importance and functions of retinol and retinoic acid

Vitamin D (see Chapter 14)

1645	Rickets described (Daniel Whistler)
18th century	Cod liver oil used as cure
1838	Experimental rickets produced in puppies (Jules Guerin)
1918	Rickets in puppies shown to be due to dietary deficiency and cured by certain fats (Mellanby)
1922	Anti-rachitic factor in fats distinguished from vitamin A (McCollum *et al.*)
1923	Shown that rickets cured by ultraviolet light, sunlight or cod liver oil (Hume)
1925	Named vitamin D (McCollum *et al.*)
1926	Ergosterol in plants converted into vitamin D and called D_2 (Windhaus and Hess; Rosenheim and Webster)
1932	Structure of D determined (Windhaus; Askew)
1934	7-dehydrocholesterol converted into D_3 (cholecalciferol) (Waddell; Windhaus)
1936	Structure of D_3 elucidated (Windhaus)
1963	Anti-rachitic metabolites of vitamin D detected (Norman *et al.*)
1970	Conversion of D_3 to active metabolites (1,25-dihydroxy vitamin D, calcitriol) shown to take place in the kidney (Fraser and Kodicek) and so vitamin D shown to be analogous to a hormone
1980s	Elucidation of role of calcitriol in gene expression
1990s	Discovery of calcitriol receptors in a variety of tissues not known to be vitamin D-responsive

Vitamin E (see Chapter 15)

1922	Factor in lettuce leaves and butter (distinct from A and B) that prevented resorption of foetus and infertility in female rats (Evans and Bishop)
1925	Named vitamin E
1927	Essentiality for reproduction confirmed by cure of testicular atrophy in male rats
1936	Isolated from wheat germ oil and identified as α-tocopherol (Evans *et al.*)
1938	Structure established (Fernholz) and synthesized (Karrer)
1945	Antioxidant properties recognised (Dam)
1983	Essentiality to human beings firmly established (Muller *et al.*)

Vitamin K (see Chapter 16)

1929	Haemorrhagic disease observed in chicks fed very low fat diets (Dam)
1931	Clotting defect observed (McFarlane *et al.*)
1935	Prevented by factor in hog liver fat, hemp seed and certain vegetables; named vitamin K (Koagulation) (Dam)
1935	Extracted from alfalfa and formed by putrefaction (Almquist and Stokstad)
1939	K_1 isolated from alfalfa and K_2 from putrefied sardine meal
1939	Structure determined and K_1 and K_2 synthesized

Thiamin (vitamin B_1, see Chapter 17)

700	Beriberi described in China
1642	Beriberi described in Europe
1885	Beriberi cured by increased intake of protein foods (Takaki)
1900	Polyneuritis in chickens cured with rice bran (Eijkman and Grijns)
1911	Crystallized (Funk)

Table 1.2: (Cont'd)

1930	Elucidation of coenzyme role of thiamin diphosphate (Peters)
1936	Synthesized (Williams)
1970s	Recognition of role of thiamin triphosphate in nerve conduction

Riboflavin (vitamin B_2, see Chapter 18)

1917	Growth factor recognized in 'water-soluble B'
1932	'Yellow enzyme' described (Warburg and Christian)
1933	Isolation from various sources of pigments with growth promoting properties (flavins) (Kuhn *et al.*)
1935	Synthesized (Kuhn *et al.*)
1937	Flavins from various sources found to be identical; structure elucidated; named riboflavin

Niacin (see Chapter 20)

1735	Pellagra (*la mal de la rosa*) described (Casal)
1867	Nicotinic acid produced by oxidation of nicotine
1928	Pellagra identified as a deficiency disease
1935	Nicotinic acid isolated from Coenzyme II (NADP) (Warburg and Christian)
1935	Nicotinamide isolated from heart muscle (Kuhn and Vetter)
1937	Nicotinamide shown to cure black tongue in dogs and pellagra in human beings
1945	Tryptophan shown to be equally effective (Krehl *et al.*)
1949	Conversion of tryptophan to nicotinic acid explained (Heidelberg)
1956	Equivalence of dietary tryptophan and niacin determined (Horwitt *et al.*)
1980s	Recognition of importance of NAD in ADP-ribosyltransfer; role in cellular regulation and DNA repair

Vitamin B_6 (see Chapter 20)

1926	Dermatitis (acrodynia) produced in rats deficient in 'pellagra- preventative factor' (Goldberger and Lillie)
1934	New factor in vitamin B complex cured lesions in rats; named B_6 (Gyorgi)
1938	Isolated; named pyridoxine
1939	Synthesized
1942	Two other active forms isolated—pyridoxal and pyridoxamine
1950s	Role in amino acid metabolism elucidated (Snell, Metzler, and others)
1954	Shown to be dietary essential for infants
1981	Role in steroid hormone action proposed (Cidlowski and Thanassi)
1990	Function in glycogen phosphorylase elucidated

Folate (see Chapter 21)

1930s	Studies on factors present in liver, kidney, yeast and leafy vegetables in a variety of laboratories using human subjects, chicks, monkeys and micro-organisms resulted in the identification of a number of factors variously called vitamin M, vitamin B_c, factors U, R and S, Wills factor, *Streptococcus lactis* factor, *L. casei* factor, rhizopterin, and leucovorin by their investigators. All were subsequently shown to be derivatives of pteroyl glutamic acid—folic acid
1946	Folic acid synthesized
1990s	Role of folate in preventing neural tube defect discovered

Vitamin B_{12} (see Chapter 21)

1855	Pernicious anaemia described (Addison)
1926	Treated with liver (Minot and Murphy)
1929	Anti-pernicious anaemia principle shown to consist of an extrinsic factor in liver and an intrinsic factor secreted by the stomach needed for its absorption (Castle)
1948	Isolated (Rickes *et al.;* L. Smith)
1958	Shown to exist as several derivatives of cobalamin (Barker *et al.*; Weissbach *et al.*)
1965	Molecular structure determined (Hodgkin)

Biotin (vitamin H, see section 23.1)

1900	Growth factor for yeast discovered and called bios (Wildiers) Subsequently bios I (myoinositol), bios IIA (β-alanine plus pantothenate) and bios II B (biotin)
1927	Dermatitis and hair loss in rats fed large doses of egg white (egg-white injury factor) cured by liver extract
1931	Factor named vitamin H (Haut = skin) (Gyorgi)
1936	Isolated from egg yolk and named biotin (Kogl and Tonnis)
1940-43	Structure elucidated; vitamin H identical with biotin
1942	Egg white injury created in human volunteers and cured with biotin
1942-45	Synthesized

Table 1.2: (Cont'd)

Pantothenic acid (see section 23.2)

1933	Recognized as a growth factor for yeast cells and named (Williams)
1940	Structure established and synthesized (Stiller *et al.*; Williams and Major)
1945	Metabolic role as part of coenzyme A demonstrated (Lipmann)

Ascorbic acid (vitamin C see Chapter 22)

1500 BC	Scurvy described in Eber's Papyrus; and by Hippocrates (400 BC)
1535	Scurvy treated with infusion of swamp spruce by Jacques Cartier
1570	Captain James Lancaster prevented scurvy with lemon juice
1754	Dr James Lind carried out controlled clinical trials at sea and showed curative effect of lemon juice
1907	Guinea pigs used as experimental animals (Holst and Fröhlich)
1928	Pure substance isolated (Szent-Györgi)
1932	Isolated substance shown to be the anti-scorbutic factor (Waugh and King)
1933	Synthesized (Hirst *et al.*; Reichstein *et al.*)

Body composition

In order to determine appropriate levels of energy and nutrient intake, a number of different authorities have defined 'Reference Man and Woman', intended to be a sensible average of the diverse human population. The United Nations Food and Agriculture Organization reference man is aged 25, living in a temperate climate and performing moderate physical work. He weighs 65 kg, while the FAO reference woman weighs 55 kg. These body weights are a mean of the lower weights in less-developed countries (which are generally tropical rather than temperate) and those in western Europe and north America, which are significantly higher on average. The International Commission on Radiological Protection Reference Man weighs 70 kg, and the Reference Woman 58 (see Table 2.4), while the Scientific Committee for Food of the European Union (1993) based its estimates of requirements on both desirable weights (66 kg for men and 57 kg for women) and observed mean weights (75 kg for men and 62 kg for women). The US Recommended Dietary Allowances (National Research Council 1989) are based on the median weights for age, 79 kg for men and 63 kg for women).

Simple measurement of body weight alone does not give useful information without making an allowance for height. As shown in Table 2.1, a number of different indices have been used to express weight for height. The most widely used such index is the Body Mass Index (BMI, Quetelet's index, weight/height^2), first introduced in 1869 by the Belgian statistician Lambert Quetelet (1796–1874), on the basis that there was an approximately linear relationship between weight and height^2. Benn (1971) calculated the regression of log(weight) on log(height) from a number of studies, and suggested that the best height-independent index of relative weight was given by the ratio of weight/height^p, with values of p ranging from 1.8–1.9. Coles (1986) extended Benn's index to apply to children, calculating values of p from the regression of log(weight-for-age) on log(height-for-age). He showed that the best value

of p was 2.0 for preschool children (i.e. the same as BMI), increasing to 3.0 at age 11 and falling back to 2.0 after puberty, and proposed that for any age p could be calculated from $p = 2 + \exp(-0.5 \times (\text{age} - 11)^2)$.

The interpretation of ranges of BMI is shown in Table 2.2; as discussed in section 11.1, the desirable range is based on life expectancy. Ranges of desirable weight for height (based on BMI = 20–25) are given in Tables 11.8–11.10. Ranges of weight for height and age for children are discussed in section 3.3.1

2.1 Chemical composition of the body

It is perhaps surprising that full data for the proximate analysis of the human body (water, fat, protein and ash) have been reported for only six subjects, most of whom died of disease, and therefore may not accurately reflect the composition of the healthy body. The results are shown in Table 2.3. The International Commission on Radiological Protection (Snyder *et al.* 1975) has defined Reference Man and Woman, with the body composition shown in Table 2.4, based on interpretation of, and extrapolation from, such data as are available. Table 2.5 shows the distribution of total body fat.

Analysis of the major minerals was performed on four of the subjects reported in Table 2.3; the results are shown in Table 2.5, expressed per kg fat-free body mass. Table 2.6 shows the total body content of the major minerals of the ICRP Reference Man; estimated body contents of other minerals are shown in Table 25.2

2.1.1 Organs of the body

Table 2.8 shows the percentage of total body weight of the major organs of the body in the four subjects shown in Table 2.3, Table 2.9 the average proportion of adipose tissue, muscle, bone and skin, and Table 2.10 the weights and percentage of body weight of the organs of the ICRP Reference Man and Woman. Table 2.11 shows the proximate composition and DNA and RNA content of individual organs; see Table 5.7 for the contribution of different organs to Basal Metabolic Rate.

2.1.2 Body water and fluid balance

The total water content of the body is 600 mL /kg body weight (men) or 500 mL /kg body weight (women). As shown in Table 2.12, 57 per cent of this is intracellular and 43 per cent extracellular, mainly in the plasma and interstitial lymph. The concentrations of the principal intra- and extracellular electrolytes are shown in Table 2.13; Table 2.14 shows the distribution of blood throughout the body.

Total body water is determined by the dilution of a test dose of isotopically labelled water, which is assumed to equilibrate uniformly in all body water pools. Alternatively, determination of total body potassium, by measurement of the radioactivity of naturally occurring ^{40}K by whole body scintillation counting, can be used to estimate total body water (see section 2.2.1.2). Extracellular water is determined by measuring the dilution of a substance such as inulin (see section 7.3.1), thiosulphate, or thiocyanate, that does not cross cell membranes, and hence equilibrates only in extracellular pools. Intracellular water is then calculated from the difference between total and extracellular water. Table 2.15 shows formulae for estimating total body water, extracellular water and plasma volume from body weight, height and age.

As shown in Table 2.16, 65–70 per cent of total water intake is as visible fluids, with 20–23 per cent as 'hidden' water in foods; the remaining 10–12 per cent is metabolic water, arising from the oxidation of metabolic fuels (see section 5.5). Urine accounts for 47–50 per cent of water output, varying with total fluid intake, and decreasing when sweat losses are higher than normal. Altogether there are some 2–5 x 10^6 sweat glands in the body; a constant number throughout life, so that in an infant the density per cm^2 of skin is 8–10 times that in an adult (see Table 2.18). Most, but not all, of the sweat glands are stimulated to higher activity by heat. The highest density of sweat glands is on the palms of the hand (424 / cm^2 in an adult) and the soles of the feet (416 /cm^2); see section 25.26.3 for a discussion of losses of zinc in sweat on the feet.

2.1.3 Body surface area

The major loss of heat from the body is from the skin; body surface area is an important determinant of heat loss and hence energy requirement. Inter-species comparisons show that while basal metabolic rate (see section 5.3.1) is not related to body weight, it is highly correlated with body surface area. As shown in Table 2.17, there are a number of formulae for the calculation of body surface area, the earliest of which (the Vierordt formula) dates back to 1906; the most widely used formula is that of DuBois and DuBois (dating back to 1916). Martin *et al.* (1984) showed that the various formulae based only on weight and height gave values that were not significantly different from those determined by dissection.

Takai and Shimaguchi (1986) refined the precision with which surface area can be estimated by making an allowance for head circumference as well as weight and height. As can be seen from Table 2.18, correction for head circumference will be more important in young children than adults.

2.1.4 The skeleton

Tables 2.19 and 2.20 show the composition and proximate analysis of the skeleton. See section 14.3.3.3 for a discussion of the turnover of bone mineral, and section 22.4.3 for collagen synthesis. Body weight, and hence estimation of the degree of adiposity, are affected by the size of the skeleton. The breadth of the elbow joint (the distance between the epicondyles of the humerus), measured with the arm flexed upwards, gives an index of skeletal breadth that is not significantly affected by adiposity. Overall frame size is classified as small, medium or large, as shown in Table 2.21.

2.1.5 Skeletal muscle

Skeletal muscle makes up 40 per cent of the adult male body weight and 29 per cent of the adult female. Muscle mass can be estimated by measurement of urinary excretion of creatinine, which is formed by non-enzymic cyclization of creatine and creatine phosphate. Creatinine is metabolically useless, and is excreted in the urine. The amount excreted therefore reflects the total body content of creatine, which in turn is a reflection of skeletal muscle mass, since about 98 per cent of total body creatine is in skeletal muscle. A reasonable approximation of the total mass of skeletal muscle can be calculated from (Forbes and Bruining 1976):

Muscle mass (in kg) = 1.85 x g creatinine excreted /kg body weight /day;

Muscle mass (in kg) = 16.4 x mmol creatinine excreted /kg body weight /day.

Dietary creatine (from meat) also gives rise to urinary creatinine, so subjects should abstain from meat for two days before determination of creatinine excretion, and the collection of a precise 24 hour urine sample is obviously important. Creatinine excretion increases somewhat after moderately severe exercise, followed by a period of lower excretion, in compensation.

Table 2.22 shows the distribution of skeletal muscle and its composition.

2.1.5.1 Anthropometry of limb muscle

Skeletal muscle, and especially limb muscle, acts as a source of amino acids that are metabolized as metabolic fuel during the fasting state (see section 5.5). As discussed in section 10.8.3.3, there is a normal cycling between muscle protein synthesis (in the fed state) and its catabolism in the fasting state. More importantly, measurement of the diameter, circumference or area of limb muscle provides a useful index of the general state of nutrition, falling significantly in protein-energy malnutrition (see section 12.2).

Table 2.23 shows the formulae used to calculate parameters of arm muscle from the limb circumference and skinfold thickness (a measure of subcutaneous adipose tissue, see section 2.2.1.7). The formulae make allowance for the diameter of the bone. However, Heymsfield *et al.* (1982) reported that the formulae for arm muscle area over-estimated the values obtained by computerized axial tomography (CAT) scanning by 20–25 per cent. They proposed the modified formulae shown in the last two rows of Table 2.23. Reference ranges and median values of arm muscle size at different ages are shown in Tables 3.28–3.30.

2.2   Body fat

The total body weight can be considered to consist of either lean body mass plus adipose tissue, or fat-free mass plus fat. Lean body mass differs from fat-free mass in that it contains essential body fat. The lean body or fat-free mass, in turn, consists of bone mineral and metabolically active tissue.

Clinically, what is needed is an assessment of adipose tissue, as an index of the adequacy or otherwise of body energy reserves. Experimentally, what can be determined is the fat content of the body and/or the fat-free mass. Garrow (1983) noted that fat and adipose tissue are not synonymous, and while the non-fat component of adipose tissue (see Table 2.24) may be negligible in lean subjects, in obese people it makes a significant contribution to basal metabolic rate (see Chapter 11 and section 5.4).

All of the methods for indirect estimation of lean body mass or fat-free mass described below involve the following assumptions, none of which is wholly strictly justified.

1.   Lean body mass contains a constant proportion of water, is of constant composition, and has a constant density.

2.   Bone is a constant proportion of lean body mass (but bone density decreases significantly with age, see section 14.5).

3.   Cell water is a constant proportion of cell mass.

2.2.1 Methods for the estimation of body fat

A number of different methods are available for estimation of the fat content of the body; of these only two—determination of skinfold thickness (see section 2.2.1.7) and methods based on the electrical conductivity of the body (see section 2.2.1.8)—can be considered routine procedures; the other methods, while of value in research, cannot, for various reasons, be performed routinely.

2.2.1.1 Direct determination of body density

The density of body fat is 0.90, while that of the fat-free body mass is 1.10. Direct determination of the density of the body therefore permits calculation of the proportions of fat-free and fat mass. Considerable precision is required, since the density of the body at 10 per cent fat (below an acceptable range) is 1.08, while at 50 per cent fat (severe obesity) the density is 1.00.

The original method of determining body density is by weighing in air and in water—a procedure that requires total immersion, and therefore cannot be considered a routine procedure. An allowance must be made for the air in the lungs and gastrointestinal tract. Lung volume can be determined by gas washout techniques, but there are no reliable methods for estimation of the gas content of the gastrointestinal tract; a volume of 100 mL is generally assumed.

An alternative method of determining body density is by measurement of the volume of the body by plethysmography. The plethysmograph chamber is filled with water, then a weight of water equal to the subject's body weight is removed, and the subject is immersed up to the neck, with the head covered by a clear plastic dome. The rise in the water level gives the volume of the body. The volume of air surrounding the head and in the lungs and gastrointestinal tract is then determined by measuring the change in pressure produced by a pump of known stroke volume (Garrow *et al.* 1979; Gundlach *et al.* 1980).

The percentage body fat can be calculated from density using the following formulae:

percentage fat = (4.950/density)−4.50 (Siri 1956)

percentage fat = (4.570/density)−4.142 (Brozek *et al.* 1963).

For densities between 1.03–1.09 these two formulae yield results that agree to within about 1 per cent; for more than about 30 per cent of body weight as fat, the Siri formula yields higher values of density that that of Brozek *et al.*

If total body water is also determined (see section 2.2.1.2) then a more precise estimate can be obtained from

percentage fat = (2.118/density)−0.78 x total body water−1.354 (Siri 1961)

Although direct determination of body density is not a routine procedure, it is the standard against which all alternative, indirect, methods must be calibrated. The standard error of fat determination by densitometric methods is of the order of ±2 per cent of body weight or ±10 per cent of the weight of fat.

2.2.1.2 Determination of total body water

As discussed in section 2.1.2, total body water can be determined by the dilution of isotopically labelled water. This is a non-invasive procedure, since the water is given by mouth, and the isotopic dilution can be measured in urine or saliva, although plasma gives better reproducibility and precision. It is assumed that the tracer equilibrates throughout body water pools within 2 hours, and that there is constant dilution over the next 2–3 hours.

If stable isotopes are to be used (^2H_2O or $H_2^{18}O$) then a relatively large amount of (costly) isotope is required to achieve adequate sensitivity; although greater sensitivity is possible using radioactive ^3H_2O, this cannot, for obvious reasons, be considered a routine procedure; indeed it is unlikely that an experimental procedure using ^3H_2O would receive ethical permission in most countries.

Allowance must be made for isotope exchange, and hence loss of label from the water into other metabolic pools.

1. Both ^3H and ^2H will exchange with various ionizable compounds; 5.22 per cent of total body exchangeable hydrogen is in solutes rather than water. In animals the tritium space overestimates total body water, as determined by desiccation, by 1.7 perccent (Culebras *et al.* 1977; Culebras and Moore 1977).

2. Label from ^{18}O will be lost slowly as carbon dioxide (see section 5.2.2.3), although within the time-course of determination of total body water this is probably negligible.

The water content of fat mass is zero, while that of the fat-free mass is 73 per cent; therefore

fat-free mass = total body water / 0.73,

fat = body weight-fat − free mass.

2.2.1.3 Determination of total body potassium

There is no significant potassium in fat, and therefore determination of total body potassium is an index of the fat-free mass. Since potassium is primarily an intracellular cation (see Table 2.13), total body potassium reflects body cell mass. The potassium content of fat-free mass has been estimated by various authors as: 63, 64, 66 or 68 mmol/kg in men and 58, 59, 60 and 63 mmol/kg in women (Lukaski 1987). Morgan and Burkinshaw (1983) have suggested that the potassium content of fat-free mass varies with the fat-free mass of the body, ranging from 54 mmol/kg with a fat-free mass of 30 kg, to 61 mmol/kg with a fat-free mass of 80 kg.

Potassium can be determined by measuring the γ-emission due to the naturally occurring radioactive isotope ^{40}K, which has a natural abundance of 0.012 per cent (see Table 29.6). The procedure requires enclosure in a shielded whole body counter for approximately 15 minutes to achieve a precision of ±3 per cent; quite apart from the capital cost of a whole body counter, it is hardly a procedure that will appeal to many subjects.

Garrow (1982, 1983) notes that measurement of total body potassium will over estimate fat in obese subjects, whereas determination of total body water under estimates fat; he suggests that the mean of both methods is the best approximation.

2.2.1.4 Determination of total body nitrogen, calcium and chlorine by neutron activation analysis

On exposure to a neutron beam, a number of elements will capture neutrons into the atomic nucleus, leading to the production of unstable (radioactive) isotopes, which can then be measured by the γ-radiation emitted on radioactive decay. Physiologically the important elements that can be determined in this way are nitrogen, calcium, and chlorine.

Measurement of whole body nitrogen permits estimation of total protein content, while whole body calcium reflects the mass of bone mineral, and chlorine the extracellular fluid, since chloride is largely an extracellular ion (see Table 2.13).

Neutron activation analysis, together with determination of whole body potassium (see section 2.2.1.3) permits partition of the fat-free body mass into separate intracellular and extracellular water, protein and bone mineral, thus permitting more precise estimation of fat by difference. There is a problem that the activation of bone calcium is not uniform, so bone mineral may well be under estimated. It is not a routine technique; world-wide only seven centres are equipped to perform whole body neutron activation analysis (Cohn 1991, 1992).

On average, muscle contains 91 mmol (3.55 g) potassium and 2.14 mol (30 g) nitrogen /kg, whereas non-muscle lean tissue contains 48 mmol (1.87 g) potassium and 2.57 mol (36 g) nitrogen /kg. Therefore, determination of total body potassium and nitrogen should permit separate estimation of muscle and non-muscle lean tissue (Burkinshaw *et al.* 1981). However, Garrow (1982, 1983) has reported that the nitrogen:potassium ratio in various organs differs widely, and none approaches the theoretical non-muscle value.

2.2.1.5 Direct estimation of fat using krypton

A number of gases, including anaesthetics (see section 11.2.3) and inert gases such as krypton, are considerably more soluble in fat than in water. This can be exploited to estimate the body fat content. The subject rebreathes air containing ^{85}Kr for a period of about 2 hours, by which time it is assumed that equilibrium has been achieved, and the disappearance of krypton from the respirometer circuit represents that which has been dissolved in the fat, water and protein in the body. The volume of the lungs and respirometer circuit is measured by dilution of helium, total body water is determined by dilution of isotopically labelled water, and the protein content of the body is estimated on the basis that protein equals 25 per cent of total body water. This method determines the volume of fat in the body; fat mass is calculated from the density of body fat (Hytten *et al.* 1966).

The volume of fat in the body can be calculated as follows:

total disappearance of krypton $(V \times (Kr_i\text{-}Kr_f)) / Kr_f$ = gas + water $\times S_w$ + fat $\times S_f$ + protein x S_p

Hence

fat volume = $((V \times (Kr_i/Kr_f\text{-}1) - \text{gas} - \text{water} \times S_w - \text{protein} \times S_p) / S_f$

where Kr_i is the initial and Kr_f the final volume of krypton in the respirometer;

water, fat and protein are the volumes occupied by these body pools;

gas is the volume of the lungs plus tubing, and V is the total respirometer volume,

S_w is the solubility coefficient of krypton in water (0.0522 at 37°C), S_f in fat (0.425) and S_p in protein (0.020).

2.2.1.6 X-ray and imaging techniques

Photon absorptiometry depends on the differential absorption of a tightly focused beam of X-rays or γ-rays at a single wavelength by different tissues. At its simplest it is thus high resolution radiography. Simultaneous use of two wavelengths permits more precise differentiation of different tissue types and higher resolution. Early dual-beam photon methods used the two γ-emissions of radioactive gadolinium (^{153}Gd); modern methods use X-ray tubes emitting two precisely defined wavelengths—dual energy, dual photon X-ray absorption (DEXA-DPX). Such techniques have proven invaluable in determination of bone density, permitting determination of bone mineral content in specific regions or the whole body with a relatively low X-ray dose (Peppler and Mazess 1981).

Three imaging techniques that are in routine clinical use can be used to visualize individual organs, and hence determine the volumes occupied by bone, muscle, fat and individual organs. Not only is it possible to determine the total volume of fat in the body, but its anatomical localization (subcutaneous or intra-abdominal) can also be determined (see section 11.3).

1. Computerized axial tomography (CAT scanning) is an X-ray technique; it is capable of giving extremely high resolution three–dimensional images, but the radiation dose to the subject is significant. The impact of CAT scanning in clinical medicine was such that Hounsfield, who developed the first scanner, and Cormack, who developed the mathematical theory, shared the Nobel Prize in Medicine in 1979 (Borkan *et al.* 1982*a*, 1983).

2. Nuclear magnetic resonance depends on the flipping of the direction of spin of atomic nuclei in response to a high frequency alternating magnetic field (typically 200–500 MHz). Like CAT scanning, magnetic resonance imaging (MRI scanning), gives high resolution three–dimensional images; there is no exposure to ionizing radiation, and the magnetic and radio-frequency fields used

are at a sufficiently low level that they are believed to have no effects on the body.

3. Ultra sound scanning depends on the differential transmission of high frequency sound waves by body organs and tissues, using either pulsed ultrasound at 20–30 kHz or continuous Doppler ultrasound at 2.5–3.5 MHz. Again it can be used to build up three–dimensional images of high resolution. Like MRI scanning, ultra sound is believed to pose no hazard to the subject and indeed is routinely used in obstetric practice (Booth *et al.* 1966; Borkan *et al.* 1982*b*). Average transmission rates for 20 kHz ultrasound are: air 331, fat 1450, and water 1495 m/sec. Average soft tissues transmit at a rate of 1540, and bone 4080 m/sec; more precisely, blood transmits at 1570, kidney 1561, and muscle 1585 m/sec (Cronk 1983).

2.2.1.7 Skinfold thickness

Measurement of the thickness of subcutaneous fat is currently the most widely used method of estimating total body fat. Standard skinfold calipers exert a pressure of 10 g/mm^2 over an area of 20–40 mm^2 — a fairly sharp 'pinch'. With a modicum of training, the method is capable of yielding highly reproducible results, although identification of the correct sites for measurement requires some practice. Lohman (1981) quotes intra-observer variation of 0.5–0.95 mm, and inter-observer variation of 0.9–1.9 mm in determination of skinfold thickness. The disadvantage of skinfold measurement is that it only measures subcutaneous fat, not internal (abdominal) fat—see section 11.3 for a discussion of the importance of adipose tissue distribution. Gray *et al.* (1990) reported that skinfold measurements significantly underestimated body fat (as determined by underwater weighing) in severely obese subjects, presumably because of a high proportion of intra-abdominal fat. They also noted that standard skinfold calipers were not large enough to measure the skinfolds at some sites in their subjects.

The four sites most commonly used for skinfold determination are the biceps, triceps, subscapular, and supra-iliac; precise locations are shown in Table 2.25. Durnin and Womersley (1974) have calculated the regression equations shown in Table 2.25 to give an age-independent estimate of body density from the sum of the skinfold thicknesses at these four sites.

The relationship between skinfold thickness and body density is not age independent. Brozek and Keys (1951) derived the regression equations shown in Table 2.26 for calculation of density from single or multiple skinfold thicknesses in young (college age) and middle-aged men.

Durnin and Womersley (1974) showed that the relationship between body density and skinfold thickness is not only age-dependent, but also non-linear. They calculated a series of logarithmic regression equations, in the form

density = gradient x log(skinfold) + intercept

for prediction of body density from single skinfolds or the sum of four-site skinfold thickness at various ages. Table 2.27 shows their approximate equations using a common, age-independent gradient for each skinfold site. They reported that they could not calculate an appropriate age-independent gradient for the subscapular skinfold in men. More precise estimation of density from single-site skinfold or the sum of all four sites is possible using age-dependent gradients and intercepts, as shown in Table 2.28.

Equations for the prediction of body density from the sums of multiple skinfold thicknesses and other parameters are shown in Table 2.29. Norgan and Ferro-Luzzi (1985) noted that these and similar empirical regression equations can only be considered to predict body density for the age and population group from whom they were determined; they concluded that generalized equations applicable to all population groups are unlikely to be achievable.

Slaughter *et al.* (1988) have calculated a series of equations to predict percentage body fat from the sum of calf and triceps skinfold thickness in children aged 8–18 years. As shown in Table 2.30, their results introduce a further complication; the intercepts of the regression equations for males show both an ethnic difference and also an effect of whether the subjects were prepubescent, pubescent or post-pubescent.

2.2.1.8 Electrical conductivity of the body

Fat is an electrical insulator, while the electrolytes in lean tissue conduct an electric current. Therefore measurement of the electrical conductivity of the body permits estimation of the relative content of fat and fat-free mass. Two methods are in use.

2.2.1.8.1 Total body electrical conductivity (TOBEC)

A high frequency (5 MHz) alternating current in a solenoid will induce a magnetic field, and hence an electric current, in a conductor placed under the solenoid; this evoked field can then be detected by a secondary coil. The intensity of the evoked field depends on both the electrolyte content of the body and its shape; the method was adapted from techniques used in the meat industry to estimate the fat content of joints and carcasses, which are of a reasonably uniform shape. However, the differences in body shape between tall and short, and lean and stout people, are a source of significant inaccuracy (Segal *et al.* 1985; van Loan and Mayclin 1987).

Fat-free mass is calculated from either the phase average of the evoked signal or the first and third Fourier transformation coefficients (FC0 and FC2 respectively):

(1) fat-free mass = 11.8 + 0.078 x phase average,

(2) fat-free mass = 22.5 + 0.119 x FC0 − 0.282 × FC2,

(3) fat-free mass = 14.0 + 0.096 x FC0 − 0.289 × FC2 + 0.057 x age + 0.013 x alc x height

(alc is the average lean circumference, equal to the mean of chest, abdomen and thigh lean circumferences).

Equation 3 gives the highest correlation with fat-free mass as determined by dilution of isotopically labelled water (Fiorotto 1991).

2.2.1.8.2 Bio-electrical impedance

The electrical resistance (or impedance for an alternating current) of the body is proportional to the square of height and inversely proportional to lean body mass. A 50 MHz alternating current (800 μA) is passed from electrodes attached to the hands to electrodes attached to the feet; the fall in voltage is measured, so permitting calculation of the impedance (Lukaski *et al.* 1985).

Heitman (1990) derived the following equation for prediction of body fat (in kg) from impedance:

fat = constant x weight − $(0.279 \times \text{height}^2)$/impedance − $0.231 \times \text{height} + 0.077 \times \text{age} + 14.941$

The constant is 0.819 for men and 0.755 for women.

Kushner *et al.* (1992) derived a gender- and age-independent equation for predicting total body water from impedance, which correlated well with total body water as determined by ^2H_2O dilution for all subjects tested except pre-school children:

total body water = $0.59 \times \text{height}^2$/impedance + $0.065 \times \text{weight} + 0.04$

Table 2.1: Indices of weight for height

weight for height	weight / height	affected by height; taller people appear to be overweight.
ponderal Index	weight / height$^{1/3}$	poorly correlated with weight; more biased by height than other indices (shorter people appear to be overweight); lower values with increasing body weight for height.
body mass index (Quetelet's index)	weight / height^2	relatively independent of height, no bias towards apparent obesity at extremes of height; the most commonly used index (see Table 2.2).
Benn's Index	weight / height^p	p is derived from weight/height ratio and the regression coefficient of log (weight) on log(height) for the specific age, gender and population group; relatively unaffected by height. Values of p range between 1.6–1.83.

Table 2.2: Interpretation of Body Mass Index (weight / height^2) in adults

BMI	
< 16	severe protein-energy malnutrition
16 – 17	moderately severe protein-energy malnutrition
17 – 18.4	moderate protein-energy malnutrition
18.4 – 20	underweight
20 – 25	acceptable / desirable range
25 – 30[1]	overweight
30 – 40	obesity
> 40	severe obesity

(1) A range of body mass index from 25–27 is sometimes considered as a 'grey' area — acceptable but not desirable.

Table 2.3: Chemical analysis of the human body

	weight	height	% of body weight				% of fat free mass		
	kg	cm	water	fat	protein	ash	water	protein	ash
(1) female age 42 y	45.1	169	56.0	23.6	14.4	-	73.2	18.8	7.6
(2) male age 25 y	71.8	179	61.8	14.9	16.6	-	72.6	17.5	7.5
(3) male age 48 y	63.8	-	81.5	1.1	12.8	-	82.4	12.9	4.9
(4) boy age 4.5 y	14.0	107	53.8	22.7	18.5	-	69.5	23.8	6.4
(5) male age 46 y	53.8	168.5	55.1	19.4	18.6	5.4	68.4	23.1	6.7
(6) male age 35 y	70.6	183	67.9	12.5	14.4	4.8	77.6	16.5	5.5

Source: from data reported by (1–4) Widdowson *et al.* 1951; (5) Forbes *et al.* 1953; (6) Mitchell *et al.* 1945.

Table 2.4: Body composition of the ICRP reference man and woman

	male	female
body weight (kg)	70	58
body length or height (cm)	170	160
body surface area (cm^2)	18 000	16 000
specific gravity (g /cm^3)	1.07	1.04
total body water (L)	42 (600 mL /kg bw)	29 (500 mL /kg bw)
extracellular water (L)	18.2 (260 mL /kg bw)	11.6 (200 mL /kg bw)
intracellular water (L)	23.8 (340 mL/kg bw)	17.4 (300 mL/kg bw)
total blood volume (L)	5.2	3.9
total red blood cell volume (L)	2.2	1.35
plasma volume (L)	3	2.5
total connective tissue (kg)	5.05	4.1
cartilage (kg)	2.5	2.0
tendons and fascia (kg)	0.85	0.7
total skin weight (kg)	2.6	1.79
total skin thickness (mm)	1300	1300
epidermis (mm)	50	50
dermis (mm)	1250	1250
hypodermis (mm)	2750	6600
total body fat (kg)	13.5	16
non-essential body fat (kg)	12	15
essential body fat (kg)	1.5	1
subcutaneous adipose tissue (kg)	7.5	13.0
separable adipose tissue (kg)	5.0	4.0
yellow marrow adipose tissue (kg)	1.5	1.3
interstitial adipose tissue (kg)	1.0	0.7

Source: Snyder *et al.* 1975.

Table 2.5: Estimation of body fat from body mass index (BMI) and distribution of body fat as percentage of total

		male	female
% body fat	(Blaxter 1989)	0.12 x BMI − 1.01	1.48 x BMI − 7.0
	(Sutcliffe *et al.* 1993)	1.962 x BMI − 34.0	2.670 x BMI − 27.7
body fat as % body weight		14.7	26.9
% of total fat as			
	essential fat[1]	20	32
	storage fat	80	68
% of storage fat			
	subcutaneous	38	49
	intermuscular	40	34
	intramuscular	10	5
	thoracic and abdominal cavity	12	12

(1) Essential fat is that in cell membranes, bone marrow, nervous system, and mammary glands.
Source: from data reported by Lohman 1981.

Table 2.6: Mineral composition of the human body

(figures show content /kg fat-free body mass for subjects 1–4 shown in Table 2.3)

	(1) female age 42		(2) male age 25		(3) male age 48		(4) male age 4.5	
	g	mmol	g	mmol	g	mmol	g	mmol
sodium	2.22	96.6	2.12	92.3	2.70	117	2.29	99.6
potassium	2.84	72.6	2.78	71.1	1.36	34.8	2.53	64.7
calcium	24.8	619	21.3	531	16.2	404	21.1	526
magnesium	0.427	17.6	0.482	19.8	0.43	17.7	0.358	14.7
phosphorus	12.9	416	14.0	452	7.9	255	10.5	339
iron	0.060	1.07	0.0875	1.57	0.0605	1.08	0.0642	1.15
copper	0.0018	0.028	0.0016	0.025	0.0027	0.042	0.0033	0.052
zinc	0.022	0.34	0.0333	0.51	0.0194	0.29	0.0223	0.34

Source: from data reported by Widdowson *et al.* 1951.

Table 2.7: Elemental composition of the ICRP reference man

	total body content	
	mol	g
hydrogen	7000	7000
oxygen	2687	4300
carbon	1333	1600
nitrogen	129	1800
calcium	25	1000
phosphorus	25	780
sulphur	4.36	140
sodium	4.35	100
potassium	3.58	140
chlorine	2.67	95
magnesium	0.780	19
fluorine	0.136	2.6
iron	0.075	4.2
zinc	0.035	2.3

For more detailed information on the mineral content of the body, see Table 25.2.
Source: Snyder *et al.* 1975.

Table 2.8: Major organs of the body as percent of body weight
(for subjects 1-4 in Table 2.3)

	(1) female age 42	(2) male age 25	(3) male age 48	(4) male age 4.5
brain	2.90	1.88	2.23	9.30
heart	0.62	0.91	1.04	0.54
lungs	2.22	2.66	2.87	1.76
kidneys	0.56	0.25[1]	0.67	0.69
liver	2.68	3.48	3.43	3.27
spleen	0.28	0.38	1.48[2]	0.30
gastro-intestinal tract	3.83	4.73	3.83	4.52

(1) The kidneys were small and fibrous in this subject, who died of uraemia.
(2) The spleen was enlarged in this subject, who died of infective endocarditis.
Source: Widdowson *et al.* 1951.

Table 2.9: Proportion of body weight as adipose tissue, muscle, bone and skin

| | % of body weight | | % of adipose tissue free weight | |
	male	female	male	female
adipose tissue	28.1 ± 6.4	34.6 ± 9.3	-	-
muscle	37.4 ± 4.9	32.9 ± 6.3	52.0 ± 4.3	50.0 ± 4.4
bone	14.3 ± 2.0	13.4 ± 2.2	19.9 ± 2.4	20.6 ± 2.6
skin	5.6 ± 0.6	5.5 ± 0.7	7.8 ± 0.8	8.5 ± 1.2

Source: Clarys *et al.* 1984.

Table 2.10: Organ weights for the ICRP reference man and woman

| | male | | female | |
	g	% body weight	g	% body weight
skeletal muscle	28000	40.0	17000	29.3
liver	1800	2.57	1400	2.41
brain	1400	2.00	1200	2.07
cerebrospinal fluid	120	0.17	100	0.17
gastrointestinal tract (empty)	1200	1.71	1100	1.89
lungs	1000	1.43	800	1.38
intestine (small + large)	1000	1.43	950	1.64
kidneys (both)	310	0.44	275	0.47
spleen	180	0.26	150	0.26
stomach	150	0.21	140	0.24
pancreas	100	0.14	85	0.15
salivary glands	85	0.12	70	0.12
uterus	-	-	80	0.14
tongue	70	0.10	60	0.10
oesophagus	40	0.057	34	0.059
testes (both)	35	0.050	-	-
ovaries (both)	-	-	11	0.019
spinal cord	30	0.043	28	0.048
larynx	28	0.040	19	0.033
breasts (both)[1]	26	0.037	360	0.62
thyroid gland	20	0.029	17	0.029
prostate gland	16	0.023	-	-
adrenal glands (both)	14	0.020	14	0.024
trachea	10	0.014	8	0.014
gall bladder	10	0.014	8	0.014
pituitary gland	0.6	-	0.7	-
pineal gland	0.18	-	0.15	-
parathyroid glands (four)	0.12	-	0.14	-

(1) Breasts enlarge to between 560—1800 g during lactation.
Source: Snyder *et al.* 1975.

Table 2.11: Composition of the major organs

(Figures show mean values or ranges reported in the literature.)

| | % by weight | | | | mg /g protein | |
	water	fat	protein	ash	DNA	RNA
brain	77.4 (76.3–78.5)	11 (9–17)	8	1.5 (1.4–2)	0.12–0.31	0.27–0.63
heart	72	2.6	14–19	1.1	-	-
kidneys	76 (70.6–81)	5 (1.8–7.2)	17 (14.7–19.3)	1.1 (0.99–1.3)	1.1–1.2	1.4–1.5
large intestine	79	6.2	13	0.8	0.49–0.94	0.55–0.97
liver[1]	71	6.9 (1.1–11.5)	18 (16–22)	1.3 (1–1.7)	0.77–1.29	2.83–4.13
lung[2]	71–84	1–1.5	16.4–19.2	1.1 (0.98–1.63)	-	-
ovaries	78	1.6 (1.3–2.3)	14	0.97 (0.8–1.4)	0.25	0.18
pancreas	71	8 (2.9–20.4)	13	1.2 (0.7–1.5)	1.3–2.4	1.8–8
skeletal muscle	79	2.2–9.4	17.2	1.2	1.9	3.5
small intestine	79	6.2	13	0.8	1.14–1.91	1.26–1.63
spleen	77	1.6	19.5	1.4	3.83	1.95
stomach	75	—	—	0.8	1.3	1.57
testes	81	3	12	1.1	1.35–1.7	0.72–1.92
thyroid gland	72–78	—	14	1.1 (0.81–1.8)	0.9 (0.58–1.63)	1.1 (0.86–1.58)
tongue	60–72	15–24	16–18	1	-	-

(1) Liver contains 10 mg DNA /10^6 cells.
(2) Lung contains: 8.1 ± 1.4 (male) or 9.5 ± 1.2 % (female) elastin on a dry weight basis.
See also Table 5.7 for the relative contribution of different organs to basal metabolic rate.
Source: Snyder *et al.* 1975.

Table 2.12: Distribution of total body water in the adult male

	mL /kg bw	% total	total (L)
total body water	600	-	42
intracellular water	340	57	23.8
extracellular water	260	43	18.2
plasma	41	7	2.87
interstitial lymph	121	20	8.47
dense connective tissue and cartilage	41	7	2.87
inaccessible bone water	41	7	2.87
transcellular water	15	2.5	1.05
intraluminal in gastrointestinal tract	8.4	1.4	0.58

Source: Snyder *et al.* 1975.

Table 2.13: Intracellular and extracellular electrolytes

| | mmol /L | |
	intracellular	extracellular
sodium	10	140
potassium	150	5
calcium	2	3
magnesium	15	2
chloride	5	100
bicarbonate	10	25
phosphate	120	6

Table 2.14: Distribution of blood throughout the body

	volume (mL)		% of total
	male	female	
total	5200	3900	-
arterial system	1000	750	19.2
venous system	3200	2400	61.5
pulmonary system	500	400	9.6
heart chambers (average)	500	350	9.6
cerebral pool	156	117	3
thoracic pool	2700	1950	52
splanchnic pool	1040–1090	780–820	20–21
liver	310	230	6
spleen	310	230	6
mesenteric vessels	420–470	310–350	8–9

Source: Snyder *et al.* 1975.

Table 2.15: Formulae for estimating total body water, extracelllular water, and plasma volume

total body water		males	females
	prepubertal[1] (L)	$0.135 \times W^{0.666} \times H^{0.535}$	$0.135 \times W^{0.666} \times H^{0.535}$
	birth to adulthood (L)	$0.6111 \times W + 0.251$	$0.511 \times W + 1.244$
	adults (% body weight)	$79.45 - 0.24 \times W - 0.15 \times A$	$69.81 - 0.26 \times W - 0.12 \times A$
extracellular water			
	1m–4y[1] (L)	$0.239 \times W + 0.325$	$0.239 \times W + 0.325$
	children (L)	$0.227 \times W + 0.916$	$0.211 \times W + 0.989$
	adults (L)	$0.135 \times W + 7.35$	$0.135 \times W + 5.27$
plasma volume			
	adults (mL)	$23.7 \times H + 9.0 \times W - 1709$	$40.5 \times H + 8.4 \times W - 4811$
	adults[1] (mL /kg body weight)	$49.6 \times W - 0.0348$	$49.6 \times W - 0.0348$

Where W = body weight (kg), H = height (cm) and A = age (y).
(1) No gender difference.

Table 2.16: Average fluid balance

		mL /day		
		adult man	adult woman	child (10y)
intake	fluids	1950	1400	1400
	water in food	700	450	400
	metabolic water	350	250	200
output	urine	1400	1000	1000
	exhaled air	320	320	-
	insensible loss[1]	530	280	580[1]
	sweat loss	650	420	350
	faecal water	100	90	70
total intake or output		3000	2100	2000

(1) Insensible loss includes losses in exhaled air.
Source: Snyder *et al.* 1975.
See Table 10.2 for nitrogenous compounds in urine and Table 6.11 for the composition of faeces.

Table 2.17: Formulae for calculation of body surface area

	date	surface area (cm^2) =
Bardeen	1920	$1.43 \times (2 \times weight \times (1000/height)) + 4 \times height \times (weight \times 1000/height)^{0.5}$
Behnke *et al.*	1959	$1.138 \times gluteal\ girth \times height$
Biering	1931	$1090 \times weight^{2/3}$
Boyd	1939	$3.207 \times weight^{(0.728-0.0188 \times log(weight \times 1000)} \times height^{0.03}$
Breitman	1932	$0.0087 \times (height + weight) - 2600$
DuBois & DuBois	1916	$71.84 \times weight^{0.425} \times height^{0.725}$
Haycock	1978	$242.65 \times weight^{0.5378} \times height^{0.3964}$
Meeh	1931	$1190 \times weight^{2/3}$
Takai & Shimaguchi	1986	$-2142 + 617 \times weight^{2/3} + 0.2453 \times height^2 + 0.6825 \times head\ circumference^2$
Vierordt	1906	$1230 \times weight^{2/3}$
von Schelling	1954	$531.75 \times (height \times 10)^{0.5} \times weight$

Height, gluteal girth and head circumference in cm, weight in kg.
Source: from data reported by Martin *et al.* 1984; Takai and Shimaguchi 1986.

Table 2.18: Surface area of the body and the four major subdivisions as percent of total

age (years)	area (cm^2)	% of total surface area			
		head	trunk	arms	legs
birth	2115	20.8	31.9	16.8	30.5
1	3925	17.2	34.4	17.8	30.6
2	5275	15.2	33.6	18.5	32.7
3	6250	14.4	33.6	18.8	33.2
4	6950	13.7	33.1	19.4	33.8
5	7510	13.1	33.0	19.6	34.3
6	7925	12.6	33.4	19.6	34.4
7	8275	12.4	33.5	19.3	34.7
8	8690	12.0	33.4	19.6	35.1
9	9100	11.5	33.5	19.2	35.7
10	9610	10.9	33.6	19.4	36.2
11	10165	10.4	33.4	19.5	36.6
12	10750	10.0	33.3	19.5	37.2
13	11425	9.6	33.0	19.7	37.6
14	12290	9.2	32.5	20.3	38.0
15	13325	8.8	31.9	21.4	37.9
16	14300	8.4	31.6	21.5	38.5
17	15200	8.2	31.7	21.2	38.8
18	15850	7.9	32.5	20.8	38.8
19	16435	7.7	33.5	20.5	38.3
20	16800	7.6	33.9	20.2	38.2
21	17050	7.5	34.3	19.9	38.3
22	17255	7.5	34.4	19.7	38.3
23	17415	7.5	34.5	19.5	38.5
24	17535	7.5	34.6	19.4	38.5

Source: Snyder *et al.* 1975.

Table 2.19: Composition of the skeleton

	newborn	adult male	adult female
wet weight (kg)	0.35	10	6.8
fat-free wet weight (kg)	0.34	8	5.8
dry weight (kg)	0.15	5	3.4
ash (% wet weight)	15	28	28
total bone marrow (kg)	0.04	3	2.6
red bone marrow (kg)	0.04	1.5	1.3
yellow bone marrow (kg)	0	1.5	1.3
skeletal cartilage	–	1100	900
tendons and deep fascia	–	850	700
superficial fascia	–	500	400
total periarticular tissue	–	1500	1200
other connective tissue	–	500	400

Source: Snyder *et al.* 1975.

Table 2.20: Composition of the adult male skeleton

	mass (kg)	water %	ash %	fat %	protein %
total skeleton	10	33	28	19	19
total bone	5	17	54	1	25
cortical bone	4	15	55	1	25
trabecular bone	1	23	50	1	24
red marrow	1.5	40	0.6	40	20
yellow marrow	1.5	15	0.2	80	4
skeletal cartilage	1.1	78	4.1	1.3	16
periarticular tissue	0.9	78	4.1	1.3	16

Source: Snyder *et al.* 1975.

Table 2.21: Elbow breadth as an indicator of frame size

| | elbow breadth (cm) | | | |
| | males | | females | |
age (years)	small	large	small	large
18-25	< 6.6	> 7.7	< 5.6	> 6.5
25-35	< 6.7	> 7.9	< 5.7	> 6.8
35-45	< 6.7	> 8.0	< 5.7	> 7.1
45-55	< 6.7	> 8.1	< 5.7	> 7.2
55-65	< 6.7	> 8.1	< 5.8	> 7.2
65-75	< 6.7	> 8.1	< 5.8	> 7.2

Source: Frisancho 1984

Table 2.22: Distribution and composition of skeletal muscle

(Figures show mean and extreme ranges).

		newborn	4-7 m	adult
% of skeletal muscle in	head and trunk	40	-	25-30
	arms	18-20	-	18-20
	legs	40	-	55
composition of skeletal muscle (%)	water	80.4 (79.3-81.2)	78.5 (78.2-79)	79 (68.9-80.3)
	extracellular water	35	29.3	18.3
	protein	11.6-12.9	16.1 (15.8-16.3)	17.2 (12.9-20)
	collagen	1.8	1.8 (1.6-1.9)	0.6 (1.4-0.8)
	sarcoplasmic protein	2.4 (2.3-2.6)	3.1 (2.9-3.4)	4.2 (3.8-4.7)
	fibrillar protein	6.8 (6.5-7.1)	10.6 (9.6-11.6)	12.4 (12.3-12.7)
	fat	2.0 (0.67-2.2)	2.0	male 2.2 (2.2-9.4) female 2.9 (2.2-9.4)
	carbohydrate	4	-	0.2-1.8

Source: Snyder *et al.* 1975.

Table 2.23: Calculation of limb muscle circumference and area

limb muscle circumference	mid-limb circumference$-\pi$ x skinfold
limb fat area	0.5 x (mid-limb circumference x skinfold)-0.25 x. π x skinfold^2
calf muscle area	0.25 x (mid-calf circumference$-\pi$ x skinfold^2)
arm muscle area, men	0.25 x (mid-arm circumference$-\pi$ x skinfold^2)-10 ((mid-arm circumference$-\pi$ x skinfold)^2 / (4 x π)) -10
arm muscle area, women	0.25 x (mid-arm circumference$-\pi$ x skinfold^2)-6.5 ((mid-arm circumference$-\pi$ x skinfold)^2 / (4 x π)) -6.5

See also Table 3.30 for arm muscle anthropometry at various ages.
Source: from data reported by Jelliffe 1966; Heymsfield *et al.* 1982.

Table 2.24: Composition of adipose tissue

| | abdominal subcutaneous adipose tissue | | | | perirenal adipose tissue | | | |
| | % composition | | | cells | % composition | | | cells |
	lipid	water	protein	$(\times 10^6 /g)$	lipid	water	protein	$(\times 10^6 /g)$
infants, stillborn at term	45.3	50.3	4.4	108	35.9	57.7	6.4	193
infants, birth–48 h	46.8	46.6	6.6	206	45.1	48.4	6.5	270
infants, 6m–10 m	68.7	87.6	3.7	101	57.7	39.2	3.1	138
children, 2.5–4 y	64.0	31.4	4.6	79	48.8	47.1	4.1	135
children, 9–17 y	70.6	25.4	4.0	62	62.0	34.6	3.4	93
adults, 19–25 y	78.4	19.7	1.9	32	72.5	26.1	1.4	40
adults, 38–71 y	78.9	19.0	2.1	29	71.5	26.2	2.3	46

Source: from data reported by Baker 1969.

Table 2.25 Standard skinfold sites and prediction of body density from four-site skinfold thickness

(Using calipers exerting a pressure of 10 g /mm^2 over an area of 20–40 mm^2.)

site	
biceps	a vertical fold on the front of the upper arm, at the midpoint of the muscle, directly above the centre of the cubital fossa, opposite the site of the triceps skinfold, with arm hanging vertically.
triceps	at the back of the arm upper, at a point equidistant between the tip of acromion and olecranon, with the arm hanging vertically.
subscapular	just below, and laterally to, the tip of the inferior angle of the scapula, with the shoulder and arm relaxed or placed behind the subject's back, at an angle of 45°, in the same direction as the inner border of the scapula.
suprailiac	over iliac crest in midaxillary line, parallel to the cleavage lines of the skin

| men aged 17—72 | density $\times 10^3$ = -0.0744 x log Σ(skinfold) + 1.1765 |
| women aged 16—68 | density $\times 10^3$ = -0.0717 x log Σ(skinfold) + 1.1567 |

Source: from data reported by Gibson 1990; Durnin and Womersley 1974.

Table 2.26 Prediction of body density from single site skinfold, relative body weight or combined data

	college age males	males aged 45-55
abdomen skinfold (sf)	-0.001398 x sf + 1.0996	-0.000851 x sf + 1.0783
chest skinfold	-0.001586 x sf + 1 .0984	-0.001039 x sf + 1.0810
back skinfold	-0.001770 x sf + 1.1012	-0.001148 x sf + 1.0791
upper arm skinfold	-0.002313 x sf + 1.1034	-0.001840 x sf + 1.0824
thigh skinfold	-0.003209 x sf + 1.0155	-0.002172 x sf + 1.0789
relative body weight[1]	-0.000787 x rel weight + 1.1588	-0.000605 x rel weight + 1.1168

college age males	1.1125 – 0.000292 x abdomen sf – 0.000661 x chest sf + 0.000181 x back sf – 0.000711 x upper arm sf - 0.000375 x thigh sf – 0.000122 x relative weight
	1.1017 - 0.000282 x abdomen sf – 0.000736 x chest sf - 0.00883 x upper arm sf
males ages 45-55	1.0967 + 0.000042 x abdomen sf - 0.000423 x chest sf - 0.00032 x back sf - 0.000511 x upper arm sf - 0.000247 x thigh sf - 0.000156 x relative weight
	1.0967 - 0.000393 x chest sf - 0.000315 x back sf - 0.000598 x upper arm sf - 0.00017 x relative weight

(1) body weight as % of reference weight for height, see Table 11.8.
Source: Brozek and Keys 1951

Table 2.27 Prediction of body density from single-site skinfold thickness, using age-independent gradients
density x 10^3 = gradient x log(skinfold) + intercept

	biceps	triceps	subscapular	supra-iliac	$\sum$(skinfolds)
males					
common gradient	-0.05731	-0.05523	[1]	-0.04564	-0.06496
			intercept		
16—19y	1.0998	1.1183	-	1.1131	1.1653
20—29y	1.0989	1.1155	-	1.1145	1.1659
30—39y	1.0923	1.1030	-	1.1080	1.1607
40—49y	1.0881	1.0984	-	1.0995	1.1533
50—59y	1.0800	1.0917	-	1.0944	1.1490
females					
common gradient	-0.05492	-0.07284	-0.06248	-0.04765	-0.06711
			intercept		
16—19y	1.0884	1.1253	1.1085	1.0938	1.1537
20—29y	1.0855	1.1259	1.1076	1.0886	1.1518
30—39y	1.0832	1.1233	1.1054	1.0835	1.1495
40—49y	1.0798	1.1171	1.1015	1.0775	1.1443
50—59y	1.0725	1.1115	1.0952	1.0730	1.1389

(1) For males, the gradient of the regression of body density on log(subscapular skinfold thickness) varies significantly with age, and hence no age-independent gradient is quoted.
Source: Durnin and Womersley 1974.

Table 2.28 Prediction of body density from single-site skinfold thickness, using best estimates of gradient at each age
density x 10^3 = gradient x log(skinfold) + intercept

	biceps		triceps		subscapular		supra-iliac		$\sum$(skinfolds)	
	gradient	intercept	gradient	intercept	gradient	intercept	gradient	intercept	gradient	intercept
males										
17—19y	-0.0686	1.1066	-0.0625	1.1252	-0.0670	1.1312	-0.0420	1.1092	-0.0630	1.1620
20—29y	-0.0616	1.1015	-0.0530	1.1131	-0.0700	1.1360	-0.0431	1.1117	-0.0632	1.1631
30—39y	-0.0396	1.0781	-0.0361	1.0834	-0.0416	1.0978	-0.0432	1.1047	-0.0544	1.1422
40—49y	-0.0508	1.0829	-0.0609	1.1041	-0.0686	1.1246	-0.0483	1.029	-0.0700	1.1620
› 50 y	-0.0617	1.0833	-0.0662	1.1027	-0.0760	1.1334	-0.0652	1.1193	-0.0779	1.1715
17—72 y	-0.0659	1.0997	-0.0618	1.1143	-0.0741	1.1369	-0.0530	1.1171	-0.0744	1.1765
females										
16—19y	-0.0553	1.0889	-0.0648	1.1159	-0.0621	1.1081	-0.0470	1.0931	-0.0678	1.1549
20—29y	-0.0601	1.0903	-0.0776	1.1319	-0.0716	1.1184	-0.0509	1.0923	-0.0717	1.1599
30—39y	-0.0511	1.0794	-0.0686	1.1176	-0.0567	1.0979	-0.0497	1.0860	-0.0632	1.1423
40—49y	-0.0492	1.0736	-0.0691	1.1121	-0.0505	1.0860	-0.0407	1.0691	-0.0612	1.1333
› 50 y	-0.0510	1.0682	-0.0762	1.1160	-0.0590	1.0899	-0.0419	1.0656	-0.0645	1.1339
16—68y	-0.0593	1.0871	-0.0775	1.1278	-0.0669	1.1100	-0.0514	1.0884	-0.0717	1.1567

Source: Durnin and Womersley 1974.

Table 2.29 Prediction of body density from multiple skinfolds, for men aged between 20-60 years

---

$\sum$(chest + axilla + triceps + subscapular + abdomen + supra-iliac + thigh skinfolds)
    $1.112 - 0.00043499 \times (\sum\text{skinfolds}) + 0.00000055 \times (\sum\text{skinfolds})^2 - 0.00028826 \times \text{age}$
    $1.101 - 0.0004115 \times (\sum\text{skinfolds}) + 0.00000069 \times (\sum\text{skinfolds})^2 - 0.00022631 \times \text{age} - 0.0059239 \times (\text{waist circumference}) +$
    $0.0190632 \times (\text{forearm circumference})$
    $1.21394 - 0.03101 \times \log(\sum\text{skinfolds}) - 0.00029 \times \text{age}$
    $1.17915 - 0.02394 \times \log(\sum\text{skinfolds}) - 0.00022 \times \text{age} - 0.007 \times (\text{waist circumference}) + 0.02120 \times (\text{forearm circumference})$
$\sum$(chest + abdomen + thigh skinfolds)
    $1.10938 - 0.0008267 \times (\sum\text{skinfolds}) + 0.0000016 \times (\sum\text{skinfolds})^2 - 0.0002574 \times \text{age}$
    $1.0990750 - 0.0008209 \times (\sum\text{skinfolds}) + 0.0000026 \times (\sum\text{skinfolds})^2 - 0.0002017 \times \text{age} - 0.005675 \times (\text{waist circumference}) +$
    $0.018586 \times (\text{forearm circumference})$
    $1.1886 - 0.03049 \times \log(\sum\text{skinfolds}) - 0.00027 \times \text{age}$
    $1.15737 - 0.02288 \times \log(\sum\text{skinfolds}) - 0.00019 \times \text{age} - 0.0075 \times (\text{waist circumference}) + 0.0223 \times (\text{forearm circumference})$
$\sum$(thorax + triceps skinfolds)
    $1145.5 - 59.69 \times \log(\sum\text{skinfolds}) - 1.529 \times \text{age}$
$\sum$(biceps + triceps + subscapular + supra-iliac skinfolds)
    $1163.9 - 57.15 \times (\sum\text{skinfolds}) - 0.607 \times \text{age}$
$\sum$(pectoral + thorax + abdominal + thigh skinfolds)
    $1161.4 - 55.47 \times \log(\sum\text{skinfolds}) - 03582 \times \text{age}$
$\sum$(biceps + triceps + subscapular + supra-iliac+ pectoral + abdominal + thigh + thorax skinfolds)
    $1181 - 57.58 \times \log(\sum\text{skinfolds}) - 0.588 \times \text{age}$

Source: from data reported by Jackson and Pollock 1978; Norgan and Ferro-Luzzi 1985.

Table 2.30: Prediction of percent body fat from skinfold thickness, ages 8—18 years

---

	males	females
	$0.735 \times \sum(\text{triceps + calf skinfold}) + 1.0$	$0.610 \times \sum(\text{triceps + calf skinfold}) + 5.1$ $1.33 \times \sum(\text{triceps + subscapular skinfold}) - 0.13 \times (\text{skinfold})^2 - 2.5$
prepubescent white	$1.21 \times (\text{triceps + subscapular skinfold}) - 0.008 \times (\text{skinfold})^2 - 1.7$	
prepubescent black	$1.21 \times (\text{triceps + subscapular skinfold}) - 0.008 \times (\text{skinfold})^2 - 3.2$	
pubescent white	$1.21 \times (\text{triceps + subscapular skinfold}) - 0.008 \times (\text{skinfold})^2 - 3.4$	
pubescent black	$1.21 \times (\text{triceps + subscapular skinfold}) - 0.008 \times (\text{skinfold})^2 - 5.2$	
post-pubescent white	$1.21 \times (\text{triceps + subscapular skinfold}) - 0.008 \times (\text{skinfold})^2 - 5.5$	
post-pubescent black	$1.21 \times (\text{triceps + subscapular skinfold}) - 0.008 \times (\text{skinfold})^2 - 6.8$	
if $\sum$ (triceps + subscapular skinfold) > 35mm		
	$0.783 \times \sum(\text{triceps + subscapular skinfold}) + 1.6$	$0.546 \times \sum(\text{triceps + subscapular skinfold}) + 9.7$

Source: Slaughter *et al.*, 1988.

3

Growth and development

As discussed in Chapter 12, children are most at risk from undernutrition, and assessment of growth provides a sensitive index of their nutritional status, albeit confounded by the effects of infection and emotional and metabolic stress.

For individual assessment, the child's measurements are compared with standards for the weight or height achieved at a given age, or weight for height. For population studies, the distribution of weight, height or height for age in the group being studied should be compared with the distribution in a reference population.

3.1 Foetal development, intra-uterine growth and birth measurements

Through pregnancy, the foetus develops from a single cell (the fertilized ovum) to contain, at birth, some 2×10^{12} cells; as shown in Table 3.1, from birth to adulthood the cell number increases by only a further 30-fold.

The stages in foetal development are shown in Table 3.2. A severe nutritional or metabolic insult at a given time will result in impairment of those systems that are developing, with little or no possibility of catch-up at a later stage. Intra-uterine sub-optimal nutrition results in lower birth weight, length and head circumference. Lower birth weight is associated with higher peri-natal and infant mortality, and may persist throughout life as smaller stature. There is a considerable body of evidence that low birth weight due to maternal undernutrition is a major factor in the later development of cardiovascular disease (Barker et al. 1989a, b, c).

Table 3.3 shows body size and composition at birth for the International Commission on Radiological Protection Reference Infant, together with equations for estimating weight and body surface area from length, and length from gestational age.

Table 3.4 shows the distribution of birth weights in American and British infants born at full term, and Table 3.5 the distribution of birth weight according to gestational age for American and German infants. WHO defines low birth weight as below 2.5 kg for full-term infants; in developing countries about 80 per cent of low birth weight infants are small for gestational age, rather than premature, reflecting poor maternal nutrition.

Table 3.6 shows the distribution of body length at birth in American and British infants born at full term, and Table 3.7 the distribution of body length at birth according to gestational age for American and German infants.

Head circumference provides a valuable index of brain size, and hence brain development. The development of brain cell numbers is more or less complete at birth, and post-natal brain development is largely a matter of formation of inter-neuronal connections. Intra-uterine undernutrition will result in fewer brain cells, and presumably impaired intelligence throughout life, although the evidence is disputed. Table 3.8 shows the distribution of head circumference at birth.

3.2 Changes in body composition with age

There are considerable changes in body composition with growth. Table 3.9 shows the ratio of protein: water in various tissues; overall there is a doubling of the protein content of tissues from birth to adulthood. Tables 3.10 and 3.11 show the changes in body composition with age.

Table 3.12 shows the growth of the major organs from birth to age 10, based on post mortem reports where the weights of one or more healthy organs were recorded (Coppoletta and Wolbach 1933), so that not all the organs from any one child were included in the published data. The original report did not include any information on body weight or the percentage of body weight contributed by each organ; in Table 3.12 organ weights relative to body weights have been calculated from the reference body weights reported by Fomon *et al.* (1982).

3.3 Reference standards for growth

It is debatable whether growth standards should be established for the ethnic or national group under consideration, or whether a single set of growth standards can be applied to all ethnic groups. However, the apparent ethnic differences in growth potential may be nutritional and environmental rather than genetic.

The head circumference of Japanese infants is significantly lower than the American standards (see Table 3.8), but if head circumference is expressed relative to body length then there is no difference—i.e. the difference is one of stature. Furthermore, as the body length of Japanese infants, and the stature of Japanese children, have increased over the last 50 years, as a result of improved nutrition, so the difference in head circumference from the American standards has become smaller (Tsuzaki *et al.* 1990).

Habicht *et al.* (1974) compared growth data from six developed and seven less developed countries, and suggested that in urban areas with well-nourished populations only 3 per cent of the differences in height and 6 per cent of the differences in weight could be attributed to ethnicity. By contrast, differences in socio-economic and nutritional status between urban and rural areas accounted for 12 per cent of the difference in height, and 30 per cent of the difference in weight, in the same ethnic group.

Longitudinal growth data are obtained by repeated measurement of the same individuals throughout life. For obvious reasons, little such information is available, and most growth data are from cross-sectional studies, where different individuals at different ages are measured at the same time. Such data will include both true longitudinal growth and also secular trends. The US National Center for Health Statistics (NCHS) growth standards (see below) are primarily cross-sectional, but include some longitudinal data as well.

During the 1960s and 1970s, two sets of data were generally used as growth references.

1. The Harvard standards for growth, which were based on measurements of relatively small numbers of children in Iowa and Boston in the 1930s;

there were few individuals at the extremes of the distribution curves (the 5th and 95th centiles).

2. The Tanner standards are based on a larger number of measurements of children in Britain during the 1960s (see Tables 3.15 and 3.17).

During the late 1970s and early 1980s new standards were established from data of the US National Center for Health Statistics (NCHS), which include both cross-sectional and longitudinal data, and have significant numbers of measurements at all ages. The NCHS data have been adapted to provide the WHO standards (Dibley *et al.* 1987a). The Tanner and NCHS standards are expressed in centile ranges around the median (50th centile), and individual results are expressed as either percentage above or below the median or, preferably, the centile bands. By contrast, the WHO standards are expressed as a Z-score—the number of standard deviations above or below the reference mean (Dibley *et al.* 1987b; Waterlow *et al.* 1977). This permits greater precision in evaluating very low results (those below the 5th or 3rd centile).

3.3.1 Weight and height for age

Tables 3.13 and 3.14 show the Tanner and NCHS standards for body weight from birth to age 18; the NCHS standards are plotted in Fig. 3.1.

Tables 3.15 and 3.16 show the Tanner and NCHS standards for body length of infants. For older children, height is measured rather than body length; there is a difference between the length at age 3 in the NCHS standards and age 2 in the Tanner standards, and height at the same age shown in Tables 3.17 and 3.18. The NCHS standards for length (up to 3 years of age) and height (from age 3 to 18 years) are plotted in Fig. 3.2.

Table 3.19 shows the WHO standards for weight and height with age from birth to 5 years, as standard deviations below the reference mean. Up to 24 months the measure of stature is length; thereafter it is height. Table 3.20 shows the 95 per cent reference ranges (i.e. ±2 SD either side of the mean) for the WHO standards for weight and height from age 10–18.

3.3.2 Weight for stature

Wasting (or thinness) indicates a lack of muscle tissue and fat reserves compared with an adequately nourished subject; it may develop rapidly as a result of acute food lack or infection, and under favourable conditions is readily and rapidly reversible. By con-

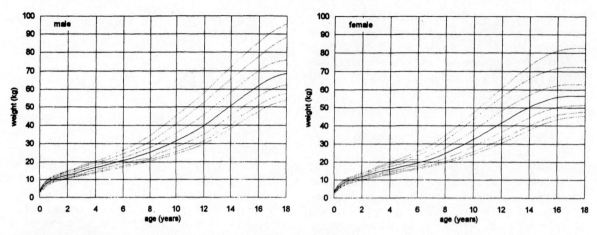

Figure 3.1 Weight from birth to age 18 years, NCHS data
Curves show the 5th, 10th, 25th, 50th, 75th, 90th, and 95th centiles: the 50th centile is shown as a solid line. (Plotted from data in Table 3.14)

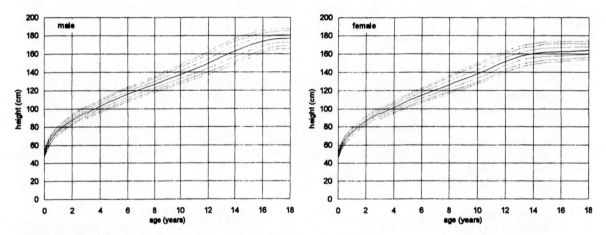

Figure 3.2 Height from birth to age 18 years, NCHS data
Curves show the 5th, 10th, 25th, 50th, 75th, 90th, and 95th centiles: the 50th centile is shown as a solid line. The discontinuity at age 3 is because up to 3 years of age it is length rather than height that is measured. (Plotted from data in Table 3.16 and 3.1)

trast, stunting or shortness is a failure to achieve the height expected in an adequately nourished child. Linear growth is slower than weight gain, and is, of course, irreversible. Therefore stunting is generally considered to be the result of more prolonged food shortage. Catch-up linear growth, even under favourable circumstances, is considerably slower than replacement of wasted tissue.

Attainment of stature for age is used to assess stunting (see section 3.3.1); wasting is assessed by attainment of reference weight for stature, rather than for age. The NCHS standards of weight for body length for infants under 4 years of age are shown in Table 3.21, and weight for height for prepubescent children in Table 3.22. Table 3.23 shows the WHO standards of weight for height.

3.3.3 Head circumference

Head circumference reflects brain growth, and provides a useful indication of nutrition during the first two years of life. Table 3.24 shows the NCHS standards for head circumference from birth to 3 years of age, and Table 3.25 the 95 per cent reference range from birth to age 18.

3.3.4 Skinfold thickness and arm muscle circumference

Tables 3.26 and 3.27 show reference ranges of triceps and subscapular skinfold thickness with age. The gender difference in skinfold thickness is established by the age of 3 years, and in adulthood females have approximately an 83 per cent greater mean or total skinfold thickness than males.

Table 3.28 shows references of mid-upper arm circumference with age, Table 3.29 the reference range of calculated mid-upper arm muscle circumference with age (see section 2.1.5.1), and Table 3.30 the reference ranges of arm muscle diameter, circumference and area with age. The gender difference in mid-upper arm muscle circumference is established by age 13; adult males have 56 per cent higher values than females (McDowell and Savage-King 1982).

Reviews and further reading

Falkner, F. and Tanner J. M. (1986). *Human Growth: A Comprehensive Treatise*. Plenum Press, New York.

Garn, S. M. (1962). Anthropometry in clinical appraisal of nutritional status. *American Journal of Clinical Nutrition* **11**: 418–32.

Gibson, R. S. (1990). *Principles of Nutritional Assessment*. Oxford University Press, New York.

Hall, J. G., Frosker-Iskenius, U. G., and Allanson, J. E. (1989). *Handbook of Normal Physical Measurements*. Oxford University Press.

Preese, M. A. and Baines, M. J. (1978). A new family of mathematical models describing the human growth curve. *Annals of Human Biology*, 5, 1–24.

WHO Working Group (1986). Use and interpretation of anthropometric indicators of nutritional status. *Bulletin of the World Health Organization*, **64**, 929–41.

World Health Organization (1983). *Measuring Change in Nutritional Status. Guidelines for Assessing the Impact of Supplementary Feeding Programmes for Vulnerable Groups*. WHO, Geneva.

Table 3.1: Cell numbers in the human body

age	cell number
4 d foetus (blastocyst)	58
7 w foetus	1.3×10^9
21 w foetus	2.2×10^{11}
newborn	2.0×10^{12}
adult	6.0×10^{13}

Table 3.2 Stages in embryological development

age	nervous system	eye	ear	skeleton and limbs	organs
4d	Early blastocyst (58 cells) free in uterine cavity				
8d	Implantation, trophoblast invasion				
12d	Early amnion sac, chorionic gonadotrophin secretion				
19d	Primitive streak, notochord, blood cells in yolk sac, stomatomedium and cloaca formed				
23d	partial fusion of folds	optic evagination			foregut develops, single heart tube.
28d	closure of neural tube	optic cup	otic placode otic invagination	arm buds form	evagination of thyroid, liver and dorsal pancreas from gut, lung bud forms, ventricular outpunching in heart, mesonephric duct enters cloaca, migration of myotomes from somites.
34d	cerebellar plate, cervical and mesencephalic flexures	lens invagination	otic vesicle	leg buds form	pharyngeal pouches yield parathyroids, thyroid and thymus, stomach broadens, auricular outpunching in heart, bronchi form, ureteral evagination, germ cells and gonadal ridge develop.
38d	basal lamina, cerebral evagination, neural hypophysis	lens separate, pigmented retina	endolymphatic sac, external auditory meatus, tubotympanic recess	hand plates form, innervation begins	intestinal loop into yolk sac, caecum, gall bladder, hepatic ducts, spleen develop, fusion mid auricular-ventricular canal, muscular septum formed in heart, main lobes of lungs formed, adrenal cortex invaded by sympathetic cells forming medulla.
45d	olfactory evagination, cerebral hemispheres apparent	lens fibres, migration of retinal cells	finger rays form,	elbow develops	caecum rotates right, appendix formed, aorta, pulmonary artery, heart valves and membrane ventricular septum form, tracheal cartillage, opening of urogenital membrane, early muscle. S-shaped vesicles in nephron connect with collecting tubes.
51d	optic nerve to brain	corneal body		cartillaginous models of bones	
8w	olfactory lobes, dura and pia mater formed	eyelids form	ear canals, spiral cochlear duct	ossification centres in bones	a few large glomeruli in kidney, testicles have interstitial cells, ovaries distinguishable and Mullerian ducts fusing, thyroid follicles develop.

Table 3.2 (Cont'd)

age	nervous system	eye	ear	skeleton and limbs	organs
10w	cerebellum apparent	iris, lachrymal gland developed			bladder sac forms, renal excretion begins, anal canal formed, enucleated red blood cells circulate, thoracic duct and lymph nodes form, adrenaline, noradrenaline and testosterone secreted.
12w	cervical and lumbar spinal cord enlarged	retina layered, eye axis forward		tail and notochord degenerated	gut muscle layers and pancreatic islets, bile secretion begins, nails beginning, palm creases formed, sebaceous glands develop, primary follicles in ovary, Leydig cells in testicle.
16w	cerebellum prominent, corpora quadrigemina, spinal cord myelination			distinct bones	typical kidney, uterus and vagina present, hand creases and sweat glands develop, keratinisation begins.
20w			inner ear ossified		hair at eyebrow, nail plates formed.
24w	typical layers in cerebral cortex				
28w	cerebral fissures and convolutions form	eyelids open, retinal layers complete, light perceived			testes descend.
32w			auricular cartilage		
36w					nails to fingertips
38w	brain myelination begins				eccrine sweat, nails to toe tips.

Table 3.3: Body size at birth
Figures show mean ± SD for the ICRP reference newborn infant

	calculation from	male	female
body weight (kg)	$((0.26 \times length)^{3.108} + 4.6)/1000$	3.5 ± 0.59	3.4 ± 0.59
body length (cm)	$107.3 \times e^{-(208.2/gestational\ age,\ days)}$	50.8 ± 2.5	50.0 ± 2.5
body surface area (cm^2)	$0.2808 \times length^{2.278}$	2200	2200
total body water (L)	757 mL /kg bw, range 700—810	2.65	2.57
density (g/cm^3)	-	1.026	1.022

Source: Snyder *et al.* 1975.

Table 3.4: Birth weight at term

	birth weight centiles (kg)								
	3	5	10	25	50	75	90	95	97
USA									
male	-	2.54	2.78	3.00	3.27	3.64	3.82	4.15	-
female	-	2.36	2.58	2.93	3.23	3.52	3.64	3.81	-
UK									
male	2.6	-	2.9	3.2	3.5	3.8	4.2	-	4.4
female	2.5	-	2.8	3.0	3.4	3.6	4.0	-	4.2

Source: from data reported by Lubchenko *et al.* 1963, 1966; Tanner and Whitehouse 1973.

Table 3.5: Birth weight according to gestational age

| gestational age (weeks) | birth weight centiles (kg) | | | | | | |
	3	10	25	50	75	90	97
USA, both genders							
27	-	0.75	0.91	1.03	1.21	1.42	-
28	-	0.82	0.96	1.12	1.33	1.55	-
29	-	0.89	1.08	1.21	1.45	1.64	-
30	-	0.96	1.21	1.33	1.58	1.78	-
31	-	1.12	1.33	1.47	1.74	1.95	-
32	-	1.24	1.48	1.62	1.94	2.19	-
33	-	1.39	1.62	1.83	2.17	2.45	-
34	-	1.53	1.79	2.04	2.45	2.79	-
35	-	1.71	1.99	2.20	2.74	3.08	-
36	-	1.90	2.24	2.61	2.97	3.29	-
37	-	2.17	2.49	2.83	3.16	3.48	-
38	-	2.38	2.67	3.00	3.32	3.61	-
39	-	2.51	2.81	3.13	3.39	3.69	-
40	-	2.61	2.92	3.24	3.50	3.80	-
41	-	2.67	2.97	3.29	3.56	3.86	-
Germany, male							
33	1.18	1.52	1.84	2.05	2.40	2.82	3.08
34	1.39	1.76	2.05	2.40	2.73	3.12	3.41
35	1.60	2.03	2.37	2.65	3.00	3.39	3.68
36	1.82	2.23	2.61	2.91	3.25	3.61	3.89
37	2.09	2.42	2.83	3.16	3.49	3.82	4.11
38	2.22	2.63	3.06	3.33	3.68	3.99	4.39
39	2.40	2.83	3.19	3.53	3.86	4.15	4.44
40	2.54	2.96	3.35	3.67	3.99	4.31	4.56
41	2.69	3.11	3.47	3.78	4.07	4.37	4.66
Germany, female							
33	0.94	1.49	1.76	1.99	2.21	2.51	2.95
34	1.21	1.67	1.94	2.19	2.42	2.72	3.20
35	1.48	1.87	2.14	2.38	2.62	2.99	3.43
36	1.71	2.03	2.31	2.56	2.81	3.13	3.63
37	1.94	2.24	2.49	2.76	2.99	3.35	3.84
38	2.12	2.40	2.65	2.92	3.17	3.52	3.99
39	2.31	2.59	2.83	3.15	3.36	3.70	4.15
40	2.46	2.70	2.99	3.26	3.52	3.84	4.23
41	2.54	2.88	3.13	3.38	3.67	3.95	4.27

Source: from data reported by Lubchenko *et al.* 1963; Hohenauer 1980.

Table 3.6: Body length at birth, full-term infants

| | body length centiles (cm) | | | | | | | | |
	3	5	10	25	50	75	90	95	97
USA									
male	-	46.4	47.5	49.0	50.5	51.8	53.5	54.4	-
female	-	45.4	46.5	48.2	49.9	51.0	52.0	52.9	-
UK									
male	47.0	-	48.5	49.8	51.0	52.7	53.7	-	55.0
female	46.0	-	47.8	48.8	50.0	51.9	53.0	-	54.5

Source: from data reported by Lubchenko *et al.* 1963, 1966; Tanner and Whitehouse 1973.

Table 3.7: Body length at birth according to gestational age

| | | body length centiles (cm) | | | | | | |
Gestational age (weeks)		3	10	25	50	75	90	97
USA	26	-	30.8	32.9	35.5	37.5	39.9	-
	27	-	31.8	34.1	36.6	38.6	41.0	-
	28	-	33.0	35.5	37.8	39.8	42.2	-
	29	-	34.4	36.8	39.0	40.9	43.1	-
	30	-	36.1	38.3	40.3	42.2	44.5	-
	31	-	37.5	39.7	41.6	43.5	45.9	-
	32	-	38.8	41.1	43.2	45.0	47.2	-
	33	-	39.9	42.3	44.7	46.2	48.4	-
	34	-	41.0	43.4	45.8	47.3	49.4	-
	35	-	42.0	44.6	46.7	48.1	50.2	-
	36	-	43.1	45.6	47.4	48.8	50.9	-
	37	-	44.1	46.5	48.0	49.3	51.3	-
	38	-	44.9	47.1	48.4	49.8	51.7	-
	39	-	45.5	47.6	48.8	50.1	52.0	-
	40	-	45.8	47.9	49.2	50.5	52.3	-
	41	-	46.1	48.1	49.5	50.8	52.6	-
	42	-	46.2	48.2	49.7	51.0	52.8	-
Germany	33	38.6	39.8	41.9	43.7	45.4	47.5	48.5
	34	39.9	41.5	43.3	45.0	46.7	48.7	49.8
	35	41.2	43.2	44.9	46.4	48.1	49.8	51.1
	36	42.3	44.3	46.0	47.5	49.2	50.7	52.0
	37	43.6	45.6	47.1	48.5	50.4	51.8	53.2
	38	44.4	46.6	48.1	49.5	51.2	52.5	53.8
	39	45.4	47.5	4839	50.4	52.1	53.1	54.6
	40	46.4	48.3	49.4	50.8	52.5	53.6	54.9
	41	46.9	48.4	49.4	50.8	52.5	53.9	55.5

Source: from data reported by Lubchenko *et al.* 1963; Hohenauer 1980.

Table 3.8: Head circumference at birth

Gestational age (weeks)	head circumference centiles (cm)						
	5	10	25	50	75	90	95
26	-	22.4	23.6	25.5	26.6	28.5	-
27	-	23.2	24.4	25.8	27.2	28.9	-
28	-	24.3	25.4	26.7	28.0	29.4	-
29	-	25.3	26.4	27.6	28.8	30.2	-
30	-	26.2	27.4	28.6	29.7	31.1	-
31	-	26.9	28.2	29.6	30.5	31.9	-
32	-	27.6	29.0	30.4	31.4	32.7	-
33	-	28.4	29.8	31.2	32.1	33.4	-
34	-	29.2	30.6	31.9	32.9	34.0	-
35	-	30.0	31.3	32.5	33.4	34.5	-
36	-	30.6	31.8	32.9	33.8	34.9	-
37	-	31.1	32.3	33.2	34.1	35.2	-
38	-	31.4	32.5	33.4	34.3	35.4	-
39	-	31.6	32.8	33.7	34.6	35.7	-
40	-	31.8	33.0	34.0	34.8	35.9	-
41	-	32.0	33.2	34.2	35.0	36.0	-
42	-	32.1	33.4	34.3	35.1	36.2	-
full term (NCHS standards)							
boys	32.6	33.0	33.9	34.8	35.6	36.6	37.2
girls	32.1	32.9	33.5	34.3	34.8	35.5	35.9

Source: from data reported by Lubchenko *et al.* 1963, 1966.

Table 3.9: Changes in tissue protein content with age

	newborn	2-9 months old	adult
		ratio protein:water	
skeletal muscle	0.16	0.23	0.27
adipose tissue	0.11	0.14	0.05
skin	0.20	0.51	0.48
bone	0.27	0.30	1.10
liver	0.18	0.20	0.25
heart	0.15	0.16	0.17
mean of tissues reported	0.17	0.26	0.39

Source: Fomon 1967.

Table 3.10: Changes in body composition with age

age	fat %body weight	protein	water	sodium	potassium g/kg fat-free mass	calcium	magnesium	phosphorus
foetus, 1.5kg	3.5	111	856	105	49.6	354	19.7	126
foetus, 2.5kg	7.6	126	837	101	52.1	413	20.4	152
birth	16.2	137	822	97	50.8	464	20.6	171
1 year	20	170	780	95	58.0	698	24.7	226
4.5 years	22.7	238	697	99.9	65.0	1050	29.6	338
adult, mean	19.7	205	723	87	69	1064	38.4	375
adult, range	12.5–27.9	165-238	674-775	78-96	66.5-73.0	912-1240	35.4-40.3	284-452

Source: from data reported by Garrow *et al.* 1965 and the calculated means and ranges of data for adults cited in that paper.

Table 3.11: Changes in body composition with age

age	weight	fat kg	fat % bw	ffbm kg	protein	tbw	ecf % bw	icw	bone	protein	tbw	ecf % ffm	icw	bone	tbk mmol/kg ffm	density ffm
males																
birth	3.54	0.49	13.7	3.06	12.9	69.6	42.5	27.0	2.6	15.0	80.6	49.3	31.3	3.0	49.0	1.063
1 m	4.45	0.67	15.1	3.78	12.9	68.4	41.1	27.3	2.6	15.1	80.5	48.4	32.1	3.0	50.1	1.064
2 m	5.51	1.09	19.9	4.41	12.3	64.3	38.0	26.3	2.4	15.4	80.3	47.4	32.9	3.0	51.2	1.065
3 m	6.43	1.49	23.2	4.94	12.0	61.4	35.7	25.8	2.3	15.6	80.0	46.4	33.6	3.0	52.2	1.065
4 m	7.06	1.74	24.7	5.31	11.9	60.1	34.5	25.7	2.3	15.8	79.9	45.8	34.1	3.0	53.0	1.066
5 m	7.58	1.91	25.3	5.66	11.9	59.6	33.8	25.8	2.3	15.9	79.7	45.2	34.5	3.0	53.6	1.066
6 m	8.03	2.04	25.4	5.99	12.0	59.4	33.4	26.0	2.3	16.0	79.6	44.7	34.9	3.0	54.1	1.066
9 m	9.18	2.19	24.0	6.98	12.4	60.3	33.0	27.2	2.3	16.4	79.3	43.5	35.8	3.0	55.5	1.068
1 y	10.15	2.29	22.5	7.86	12.9	61.2	32.9	28.3	2.3	16.6	79.0	42.5	36.5	3.0	56.5	1.068
1.5 y	11.47	2.38	20.8	9.09	13.5	62.2	32.3	29.9	2.5	17.1	78.5	40.8	37.7	3.1	58.2	1.070
2 y	12.59	2.46	19.5	10.13	14.0	62.9	31.9	31.0	2.6	17.4	78.1	39.6	38.5	3.2	59.3	1.072
3 y	14.68	2.58	17.5	12.10	14.7	63.9	31.1	32.8	2.8	17.8	77.5	37.8	39.7	3.3	61.1	1.074
4 y	16.69	2.66	15.9	14.03	15.3	64.8	30.5	34.2	2.9	18.2	77.0	36.3	40.7	3.5	62.5	1.076
5 y	18.67	2.72	14.6	15.95	15.8	65.4	30.0	35.4	3.1	18.5	76.6	35.2	41.4	3.6	63.6	1.078
6 y	20.69	2.79	13.5	17.89	16.2	66.0	29.6	36.4	3.2	18.7	76.3	34.2	42.0	3.7	64.4	1.080
7 y	22.85	2.93	12.8	19.92	16.5	66.2	29.1	37.1	3.3	18.9	75.9	33.4	42.6	3.8	65.2	1.081
8 y	25.30	3.29	13.0	22.00	16.6	65.8	28.3	37.5	3.4	19.1	75.7	32.6	43.1	3.9	65.9	1.082
9 y	28.13	3.72	13.2	24.41	16.8	65.4	27.6	37.8	3.5	19.3	75.4	31.8	43.6	4.0	66.7	1.084
10 y	31.44	4.32	13.7	27.12	16.8	64.8	26.7	38.0	3.5	19.5	75.1	31.0	44.1	4.1	67.4	1.085
females																
birth	3.33	0.49	14.9	2.83	12.8	68.6	42.0	26.7	2.6	15.0	80.6	49.3	31.3	3.0	49.0	1.064
1 m	4.13	0.67	16.2	3.46	12.7	67.5	40.5	26.9	2.5	15.2	80.5	48.3	32.1	3.0	50.2	1.064
2 m	4.99	1.05	21.1	3.94	12.2	63.2	37.1	26.1	2.5	15.5	80.2	47.1	33.1	3.0	51.5	1.065
3 m	5.74	1.37	23.8	4.38	12.0	60.9	35.1	25.8	2.3	15.8	79.9	46.0	33.9	3.0	52.7	1.066
4 m	6.30	1.59	25.2	4.72	11.9	59.6	33.8	25.8	2.3	15.9	79.7	45.2	34.5	3.0	53.5	1.066
5 m	6.80	1.77	26.0	5.03	11.9	58.8	33.0	25.9	2.2	16.1	79.5	44.6	34.9	3.0	54.2	1.067
6 m	7.25	1.92	26.4	5.34	12.0	58.4	32.4	26.0	2.2	16.3	79.4	44.0	35.4	3.0	54.8	1.067
9 m	8.27	2.07	25.0	6.20	12.5	59.3	32.0	27.3	2.3	16.6	79.0	42.7	36.4	3.0	56.3	1.068
1 y	9.18	2.18	23.7	7.01	12.9	60.1	31.8	28.3	2.3	16.9	78.8	41.6	37.1	3.0	57.4	1.069
1.5 y	10.78	2.35	21.8	8.43	13.5	61.3	31.5	29.8	2.4	17.2	78.4	40.3	38.1	3.0	58.8	1.070
2 y	11.91	2.43	20.4	9.48	13.9	62.2	31.5	30.8	2.4	17.4	78.2	39.5	38.7	3.0	59.6	1.071
3 y	14.10	2.61	18.5	11.49	14.4	63.5	31.3	32.2	2.5	17.7	77.9	38.4	39.5	3.0	60.8	1.071
4 y	15.96	2.76	17.3	13.20	14.8	64.3	31.2	33.1	2.5	17.9	77.7	37.8	40.0	3.0	61.5	1.072
5 y	17.66	2.95	16.7	14.71	15.0	64.6	31.0	33.6	2.5	18.0	77.6	37.3	40.3	3.0	62.0	1.073
6 y	19.52	3.21	16.4	16.31	15.2	64.7	30.8	34.0	2.6	18.1	77.5	36.8	40.7	3.1	62.5	1.073
7 y	21.84	3.66	16.8	18.18	15.2	64.4	30.3	34.1	2.5	18.3	77.3	36.3	41.0	3.1	62.9	1.073
8 y	24.84	4.32	17.4	20.52	15.2	63.8	29.6	34.2	2.5	18.4	77.2	35.8	41.4	3.1	63.4	1.074
9 y	28.46	5.21	18.3	23.25	15.1	63.0	28.9	34.1	2.5	18.5	77.1	35.4	41.7	3.1	64.0	1.074
10 y	32.55	6.32	19.4	26.23	15.0	62.0	28.1	33.9	2.5	18.7	76.9	34.9	42.0	3.1	64.5	1.075

ffm = fat-free mass, tbw = total body water, ecf = extra-cellular fluid, icw = intracellular water, bone = bone mineral. Extra-osseous mineral comprises 0.5—0.6 of fat-free body mass, and carbohydrate 0.4-0.5%.

Source: Fomon et al. 1982.

Table 3.12: Changes in organ weight with age

age	heart	lungs	spleen	liver	kidneys	brain	heart	lungs	spleen	liver	kidneys	brain
			weight (g)						g /kg body weight			
birth	17	39	8	78	27	335	4.80	11.00	2.26	22.00	7.62	94.50
3-5 w	20	58	12	127	32	413	4.49	13.03	2.70	28.53	7.19	92.77
5-7 w	21	60	13	133	37	422	4.22	12.05	2.61	26.70	7.43	84.73
7-9 w	23	61	13	136	37	489	4.17	11.07	2.36	24.69	6.72	88.76
3 m	23	65	14	140	39	516	3.57	10.10	2.18	21.76	6.06	80.19
4 m	27	70	16	160	43	540	3.82	9.92	2.27	22.66	6.09	76.49
5 m	29	73	16	188	50	644	3.83	9.64	2.11	24.82	6.60	85.02
6 m	31	81	17	200	51	660	3.86	10.09	2.12	24.91	6.35	82.19
9m	37	100	20	260	61	750	4.03	10.89	2.18	28.32	6.64	81.70
12m	44	121	26	288	71	925	4.33	11.92	2.56	28.37	7.00	91.13
18m	52	137	32	345	83	1042	4.53	11.94	2.79	30.08	7.24	90.85
24m	56	164	33	394	93	1064	4.45	13.03	2.62	31.29	7.39	84.51
3y	59	166	37	418	97	1141	4.02	11.31	2.52	28.48	6.61	77.75
4y	73	175	39	516	114	1191	4.37	10.49	2.34	30.92	6.83	71.36
5y	85	211	47	596	129	1237	4.55	11.30	2.52	31.92	6.91	66.26
6y	94	243	58	642	135	1243	4.54	11.74	2.80	31.03	6.52	60.08
7y	100	253	66	680	139	1263	4.38	11.07	2.89	29.76	6.08	55.27
8y	110	290	69	736	149	1273	4.35	11.46	2.73	29.09	5.89	50.32
9y	115	326	73	756	165	1275	4.09	11.59	2.60	26.88	5.87	45.33
10y	116	343	85	852	187	1290	3.69	10.91	2.70	27.10	5.95	41.03

Source: calculated from organ weights reported by Coppoletta and Wolbach 1933 and reference body weights reported by Fomon *et al.* 1982.

Table 3.13: Body weight from birth to 18 years of age, Tanner standards

| | body weight centiles (kg) | | | | | | | | | | | | |
| | males | | | | | | | females | | | | | |
age (years)	3	10	25	50	75	90	97	3	10	25	50	75	90	97
birth	2.50	2.80	3.10	3.50	3.80	4.10	4.40	2.55	2.85	3.15	3.40	3.65	3.95	4.35
0.25	4.65	5.01	5.43	5.93	6.45	6.99	7.43	4.36	4.81	5.18	5.56	6.02	6.41	6.90
0.5	6.38	6.80	7.32	7.90	8.58	9.2	9.90	5.89	6.44	6.90	7.39	7.99	8.49	9.08
0.75	7.48	7.98	8.55	9.20	9.95	10.63	11.45	6.99	7.58	8.13	8.72	9.42	10.02	10.64
1.0	8.3	8.8	9.5	10.2	11.0	11.7	12.6	7.8	8.4	9.0	9.7	10.5	11.2	11.8
1.25	8.9	9.6	10.2	11.0	11.8	12.6	13.5	8.3	9.0	9.6	10.4	11.3	12.0	12.7
1.5	9.4	10.1	10.7	11.6	12.5	13.3	14.3	8.9	9.5	10.2	11.1	12.0	12.8	13.5
1.75	9.8	10.5	11.2	12.2	13.1	13.9	14.9	9.3	10.0	10.8	11.7	12.6	13.5	14.3
2.0	10.2	11.0	11.8	12.7	13.7	14.6	15.6	9.7	10.4	11.3	12.2	13.2	14.1	14.9
2.25	10.5	11.4	12.2	13.2	14.2	15.1	16.2	10.0	10.8	11.7	12.7	13.7	14.6	15.5
2.5	10.9	11.9	12.7	13.7	14.8	15.8	16.9	10.5	11.3	12.2	13.3	14.3	15.3	16.3
2.75	11.2	12.2	13.1	14.2	15.3	16.3	17.4	10.9	11.8	12.7	13.7	14.8	15.8	16.9
3	11.6	12.7	13.6	14.7	15.8	16.9	18.0	11.4	12.3	13.2	14.3	15.3	16.4	17.6
3.5	12.3	13.4	14.5	15.6	16.8	18.0	19.2	12.2	13.2	14.2	15.2	16.3	17.6	18.9
4	13.0	14.3	15.3	16.6	17.9	19.1	20.4	13.1	14.1	15.2	16.3	17.5	18.8	20.3
4.5	13.7	15.0	16.1	17.5	19.0	20.2	21.8	13.8	15.0	16.1	17.2	18.6	20.1	21.8
5	14.4	15.7	16.9	18.5	20.0	21.5	23.2	14..6	15.9	17.0	18.3	19.8	21.4	23.3
5.5	15.1	16.5	17.7	19.5	21.2	22.8	24.8	15.4	16.7	18.0	19.3	20.9	22.9	25.0
6	15.9	17.3	18.6	20.5	22.4	24.0	26.5	16.2	17.6	18.9	20.4	22.2	24.4	26.8
6.5	16.6	18.1	19.5	21.5	23.6	25.4	28.3	17.0	18.4	19.8	21.5	23.5	26.0	28.5
7	17.4	19.0	20.6	22.6	24.9	26.9	30.3	17.8	19.2	20.8	22.6	25.0	27.7	30.6
7.5	18.2	19.9	21.6	23.7	26.1	28.4	32.3	18.6	20.1	21.9	23.8	26.4	29.3	32.6
8	19.1	20.9	22.7	25.0	27.5	30.0	34.4	19.4	21.0	22.9	25.1	28.0	31.2	35.0
8.5	20.0	21.9	23.9	26.2	28.9	31.6	36.5	20.2	21.9	24.0	26.4	29.5	33.2	37.7
9	21.0	22.9	25.0	27.5	30.3	33.4	38.8	21.0	23.0	25.2	27.7	31.4	35.4	40.6
9.5	21.9	24.0	26.2	28.9	31.9	35.3	41.0	21.8	24.0	26.4	29.3	33.4	38.0	43.8
10	23..0	25.2	27.5	30.3	33.6	37.3	43.3	22.7	25.1	27.7	31.1	35.7	41.0	47.7
10.5	24.0	26.3	28.7	31.9	35.6	39.7	46.3	23.6	26.4	29.2	33.0	38.3	44.1	51.7
11	24.9	27.4	30.1	33.6	37.7	42.6	49.5	24.7	27.8	31.0	35.2	41.0	47.7	55.7
11.5	26.0	28.6	31.6	35.5	40.2	45.4	53.5	26.2	29.6	33.2	37.7	43.7	51.2	59.6
12	27.1	29.9	33.2	37.7	42.7	49.0	57.2	27.8	31.6	33.5	40.5	46.7	54.7	63.3
12.5	28.1	31.3	35.0	40.0	45.7	52.5	61.0	29.7	33.9	38.0	43.1	49.5	57.6	66.5
13	29.6	33.0	37.1	42.6	49.0	56.0	64.4	32.0	36.3	40.7	45.8	52.3	60.0	69.3
13.5	31.2	35.1	39.7	45.	52.2	59.4	67.8	34.5	38.7	43.3	48.6	54.8	62.3	71.1
14	33.3	37.7	42.6	48.8	55.4	62.5	70.9	37.0	41.2	45.5	51.0	57.0	63.9	72.3
14.5	36.0	40.6	45.7	51.9	58.4	65.4	73.7	39.5	43.3	47.4	52.9	58.6	65.3	73.2
15	39.0	43.7	48.7	54.7	60.9	68.0	75.9	41.7	45.1	49.0	54.4	59.8	66.3	73.7
15.5	42.7	47.0	51.7	57.4	63.0	70.1	77..5	43.5	46.6	50.2	55.2	60.6	67.1	74.1
16	45.7	49.6	54.1	59.6	65.0	71.7	78.6	44.6	47.6	51.0	55.8	61.1	67.5	74.5
16.5	47.5	51.3	55.6	61.0	66.2	72.8	79.5	45.7	48.6	51.9	56.4	61.6	67.9	74.9
17	48.6	52.3	56.6	61.9	67.1	73.6	80.2	46.0	48.8	52.1	56.6	6138	68.0	75.0
18	50.0	53.5	57.8	63.0	68.0	74.5	81.0	-	-	-	-	-	-	-
19	50.4	53.7	58.1	63.3	68.3	75.0	81.6	46.1	48.9	52.2	56.7	61.9	68.1	75.1

Source: Tanner *et al.* 1966.

Table 3.14: Body weight from birth to 18 years of age, NCHS standards

age			male							female				
	5	10	25	50	75	90	95	5	10	25	50	75	90	95
birth	2.54	2.78	3.00	3.27	3.64	3.82	4.15	2.36	2.58	2.93	3.23	3.52	3.64	3.81
1 m	3.16	3.43	3.82	4.29	4.75	5.14	5.38	2.97	3.22	3.59	3.98	4.36	4.65	4.92
3 m	4.43	4.78	5.32	5.98	6.56	7.14	7.37	4.18	4.47	4.88	5.40	5.90	6.39	6.74
6 m	6.20	6.61	7.20	7.85	8.49	9.10	9.46	5.79	6.12	6.60	7.21	7.83	8.38	8.73
9 m	7.52	7.95	8.56	9.18	9.88	10.49	10.93	7.00	7.34	7.89	8.56	9.24	9.83	10.17
1 y	8.43	8.84	9.49	10.15	10.91	11.54	11.99	7.84	8.19	8.81	9.53	10.23	10.87	11.24
1.5 y	9.59	9.92	10.67	11.47	12.31	13.05	13.44	8.92	9.30	10.04	10.82	11.55	12.30	12.76
2 y	10.54	10.85	11.65	12.59	13.44	14.29	14.7	9.87	10.26	11.10	11.90	12.74	13.57	14.08
2.5 y	11.44	11.80	12.63	13.27	14.51	15.47	15.97	10.78	11.21	12.11	12.93	13.93	14.81	15.35
3 y	12.1	12.6	13.1	14.6	15.8	16.9	17.8	11.6	12.3	13.1	14.1	15.5	16.5	17.2
3.5 y	12.8	13.4	14.5	15.7	16.9	18.2	18.9	12.4	13.1	14.0	15.1	16.6	17.8	18.6
4 y	13.6	14.2	15.4	16.7	18.0	19.3	20.3	13.1	13.8	14.8	16.0	17.6	18.9	19.9
4.5 y	14.5	15.1	16.3	17.7	19.1	20.5	21.6	13.8	14.6	15.6	16.8	18.5	20.1	21.2
5 y	15.3	15.9	17.2	18.7	20.1	21.7	23.1	14.6	15.3	16.3	17.7	19.4	21.2	22.6
5.5 y	16.1	16.8	18.1	19.7	21.3	23.0	24.7	15.3	15.9	17.5	18.6	21.4	22.5	24.1
6 y	16.9	17.7	19.1	20.7	22.4	24.3	26.3	16.1	16.7	17.9	19.5	21.4	23.9	25.8
6.5 y	17.8	18.6	20.0	21.7	23.6	25.8	28.2	16.9	17.5	18.8	20.6	22.7	25.5	27.6
7 y	18.6	19.5	21.0	22.9	24.9	27.4	30.1	17.7	18.4	19.8	21.8	24.2	27.4	29.7
7.5 y	18.6	19.5	21.0	22.9	24.9	27.4	30.1	18.6	19.4	21.0	23.3	25.9	29.6	32.1
8 y	20.4	21.4	22.1	25.3	27.9	31.1	34.5	19.6	20.5	22.3	24.8	27.9	32.0	34.7
8.5 y	21.3	22.3	24.2	26.7	29.6	33.2	37.0	20.7	21.6	23.7	26.6	30.1	34.7	37.6
9 y	22.3	23.3	25.4	28.1	31.5	35.6	39.6	21.8	22.9	25.3	28.5	32.4	37.6	40.6
9.5 y	23.3	24.4	26.9	29.7	33.5	38.1	42.4	23.1	24.3	26.9	30.5	34.9	40.6	43.9
10 y	24.3	25.5	28.1	31.4	35.6	40.8	45.3	24.4	25.8	28.7	32.6	37.5	43.7	47.2
10.5 y	25.5	26.8	29.6	33.3	37.9	43.6	48.3	25.8	27.3	30.6	34.7	40.2	46.8	50.6
11 y	26.8	28.2	31.3	35.3	40.4	46.6	51.5	27.2	29.0	32.5	37.0	42.8	50.0	54.0
11.5 y	28.2	29.7	33.1	37.5	43.0	49.6	54.7	28.8	30.7	34.5	39.2	45.5	53.0	57.4
12 y	29.9	31.4	35.1	39.8	45.8	52.7	58.1	30.5	32.5	36.5	41.5	48.1	56.0	60.8
12.5 y	31.6	33.4	37.3	42.3	48.7	55.9	61.5	32.3	34.4	38.6	43.8	50.6	58.8	64.1
13 y	33.6	35.6	39.7	45.0	51.8	59.1	65.0	34.1	36.4	40.6	46.1	52.9	61.5	67.3
13.5 y	35.9	38.0	42.4	47.8	55.0	62.4	68.5	36.0	38.3	42.7	48.3	55.1	63.9	70.3
14 y	38.2	40.0	45.2	50.8	58.3	65.6	72.1	37.8	40.1	44.5	50.3	57.1	66.0	73.1
14.5 y	40.7	43.3	48.1	53.8	61.6	68.8	75.7	39.5	41.8	46.3	52.1	58.8	68.0	75.6
15 y	43.1	46.1	50.9	56.7	64.7	71.9	79.1	41.0	43.4	47.8	53.7	60.3	69.5	77.8
15.5 y	45.5	48.7	53.6	59.5	67.6	75.0	82.5	42.3	44.7	49.1	55.0	61.5	70.8	79.6
16 y	47.4	51.2	56.2	62.1	70.3	78.0	85.6	43.4	5.8	50.1	55.9	62.3	71.7	81.0
16.5 y	49.8	53.4	58.4	64.4	72.5	80.8	88.6	44.2	46.5	50.8	56.4	62.8	72.2	81.9
17 y	51.5	55.3	60.2	66.3	74.2	83.6	91.3	44.7	47.0	51.1	56.7	62.9	72.4	82.5
17.5 y	52.9	56.8	61.6	67.8	75.3	86.1	93.7	45.1	47.3	51.3	56.7	62.9	72.4	82.6
18 y	54.0	57.9	62.6	68.9	76.0	88.4	95.8	45.3	47.5	51.4	56.6	62.8	72.3	82.5

Source: Hamill *et al.* 1979.

Table 3.15: Body length from birth to 2 years, Tanner standards

age (years)	body length centiles (cm)													
	male							female						
	3	10	25	50	75	90	97	3	10	25	50	75	90	97
0.08	50.2	51.4	52.7	54.0	55.4	56.6	57.8	49.2	50.4	51.6	53.0	54.4	55.6	56.8
0.25	56.6	57.9	59.2	60.7	62.1	63.4	64.7	54.9	56.2	57.5	59.0	60.5	61.8	63.1
0.50	63.8	65.2	66.6	68.2	69.7	71.2	72.6	61.1	62.5	63.9	65.5	67.1	68.5	69.9
0.75	67.9	69.4	71.0	72.7	74.4	75.9	77.4	65.5	67.0	68.6	70.2	72.0	73.5	74.9
1.00	71.2	72.8	74.5	76.3	78.1	79.7	81.4	69.1	70.8	72.4	74.2	76.0	77.7	79.3
1.25	74.0	75.7	77.4	79.4	81.3	83.0	84.7	72.2	73.9	75.7	77.6	79.5	81.2	82.9
1.50	76.5	78.3	80.1	82.1	84.2	86.0	87.8	74.9	76.7	78.5	80.5	82.6	84.4	86.2
1.75	78.7	80.6	82.5	84.6	86.7	88.7	90.5	77.2	79.1	81.1	83.2	85.3	87.2	89.1
2.00	80.7	82.7	84.7	86.9	89.1	91.1	93.1	79.4	81.3	83.4	85.6	87.8	89.8	91.8

Source: Tanner *et al.* 1966.

Table 3.16: Body length from birth to 3 years, NCHS standards

age (months)	body length centiles (cm)													
	males							females						
	5	10	25	50	75	90	95	5	10	25	50	75	90	95
birth	46.4	47.5	49.0	50.5	51.8	53.5	54.4	45.4	46.5	48.2	49.9	51.0	52.0	52.9
1	50.4	51.3	53.0	54.6	56.2	57.7	58.6	49.2	50.2	51.9	53.5	54.9	56.1	56.9
3	56.7	57.7	59.4	61.1	63.0	64.5	65.4	55.4	56.2	57.8	59.5	61.2	62.7	63.4
6	63.4	64.4	66.1	67.8	69.7	71.3	72.3	61.8	62.6	64.2	65.9	67.8	69.4	70.2
9	68.0	69.1	70.6	72.3	74.0	75.9	77.1	66.1	67.0	68.7	70.4	72.4	74.0	75.0
12	71.7	72.8	74.3	76.1	77.7	79.8	81.2	69.8	70.8	72.4	74.3	76.3	78.0	79.1
18	77.5	78.7	80.5	82.4	84.3	86.6	88.1	76.0	77.2	78.8	80.9	83.0	85.0	86.1
24	82.3	83.5	85.6	87.6	89.9	92.2	93.8	81.3	82.5	84.2	86.5	88.7	90.8	92.0
30	87.0	88.2	90.1	92.3	94.6	97.0	98.7	86.0	87.0	88.9	91.3	93.7	95.6	96.9
36	91.2	92.4	94.2	96.5	98.9	101.4	103.1	90.0	91.0	93.1	95.6	98.1	100.0	101.5

Source: Hamill *et al.* 1979.

Table 3.17: Height from 2–18 years, Tanner standards

age (years)	height centiles (cm)													
	males							females						
	3	10	25	50	75	90	97	3	10	25	50	75	90	97
2	79.7	81.7	83.7	85.9	88.1	90.1	95.1	78.4	80.3	82.4	84.6	86.8	88.8	90.8
2.5	83.5	85.6	87.8	90.2	92.6	94.8	96.9	82.2	84.3	86.5	88.9	91.3	93.5	95.6
3	87.0	89.3	91.6	94.5	96.8	99.1	101.4	85.7	88.1	90.4	93.0	95.6	97.9	100.2
3.5	90.4	92.8	95.3	98.0	100.8	103.2	105.7	89.2	91.6	94.1	96.8	99.6	102.0	104.5
4	93.5	96.1	98.7	101.6	104.5	107.1	109.7	92.3	94.9	97.5	100.4	103.3	105.9	108.5
4.5	96.5	99.2	102.0	105.0	108.1	110.8	113.5	95.4	98.1	100.8	103.8	106.9	109.7	112.4
5	99.4	102.2	105.1	108.3	111.5	114.4	117.2	98.2	101.1	104.0	107.2	110.3	113.2	116.1
5.5	102.2	105.2	108.2	111.5	114.8	117.8	120.8	101.0	104.0	107.0	110.3	113.7	116.7	119.6
6	104.9	108.0	111.1	114.6	118.1	121.2	124.3	103.8	106.8	110.0	113.4	116.9	120.0	123.1
6.5	107.6	110.8	114.0	117.6	121.2	124.2	127.6	106.4	109.6	112.8	116.4	120.0	123.2	126.4
7	110.3	113.5	116.8	120.5	124.2	127.5	130.8	109.1	112.4	115.7	119.3	123.0	126.3	129.6
7.5	112.9	116.2	119.6	123.4	127.2	130.6	133.9	111.7	115.0	118.4	122.2	126.0	129.4	132.8
8	115.4	118.8	122.3	126.2	130.0	133.5	137.0	114.2	117.6	121.1	125.0	128.9	132.4	135.8
8.5	117.9	121.4	125.0	128.9	132.9	136.4	139.9	116.7	120.3	123.8	127.8	131.8	135.3	138.8
9	120.4	124.0	127.6	131.6	135.7	139.3	142.9	119.3	122.9	126.6	130.6	134.6	138.3	141.9
9.5	122.8	126.5	130.2	134.3	138.4	142.1	145.8	121.9	125.6	129.3	133.5	137.6	141.3	145.0
10	125.1	128.8	132.6	136.8	141.0	144.8	148.5	124.5	28.3	132.1	136.4	140.6	144.5	148.3
10.5	127.2	131.0	135.0	139.3	143.6	147.6	151.4	127.1	131.1	135.0	139.5	143.9	147.9	151.8
11	129.4	133.3	137.4	141.9	146.4	150.4	154.4	129.5	133.7	138.0	142.7	147.4	151.6	155.8
11.5	131.7	135.8	140.0	144.7	149.4	153.6	157.8	132.0	136.5	141.0	146.1	151.1	155.6	160.1
12	133.7	138.0	142.4	147.3	152.2	156.6	160.9	135.0	139.6	144.2	149.3	154.4	159.1	163.6
12.5	136.3	140.7	145.3	150.3	155.4	159.9	164.4	139.0	143.3	147.7	152.5	157.4	161.8	166.1
13	138.7	143.4	148.2	153.4	158.7	163.5	168.2	142.6	146.7	150.9	155.5	160.2	164.4	168.5
13.5	141.5	146.4	151.3	156.8	162.3	167.2	172.0	145.4	149.4	153.4	157.9	162.3	166.3	170.3
14	145.0	150.0	155.0	160.7	166.3	171.2	176.2	147.6	151.4	155.3	159.6	163.9	167.8	171.6
14.5	148.4	153.4	158.4	164.0	169.6	174.6	179.6	149.4	153.1	156.9	161.1	165.3	169.0	172.7
15	152.3	157.1	161.9	167.3	172.7	177.6	182.4	150.3	153.9	157.6	161.7	165.8	169.5	173.2
15.5	155.9	160.4	165.0	170.1	175.2	179.8	184.3	150.6	154.2	157.9	162.0	166.1	169.7	173.4
16	158.9	163.1	167.4	172.2	177.0	181.3	185.5	150.9	154.5	158.2	162.2	166.2	169.9	173.5
16.5	160.7	164.8	168.9	173.5	178.0	182.1	186.2	-	-	-	-	-	-	-
17	161.7	165.7	169.8	174.3	178.8	182.8	186.8	-	-	-	-	-	-	-
17.5	162.0	166.0	170.0	174.5	179.0	183.0	187.0	-	-	-	-	-	-	-
18	162.2	166.2	170.2	174.7	179.2	183.2	187.2	-	-	-	-	-	-	-

Source: Tanner *et al. 1966.*

Table 3.18: Height from 3–18 years of age, NCHS standards

age	height centiles (cm)												
(years)	male							female					
	5	10	25	50	75	90	95	5	10	25	50	75	90	95
3	89.0	90.3	92.6	94.9	97.5	100.1	102.0	88.3	89.3	91.4	94.1	96.6	99.0	100.6
3.5	92.5	93.9	96.4	99.1	101.7	104.3	106.1	91.7	93.0	95.2	97.9	100.5	102.8	104.5
4	95.8	97.3	100.0	102.9	105.7	108.2	109.9	95.0	96.4	98.8	101.6	104.3	106.6	108.3
4.5	98.9	100.6	103.4	106.6	109.4	111.9	113.5	98.1	99.7	102.2	105.0	107.9	110.2	112.0
5	102.0	103.7	106.5	109.9	112.8	115.4	117.0	101.1	102.7	105.4	108.4	111.4	113.8	115.6
5.5	104.9	106.7	109.6	113.1	116.1	118.7	120.3	103.9	105.6	108.4	111.6	114.8	117.4	119.2
6	107.7	109.6	112.5	116.1	119.2	121.9	123.5	106.6	108.4	111.3	114.6	118.1	120.8	122.7
6.5	110.4	112.3	115.3	119.0	122.2	124.9	126.6	109.2	111.0	114.1	117.6	121.3	124.2	126.1
7	113.0	115.0	118.0	121.7	125.0	127.9	129.7	111.8	113.6	116.8	120.6	124.4	127.6	129.5
7.5	115.6	117.6	120.6	124.4	127.8	130.8	132.7	114.4	116.2	119.5	125.5	127.5	130.9	132.9
8	118.1	120.2	123.2	127.0	130.5	133.6	135.7	116.9	118.7	122.2	126.4	130.6	134.2	136.2
8.5	120.5	122.7	125.7	129.6	133.2	136.5	138.8	119.5	121.3	124.9	129.3	133.6	137.4	139.6
9	122.9	125.2	128.2	132.2	136.0	139.4	141.8	122.1	123.9	127.7	132.2	136.7	140.7	142.9
9.5	125.3	127.6	130.8	134.8	138.8	142.4	144.9	124.8	126.6	130.6	135.2	139.8	143.9	146.2
10	127.7	130.1	133.4	137.5	141.6	145.5	148.1	127.5	129.5	133.6	138.3	142.9	147.2	149.5
10.5	130.1	132.6	136.0	140.3	144.6	148.7	151.5	130.4	132.5	136.7	141.5	146.1	150.4	152.8
11	132.6	135.1	138.7	143.3	147.8	152.1	154.9	133.5	135.6	140.0	144.8	149.3	153.7	156.2
11.5	135.0	137.7	141.5	146.4	151.1	155.6	158.5	136.6	139.0	143.5	148.2	152.6	156.9	159.5
12	137.6	140.3	144.4	149.7	154.6	159.4	162.3	139.8	142.3	147.0	151.5	155.8	160.0	162.7
12.5	140.2	143.0	147.4	153.0	158.2	163.2	166.1	142.7	145.4	150.1	154.6	158.8	162.9	165.6
13	142.9	145.8	150.5	156.5	161.8	167.0	169.8	145.2	148.0	152.8	157.1	161.3	165.3	168.1
13.5	145.7	148.7	153.6	159.9	165.3	170.5	173.4	147.2	150.0	154.7	159.0	163.2	167.3	170.0
14	148.8	151.8	156.9	163.1	168.5	173.8	176.7	148.7	151.2	155.9	160.4	164.6	167.8	171.3
14.5	152.0	155.0	160.1	166.2	171.5	176.1	179.5	149.7	152.5	158.8	161.2	165.6	169.8	172.2
15	155.2	158.2	163.3	169.0	174.1	178.9	181.9	150.5	153.2	157.2	161.8	166.3	170.5	172.8
15.5	158.3	161.2	166.2	171.5	176.3	180.8	183.9	151.1	153.6	157.5	162.1	166.7	170.9	173.1
16	161.1	163.9	168.7	173.5	178.1	182.4	185.4	151.6	154.1	157.8	162.4	166.9	171.1	173.3
16.5	163.4	166.1	170.6	175.2	179.5	183.6	186.6	152.2	154.6	158.2	162.7	167.1	171.2	173.4
17	164.9	167.7	171.9	176.2	180.5	184.5	187.3	152.7	155.1	158.7	163.1	167.3	171.2	173.5
17.5	165.6	168.5	172.4	176.7	181.0	185.0	187.6	153.2	155.6	159.1	163.4	167.5	171.1	173.5
18	165.7	168.7	172.3	176.8	181.2	185.3	187.6	153.6	156.0	159.6	163.7	167.6	171.0	173.6

Source: Hamill *et al. 1979.*

Table 3.19: Weight and length or height for age; standard deviations below reference values, NCHS/WHO standards

age, months	weight (kg)						length or height (cm)				
	reference	-1 SD	-2 SD	-3 SD	-4 SD	-5 SD	reference	-1 SD	-2 SD	-3 SD	-4 SD
birth	3.2	2.8	2.3	1.9	1.4	1.0	50.2	48.0	45.7	43.5	41.2
1	4.1	3.5	2.9	2.3	1.7	1.1	54.1	51.7	49.3	46.9	44.5
2	4.9	4.2	3.4	2.7	1.9	1.2	57.4	54.9	52.4	49.9	47.4
3	5.7	4.9	4.0	3.2	2.3	1.4	60.3	57.8	55.2	52.7	50.1
4	6.4	5.5	4.6	3.7	2.8	1.9	62.8	60.2	57.6	55.0	52.4
5	7.0	6.1	5.2	4.3	3.4	2.5	65.0	62.4	59.7	57.1	54.4
6	7.5	6.6	5.7	4.8	3.9	3.0	66.9	64.2	61.5	58.8	56.1
7	8.0	7.1	6.2	5.3	4.4	3.5	68.5	65.9	63.2	60.6	57.9
8	8.5	7.6	6.6	5.7	4.7	3.8	70.0	67.4	64.7	62.1	59.4
9	8.9	7.9	6.9	5.9	5.0	4.1	71.4	68.7	66.0	63.3	60.6
10	9.2	8.3	7.3	6.4	5.3	4.3	72.7	70.0	67.3	64.6	61.9
11	9.6	8.6	7.5	6.5	5.6	4.5	74.0	71.3	68.5	65.8	63.0
12	9.8	8.8	7.8	6.8	5.8	4.8	75.2	72.5	69.7	67.0	64.2
13	10.1	9.1	8.0	7.0	5.9	4.9	76.4	73.6	70.8	68.0	65.2
14	10.3	9.3	8.2	7.2	6.1	5.0	77.5	74.7	71.8	69.0	66.1
15	10.6	9.5	8.4	7.3	6.2	5.1	78.6	75.7	72.8	69.9	67.0
16	10.8	9.7	8.5	7.4	6.3	5.2	79.7	76.8	73.8	70.9	67.9
17	11.0	9.9	8.7	7.6	6.4	5.3	80.7	77.7	74.7	71.7	68.7
18	11.2	10.0	8.8	7.6	6.5	5.4	81.7	78.7	75.6	72.6	69.5
19	11.4	10.2	8.9	7.7	6.6	5.5	82.6	79.5	76.4	73.3	70.2
20	11.5	10.3	9.1	7.9	6.7	5.5	83.6	80.4	77.2	74.0	70.8
21	11.7	10.5	9.2	8.0	6.8	5.6	84.5	81.3	78.1	74.9	71.7
22	11.8	10.6	9.4	8.2	7.0	5.8	85.4	82.2	78.9	75.7	72.4
23	12.0	10.8	9.5	8.4	7.1	5.9	86.2	82.9	79.6	76.3	73.0
24	12.1	11.0	9.8	8.7	7.2	6.0	85.0	81.8	78.6	75.4	72.2
25	12.3	11.1	9.9	8.7	7.3	6.1	85.9	82.7	79.4	76.2	72.9
26	12.5	11.3	10.0	8.8	7.4	6.1	86.7	83.4	80.1	76.8	73.5
27	12.7	11.5	10.2	9.0	7.5	6.2	87.6	84.2	80.8	77.4	74.0
28	12.9	11.6	10.3	9.0	7.6	6.2	88.4	85.0	81.5	78.1	74.6
29	13.1	11.8	10.4	9.1	7.7	6.3	89.2	85.7	82.2	78.7	75.2
30	13.3	11.9	10.5	9.1	7.8	6.4	89.8	86.4	82.9	79.5	76.0
31	13.5	12.1	10.7	9.3	7.9	6.5	90.7	87.2	83.6	80.1	76.5
32	13.6	12.2	10.8	9.4	8.0	6.6	91.5	87.9	84.3	80.7	77.1
33	13.8	12.4	10.9	9.5	8.1	6.6	92.2	88.6	84.9	81.3	77.6
34	14.0	12.5	11.0	9.5	8.1	6.6	93.0	89.3	85.6	81.9	78.2
35	14.2	12.7	11.2	9.7	8.2	6.7	93.7	90.0	86.3	82.6	78.9
36	14.4	12.9	11.3	9.8	8.2	6.7	94.4	90.7	86.9	83.2	79.4
37	14.5	13.0	11.4	9.9	8.3	6.8	95.1	91.3	87.5	83.7	79.9
38	14.7	13.1	11.5	9.9	8.4	6.8	95.8	92.0	88.2	84.4	80.6
39	14.9	13.3	11.7	10.1	8.4	6.9	96.5	92.7	88.8	85.0	81.1
40	15.0	13.4	11.8	10.2	8.5	6.9	97.2	93.3	89.4	85.5	81.6
41	15.2	13.6	11.9	10.3	8.6	7.0	97.8	93.9	90.0	86.1	82.2
42	15.4	13.7	12.0	10.3	8.6	7.0	98.5	94.6	90.6	86.7	82.7
43	15.5	13.8	12.1	10.4	8.7	7.1	99.2	95.2	91.2	87.2	83.2
44	15.7	14.0	12.3	10.6	8.8	7.1	99.8	95.8	91.7	87.7	83.6
45	15.9	14.2	12.4	10.7	838	7.2	100.4	96.4	92.3	88.3	84.2
46	16.0	14.3	12.5	10.8	8.9	7.2	101.1	97.0	92.9	88.8	84.7
47	16.2	14.4	12.6	10.8	9.0	7.3	101.7	97.6	93.4	89.3	85.1
48	16.3	14.5	12.7	10.9	9.0	7.3	102.3	98.2	94.0	89.9	85.7
49	16.5	14.7	12.8	11.0	9.1	7.4	102.9	98.7	94.5	90.3	86.1
50	16.6	14.8	13.0	11.2	9.2	7.4	103.5	99.3	95.1	90.9	86.7
51	16.8	15.0	13.1	11.3	9.3	7.5	104.1	99.9	95.6	91.4	87.1
52	16.9	15.1	13.2	11.4	9.4	7.5	104.7	100.4	96.1	91.8	87.5
53	17.1	15.2	13.3	11.4	9.5	7.6	105.2	101.0	96.7	92.5	88.2

Table 3.19 (Cont'd)

54	17.2	15.3	13.4	11.5	9.6	7.7	105.8	101.5	97.2	92.9	88.6
55	17.4	15.5	13.5	11.6	9.7	7.7	106.4	102.1	97.7	93.4	89.0
56	17.6	15.7	13.7	11.8	9.8	7.8	106.9	102.6	98.2	93.9	89.5
57	17.7	15.8	13.8	11.9	9.9	7.9	107.5	103.1	98.7	94.3	89.9
58	17.8	15.9	13.9	12.0	10.0	8.0	108.1	103.7	99.2	94.8	90.3
59	18.0	16.0	14.0	12.0	10.0	8.0	108.6	104.2	99.7	95.3	90.8
60	18.2	16.2	14.1	12.1	10.1	8.1	109.2	104.7	100.1	95.6	91.0

Source: Jelliffe & Jelliffe 1989.

Table 3.20: Weight and height for age 10–18 years, as standard deviations, NCHS/WHO standards

age (years)	weight (kg)						height (cm)					
	+2 SD	male reference	-2 SD	+2 SD	female mean	-2SD	+2 SD	male mean	-2SD	+2 SD	female reference	-2SD
10	46.0	31.4	22.1	49.2	32.5	21.9	149.7	137.5	125.3	152.0	138.3	124.6
10.5	49.3	33.3	23.1	52.8	34.7	23.1	153.1	140.3	127.6	155.3	141.5	127.6
11	52.7	35.3	24.1	56.4	37.0	24.5	156.7	143.3	129.9	158.7	144.8	130.9
11.5	56.3	37.5	25.4	60.0	39.2	25.9	160.5	146.4	132.2	162.0	148.2	134.4
12	59.9	39.8	26.8	63.3	41.5	27.4	164.7	149.7	134.6	165.2	151.5	137.9
12.5	63.5	42.3	28.4	66.5	43.8	29.1	168.9	153.0	137.2	168.0	154.6	141.1
13	67.2	45.0	30.4	69.4	46.1	30.8	173.0	156.5	139.9	170.5	157.1	143.8
13.5	70.9	47.8	32.5	72.1	48.3	32.5	176.9	159.9	142.8	172.4	159.0	145.7
14	74.6	50.8	34.9	74.5	50.3	34.2	180.2	163.1	146.0	173.7	160.4	147.0
14.5	78.2	53.8	37.4	76.5	52.1	35.9	183.0	166.2	149.4	174.7	161.2	147.8
15	81.6	56.7	39.9	78.3	53.7	37.4	185.1	169.0	152.9	175.3	161.8	148.3
15.5	84.9	59.5	42.4	79.6	55.0	38.7	186.7	171.5	156.2	175.6	162.1	148.7
16	87.9	62.1	44.7	80.6	55.9	39.8	187.9	173.5	159.2	175.7	162.4	149.1
16.5	90.7	64.4	46.8	81.2	56.4	40.7	188.8	175.2	161.5	175.8	162.7	149.7
17	93.2	66.3	48.6	81.5	56.7	41.3	189.4	176.2	163.1	175.7	163.1	150.4
17.5	95.3	67.8	49.9	81.5	56.7	4138	189.8	176.7	163.7	175.7	163.4	151.1
18	97.0	68.9	50.9	81.3	56.6	42.1	190.0	176.8	163.6	175.6	163.7	151.8

Source: Jelliffe and Jelliffe 1989.

Table 3.21: Body weight for length, children under 4 years of age, NCHS standards

| | body weight centiles (kg) | | | | | | | | | | | | | |
| | males | | | | | | | females | | | | | | |
length cm	5	10	25	50	75	90	95	5	10	25	50	75	90	95
48–50	-	-	2.9	3.2	3.5	-	-	-	-	3.0	3.3	3.6	-	-
50–52	-	-	3.2	3.5	3.9	-	-	-	-	3.3	3.6	3.9	-	-
52–54	-	-	3.5	3.9	4.3	-	-	-	-	3.6	3.9	4.3	-	-
54–56	3.5	3.7	4.0	4.3	4.8	5.1	5.3	3.5	3.6	3.9	4.3	4.7	5.0	5.2
56–58	3.9	4.1	4.4	4.8	5.3	5.7	5.9	3.9	4.1	4.4	4.8	5.2	5.6	5.8
58–60	4.4	4.6	4.9	5.4	5.8	6.3	6.5	4.4	4.5	4.9	5.3	5.7	6.1	6.4
60–62	4.9	5.1	5.5	5.9	6.4	6.9	7.1	4.9	5.0	5.4	5.8	6.3	6.7	7.0
62–64	5.4	5.7	6.1	6.5	7.0	7.5	7.7	5.4	5.5	5.9	6.4	6.9	7.3	7.6
64–66	6.0	6.2	6.6	7.1	7.6	8.1	8.4	5.9	6.0	6.5	7.0	7.5	7.9	8.2
66–68	6.6	6.8	7.2	7.7	8.2	8.8	9.0	6.4	6.6	7.0	7.6	8.1	8.5	8.8
68–70	7.1	7.3	7.8	8.3	8.8	9.4	9.6	6.9	7.1	7.6	8.1	8.6	9.1	9.3
70–72	7.6	7.8	8.3	8.8	9.4	9.9	10.2	7.4	7.6	8.1	8.6	9.2	9.6	9.9
72–74	8.1	8.3	8.8	9.3	9.9	10.5	10.8	7.8	8.1	8.6	9.1	9.7	10.2	10.4
74–76	8.6	8.8	9.2	9.8	10.4	11.0	11.3	8.2	8.5	9.0	9.6	10.1	10.6	10.9
76–78	9.0	9.2	9.7	10.3	10.9	11.5	11.8	8.6	8.9	9.4	10.0	10.6	11.1	11.4
78–80	9.4	9.6	10.1	10.7	11.4	11.9	12.3	9.0	9.3	9.8	10.4	11.0	11.5	11.9
80–82	9.8	10.0	10.5	11.1	11.8	12.4	12.7	9.3	9.7	10.2	10.8	11.4	11.9	12.3
82–84	10.1	10.4	10.9	11.5	12.2	12.8	13.1	9.7	10.0	10.6	11.2	11.8	12.4	12.7
84–86	10.5	10.8	11.3	11.9	12.7	13.3	13.6	10.0	10.4	10.9	11.6	12.2	12.8	13.2
86–88	10.9	11.1	11.7	12.3	13.1	13.7	14.0	10.4	10.8	11.3	12.0	12.6	13.2	13.6
88–90	11.2	11.5	12.1	12.8	13.5	14.1	14.4	10.8	11.2	11.7	12.4	13.0	13.6	14.0
90–92	11.6	11.9	12.5	13.2	13.9	14.6	14.9	11.2	11.6	2.2	12.8	13.5	14.1	14.5
92–94	12.0	12.4	13.0	13.7	14.4	15.1	15.4	11.6	12.0	12.6	13.3	14.0	14.6	14.9
94–96	12.4	12.8	13.5	14.1	14.9	15.5	15.9	12.1	12.5	13.1	13.8	14.5	15.1	15.4
96–98	12.9	13.3	14.0	14.7	15.4	16.1	16.4	12.6	12.9	13.6	14.3	15.0	15.7	16.0
98–100	13.4	13.8	14.5	15.2	15.9	16.6	17.0	13.1	13.5	14.2	14.9	15.6	16.3	16.6
100–102	13.9	14.3	15.1	15.8	16.5	17.2	17.6	13.7	14.1	14.8	15.5	16.3	17.0	17.4
102–104	14.5	14.9	15.7	16.5	17.2	17.9	18.2	-	-	-	-	-	-	-

Source: Hamill *et al.* 1979.

Table 3.22: Weight for height, prepubescent children, NCHS standards

height														
	weight centiles (kg)													
	males							females						
(cm)	5	10	25	50	75	90	95	5	10	25	50	75	90	95
90–92	11.7	12.0	12.6	13.4	14.4	15.3	15.7	11.5	11.7	12.3	13.1	14.1	15.0	15.7
92–94	10.1	12.4	13.0	13.9	14.8	15.9	16.4	11.9	12.1	12.7	13.6	14.6	15.6	16.4
94–96	12.5	12.8	13.5	14.4	15.3	16.5	17.1	12.3	12.5	13.2	14.1	15.1	16.1	17.1
96–98	12.9	13.2	14.0	14.9	15.9	17.0	17.7	12.7	13.0	13.7	14.6	15.7	16.7	17.7
98–100	13.3	13.7	14.5	15.4	16.4	17.6	18.3	13.1	13.4	14.2	15.1	16.2	17.2	18.2
100–102	13.8	14.2	15.0	16.0	17.0	18.1	18.9	13.5	13.9	14.7	15.7	16.7	17.8	18.8
102–104	14.3	14.7	15.5	16.7	17.6	18.7	19.5	13.9	14.4	15.2	16.2	17.3	18.4	19.4
104–106	14.8	15.2	16.1	17.1	18.2	19.3	20.1	14.4	14.9	15.8	16.8	17.9	19.0	20.0
106–108	15.3	15.7	16.7	17.7	18.8	19.9	20.8	14.8	15.4	16.3	17.3	18.5	19.6	20.6
108–110	15.9	16.3	17.3	18.4	19.5	20.5	21.5	15.4	15.9	16.9	17.9	19.1	20.3	21.3
110–112	16.4	16.9	17.9	19.0	20.2	21.2	22.2	15.9	16.5	17.5	18.6	19.8	21.0	22.0
112–114	17.0	17.5	18.5	19.7	20.9	22.0	23.0	16.5	17.1	18.1	19.2	20.5	21.8	22.8
114–116	17.7	18.2	19.2	20.4	21.7	22.8	23.9	17.1	17.7	18.7	19.9	21.2	22.7	23.7
116–118	18.3	18.9	20.0	21.1	22.5	23.7	24.8	17.8	18.4	19.4	20.6	22.0	23.6	24.7
118–120	19.0	19.6	20.6	21.9	23.3	24.7	25.8	18.5	19.1	20.1	21.4	22.9	24.6	25.8
120–122	19.7	20.3	21.3	22.6	24.2	25.8	27.0	19.2	19.9	20.9	22.3	23.9	25.7	27.0
122–124	20.4	21.0	22.1	23.5	25.1	27.0	28.2	20.0	20.6	21.7	23.1	24.9	26.9	28.4
124–126	21.2	21.8	22.9	24.3	26.1	28.2	29.5	20.8	21.5	22.5	24.1	26.1	28.3	29.9
126–128	22.0	22.6	23.8	25.2	27.1	29.4	30.9	21.7	22.3	23.5	25.1	27.3	29.7	31.5
128–130	22.8	23.5	24.7	26.2	28.2	30.9	32.4	22.5	23.3	24.5	26.2	28.6	32.3	33.3
130–132	23.7	24.6	25.6	27.3	29.4	32.3	34.1	23.4	24.2	25.5	27.4	30.1	33.0	35.3
132–134	24.6	25.3	26.6	28.4	30.7	33.8	35.8	24.4	25.2	26.7	28.7	31.7	34.8	37.5
134–136	25.5	26.3	27.7	29.6	32.1	35.4	37.7	25.4	26.3	27.9	30.1	33.4	36.8	40.0
136–138	26.5	27.3	28.8	30.9	33.5	37.1	39.7	26.3	27.4	29.2	31.5	35.3	39.0	42.5
138–140	27.5	28.4	30.0	32.2	35.1	38.8	41.7	-	-	-	-	-	-	-
140–142	28.6	29.5	31.3	33.7	36.8	40.6	44.0	-	-	-	-	-	-	-
142–144	29.7	30.6	32.6	35.3	38.5	42.4	46.3	-	-	-	-	-	-	-
144–146	30.9	31.9	34.0	37.0	40.5	44.3	48.8	-	-	-	-	-	-	-

Source: Hamill *et al.* 1979.

Table 3.23: Weight for height as standard deviations above and below reference mean, NCHS/WHO standards

height (cm)	+2 SD	+1 SD	reference	-1 SD	-2 SD	-3 SD
49	4.1	3.7	3.2	2.9	2.5	2.2
50	4.3	3.9	3.4	3.0	2.6	2.2
51	4.5	4.0	3.5	3.1	2.7	2.3
52	4.7	4.2	3.7	3.3	2.8	2.4
53	5.0	4.5	3.9	3.4	2.9	2.4
54	5.2	4.7	4.1	3.6	3.1	2.6
55	5.5	4.9	4.3	3.8	3.3	2.8
56	5.8	5.2	4.6	4.1	3.5	3.0
57	6.1	5.5	4.8	4.3	3.7	3.2
58	6.4	5.8	5.1	4.5	3.9	3.3
59	6.7	6.0	5.3	4.7	4.1	3.5
60	7.0	6.3	5.6	5.0	4.3	3.7
61	7.3	6.6	5.9	5.3	4.6	3.9
62	7.6	6.9	6.2	5.5	4.8	4.1
63	7.9	7.2	6.5	5.8	5.1	4.4
64	8.2	7.5	6.7	6.1	5.4	4.7
65	8.5	7.8	7.0	6.3	5.6	4.9
66	8.9	8.1	7.3	6.6	5.9	5.2
67	9.2	8.4	7.6	6.9	6.1	5.4
68	9.5	8.7	7.9	7.2	6.4	5.7
69	9.8	9.0	8.2	7.5	6.7	6.0
70	10.1	9.3	8.5	7.7	6.9	6.2
71	10.4	9.6	8.7	8.0	7.2	6.4
72	10.6	9.8	9.0	8.2	7.4	6.6
73	10.9	10.1	9.2	8.4	7.6	6.8
74	11.2	10.4	9.5	8.7	7.8	7.0
75	11.4	10.6	9.7	8.9	8.1	7.2
76	11.7	10.8	9.9	9.1	8.3	7.4
77	11.9	11.0	10.1	9.3	8.5	7.6
78	12.1	11.3	10.4	9.5	8.6	7.7
79	12.4	11.5	10.6	9.7	8.8	7.9
80	12.6	11.7	10.8	9.9	9.0	8.1
81	12.8	11.9	11.0	10.1	9.2	8.3
82	13.0	12.1	11.2	10.3	9.4	8.5
83	13.3	12.4	11.4	10.5	9.6	8.7
84	13.5	12.5	11.5	10.6	9.7	8.8
85	13.7	12.7	11.7	10.8	9.9	9.0
86	13.9	12.9	11.9	11.0	10.1	9.2
87	14.1	13.1	12.1	11.2	10.3	9.4
88	14.4	13.4	12.4	11.5	10.5	9.6
89	14.6	13.6	12.6	11.7	10.7	9.8
90	14.8	13.8	12.8	11.8	10.8	9.9
91	15.1	14.1	13.0	12.1	11.1	10.2
92	15.3	14.3	13.2	12.3	11.3	10.4
93	15.6	14.6	13.5	12.5	11.5	10.5
94	15.8	14.8	13.7	12.7	11.7	10.7
95	16.1	15.1	14.0	13.0	11.9	10.9
96	16.4	15.3	14.2	13.2	12.2	11.2
97	16.6	15.6	14.5	13.5	12.4	11.4
98	16.9	15.9	14.8	13.7	12.6	11.6
99	17.2	16.1	15.0	14.0	12.9	11.9

Table 3.19 (Cont'd)

height (cm)	+2 SD	+1 SD	reference	-1 SD	-2 SD	-3 SD
100	17.6	16.5	15.3	14.3	13.2	12.2
101	19.0	17.4	15.8	14.4	13.0	11.6
102	19.3	17.7	16.1	14.7	13.3	11.9
103	19.7	18.1	16.4	15.0	13.5	12.1
104	20.0	18.4	16.7	15.2	13.7	12.2
105	20.3	18.6	16.9	15.5	14.0	12.6
106	20.7	19.0	17.2	15.7	14.2	12.7
107	21.1	19.3	17.5	16.0	14.5	13.0
108	21.4	19.6	17.8	16.3	14.7	13.2
109	21.8	20.0	18.1	16.6	15.0	13.5
110	22.2	20.3	18.4	16.8	15.2	13.6
111	22.6	20.7	18.8	17.2	15.5	13.9
112	23.0	21.1	19.1	17.5	15.8	14.2
113	23.4	21.4	19.4	17.8	16.1	14.5
114	23.9	21.9	19.8	18.1	16.4	14.7
115	24.4	22.3	20.1	18.4	16.7	15.0
116	24.8	22.7	20.5	18.8	17.0	15.3
117	25.4	23.1	20.8	19.1	17.3	15.6
118	25.9	23.6	21.2	19.4	17.6	15.8
119	26.4	24.0	21.6	19.8	18.0	16.2
120	27.0	24.5	22.0	20.2	18.3	16.5

Source: Jelliffe and Jelliffe 1989.

Table 3.24: Head circumference from birth to 36 months

age (months)	head circumference centiles (cm)													
	males							females						
	5	10	25	50	75	90	95	5	10	25	50	75	90	95
birth	32.6	33.0	33.9	34.8	35.6	36.6	37.2	32.1	32.9	33.5	34.3	34.8	35.5	35.9
1	34.9	35.4	36.2	37.2	38.1	39.0	39.6	34.2	34.8	35.6	36.4	37.1	37.8	38.3
3	38.4	38.9	39.7	40.6	41.7	42.5	43.1	37.3	37.8	38.7	39.5	40.4	41.2	41.7
6	41.5	42.0	42.8	43.8	44.7	45.6	46.2	40.3	40.9	41.6	42.4	43.3	44.1	44.6
9	43.5	44.0	44.8	45.8	46.6	47.5	48.1	42.3	42.8	43.5	44.3	45.1	46.0	46.4
12	44.8	45.3	46.1	47.0	47.9	48.8	49.3	43.5	44.1	44.8	45.6	46.4	47.2	47.6
18	46.3	46.7	47.4	48.4	49.3	50.1	50.6	45.0	45.6	46.3	47.1	47.9	48.6	49.1
24	47.3	47.7	48.3	49.2	50.2	51.0	51.4	46.1	46.5	47.3	48.1	48.8	49.6	50.1
30	48.0	48.4	49.1	49.9	51.0	51.7	52.2	47.0	47.3	48.0	48.8	49.4	50.3	50.8
36	48.6	49.0	49.7	50.5	51.5	52.3	52.8	47.6	47.9	48.5	49.3	50.0	50.8	51.4

Source: US National Center for Health Statistics.

Table 3.25: Head circumference from birth to 18 years of age

	Head circumference (cm)					
	males			females		
Age	-2 SD	mean	+2 SD	-2 SD	mean	+2SD
birth	32.0	33.0	37.5	31.8	34.0	36.5
2m	36.3	39.0	42.0	35.7	38.0	40.1
4m	39.5	42.0	44.0	38.1	41.0	43.2
6m	41.3	44.0	46.2	40.0	42.8	45.5
8m	42.5	45.2	48.0	41.3	44.0	46.5
10m	43.5	46.2	48.7	42.5	45.0	48.0
12m	44.5	47.0	49.5	43.2	45.9	48.3
14m	45.0	47.5	50.1	43.9	46.3	48.9
16m	45.4	48.0	50.5	44.1	46.8	49.5
18m	47.5	48.5	51.0	44.5	47.1	50.0
20m	45.9	48.5	51.2	45.0	47.5	50.4
22m	46.0	48.7	51.5	45.1	47.8	50.5
2y	46.8	49.3	52.0	45.6	48.0	50.8
3y	47.9	50.5	53.2	46.3	49.0	51.9
4y	48.2	53.0	53.8	47.5	50.0	52.9
5y	48.5	51.3	54.1	48.0	50.5	53.1
6y	48.8	51.6	54.1	48.0	50.5	53.1
7y	49.1	52.0	55.0	48.8	51.5	54.0
8y	49.5	52.3	53.2	49.0	51.6	54.4
9y	49.8	52.7	55.5	49.1	51.9	54.6
10y	50.1	53.0	55.9	49.2	52.1	55.0
11y	50.2	53.5	56.2	49.7	52.5	55.5
12y	50.7	53.9	56.9	50.0	53.0	56.0
13y	51.0	54.0	57.1	51.0	53.5	56.4
14y	52.0	54.6	57.4	51.2	54.0	56.8
15y	52.0	55.0	58.0	51.8	54.3	57.0
16y	53.2	55.5	58.0	52.0	54.5	57.0
17y	53.2	55.9	58.2	52.1	54.8	57.5
18y	53.2	56.0	58.5	52.1	55.0	57.9

Source: Nellhaus 1968.

Table 3.26: Triceps skinfold thickness with age

age (y)														
							triceps skinfold centiles (mm)							
			males							females				
	5	10	25	50	75	90	95	5	10	25	50	75	90	95
1	6	7	8	10	12	14	16	6	7	8	10	12	14	16
2	6	7	8	10	12	14	15	6	8	9	10	12	15	16
3	6	7	8	10	11	14	15	7	8	9	11	12	14	15
4	6	6	8	9	11	12	14	7	8	8	10	12	14	16
5	6	6	8	9	11	14	15	6	7	8	10	12	15	18
6	5	6	7	8	10	13	16	6	7	8	10	12	14	16
7	5	6	7	9	12	15	17	6	7	9	11	13	16	18
8	5	6	7	8	10	13	16	6	8	9	12	15	18	24
9	6	6	7	10	13	17	18	8	9	10	13	16	20	22
10	6	6	8	10	14	18	21	7	8	10	12	17	23	27
11	6	6	8	11	16	20	24	7	8	10	13	18	24	28
12	6	6	8	11	14	22	28	8	9	11	14	18	23	27
13	5	5	7	10	14	22	26	8	9	12	15	21	26	30
14	4	5	7	9	14	21	24	9	10	13	16	21	26	28
15	4	5	6	8	11	18	24	8	10	12	17	21	25	32
16	4	5	6	8	12	16	22	10	12	15	18	22	26	31
17	5	5	6	8	12	16	19	10	12	13	19	24	30	37
18	4	5	6	9	13	20	24	10	12	15	18	22	26	30
19-25	4	5	7	10	15	20	22	10	11	14	18	24	30	34
25-35	5	6	8	12	16	20	24	10	12	16	21	27	34	37
35-45	5	6	8	12	16	20	23	12	14	18	23	29	35	38
45-55	6	6	8	12	15	2(	25	12	16	20	25	30	36	40
55-65	5	6	8	11	14	19	22	12	16	20	25	31	36	38
65-75	4	6	8	11	15	19	22	12	14	18	24	29	34	36

Source: Frisancho 1981.

Table 3.27: Subscapular skinfold thickness with age

age (y)														
							subscapular skinfold centiles (mm)							
			males							females				
	5	10	25	50	75	90	95	5	10	25	50	75	90	95
1	4.0	4.0	5.0	6.0	7.0	8.5	10.0	4.0	4.0	5.0	6.0	8.0	9.0	9.0
2	3.0	4.0	4.5	5.0	6.5	8.0	10.0	4.0	4.0	5.0	6.0	7.0	9.0	10.0
3	3.5	4.0	4.0	5.0	6.0	7.0	9.5	4.0	4.0	4.5	5.5	6.5	8.0	9.0
4	3.0	3.5	4.0	5.0	6.0	7.0	7.0	3.5	4.0	4.5	5.0	6.0	8.0	9.0
5	3.0	3.5	4.0	5.0	6.0	7.0	8.0	3.5	4.0	4.0	5.0	6.5	9.0	15.0
6	3.0	3.0	4.0	4.5	5.0	7.0	9.0	3.0	4.0	4.5	5.5	6.5	8.0	10.0
7	3.0	3.0	4.0	4.5	6.0	9.0	11.0	3.0	4.0	4.5	5.0	7.0	10.5	11.5
8	3.0	3.0	4.0	4.5	6.0	7.5	9.0	3.5	4.0	4.5	5.5	8.0	14.5	19.5
9	3.5	3.5	4.0	5.0	8.0	14.0	14.0	4.0	4.0	5.0	7.0	10.0	17.0	19.0
10	3.5	4.0	4.0	5.5	7.0	12.0	18.0	4.0	4.5	5.5	6.5	10.0	18.0	20.0
11	4.0	4.0	4.5	6.0	8.5	15.0	19.0	4.0	5.0	6.0	8.0	13.0	19.0	25.5
12	3.5	4.0	5.0	6.0	9.0	14.0	20.5	5.0	5.0	6.0	9.5	13.0	20.0	25.0
13	3.5	4.0	5.0	6.5	9.0	17.0	26.0	5.0	6.0	7.0	9.5	15.0	23.4	26.0
14	4.0	4.5	5.0	6.5	9.0	16.0	20.0	5.0	6.0	8.0	10.0	16.0	24.0	28.0
15	4.0	5.0	5.5	7.0	10.0	15.5	23.0	6.0	6.5	7.5	10.0	14.0	20.0	27.0
16	5.0	5.5	6.5	8.0	10.5	16.5	23.5	6.0	7.0	8.0	10.5	15.0	25.5	29.0
17	5.0	5.5	7.0	8.0	10.0	16.0	23.0	6.5	7.0	9.0	12.5	20	27.0	34.1

Source: Frisancho 1981.

Table 3.28: Mid-upper arm circumference with age

| age (y) | mid-upper arm circumference centiles (mm) | | | | | | | | | | | | | |
| | males | | | | | | | females | | | | | | |
	5	10	25	50	75	90	95	5	10	25	50	75	90	95
1	142	146	150	159	170	176	183	138	142	148	156	164	172	177
2	141	145	153	162	170	178	185	142	145	152	160	167	176	184
3	150	153	160	167	175	184	190	143	150	158	167	175	183	189
4	149	154	162	171	180	186	192	149	154	160	169	177	184	191
5	153	160	167	175	185	195	204	153	157	165	175	185	203	211
6	155	159	167	179	188	209	228	156	162	170	176	187	204	211
7	162	167	177	187	201	223	230	164	167	174	183	199	216	231
8	162	170	177	190	202	220	245	168	172	183	195	214	247	261
9	175	178	187	200	217	249	257	178	182	194	211	224	251	260
10	181	184	196	210	231	262	274	174	182	193	210	228	251	265
11	186	190	202	223	244	261	280	185	194	208	224	248	276	303
12	193	200	214	232	254	282	303	194	203	216	237	256	282	294
13	194	211	228	247	263	286	301	202	211	223	243	271	301	338
14	220	226	237	253	283	303	322	214	223	237	252	272	304	322
15	222	229	244	264	284	311	320	208	221	239	254	279	300	322
16	244	248	262	278	303	324	343	218	224	241	258	283	318	334
17	246	253	267	285	308	336	347	220	227	241	264	295	324	350
18	245	260	276	297	321	353	379	222	227	241	258	281	312	325
19-25	262	272	288	308	331	355	372	221	230	247	265	290	319	345
25-35	271	282	300	319	342	362	375	233	240	256	277	304	342	368
35-45	278	287	305	326	345	363	374	241	251	267	290	317	356	378
45-55	267	281	301	322	342	362	376	242	256	274	299	328	362	384
55-65	258	273	296	317	336	355	369	243	257	280	303	335	367	385
65-75	248	263	285	307	325	344	355	240	252	274	299	326	356	373

Source: Frisancho 1981.

Table 3.29: Mid-upper arm muscle circumference with age

| age (y) | mid-upper arm muscle circumference centiles (mm) | | | | | | | | | | | | | |
| | males | | | | | | | females | | | | | | |
	5	10	25	50	75	90	95	5	10	25	50	75	90	95
1	110	113	119	127	135	144	147	105	111	117	124	132	139	143
2	111	114	122	130	140	146	150	111	114	119	126	133	142	147
3	117	123	131	137	143	148	153	113	119	124	132	140	146	152
4	123	126	133	141	148	156	159	115	121	128	136	144	152	157
5	128	133	140	147	154	162	169	125	128	134	142	151	159	165
6	131	135	142	151	161	170	177	130	133	138	145	154	166	171
7	137	139	151	160	168	177	190	129	135	142	151	160	171	176
8	140	145	154	162	170	182	187	138	140	151	160	171	183	194
9	151	154	161	170	183	196	202	147	150	158	167	180	194	198
10	156	160	166	180	191	209	221	148	150	159	170	180	190	197
11	159	165	173	183	195	205	230	150	158	171	181	196	217	223
12	167	171	182	195	210	223	241	162	166	180	191	201	214	220
13	172	179	196	211	226	238	245	169	175	183	198	211	226	240
14	189	199	212	223	240	260	264	174	179	190	201	216	232	247
15	199	204	218	237	254	266	272	175	178	189	202	215	228	244
16	213	225	234	249	269	287	296	170	180	190	202	216	234	249
17	224	231	245	258	273	294	312	175	183	194	205	221	239	257
18	226	237	252	264	283	298	324	174	179	191	202	215	237	245
19-25	238	245	257	273	289	309	321	179	185	195	207	221	236	249
25-35	243	250	264	279	298	314	326	183	188	199	212	228	246	264
35-45	247	255	269	286	302	318	327	186	192	205	218	236	257	272
45-55	239	249	265	281	300	315	326	187	193	206	220	238	260	274
55-65	236	245	260	278	295	310	320	187	196	209	225	244	266	280
65-75	223	235	251	268	284	298	306	185	195	208	225	244	264	279

Source: Frisancho 1981.

Table 3.30: Arm anthropometry with age

age	circumference (mm) percentile			triceps skinfold (mm) percentile			muscle diameter (mm) percentile			muscle circumference (mm) percentile			muscle area (mm²) percentile		
	5	50	95	5	50	95	5	50	95	5	50	95	5	50	95
males															
0.3	113	134	153	4	8	15	26	34	42	81	106	133	522	892	1414
1	128	152	175	5	9	15	32	39	46	100	123	146	791	1201	1690
2	141	157	180	5	10	14	35	40	46	111	127	146	978	1284	1686
3	144	161	182	6	9	14	36	42	48	114	132	152	1027	1384	1842
4	143	165	190	5	9	14	38	43	50	118	135	157	1106	1451	1973
5	146	169	199	5	8	16	39	45	53	121	141	166	1171	1579	2193
6	151	172	198	5	8	15	40	47	53	127	146	167	1275	1700	2220
7	154	176	212	4	8	14	41	48	55	130	151	173	1342	1815	2386
8	161	185	233	5	8	17	44	50	59	138	158	185	1506	1987	2729
9	165	190	262	5	9	19	44	51	64	138	161	200	1522	2074	3188
10	170	200	255	5	10	22	45	53	64	142	168	202	1608	2239	3239
11	177	208	276	6	10	25	48	55	67	150	174	211	1801	2406	3544
12	184	216	291	5	11	26	49	58	70	153	181	221	1874	2603	3902
13	186	230	297	5	10	25	51	62	77	159	195	242	2012	3013	4661
14	198	243	321	5	10	22	53	67	84	167	211	265	2231	3544	5601
15	202	253	320	4	9	26	55	70	86	173	220	271	2375	3867	5826
16	217	262	335	4	9	27	59	73	89	186	229	281	2741	4184	6266
17	230	275	326	4	8	20	66	78	92	206	245	290	3373	4771	6713
21	250	292	354	4	10	25	69	82	97	217	258	305	3748	5315	7411
30	260	310	366	4	11	28	70	86	100	220	270	315	3837	5802	7918
40	259	312	371	4	12	28	71	86	101	222	270	318	3938	5820	8041
females															
0.3	107	127	150	4	8	13	27	33	40	86	104	126	591	866	1272
1	125	146	170	6	9	15	31	37	43	97	117	135	756	1084	1460
2	136	155	180	6	10	15	34	40	46	105	125	146	885	1241	1693
3	137	157	176	6	10	14	34	41	46	108	128	143	928	1298	1628
4	145	162	184	5	10	14	36	42	48	114	132	152	1040	1390	1828
5	149	169	195	6	10	16	38	44	51	119	138	160	1119	1516	2045
6	148	170	202	6	10	15	38	45	53	121	140	165	1163	1563	2174
7	153	178	216	6	10	17	39	47	56	123	146	175	1213	1700	2433
8	158	183	231	6	10	19	41	48	59	129	151	186	1322	1818	2758
9	166	192	255	6	11	24	43	50	62	136	157	193	1473	1955	2978
10	170	203	263	6	12	24	44	52	62	139	163	196	1528	2115	3066
11	173	210	280	7	12	29	44	55	67	140	171	209	1551	2335	3486
12	185	220	275	6	13	25	48	57	68	150	179	212	1781	2588	3582
13	186	230	294	7	14	30	49	59	71	155	185	225	1905	2711	4014
14	201	240	306	8	15	28	53	61	74	166	193	234	2186	2952	4358
15	205	245	310	8	16	30	52	62	74	163	195	232	2126	3031	4279
16	211	249	322	8	15	27	54	64	83	171	200	260	2316	3198	5386
17	207	250	328	9	16	31	54	62	77	171	196	241	2316	3058	4612
21	215	260	329	9	17	31	54	65	80	170	205	253	2289	3341	5089
30	230	275	361	9	19	36	56	68	87	177	213	272	2486	3606	5889
40	232	286	374	10	22	39	57	69	89	180	216	279	2566	3724	6195

Source: Frisancho 1974.

Reference intakes, dietary goals and nutrition labelling of foods

4.1 Reference intakes

There is a 20–30 per cent range of individual variation around the mean requirement for most nutrients. For the planning of diets for populations, specific groups of the population or institutions, it is necessary to ensure that the intakes of nutrients provided are sufficient to ensure that no-one suffers deficiency or inadequacy. For any parameter that is statistically normally distributed, a range of $\pm$ 2SD around the mean includes 95 per cent of the values. Although there is little evidence, it is generally assumed that individual nutrient requirements are normally distributed around the mean—the only nutrient for which there is clear evidence that this is not so is iron, which shows a markedly skewed distribution of requirements (see section 24.2). Therefore, an appropriate level of intake for all nutrients, but not for energy, is considered to be 2 standard deviations above the mean requirement, as determined experimentally. Because energy intake in excess of requirements to meet expenditure leads to the development of obesity (see Chapter 11), appropriate levels of energy intake are considered to be the mean requirement, not a level $2 \times$ SD above the mean.

As can be seen from Fig. 4.1, a level of intake $2 \times$ SD above the mean requirement is greater than the individual requirements of 97.5 per cent of the population, and would therefore ensure freedom from deficiency for (essentially) all of the population. Over the years, various terms have been used to describe this level of intake, as shown in Table 4.1. United Nations Agencies refer to safe levels of intake, meaning safe and adequate; in the USA they are known as Recommended Dietary Allowances (RDA), while in UK the term Reference Nutrient Intake was coined in the 1991 tables. This was by parallel with clinical chemistry, where the range of ± 2 SD around the mean value of an analyte for a population group is known as a reference range. The EU Scientific Committee for Food (1993) adopted the term

Population Reference Intake, to emphasize that the values apply to population groups as a whole, and not to individuals.

For nutrients such as biotin (see section 23.1), pantothenic acid (see section 23.2), and a number of trace elements (see chapter 25), deficiency is more or less unknown, and there are insufficient data on which to base estimates of average requirements and hence reference intakes. Since the average intakes of these nutrients are apparently quite adequate, these figures are used to indicate a range of estimated safe and (more than) adequate levels of intake.

Some tables of reference intakes also consider the level $2 \times$ SD below the mean requirement—a level of intake that would theoretically be adequate to meet the requirements of only 2.5 per cent of the population. In New Zealand this is termed the Minimum Safe Intake; the UK 1991 report adopted the term Lower Reference Nutrient Intake, signifying only that this was the level at the lower end of the reference range. The EU 1993 report coined the term Lower Threshold Intake, on the basis that this is a level of intake at or below which it is highly improbable that an individual's requirement would be met, and normal metabolic homeostasis and health cannot be maintained; it is a level of intake at or below which further investigation for dietary deficiency would be deemed appropriate. For some nutrients listed in the EU report, the Lower Threshold Intake is not set at 2 $\times$ SD below the mean requirement, but rather at a level at which signs of metabolic disturbance have been observed in experimental studies or population groups with marginal intakes.

Tables of reference intakes of energy and nutrients have been published by United Nations Agencies, individual national governments and the European Union. Two major studies have compared the levels deemed appropriate by different national authorities: Truswell *et al.* (1983) compiled tables from all countries that had published them, and Trichopolou and Vassilakou (1990) compiled tables from all European countries. Since those reviews were published, new

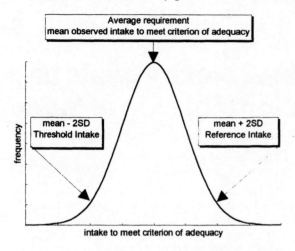

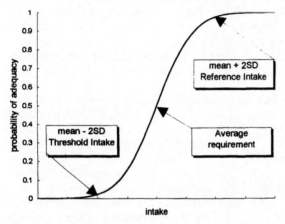

Figure 4.1 Determination of Reference and Threshold Intakes from the mean observed requirement to meet the chosen criterion of adequacy 2 standard deviations around the mean, and (below) the cumulative distribution of requirements, expressed as the probability that a given level of intake will meet an individual's requirement.

figures have been published in the USA (National Research Council / National Academy of Sciences 1989), UK (Department of Health 1991) and the EU (Scientific Committee for Food 1993). Summaries of these reference intakes are shown in Tables 4.2, 4.3 and 4.4, and more detailed information for each nutrient appears in Chapters 13–25. Most of the differences between the different tables of reference intakes can be attributed to the adoption of different criteria of adequacy, and differences of opinion in the interpretation of sometimes relatively sparse experimental evidence. In some instances the differences can be accounted for simply by the rounding of experimental data to avoid spurious precision,

and calculation of nutrient requirements that are related to energy intake on the basis of kcal (in the USA and UK tables) or MJ (in the EU tables). Average requirements for energy are discussed in section 5.3, and methods for assessing protein requirements in section 10.5

4.1.1 Determination of average requirements for vitamins and minerals

The most important problem in determining requirements is to establish appropriate criteria of adequacy. It is not an appropriate goal only to ensure that people do not suffer from clinical deficiency diseases, which may involve irreversible anatomical lesions, and may prove fatal. Furthermore, such an endpoint is not ethical in studies where requirements are determined by depriving volunteers of the nutrient under investigation until signs of deficiency are apparent.

Table 4.5 shows the stages of micronutrient deficiency, in order of decreasing severity—obviously, if an appropriate test is available then the most sensitive index of inadequacy should be used in order to determine requirements. Table 4.6 shows some clinical signs that are useful for the detection of nutrient deficiency in field studies, and Table 4.7 the tests that are available for detection of subclinical deficiency of the vitamins; many of these can also be used for assessment of nutritional status in field studies.

Once a criterion of adequacy has been selected, the most usual type of experiment is a depletion/repletion study, in which a group of people are maintained on a diet deficient in the nutrient under consideration, but otherwise adequate, until biochemical or other signs of deficiency appear. They are then repleted with graded levels of intake until the metabolic abnormality is just corrected.

For many minerals, and for protein, the simplest way of estimating requirements is to determine the level of intake that will just permit the maintenance of balance between intake and output; at this level of intake metabolic losses are obviously being replaced from the diet. Such methods are not applicable to studies of vitamin requirements. However, there have been some studies of metabolic turnover using isotopically labelled vitamins, as a means of determining physiological requirements. Such studies have given useful information about requirements for vitamins A (see section 13.2.3) and C (see section 22.1.3); studies of the turnover of vitamin B_6 (see section 20.3) have so far failed to give any useful information about requirements.

Regardless of whether requirements have been estimated by balance studies or by depletion and repletion, the biological availability of the nutrient as it occurs in foods must be taken into account in converting the results of experimental studies using purified compounds into reference intakes of nutrients to be obtained from foods. The biological availability of vitamins has been reviewed by Bates and Heseker (1994); biological availability of iron is discussed in section 24.2.3.1, of calcium in section 14.1, and of other minerals in Chapter 25.

4.1.2 Possibly desirable higher levels of intake of vitamins and minerals

To date reference intakes have always been based on levels of intake more than adequate to prevent detectable impairment of normal metabolic functioning or (subclinical) deficiency. There is evidence that higher levels of intake of some micronutrients, and especially those that act as radical trapping antioxidants, such as vitamin E (see section 15.5), carotene (see section 13.6.2), vitamin C (see section 22.4.4.4), and possibly selenium (see section 15.5.1) may provide additional protection against the development of cardiovascular disease and some forms of cancer. Given the difficulty of determining reference intakes to prevent subclinical deficiency, reflected in the differences between reference intakes published by different national authorities, it is not surprising that as yet there has been no attempt to define levels of intake that may be appropriate to meet the much less well-defined aim of optimum health.

For many minerals, and vitamins A (see section 13.7), D (section 14.6), B$_6$ (section 20.7.4), and niacin (section 19.7), high levels of intake may pose hazards, and upper levels of safe habitual intake must also be considered. For most nutrients, toxic hazards only become relevant at a level of intake that would be obtained only from supplements, and not from normal foods. However, the difference between adequate and potentially undesirable levels of intake of vitamin A, manganese, selenium, and zinc is relatively small, and injudicious selection of foods may result in undesirably high habitual intakes (Mertz 1995; Ministry of Agriculture, Fisheries and Food / Department of Health 1991).

4.1.3 Determination of requirements for infants and children

For obvious reasons, most of the direct experimental studies to determine vitamin and mineral requirements have been conducted using college students, although some studies have been conducted on older people, and a number of major studies were conducted during the 1940s–1960s using groups of prisoner volunteers and long-stay patients in mental institutions. Therefore, most of the information concerning requirements to meet the more sensitive criteria of deficiency listed in Tables 4.5 and 4.7 is derived from studies on young men (and a few young women) aged between 18–25.

It is generally assumed that breast milk from an adequately nourished mother will provide adequate amounts of nutrients to permit both metabolic turnover and the accumulation of body reserves for infants under about 3 months. The micronutrient composition of breast milk varies considerably with the mother's intake, and the published reports show a wide range of variation in the content of some nutrients (see Table 4.8). On the basis of these analyses, the standards for the formulation of breast milk substitutes (infant feeding formula) shown in Table 4.8 have been established, and provide the best estimate of infant nutrient requirements and reference intakes.

There are thus two sets of data that can be regarded as being relatively soundly based: for suckling infants and for young adults. In the absence of any further information, most expert committees preparing tables of reference intakes have estimated those for children between weaning and 18 years of age by simple linear interpolation between these two points. The report of the EU Scientific Committee for Food (1993) adopted a completely different approach. Energy requirements for children are known with reasonable precision, largely as a result of a series of studies using the dual-isotopically-labelled water technique (see section 5.2.2.3), and determination of Basal Metabolic Rate (see section 5.3.1)—such measurements show the energy cost of growth. It was assumed that the requirements for growth of other nutrients follow the same pattern as energy requirements, and reference intakes for vitamins and minerals were calculated by extrapolation from those for young adults, on the basis of the nutrient density of the diet, i.e. per MJ energy expenditure, whether or not there was any metabolic reason to associate the micronutrient requirement with energy expenditure. The reference intakes for micronutrients for children calculated by this backwards extrapolation to the age of 3–6 months match those estimated on the basis of the composition of breast milk remarkably well. Furthermore, the calculated values for nutrients such as calcium (see section 14.1) are in close agreement with those derived from balance studies.

4.2   Dietary goals

There is broad agreement among all national and international authorities as to those changes in the average diet in developed countries that are desirable in order to minimize the risks of cardiovascular disease and cancer (Department of Health 1994; James *et al.* 1988; National Research Council Committee on Diet and Health 1989; WHO 1990):

1. Energy intake should be appropriate to maintain body weight within the desirable range (see section 11.1), with a desirable level of physical activity (see section 5.3.2).

2. Fat should provide 30 per cent of energy intake, compared with about 40 per cent at present.

3. Saturated fat should provide no more than 10 per cent of energy intake compared with about 17 per cent at present.

4. The present proportions of energy from monounsaturated fats of 12 per cent and from polyunsaturated fats of 6 per cent should not change.

5. *Trans*-fatty acids should provide not more than the present 2 per cent of energy intake (see section 8.1.1.2.1).

6. Carbohydrate should provide 55 per cent of energy compared with about 43 per cent at present.

7. Sugars should provide no more than 10 per cent of energy intake compared with 14 per cent at present.

8. Starches should provide 38 per cent of energy intake compared with 24 per cent at present.

9. Non-starch polysaccharide (dietary fibre) intake should be increased from the present average of 11–13 g/day to 18 g/day (see section 7.3).

10. Alcohol should provide no more than about 7 per cent of energy intake. Prudent upper limits of habitual consumption are 21 units (= 168 g alcohol) /week for men, and 14 units (= 112 g alcohol) /week for women (see section 9.3).

11. The intake of sodium should be reduced from the present average of 3.2 g Na^+ /day to 1.6 g/day (see section 25.1).

At its simplest, advice to consumers on how to meet these goals can be summarized as follows: eat a mixed diet; reduce consumption of fatty meat and dairy fats; increase consumption of fish (and especially oily fish); increase consumption of whole grain cereal products, fruits and vegetables; reduce use of salt and sugar in cooking and at the table. In USA there is a major publicity campaign to persuade people to eat at least five servings of fruit or vegetables each day; in the Nordic countries restaurants are required to include fruit and vegetables in meals offered. In both USA and Australia a simple 'food pyramid' is used in nutrition education; the broad base of the pyramid contains those foods that should be eaten in large amounts, while the narrow apex consists of those high in fat and sugar that should be eaten sparingly.

4.3   Nutrition labelling of foods

The purpose of nutritional labelling of foods is to give the consumer information on which to base food choices and plan a sensible diet in order to meet dietary goals outlined in section 4.2. Information on the nutrient composition permits different products to be compared. In most countries packaged foods must be labelled with information on the ingredients and additives used (see section 26.2), as well as the manufacturer, importer or other responsible company, and nutritional information.

With the exception of foods intended for a specific population group (e.g. infant foods), for which a single set of reference intake values can be quoted, there is the problem of deciding what reference intake should be the basis of nutritional labelling. It is not possible to list the complete set of reference intakes for all population groups on food labelling and advertising.

To a great extent it does not matter what specific set of reference intakes is used, provided that the same figures are used for all labelling within any one country or trading bloc. Obviously, using a low reference intake as the standard will give the impression that foods are excellent sources of nutrients, and may leave some vulnerable groups inadequately supplied and at risk of deficiency. Conversely, choice of too high a reference figure will give the impression that foods are poor sources of nutrients, and may encourage unfounded fears of deficiency, and the consumption of inappropriate supplements. The reference values for use in USA are discussed in section 4.3.1.1, and in the European Union in section 4.3.2; both are shown in Tables 4.9 and 4.10.

There are two key differences between the US labelling legislation and that in the EU and most other countries, which follow the FAO/WHO Codex Alimentarius guidelines.

1. Nutrition labelling of all packaged foods is mandatory in the USA, whereas in EU and other countries nutrition labelling is only required if any nutritional claims are made. When nutrition labelling is required, then it must follow a prescribed format.

2. In USA nutrition information must be quoted per serving, and may optionally be quoted per unit weight or volume. The US Food and Drugs Administration has defined standard portions or serving sizes of 139 categories of food products (FDA 1993). In the EU nutrition information must be shown per 100 g or per 100 mL of the food, and may additionally be shown per serving; definition of serving size is left to the manufacturer.

4.3.1 Nutrition labelling legislation in USA

In the USA, new labelling legislation, under the 1990 Nutrition Education and Labelling Act, came into force in 1994, establishing a standard format for mandatory nutrition information on food labels, consisting of the following information, under the heading 'Food Facts'.

1. The serving size, in household measures (cups) and grams, together with the number of servings in the package. Optionally serving sizes may also be quoted in ounces or fluid ounces.

2. The energy yield of the food, as kcal per serving, together with calories from fat.

3. The amount per serving of each nutrient, except vitamins and minerals.

4. The amount per serving of each nutrient, including vitamins and minerals, as a percentage of the Daily Value (See section 4.3.1.1).

5. A footnote with reference values for selected nutrients based on 2000 and 2500 kcal diets.

6. A list of the energy yields /per gram of fat (9 kcal), carbohydrate (4 kcal) and protein (4 kcal).

The only foods that are exempt from this mandatory labelling are the following.

1. Food offered for sale by small businesses.

2. Food sold in restaurants and other establishments where it is served for immediate consumption, or foods that are ready to eat, but not for immediate consumption, primarily prepared on site and not offered for sale outside that location (e.g. takeaway restaurants).

3. Foods that contain insignificant amounts of nutrients (e.g. coffee and tea).

4. Dietary supplements, other than those in the form of conventional foods.

5. Infant formula.

6. Foods for special medical purposes.

8. Custom-processed fish or game.

9. Foods shipped in bulk form.

10. Donated food.

Any exempt food that makes any nutritional claim forfeits its exemption from the mandatory form of labelling.

Specific labelling provisions state the following.

1. Foods intended for children under 2 years of age must not declare information on calories from fat, fatty acids or cholesterol.

2. Foods intended for children under 4 years of age must not include Daily Value information.

3. Voluntary nutrition labelling guidelines exist for raw fruits, vegetables and nuts.

4. For foods sold from bulk containers, and for game meat, nutritional labelling is optional.

5. For foods in small packages with less than 12 square inches available for labelling, the label may omit nutrition information if an address or telephone number from which consumers may obtain nutrition information is provided.

6. Foods in packages with under 40 square inches available for labelling may:

   (i) present information in tabular or linear format if the package is of such a shape that it cannot accommodate columns,
   (ii) use specified abbreviations,
   (iii) omit the footnote and caloric conversion information,
   (iv) present the required nutrition information on any label panel.

4.3.1.1 Daily Values for nutrition labelling

Two sets of reference values have been established for nutrition labelling; together they are known as Daily

Values, and labels must show the content of the food as percentage of Daily Values.

1. Daily Reference Values (DRV) for fat, saturated fatty acids, cholesterol, carbohydrate, fibre, sodium, potassium and protein—see Table 4.9. These are intended to permit consumers to make appropriate choices to meet the dietary goals discussed in section 4.2. The Daily Values for fat, saturated fat, cholesterol, and sodium are maximum values, whereas those for carbohydrate and fibre are minimum values.

2. Reference Daily Intakes (RDI) for vitamins and minerals; these are amounts greater than the requirements of all members of the population (see Table 4.10).

The RDI are numerically the same as the US-RDA figures that were used for nutrition labelling before the implementation of the 1990 Nutrition Labelling and Education Act, and are the highest values for any age / gender group of the 1968 RDA. The Dietary Supplement Act (1992) required that these values be retained. The FDA had proposed to introduce new population-weighted RDI values for labelling purposes, based on the 1989 RDA and calculated from the proportion of the population in each age and gender group; this proposal was withdrawn after considerable protest.

4.3.1.2 Claims for foods low or high in nutrients

A food that is claimed as a 'good source' of a nutrient must provide between 10–19 per cent, and one which is claimed as 'rich in' a nutrient more than 20 per cent, of the Daily Value in a reference serving. For a food to bear a claim that it contains more or added nutrient, it must contain at least 10 per cent more of the Dietary Value of that nutrient per reference serving than a similar conventional (reference) product.

For a food to be defined as being free from a nutrient, it must contain an amount that is nutritionally insignificant; levels below which foods may be labelled as free from sodium, fat, and cholesterol are shown in Table 4.11, together with levels below which the food may be labelled as low in nutrients. If a food is naturally low in, or free from, a nutrient, this must be noted, to differentiate between such foods and those that have been specially processed to reduce that nutrient.

The terms 'reduced', 'less', and 'fewer' may only be used when the food in question contains at least 25 per cent less of the specified nutrient per reference serving than a similar conventional (reference) product.

A food may be described as 'light' or 'lite' when the reference food derives at least 50 per cent of its energy from fat and the fat content has been reduced by at least 50 per cent, or the energy yield by one-third. A product may be labelled as light in sodium if the sodium content is reduced by at least 50 per cent compared with the reference food.

4.3.1.3 Heath claims for foods

The term 'healthy' may be used to describe foods that are low in fat and saturated fat, and provide less than 480 mg sodium and less than 60 mg cholesterol per serving.

FDA regulations permit labelling to include health claims that are supported by valid and substantial scientific evidence for the following:

(1) dietary saturated fat and cholesterol and risk of coronary heart disease,

(2) dietary fat and cancer,

(3) sodium and hypertension,

(4) calcium and osteoporosis,

(5) fibre-rich grain products, fruits and vegetables and cancer,

(6) fruits, vegetables, and grain products that contain fibre, particularly soluble fibre, and risk of coronary heart disease,

(7) fruits and vegetables and cancer.

4.3.2 Nutrition labelling in the European Union

Within the EU, nutrition labelling of foodstuffs is regulated by a Council Directive (European Commission 1990) that requires labels to list the energy yield, protein, carbohydrate, fat (and proportion of saturated fat), fibre and sodium content per 100 g (or per 100 mL); the amount per serving may also be included. Nutrition labelling is optional, unless any nutritional claims are made, in which case full information must be given, including the vitamins and minerals present. Claims of health benefits (see section 4.3.1.3) are not permitted; definitions of terms such as 'free from', 'low in' and 'reduced' have not yet been agreed.

The EU Scientific Committee for Food (1993) proposed that an appropriate value for labelling would be the Population Reference Intake for adult women, which is, apart from that for iron, numerically equal to the average requirement for men. However, the EC Directive on nutritional labelling came into force before the SCF report had been published, and at present the values that are required to be used for labelling are those shown in Table 4.10. It is unlikely that the SCF figures will be adopted before 1998, when the Directive on nutritional labelling is to be reviewed.

Further reading

Department of Health (1994). *Nutritional Aspects of Cardiovascular Disease*, Report on Health and Social Subjects no 46 HMSO, London.

Gibney, M. J. (1992). Are there conflicts in dietary advice for prevention of different diseases? *Proceedings of the Nutrition Society*, 51, 35–45.

James, W. P. T., Ferro-Luzzi, A., Isaksson, B. and Szostak, W. B. (1988). *Healthy nutrition: preventing nutrition-related diseases in Europe*, WHO Regional Publications, European Series no 24 WHO, Copenhagen.

National Research Council Committee on Diet and Health (1989). *Diet and Health: Implications for Reducing Chronic Disease Risk*. National Academy Press, Washington, DC.

Oliver, M. F. (1981). Diet and coronary heart disease. *British Medical Bulletin*, 37, 49–58.

Posner, B. M., Quatromoni, P. A. and Franz, M. (1974). Nutrition and the global risk for chronic diseases: the INTERHEALTH nutrition initiative. *Nutrition Reviews*, 52, 201–7.

Rogers, A. E. and Longnecker, M. P. (1988). Dietary and nutritional influences on cancer: a review of the epidemiologic and experimental data. *Laboratory Investigation*, 59, 729–59.

Symposium Proceedings (1990). Diet and cancer. *Proceedings of the Nutrition Society*, 49, 119–83.

US Department of Agriculture and US Department of Health and Human Services (1990). *Dietary Guidelines for Americans* (3rd edn). US Government Printing Office, Washington, DC.

Various authors (1983). Diet and Cancer Prevention. *Seminars in Oncology*, 10, 257–357.

WHO (1990). *Diet, Nutrition and the Prevention of Chronic Diseases*, WHO Technical Reports Series 797, WHO, Geneva.

4.1: Terms that have been used to describe reference intakes of nutrients

RDA	Recommended Dietary Allowances	USA 1941	The name was deliberately chosen to allow the possibility of future modification of the values and was not intended to carry any connotation of minimum or optimal requirements; see Table 4.2
RDI	Recommended Dietary Intakes	UK 1969	... to emphasize that the recommendations related to foodstuffs as actually eaten
RDA	Recommended Daily Amounts	UK 1979	... to make it clear that the amounts referred to averages for a group of people and not to amounts that individuals must meet, as implied by the term "allowances"
	Safe levels of intake	UN Agencies	Means safe and adequate, but does not imply that higher intakes are unsafe
RNI	Reference Nutrient Intakes	UK 1991	By parallel with clinical chemistry reference ranges, which encompass 95% of "normal" values. To emphasize that they are not recommendations for individuals, nor are they amounts to be consumed daily; see Table 4.3
PRI	Population Reference Intakes	EU 1993	By parallel with RNI, but emphasizing that these are population ranges, and not applicable to individuals; see Table 4.4
US-RDA		USA 1973	Reference intakes for labelling purposes, the highest RDA value for any population group
RDI	Reference Daily Intakes	USA 1990	Reference intakes for labelling purposes, numerically equal to US-RDA; see Table 4.10
DRV	Daily Reference Values	USA 1990	Reference values for fat, carbohydrate, sodium, potassium and protein, for labelling purposes; see Table 4.9

4.2: US Recommended Daily Amounts of nutrients

age	protein μg	Vit A μg	Vit D μg	Vit E mg	Vit K mg	Vit C mg	Vit B_1 mg	Vit B_2 mg	niacin mg	Vit B_6 mg	folate μg	Vit B_{12} μg	calcium mg	phosp mg	magn mg	iron mg	zinc mg	iodine μg	selenium μg
0 - 6m	13	375	7.5	3	5	30	0.3	0.4	5	0.3	25	0.3	400	300	40	6	5	40	10
6 - 12m	14	375	10	4	10	35	0.4	0.5	6	0.6	35	0.5	600	500	60	10	5	50	15
1 - 3y	16	400	10	6	15	40	0.7	0.8	9	1.0	50	0.7	800	800	80	10	10	70	20
4 - 6y	24	500	10	7	20	45	0.9	1.1	12	1.1	75	1.0	800	800	120	10	10	90	20
7 - 10y	28	700	10	7	30	45	1.0	1.2	13	1.4	100	1.4	800	800	170	10	10	120	30
males																			
11 - 14y	45	1000	10	10	45	50	1.3	1.5	17	1.7	150	2.0	1200	1200	270	12	15	150	40
15 - 18y	59	1000	10	10	65	60	1.5	1.8	20	2.0	200	2.0	1200	1200	400	12	15	150	50
19 - 24y	58	1000	10	10	70	60	1.5	1.7	19	2.0	200	2.0	1200	1200	350	10	15	150	70
25 - 50y	63	1000	5	10	80	60	1.5	1.7	19	2.0	200	2.0	800	800	350	10	15	150	70
51+ y	63	1000	5	10	80	60	1.2	1.4	15	2.0	200	2.0	800	800	350	10	15	150	70
females																			
11 - 14y	46	800	10	8	45	50	1.1	1.3	15	1.4	150	2.0	1200	1200	280	15	12	150	45
15 - 18y	44	800	10	8	55	60	1.1	1.3	15	1.5	180	2.0	1200	1200	300	15	12	150	50
19 - 24y	46	800	10	8	60	60	1.1	1.3	15	1.6	180	2.0	1200	1200	280	15	12	150	55
25 - 50y	50	800	5	8	65	60	1.1	1.3	15	1.6	180	2.0	800	800	280	15	12	150	55
51+ y	50	800	5	8	65	60	1.0	1.2	13	1.6	180	2.0	800	800	280	10	12	150	55
pregnant	60	800	10	10	65	70	1.5	1.6	17	2.2	400	2.2	1200	1200	320	30	15	175	65
lactating	65	1300	10	10	65	95	1.6	1.8	20	2.1	280	2.6	1200	1200	355	15	19	200	75

Source: National Research Council / National Academy of Science 1989.

4.3: UK Reference Nutrient Intakes

age	Vit B₁ mg	Vit B₂ mg	niacin mg	Vit B₆ mg	Vit B₁₂ µg	folate µg	Vit C mg	Vit A µg	Vit D µg	calcium mg	phos mg	magn mg	sodium mg	iron mg	zinc mg	copper mg	selenium µg	iodine µg
0 - 3m	0.2	0.4	3	0.2	0.3	50	25	350	8.5	525	400	55	210	1.7	4.0	0.2	10	50
4 - m	0.2	0.4	3	0.2	0.3	50	25	350	8.5	525	400	60	280	4.3	4.0	0.3	13	60
7 - 9m	0.2	0.4	4	0.3	0.4	50	25	350	7	525	400	75	320	7.8	5.0	0.3	10	60
10-12m	0.3	0.4	5	0.4	0.4	50	25	350	7	525	400	80	350	7.8	5.0	0.3	10	60
1 - 3y	0.5	0.6	8	0.7	0.5	70	30	400	7	350	270	85	500	6.9	5.0	0.4	15	70
4 - 6y	0.7	0.8	11	0.9	0.8	100	30	500	-	450	350	120	700	6.1	6.5	0.6	20	100
7-10y	0.7	1.0	12	1.0	1.0	150	30	500	-	550	450	200	1200	8.7	7.0	0.7	30	110
males																		
11-14y	0.9	1.2	15	1.2	1.2	200	35	600	-	1000	775	280	1600	11.3	9.0	0.8	45	130
15-18y	1.1	1.3	18	1.5	1.5	200	40	700	-	1000	775	300	1600	11.3	9.5	1.0	70	140
19-50	1.0	1.3	17	1.4	1.5	200	40	700	-	700	550	300	1600	8.7	9.5	1.2	75	140
50+ y	0.9	1.3	16	1.4	1.5	200	40	700	10	700	550	300	1600	8.7	9.5	1.2	75	140
females																		
11-14y	0.7	1.1	12	1.0	1.2	200	35	600	-	800	625	280	1600	14.8	9.0	0.8	45	130
15-18y	0.8	1.1	14	1.2	1.5	200	40	600	-	800	6254	300	1600	14.8	7.0	1.0	60	140
19-50y	0.8	1.1	13	1.2	1.5	200	40	600	-	700	550	270	1600	14.8	7.0	1.2	60	140
50+ y	0.8	1.1	12	1.2	1.5	200	40	600	10	700	550	270	1600	8.7	7.0	1.2	60	140
pregnant	+0.1	+0.3	-	-	-	+100	+10	+100	10	-	-	-	-	-	-	-	-	-
lactating	+0.1	+0.5	+2	-	+0.5	+60	+30	+350	10	+550	+440	+50	-	-	+6.0	+0.3	+15	-

Source: Department of Health 1991.

4.4: EU Population Reference Intakes of nutrients

age	protein g	Vit A µg	Vit B_1 mg	Vit B_2 mg	niacin mg	Vit B_6 mg	folate µg	Vit B_{12} µg	Vit C mg	calcium mg	phosphorus mg	iron mg	zinc mg	copper mg	selenium µg	iodine µg
6 - 12 m	15	350	0.3	0.4	5	0.4	50	0.5	20	400	300	6	4	0.3	8	50
1 - 3 y	15	400	0.5	0.8	9	0.7	100	0.7	25	400	300	4	4	0.4	10	70
4 - 6 y	20	400	0.7	1.0	11	0.9	130	0.9	25	450	350	4	6	0.6	15	90
7 - 10 y	29	500	0.8	1.2	13	1.1	150	1.0	30	550	450	6	7	0.7	25	100
males																
11 - 14 y	44	600	1.0	1.4	15	1.3	180	1.3	35	1000	775	10	9	0.8	35	120
15 - 17 y	55	700	1.2	1.6	18	1.5	200	1.4	40	1000	775	13	9	1.0	45	130
18 + y	56	700	1.1	1.6	18	1.5	200	1.4	45	700	550	9	9.5	1.1	55	130
females																
11 - 14 y	42	600	0.9	1.2	14	1.1	180	1.3	35	800	625	18	9	0.8	35	120
15 - 17 y	46	600	0.9	1.3	14	1.1	200	1.4	40	800	625	17	7	1.0	45	130
18 + y	47	600	0.9	1.3	14	1.1	200	1.4	45	700	550	16[1]	7	1.1	55	130
pregnant	57	700	1.0	1.6	14	1.3	400	1.6	55	700	550	[1]	7	1.1	55	130
lactating	63	950	1.1	1.7	16	1.4	350	1.9	70	1200	950	16	12	1.4	70	160

(1) 8 mg iron post-menopausally; supplements required in latter half of pregnancy

Source: Scientific Committee for Food 1993.

4.5: Criteria for assessment of the adequacy of nutrient intake, in order of increasing sensitivity

		examples	see section
severe clinical deficiency disease	anatomical lesions, possibly irreversible	blindness due to vitamin A deficiency	13.4
mild clinical deficiency disease	functional lesions, mild, and possibly reversible, anatomical lesions	skin lesions of many nutrient deficiencies	-
		abnormal corneal cytology in vitamin A deficiency	13.4
covert deficiency disease	no lesions apparent until there is some physical or metabolic stress	impaired wound healing in vitamin C deficiency	22.5
		rickets only becomes apparent when food intake is adequate to permit growth	14.4
subclinical (biochemical) deficiency	abnormal metabolism under basal conditions	increased secretion of thyrotropin in mild iodine deficiency	25.14.4
		methylmalonic aciduria in vitamin B_{12} deficiency	21.9.3
	abnormal response to a metabolic load	abnormal tryptophan and methionine metabolism in vitamin B_6 deficiency	20.6.5, 20.6.6
		abnormal glucose metabolism in thiamin deficiency	17.5.6.1
		abnormal histidine metabolism in folate deficiency	21.9.4
depletion of body reserves	low excretion under basal conditions	the basis for estimates of riboflavin requirements	18.3.4
	low excretion of a test dose, reflecting low tissue saturation	vitamin C saturation testing	22.3.3
	low blood concentration of vitamin or active metabolite	applicable to many vitamins and minerals	-
	changes in plasma or erythrocyte enzyme activity	elevated alkaline phosphatase in vitamin D deficiency	14.4
		impaired blood clotting in vitamin K deficiency	16.6.1
	inadequate saturation of erythrocyte enzyme with coenzyme	transketolase activation with thiamin diphosphate	
		glutathione reductase activation with flavin adenine dinucleotide	18.6
		transaminase activation with pyridoxal phosphate (vitamin B_6)	20.6.3

4.6: Clinical signs of value in nutrition surveys

	signs	problem	see section
skin	xerosis, perifollicular hyperkeratosis	vitamin A deficiency	13.4
	petechial haemorrhages	vitamin C deficiency	22.5
	sunburn-like photosensitive dermatitis	niacin deficiency	19.5
	flaky paint dermatitis	kwashiorkor	12.4
	scrotal and vulval dermatitis, sebhorreic dermatitis with filiform excrescences	riboflavin deficiency	18.5
nails	concave, cracked (koilonychia)	iron deficiency	24.4
subcutaneous tissue	oedema	kwashiorkor	12.4
	little fat	marasmus, cachexia	12.2, 12.3
	excess fat	obesity	11
face	naso-labial dyssebacea	riboflavin deficiency	18.5
	moon face	kwashiorkor, iodine deficiency	12.4, 25.14.4
hair	lack of lustre, thin and sparse, poorly pigmented, easily pluckable	kwashiorkor, marasmus	12.4, 12.2
eyes	pale conjunctiva, Bitot's spots, conjunctival xerosis, corneal xerosis, keratomalacia	vitamin A deficiency	13.4
lips	angular stomatitis, angular scars, cheilosis	riboflavin deficiency	18.5
tongue	scarlet and raw tongue	niacin deficiency	19.5
	magenta tongue	riboflavin deficiency	18.5
teeth	mottled enamel	fluorosis	25.12
gums	spongy, bleeding	vitamin C deficiency	22.5
glands	thyroid enlargement	iodine deficiency	25.14.4
	parotid enlargement	starvation	12.2
muscle	wasting	marasmus, cachexia	12.2, 12.3
	calf tenderness	thiamin deficiency	17.5.2
	musculo-skeletal haemorrhages	vitamin C deficiency	22.5
heart	cardiac enlargement, tachycardia	thiamin deficiency	17.5.3, 17.5.4
liver	enlargement (hepatomegaly)	kwashiorkor	12.4
skeleton	craniotabes, frontal and parietal bossing, epiphyseal enlargement, persistently open anterior fontanelle, knock knees or bow legs	vitamin D deficiency	14.4
	thoracic rosary	vitamin C or D deficiency	22.5, 14.4
nervous system	psychomotor changes	kwashiorkor	12.4
	depressive psychosis, hallucinations	niacin deficiency	19.5
	mental confusion, psychosis, encephalopathy	thiamin deficiency	17.5.5
	sensory loss, motor weakness, loss of positional and vibrational senses, loss of ankle and knee jerks	thiamin deficiency	17.5.2

Table 4.7: Methods that are available for biochemical assessment of vitamin nutritional status and determination of requirements

vitamin	urinary excretion	saturation testing	blood concentration	blood enzyme	enzyme activation	abnormal metabolite excretion	metabolic load
A	-	dangerous	useful	-	-	-	-
D	-	dangerous	main method	alkaline phosphatase	-	-	-
E	-	-	useful	-	-	-	-
K	-	-	may be useful	blood clotting	-	-	-
thiamin	useful	may be useful	may be useful	-	transketolase	-	glucose
riboflavin	main method	-	may be useful	-	glutathione reductase	-	-
niacin	useful	-	may be useful	-	-	-	-
B_6	useful	-	useful	transaminases	transaminases	-	tryptophan, methionine
B_{12}	-	(Schilling test for absorption)	main method	-	-	methylmalonic acid	-
folate	may be useful	-	main method	-	-	-	histidine
C	-	useful	main method	-	-	-	-
biotin	-	-	-	-	-	organic acids	-

Table 4.8: Composition of breast milk and standards for breast milk substitutes

	mature human milk /100 mL			mean /100 kJ	/100 kcal	infant formula[1] /100 kJ		/100 kcal	
	min	max	mean	/100 kJ	/100 kcal	min	max	min	max
energy, kJ	270	290	315	-	-	-	-	-	-
energy, kcal	65	70	75	-	-	-	-	-	-
protein, g	0.95	1.20	1.07	0.3	1.4	0.45	0.7	1.8	3
fat, g	3.7	4.8	4.2	1.3	5.6	0.8	1.5	3.3	6.5
carbohydrates, g	7.1	7.8	7.4	2.4	9.9	1.7 g	3.4	7 g	14
sodium, mg	11	20	15	4.8	20	5	14	20	60
potassium, mg	57	62	60	19	80	15	35	60	145
chloride, mg	35	55	43	14	57	12	29	50	125
calcium, mg	32	36	35	11	47	12	-	50	-
phosphorus, mg	14	15	15	4.8	20	6	22	25	90
magnesium, mg	2.6	3.0	2.8	0.9	3.7	1.2	3.6	5	15
iron, mg	62	93	76	24	101	0.12	0.36	0.5	1.5
zinc, µg	-	-	295	94	393	120	360	500	1500
copper, µg	-	-	39	12	52	4.8	19	20	80
iodine, µg	-	-	7	2.2	9.3	1.2	-	5	-
vitamin A, µg	40	76	60	19	80	14	43	60	180
vitamin D, µg	-	-	-	-	-	0.25	0.65	1	2.5
vitamin E, mg	0.29	0.39	0.35	0.1	0.47	[2]			
vitamin K, µg	-	-	-	-	-	1	-	4	-
thiamin, µg	23	21	16	5	21	10	-	40	-
riboflavin, µg	31	31	31	9.8	41	14	-	60	-
niacin, µg	210	270	230	73	307	60	-	250	-
vitamin B_6, µg	5.1	7.2	5.9	1.9	7.9	9	-	35	-
biotin, µg	0.52	1.13	0.76	0.24	1.0	0.4	-	1.5	-
pantothenic acid, µg	220	330	260	83	111	70	-	300	-
vitamin B_{12}, µg	0.01	0.01	0.01	0.003	0.13	0.025	-	0.1	-
folate, µg	3.1	6.2	5.2	1.7	6.9	1	-	4	-
vitamin C, mg	3.1	4.5	3.8	1.2	5.1	1.9	-	8	-

(1) Energy yield of infant formula, as made up, must be between 250-315 kJ (60-75) kcal /100 mL.
(2) Minimum vitamin E must be 0.5 mg /g polyunsaturated fatty acids, and not less than 0.1 mg /100 kJ (0.5 mg /100 kcal).
Source: Dept of Health and Social Security 1977; European Commission 1991.

Table 4.9: Daily Reference Values for nutrition labelling in USA, for adults and children over 4, based on a 2000 kcal diet

fat	65 g
saturated fatty acids	20 g
cholesterol	300 mg
total carbohydrate	300 g
fibre	25 g
sodium	2,400 mg
potassium	3,500 mg
protein[1]	50 g

(1) DRV for protein does not apply to certain population groups: Reference Daily Intakes for protein have been established for the following groups: children 1-4 years, 16g; pregnant women 60 g; nursing mothers 65 g.

Table 4.11: Criteria for labelling foods low in and free from in USA

	content per reference serving for foods to be described as:	
	"low in"	"free from"
sodium[1]	not more than 140 mg	> 5 mg
calories	not more than 40 kcal	> 5 kcal
sugars	-	> 0.5 g
fat	not more than 3 g	> 0.5 g
trans-fatty acids	-	not more than 1% of total fat
saturated fat	not more than 1 g;	
	not more than 15% of energy from saturated fat	
cholesterol	not more than 20 mg	< 2 mg

(1) FDA defines very low sodium foods as those containing 35 mg or less in a standard serving.

Table 4.10: Labelling Reference Values for vitamins and minerals

	USA Reference Daily Intake	European Union Proposed by Scientific Committee for Food[1]	Required by Directive[2]
vitamin A, µg	1500	500	800
vitamin D, µg	10	5	5
vitamin E, mg	30	-	10
vitamin C, mg	60	30	60
thiamin, mg	1.5	0.8	1.4
riboflavin, mg	1.7	1.3	1.6
niacin, mg	20	15	18
vitamin B_6, mg	2.0	1.3	2.0
folate, µg	400	140	200
vitamin B_{12}, µg	6.0	1.0	1.0
biotin, µg	300	-	150
pantothenic acid, mg	10	-	6
calcium, mg	1000	550	800
copper, mg	2.0	0.8	-
iodine, µg	150	100	150
iron[1], mg	18	7, 14	14
magnesium, mg	400	-	300
phosphorus, mg	1000	-	800
selenium, µg	-	40	-
zinc, mg	15	7.5	15

(1) The Scientific Committee for Food proposed separate figures for iron for women (14 mg) and men (7 mg)
Source: (1) Scientific Committee for Food 1993; (2) EC 1990.

5

Energy balance and an overview of metabolism

The primary need of the body is for a source of metabolic fuels (fat, carbohydrate, protein and alcohol) to meet energy expenditure. Food in excess of immediate requirements for energy-yielding metabolism is stored as reserves of glycogen in muscle and liver, and as fat in adipose tissue. There is also an increase in tissue protein synthesis after a meal. In the fasting state, or when energy intake is inadequate to meet expenditure, these reserves, and labile tissue protein reserves, are used as metabolic fuels.

Normally, energy expenditure and food intake are closely balanced, at least when averaged over several days. The result of a prolonged positive energy balance (an excess of intake over expenditure) is the accumulation of excessive amounts of body fat—the development of overweight and obesity, see Chapter 11. Prolonged negative energy balance (an intake less than expenditure) is protein-energy malnutrition—wasting and emaciation, see section 12.2. As discussed in section 6.5, the physiological mechanisms by which people are able to adjust their food intake to meet energy expenditure are not known.

5.1 The energy yields of metabolic fuels

Since the overall energy yield or cost of a chemical reaction is the same regardless of the route taken, the gross energy yields of metabolic fuels can be determined by measuring the heat of combustion. For fats, carbohydrates and alcohol the products of metabolism and combustion are the same: carbon dioxide and water. For proteins allowance has to be made for the difference between combustion to nitrogen oxides and metabolism to yield urea ($CO(NH_2)_2$) or ammonia, by subtracting the heat of combustion of these nitrogenous end-products from the heat of combustion of the protein. Table 5.1 shows the gross energy yields (heats of combustion) and oxygen consumption for the major metabolic fuels.

The gross energy yield of foods must be corrected for absorption, i.e. digestible energy. On average the energy content of faeces equals 4 per cent of intake, so that 96 per cent of dietary gross energy is digestible energy. Carbohydrates are considered to be 99 per cent absorbed (but see section 7.2.2 for a discussion of resistant starch, which has lower digestibility), fats 95 per cent, and proteins 92 per cent absorbed. In the case of proteins, allowance has to be made for the urinary loss of energy in urea and ammonia, so that the metabolizable energy of protein is 25 per cent lower than the digestible energy (see Table 5.2).

The calculations of the metabolizable energy yield of metabolic fuels were originally performed by Atwater in 1899, and the final columns of Table 5.2 show the Atwater factors for calculation of metabolizable energy: carbohydrate and protein 4 kcal/g, fat 9 kcal/g, and alcohol 7 kcal/g. For food labelling purposes, and for calculation of energy intake from foods, the values shown in Table 5.3 are used.

Conventionally it is assumed that urinary and other losses of alcohol are negligible, and that the energy yield of alcohol, which is 100 per cent absorbed, is equal to the heat of combustion. However, as discussed in section 9.1, this assumption is not valid, and the true metabolic energy yield of alcohol is uncertain. More precise figures for the energy yields of individual carbohydrates are shown in Tables 7.7–7.9, of individual fatty acids in Table 8.4, and of amino acids in Table 10.8.

5.2 Measurement of energy expenditure

5.2.1 Direct calorimetry

Regardless of whether energy is being expended in physical activity, or as chemical or electrical work in the body, the end result is output of heat from the body. Given an appropriate thermally insulated chamber (a calorimeter), maintained at a constant temperature, it is possible to measure this heat output, for example by the increase in temperature of water used to cool the chamber. The (non-SI) unit of heat is the calorie; 1 cal is the heat required to raise the temperature of 1 g of water by 1°C, and the more precise 15° calorie is the heat required to raise the temperature of 1 g of water from 14.5°C to 15.5°C. Physiological and nutritional levels of energy expenditure and intake are measured in kcal (10^3 calories, the heat required to raise the temperature of 1 kg of water through 1°C).

Correctly, the unit of work or energy is the joule, a derived SI unit; 1 J is equal to a force of 1 N acting over a distance of 1 m in the direction of the force. More usefully, the specific heat of water at 15°C = 4185.5 J/kg °C, so that 1 cal = 4.1855 J. This is normally rounded to 4.186 J = 1 cal, and sometimes to 4.2 J = 1 cal.

Although the joule is the correct SI unit of energy, calories are still widely used both in the nutritional literature and in food labelling; as far as possible, both units are used in this book, with rounding off as appropriate to avoid spurious precision in converted values.

5.2.2 Indirect calorimetry

Of necessity, calorimeter chambers are relatively small, which limits the range of physical activities that can be performed for direct measurement of energy expenditure. Furthermore, measurements are usually only possible for a relatively short time (a few hours at most). In order to overcome these two problems, three techniques of indirect calorimetry have been developed, all of which must be calibrated against direct measurement of heat output:

(1) oxygen consumption and carbon dioxide production;

(2) heart rate monitoring;

(3) the dual isotopically labelled water method.

5.2.2.1 Respirometry: oxygen consumption and carbon dioxide production

As shown in Table 5.4, the mean energy yield of various metabolic fuels is 20.02 kJ (4.78 kcal)/L of oxygen consumed, with a coefficient of variation of 3.3 per cent. This means that, within the limits of experimental error, energy expenditure can be calculated from oxygen consumption, regardless of the fuel being utilized. Respirometers, with intermittent sampling of inhaled and exhaled air, are considerably less restricting than calorimeters, so that it is possible to determine energy expenditure in a wide variety of

tasks. Most of the values of energy expenditure in various activities shown in Tables 5.12 and 5.13 have been obtained by respirometry.

Table 5.5 shows the carbon dioxide produced, and oxygen consumed, for oxidation of metabolic fuels, as well as the Respiratory Quotient (RQ, L carbon dioxide produced /L oxygen consumed). If respirometry includes measurement of carbon dioxide and oxygen, as well as urinary nitrogen, then it is possible to estimate both energy expenditure and the proportions of different fuels being utilized, from the following formulae (Weir 1949):

energy expenditure (kJ) = 16.849 × mL oxygen consumed + 4.628 × mL carbon dioxide produced −9.079 × g N excreted,

energy expenditure (kcal) = 4.025 × mL oxygen consumed + 1.106 × mL carbon dioxide produced −2.168 × g N excreted.

If urinary nitrogen is not determined, and it is assumed that protein provides 15 per cent of energy, then

energy expenditure (kJ) = 16.318 × mL oxygen consumed + 4.602 × mL carbon dioxide produced,

energy expenditure (kcal) = 3.898 × mL oxygen consumed + 1.099 × mL carbon dioxide produced.

The amount of each fuel being utilized can be calculated from

grams carbohydrate oxidized = 4.706 × mL carbon dioxide produced −3.340 × mL oxygen consumed −2.714 × g N excreted,

grams fat oxidized = 1.768 × mL oxygen consumed −1.778 × mL carbon dioxide produced −2.021 × g N excreted,

grams protein oxidized = 6.25 × g N excreted.

5.2.2.2 Heart rate monitoring

Although respirometry permits estimation of energy expenditure in a wider variety of activities than does direct calorimetry, it is still limited to relatively short periods of observation. Once a subject's heart rate has been calibrated against his or her oxygen consumption, changes in heart rate with physical activity can be used to estimate oxygen utilization, and hence energy consumption. Heart rate monitors that report data by radio are small and portable, and indeed have earned the name of socially acceptable monitoring instruments (SAMI), which permit integrated estimation of energy activity over a period of days.

5.2.2.3 The dual isotopically labelled water method
Studies to determine total body water using isotopically labelled water (see section 2.2.1.2) give different results when the label is present in ^2H_2O or when $H_2{}^{18}O$ is used. This is because the label in ^2H_2O can only be lost from the body as water, while that in $H_2{}^{18}O$ can be lost either as water or as carbon dioxide, as a result of rapid equilibration between carbon dioxide (CO_2) and bicarbonate ($HCO_3{}^-$), catalysed by carbonic anhydrase (EC 4.2.1.1). The three oxygen atoms of bicarbonate are equivalent, and there is therefore label exchange between water and carbon dioxide.

This has been exploited as a non-invasive means of estimating total energy expenditure over an extended period of time, which requires minimal cooperation from the experimental subject (Schoeller and van Santen 1982; Coward 1988). Following an oral dose of $^2H_2{}^{18}O$, the isotopic enrichment of water in plasma, saliva or urine is determined at intervals over a period of 10–21 days. The rate of carbon dioxide production is then calculated from the greater rate of loss of ^{18}O than ^2H, as

carbon dioxide production rate =(0.5 × total body water) × (rate constant for ^{18}O disappearance − rate constant for ^2H disappearance).

From records of food eaten, the average RQ over the period can be estimated, and hence, allowing for any changes in body weight, the total oxygen consumption and energy expenditure can be calculated.

5.3   Components of energy expenditure

There are three components of energy expenditure:

(1) essential metabolic activity (Basal or Resting Metabolic Rate, see Table 5.6), which accounts for 60–70 per cent of total expenditure;

(2) voluntary physical activity, most usually expressed as a ratio of BMR;

(3) diet-induced thermogenesis—the increase in metabolic activity following a meal.

Total energy expenditure can be estimated by measurement or calculation of Basal Metabolic Rate, together with a record of the time spent in physical activities of different intensity (an activity diary), and an estimate of the extent of diet-induced thermogenesis. Such calculations can then be used to estimate average energy requirements for populations (see section 4.1).

5.3.1 Basal Metabolic Rate (BMR)

BMR is the energy expenditure of the body at rest, measured by direct or indirect calorimetry under rigorously standardized conditions. The subject is in the fasting state, so that there is no increased metabolic activity associated with digestion, or absorption and processing of the products of digestion, at a temperature between 26–30°C, so that metabolic energy is not being expended either to maintain body temperature or lose excess heat, and awake but completely at rest. A number of studies have shown that metabolic rate in sleep may be either higher or lower than BMR. When the conditions of measurement are less stringently controlled, the result is correctly the resting, rather than basal, metabolic rate.

BMR is the energy expended to maintain normal metabolic homeostasis and body function. The major functions are the following

(1) electrical activity of nerves and muscles—the maintenance of nerve and muscle tone;

(2) protein synthesis and other metabolic activity of all tissues, especially liver and skeletal muscle;

(3) heart and respiratory muscle contraction to permit circulation and respiration;

(4) kidney function— active resorption in the tubules of water and metabolites filtered at the glomerulus, and active secretion into the distal tubules;

(5) for children, BMR includes the energy cost of net growth (Holliday 1986).

Table 5.7 shows the relative contribution of different organs to BMR. It is apparent that both body weight and the relative proportions of fat and lean tissue (see section 2.2) will affect BMR. Therefore, for the same body weight and height, there will be a difference in BMR between men and women, since a higher proportion of body weight is fat in women. Similarly, there is a fall in BMR with increasing age, since there is an increasing proportion of fat, without any change in body weight, with increasing age. Table 5.8 shows the effects of age, body weight and gender on BMR

A number of formulae have been derived by correlation of experimentally determined BMR with weight, height and age. The simplest two such equations are those of Mifflin *et al.* (1990), shown in Table 5.9, in which a single equation, based on weight, height and age, is used for each gender.

Schofield *et al.* (1985) published a critical review of the literature, and proposed the two series of predictive equations shown in Table 5.10. There are different regression equations for males and females at each age; those which include height as well as weight give a more precise fit to the experimentally determined data. Nevertheless, the precision with which these equations predict BMR is only about ±10 per cent. The Schofield equations based on weight provided the basis for the FAO/WHO/UNU (1985) estimates of energy requirements. In turn, these United Nations figures have provided the basis for estimation of average energy requirements in the USA (National Academy of Sciences / National Research Council, 1989), the UK (Department of Health 1991) and the EU (Scientific Committee for Food 1993). Henry *et al.* (1991) proposed a different set of regression equations that provide a better fit to the experimental data for subjects living in tropical countries, shown in Table 5.11.

5.3.2 The energy cost of physical activity

The energy cost of physical activity is most usually expressed as the energy expenditure in performing a given task as a multiple of BMR—the Physical Activity Ratio (PAR). As can be seen from Table 5.12, PAR ranges from 1.0–1.4 × BMR for light, sedentary activities, to almost 8 × BMR for vigorous physical exercise. Table 5.13 lists the energy costs (as PAR) of a wide variety of physical activities; they are mean values from the literature, and in many cases only a single determination of the energy cost of the activity has been reported, from studies on a single subject.

5.3.2.1 Physical Activity Level

A person's overall Physical Activity Level (PAL) is the sum of the PAR of different types of activity performed through the day, multiplied by the time spent in that activity.

The figures for energy expenditure in various activities shown in Table 5.13 are those while the task is actually being performed, excluding the natural (and often essential) pauses in activity. James and Schofield (1980) reported that during a pause in activity energy expenditure was 1.54 × BMR in men, and 1.66 × BMR in women, regardless of the intensity of the activity. They also showed that on average pauses occupy 75 per cent of the time spent in light activities, 25 per cent of the time spent in moderate activities and 40 per cent of the time spent in heavy activity. They defined an Integrated Energy Index (IEI), based on these factors, as a true reflection of the energy cost of performing an activity, as shown in Table 5.14.

Table 5.15 shows the classification of occupational work by PAL through the working day (i.e. the IEI for occupational work) in developed and less developed countries, and Table 5.16 the classification of average PAR through the 8 hour working day used for estimation of energy requirements in UK.

Table 5.17 shows average Physical Activity Levels (i.e. occupational and leisure activities) in developed and less developed countries, and Table 5.18 a more detailed analysis for British figures, classified by intensity of occupational work and leisure activities.

Table 5.19 shows average energy requirements for children (expressed as kJ and kcal /kg body weight) with and without a desirable level of physical activity (defined by WHO as the level of physical activity associated with optimum cardiovascular and respiratory health). Table 5.20 shows average Physical Activity Levels for adolescents and adults, again with and without a desirable level of physical activity. At the simplest, these tables can be interpreted as showing, under the heading 'with desirable activity' the ideal, and under the heading 'without desirable activity' the true situation for the majority of the population of developed countries.

5.3.3 Diet-induced thermogenesis

There is a considerable increase in metabolic rate after a meal, which may be equivalent to 10–15 per cent of the energy yield of the food consumed. Part of this is the energy cost of secreting digestive enzymes, intestinal peristalsis and active transport of the products of digestion. However, this is only a small proportion of the total; Vernet *et al.* (1986) have shown that the increase in metabolic rate is not significantly different when iso-ergonic diets are fed by mouth or infused intravenously. The main contributor to diet-induced thermogenesis is the energy cost of synthesizing tissue energy reserves of protein, glycogen, and fat.

As discussed in section 10.8.3.2, the energy cost of protein synthesis is approximately 4.2 kJ /g protein, and protein turnover accounts for about 20 per cent of BMR; there is a 35–40 per cent increase in whole body protein synthesis in response to a meal (Clugston and Garlick 1982).

Glycogen synthesis is also energy requiring; if the precursor is glucose, then there is an energy cost of 2 × ATP equivalents per mol of glucose incorporated, while if glucose is to be synthesized from other monosaccharides or non-carbohydrate precursors then the energy cost of the appropriate metabolic pathway must also be accounted for. Overall the energy cost of glycogen synthesis is about 5 per cent of the energy yield of the glycogen synthesized.

As discussed in section 8.2, dietary triacylglycerols are hydrolysed in the intestinal lumen, then re-esterified in the intestinal mucosa to form triacylglycerol which is incorporated into chylomicrons. There is a cost of 2 × ATP per mol fatty acid esterified. Triacylglycerol in chylomicrons is hydrolysed by lipoprotein lipase (EC 3.1.1.34) before uptake into adipose tissue, and therefore there is a cost of 6 × ATP per mol of triacylglycerol re-esterified in adipose tissue. The synthesis of fatty acids from acetyl CoA (and hence synthesis of fatty acids from glucose and amino acids) involves a cost of 7 ATP equivalents per 2–carbon unit, or 63 × ATP per mol of palmitate synthesized (see Fig. 5.7). Overall the cost of fat synthesis is about 20 per cent of the energy yield of the fat synthesized.

5.4   The relationship between food intake, energy expenditure and body weight

There is not a simple relationship between food intake, energy expenditure and body weight. Energy expenditure depends on body weight both because body weight is the main determinant of BMR, and also because of the increased energy cost of physical activity with greater body weight. Table 5.21 shows the effects of age, body weight and physical activity on total energy expenditure.

In addition to this, the effect of positive energy balance on body weight will be attentuated to some extent by the increased diet-induced thermogenesis, and especially the relatively high energy cost of triacylglycerol synthesis. Similarly, if energy intake is inadequate to meet expenditure, there will be much reduced synthesis of fat and glycogen in the fed state, and hence reduced diet-induced thermogenesis.

The relationship is further confounded by changes in both the efficiency of physical activity, which can increase significantly in undernutrition, and fall in over nutrition, and the amount of unmeasurable activity (restlessness), which falls in undernutrition and rises with excessive food intake.

There is also evidence, albeit disputed, that overall metabolic 'efficiency' varies with energy balance. Two mechanisms have been proposed.

1. Changes in the heat output of brown adipose tissue (non-shivering thermogenesis), associated with facultative uncoupling of substrate oxidation and oxidative phosphorylation of ADP to ATP (see section 5.5). In response to noradrenaline binding to cell-surface β1–adrenergic receptors, there is stimulation of the activity of intracellular hormone-sensitive lipase (EC 3.1.1.23). The resultant long-chain fatty acids both act as substrates for increased oxidation, and also uncouple electron transport from phosphorylation of ADP to ATP, so permitting increased substrate oxidation (and heat production) without the normal limitation by the availability of ADP (respiratory control of mitochondrial activity). Fatty acids uncouple phosphorylation and electron transport in brown adipose tissue mitochondria both directly and also by binding to, and activating, the uncoupling protein thermogenin in the inner mitochondrial membrane (Bukowiecki 1984; Skulachev 1991; Wojtczack and Schonfeld 1993).

2. Changes in the extent of substrate cycling (as for example between glucose and glucose-6–phosphate, or between fructose-6–phosphate and fructose-1,6–bisphosphate, see Fig. 5.1), as a result of simultaneous activity of opposing enzymes catalysing forward and back reactions (Hers 1976). The low basal metabolic rate in hypothyroidism (see section 25.14.4) is associated with considerably reduced glucose substrate cycling, and in hyperthyroid subjects there is greater glucose substrate cycling than in euthyroid controls (Shulman *et al.* 1985).

Increased uncoupling of mitochondrial phosphorylation and increased substrate cycling in positive energy balance will 'waste' surplus food, thus reducing the amount available for fat deposition. Similarly, decreased activity in negative energy balance will spare fuel that would otherwise have been oxidized to little or no good purpose.

5.5   An overview of metabolism

The oxidation of metabolic fuels is linked to the reduction of the nicotinamide nucleotide coenzymes NAD and NADP (see section 19.2) and the flavin coenzymes (see section 18.2). The reduced coenzymes are re-oxidized in the mitochondria, by way of the electron transport chain, obligatorily linked to the phosphorylation of ADP to ATP, and the reduction of oxygen to water. Under normal conditions (i.e. in the absence of any uncoupler), electron transport can only occur as long as there is ADP available to be phosphorylated. This means that the rate of oxidation of metabolic fuels is controlled by the availability of ADP, and hence by the rate of utilization of ATP in physical work (muscle contraction), chemical work (endergonic enzyme-catalysed reactions) and the active transport of substrates and ions across cell membranes.

Tissues receive a constant supply of metabolic fuels: in the fed state this is the glucose, triacylglycerol and amino acids entering from the gut, while in the fasting state the reserves of metabolic fuel laid down after a meal are utilized. Table 5.22 shows plasma concentrations of metabolic fuels in the fed and fasting states, and after prolonged starvation.

5.5.1 The fed state: the actions of insulin

For about 3–4 hours after a meal, fuels are entering the circulation from the gut. Glucose (see section 7.2) and amino acids (see section 10.3) are absorbed into the portal circulation, and the liver controls the amounts entering the peripheral circulation for use by other tissues. Fat (see section 8.2) is absorbed into the lymphatic system incorporated in chylomicrons, entering the bloodstream at the thoracic duct, and hence is available for use by peripheral tissues without control by the liver.

The increase in glucose (and amino acids) in portal blood both stimulates insulin secretion by the β-cells of the pancreas, and suppresses glucagon secretion by the α-cells of pancreas. Insulin has five main actions:

1. Stimulation of the uptake of glucose by muscle, thus rapidly lowering the plasma concentration of glucose. As a result of this glucose becomes the main fuel for muscle metabolism, and the RQ rises to 0.9 or higher.

2. Stimulation of the activity of glycogen synthase (EC 2.4.1.11), and inhibition of the activity of glycogen phosphorylase (EC 2.4.1.1) in liver and muscle. There is thus increased synthesis of glycogen reserves in liver and muscle.

3. Stimulation of the uptake of glucose into adipose tissue, leading to increased synthesis of fatty acids and triacylglycerol.

4. Stimulation of adipose tissue lipoprotein lipase (EC 3.1.1.34), so permitting uptake of fatty acids from triacylglycerol in chylomicrons for re-esterification into adipose tissue triacylglycerols.

5. Stimulation of the uptake of amino acids into liver and muscle, leading to increased protein synthesis.

5.5.2 The fasting state: the actions of glucagon

In the normal fasting state between meals, fuels enter the circulation from the reserves of glycogen, triacylglycerol, and protein laid down in the fed state. The overall metabolic strategy in the fasting state is to provide fuels to muscle and other tissues that are used in preference to glucose, so as to spare such glucose as is available for the brain and red blood cells which, under normal conditions, can utilize only glucose.

The decrease in glucose (and amino acids) in portal blood both stimulates glucagon secretion by the α-cells of the pancreas and suppresses insulin secretion by the β-cells. Glucagon has three main actions.

1. Stimulation of the action of glycogen phosphorylase in liver, and inhibition of glycogen synthetase in both liver and muscle. The result of this is breakdown of liver glycogen to release glucose into the circulation. Muscle glycogen cannot be used directly as a source of blood glucose, but a considerable amount of alanine is formed by transamination of the pyruvate arising from glycolysis (see Fig. 5.1), and is released from muscle in the fasting state, and used in the liver for gluconeogenesis.

2. Stimulation of the activity of hormone-sensitive lipase (EC 3.1.1.23) in adipose tissue, leading to the release of fatty acids and glycerol into circulation. Muscle takes up fatty acids in preference to glucose, and in the (relative) absence of insulin the muscle glucose uptake system has low activity.

3. Stimulation of gluconeogenesis (the synthesis of glucose from amino acids, glycerol, and other non-carbohydrate precursors) in liver, kidney and small intestine. The total reserves of liver and muscle glycogen would only meet glucose requirements for about 12–18 hours. Removal of amino acids from the circulation for gluconeogenesis reduces the amounts available for protein synthesis. The breakdown of tissue protein continues at a constant rate, resulting in a net loss of tissue protein (see section 10.8).

Although muscle and other tissues can use fatty acids, they have a limited capacity for β-oxidation (see Fig. 5.3), and fatty acids alone cannot meet energy needs. By contrast, the liver has a greater capacity for β-oxidation than is required to meet its own energy needs. In the fasting state the liver exports considerable amounts of ketones (acetoacetate and β-hydroxybutyrate, formed by the pathway shown in Fig. 5.4), which are a major fuel for muscle in the fasting state, and for heart muscle at all times (see Fig. 5.5). In prolonged starvation (more than 10–14 days), the plasma concentration of ketones rises sufficiently for the brain to be able to use them as a metabolic fuel.

5.5.3 Pathways of carbohydrate and fatty acid metabolism.

Figure 5.1 shows the pathway of glycolysis and gluconeogenesis. Control over whether glucose is to be oxidized or synthesized is exerted largely by regulating the activities of phosphofructokinase (EC 2.7.1.11) in glycolysis and fructose-1,6–bisphosphatase (EC 3.1.3.54) in gluconeogenesis.

The onward metabolism of pyruvate is by way of complete oxidation—the citric acid (Krebs or tricarboxylic acid) cycle, shown in Fig. 5.2. This pathway also provides entry points for the products of amino acid metabolism, and a source of oxaloacetate for gluconeogenesis. Acetyl CoA formed from glucose can also be used for fatty acid synthesis (see Fig. 5.6).

The pathway of β-oxidation of fatty acids is shown in Fig. 5.3; the acetyl CoA resulting from β-oxidation may either undergo complete oxidation in the citric acid cycle (see Fig. 5.2), or may be used for the synthesis of ketones (see Fig. 5.4). See section 23.5.2 for the role of carnitine in the mitochondrial uptake of fatty acids for oxidation. The pathway ketone utilization is shown in Fig. 5.5, and of fatty acid synthesis from acetyl CoA in Fig. 5.6.

Further reading

Blaxter, K. and Waterlow, J. C. (1985). *Nutritional Adaptation in Man*. John Libbey, London.

FAO/WHO/UNU (1985). *Energy and protein requirements, Report of a Joint FAO/WHO/UNU Expert Consultation*, WHO Technical Report Series 724 WHO, Geneva.

James, W. P. T. and Schofield, E. C. (1980). *Human Energy Requirements: a Manual for Planners and Nutritionists*. Oxford University Press for the Food and Agriculture Organization of the UN.

Schofield, W. N., Schofield, C. and James, W. P. T. (1985). Basal metabolic rate—review and prediction, together

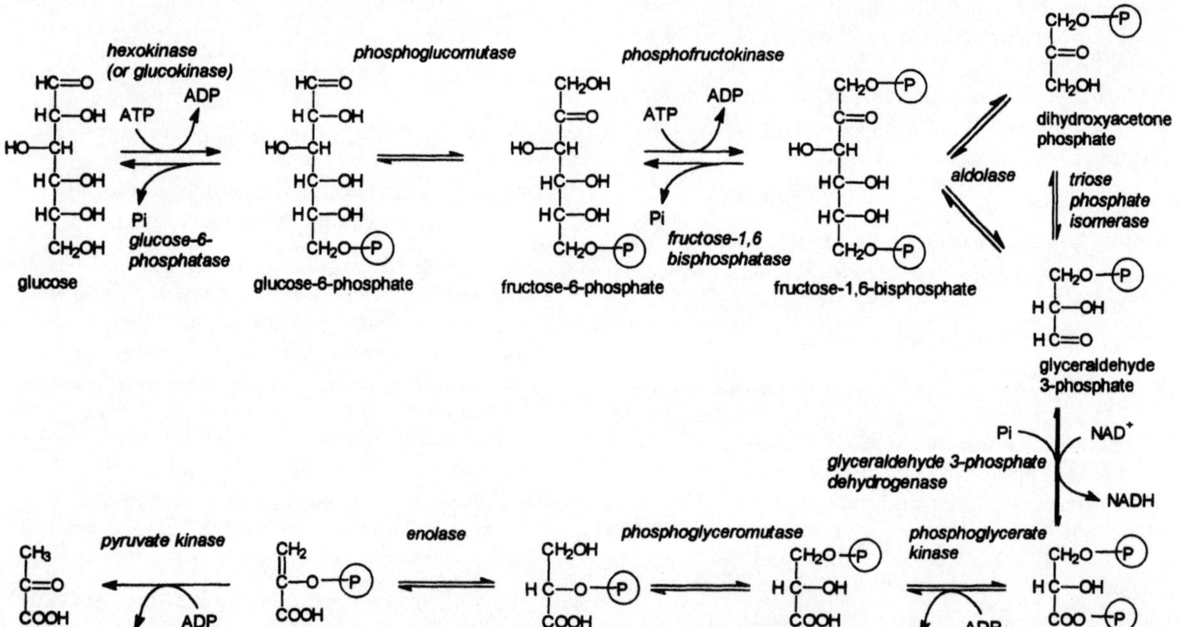

Figure 5.1 Glucose metabolism: the pathway of glycolysis and gluconeogenesis
Hexokinase and glucokinase EC 2.7.1.1; glucose-6-phosphatase EC 3.1.3.9, phosphoglucomutase EC 5.4.2.2, phosphofructokinase EC 2.7.1.11, fructose-1,6-bisphosphatase EC 3.1.3.11, aldolase EC 4.1.2.13, triose phosphate isomerase EC 5.3.1.1, glyceraldehyde 3-phosphate dehydrogenase EC 1.2.1.12, phosphoglycerate kinase EC 2.7.2.3, phosphoglyceromutase EC 5.4.2.1, phosphopyruvate hydratase (enolase)EC 4.2.1.11, pyruvate kinase EC 2.7.1.40.

with an annotated bibliography of source material. *Human Nutrition : Clinical Nutrition*, 39C, suppl 1, 5–41.

Shetty, P. S. (1990). Physiological mechanisms in the adaptive response of metabolic rates to energy restriction. *Nutrition Research Reviews*, 3, 49–74.

Symposium Proceedings (1988). Stable isotopic methods for measuring energy expenditure. *Proceedings of the Nutrition Society*, 47, 195–208.

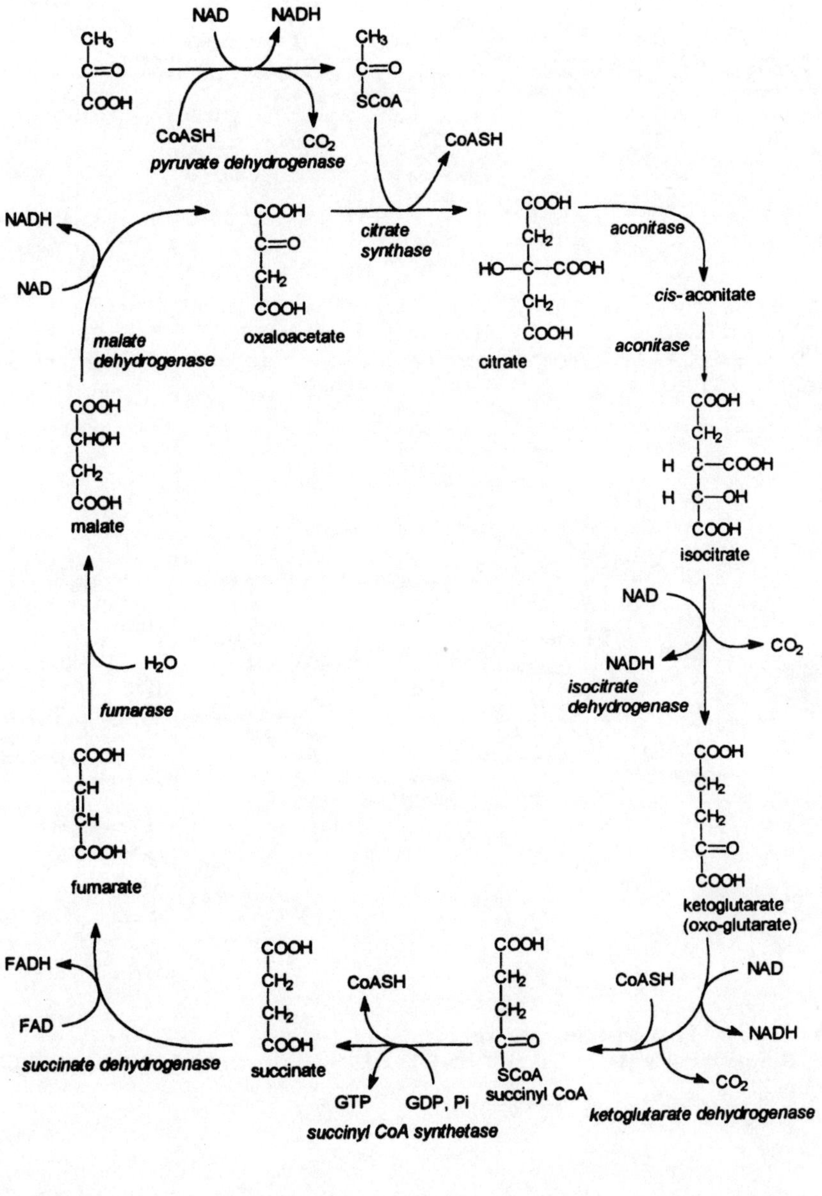

Figure 5.2 The citric acid cycle
Pyruvate dehydrogenase EC 1.2.4.1, citrate synthase EC 4.1.3.7, aconitase EC 4.2.1.3, isocitrate dehydrogenase EC 1.1.1.41, keto-glutarate dehydrogenase EC 1.2.4.2, succinyl CoA synthase EC 6.2.1.4, succinate dehydrogenase EC 1.3.5.1, fumarase EC 4.2.1.2, malate dehydrogenase EC 1.1.1.37.

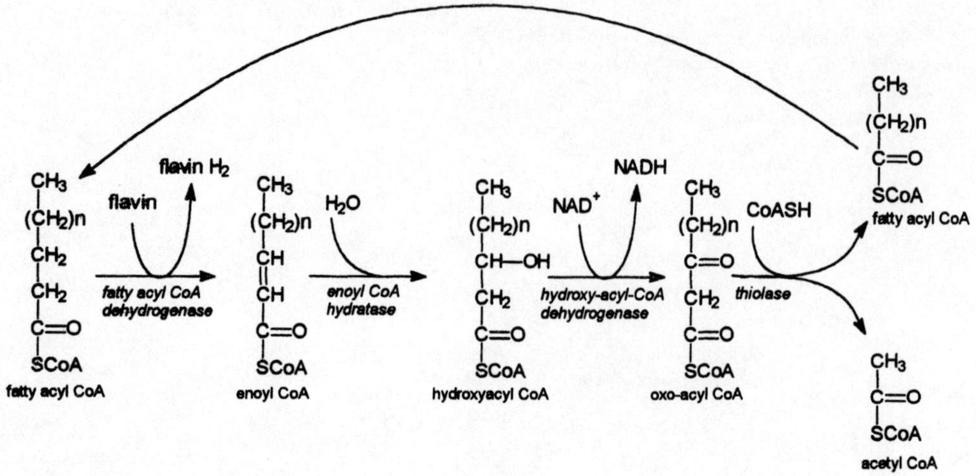

Figure 5.3 β-Oxidation of fatty acids
Fatty acyl CoA dehydrogenase EC 1.3.99.13 and EC 1.3.99.3, enoyl CoA hydratase EC 4.2.1.17 and EC 4.2.1.74, hydroxyacyl CoA dehydrogenase EC 1.1.1.35 and EC 1.1.1.211 (separate isoenzymes of each of these enzymes for short- and long-chain fatty acyl CoA derivatives), thiolase EC 2.3.1.16.

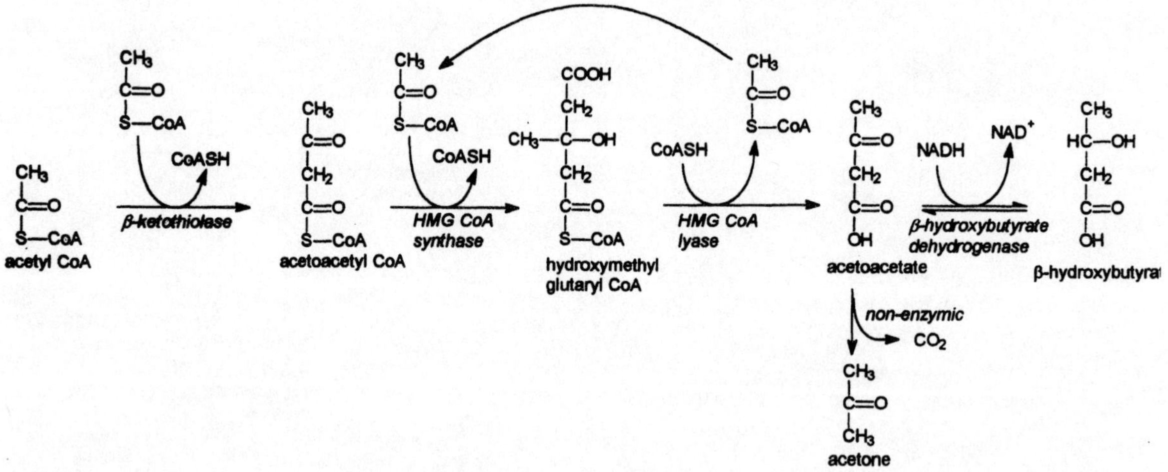

Figure 5.4 Ketogenesis, the synthesis of ketones in the liver
β-Ketothiolase EC 2.3.1.9, hydroxymethylglutaryl CoA synthase EC 4.1.3.5, hydroxymethylglutaryl CoA lyase EC 4.1.3.4, β-hydroxybutyrate dehydrogenase EC 1.1.1.30.

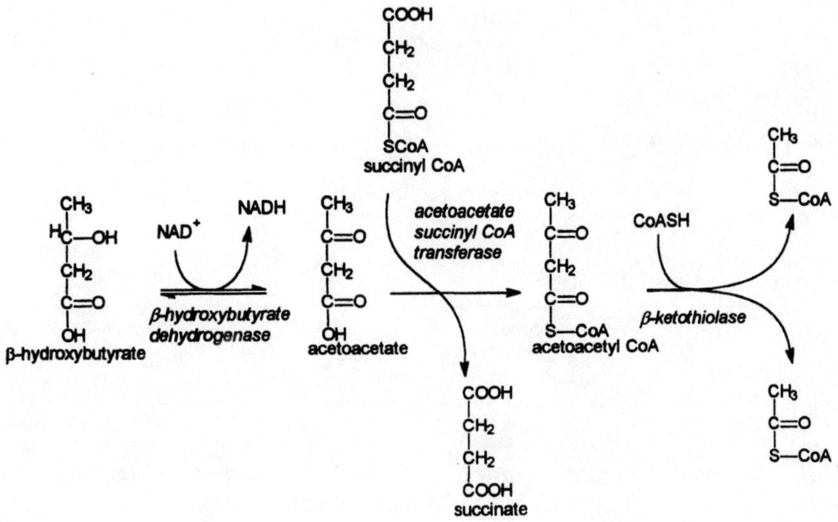

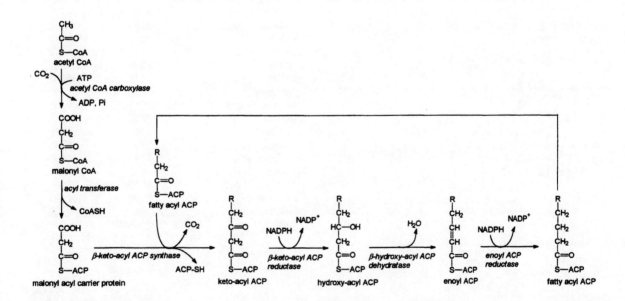

Figure 5.5 Utilization of ketones in extra-hepatic tissues
β-Hydroxybutyrate dehydrogenase EC 1.1.1.30, acetoacetate succinyl CoA transferase EC 2.8.3.7, β-ketothiolase EC 2.3.1.9.

Figure 5.6 Fatty acid synthesis
ACP = acyl carrier protein; acetyl CoA carboxylase EC 6.4.1.2, acyl transferase EC 2.3.1.39, β-keto-acyl ACP synthase EC 2.3.1.41, β-keto-acyl ACP reductase EC 1.1.1.100, enoyl ACP reductase EC 1.3.1.39.

Table 5.1: Gross energy yield of metabolic fuels

fuel	kJ /g	kcal /g	O$_2$ consumed (L /g)	kJ /L O$_2$	kcal /L O$_2$
starch	17.49	4.178	0.829	21.10	5.041
glucose	15.44	3.688	0.746	20.70	4.945
fat	39.12	9.345	1.975	19.81	4.732
protein	18.52	4.424	0.962	19.25	4.599
alcohol	29.75	7.107	1.429	20.40	4.873

Table 5.2: Metabolizable energy yield of metabolic fuels

	gross energy		absorbed	digestible energy		urine energy		metabolizable energy		Atwater factors	
	kJ /g	kcal /g	%	kJ /g	kcal /g	kJ /g	kcal /g	kJ /g	kcal /g	kJ /g	kcal /g
starch	17.49	4.178	99	17.3	4.13	-	-	17.3	4.13	16	4
glucose	15.44	3.688	99	15.4	3.68	-	-	15.4	3.68	16	4
fat	39.12	9.345	95	37.1	8.86	-	-	37.1	8.86	37	9
protein	18.52	4.424	92	21.1	5.04	5.2	1.24	15.9	3.79	17	4
alcohol	29.75	7.107	100	29.8	7.12	-	-	29.8	7.12	29	7

Table 5.3: Energy yields of metabolic fuels for labelling purposes

	kJ /g	kcal /g
fat	38	9
alcohol	29	7
carbohydrates	17	4
protein	16	4
organic acids	13	3
sugar alcohols	10	2.4

Table 5.4: Energy yield /L oxygen consumption for metabolic fuels

	kJ	kcal
acetic acid	19.74	4.716
acetoacetic acid	19.80	4.730
alcohol	20.40	4.873
butyric acid	19.55	4.670
glucose	20.70	4.945
glycerol	21.17	5.057
glycogen	21.12	5.045
3-hydroxybutyrate	19.89	4.737
lactic acid	20.33	4.857
oleic acid	19.54	4.668
palmitic acid	19.45	4.646
propionic acid	19.61	4.685
protein	19.48	4.653
starch	21.10	5.041
stearic acid	19.36	4.625
triacylglycerol	19.81	4.732
mean	20.02 ± 0.654	4.78 ± 0.156

Table 5.5: Respiratory Quotients for oxidation of metabolic fuels

	O_2 consumed (L /g)	CO_2 produced (L /g)	RQ (respiratory quotient)
starch	0.829	0.824	0.994
glucose	0.746	0.742	0.995
fat	1.975	1.402	0.710
protein	0.962	0.775	0.806
alcohol	1.429	0.966	0.663

Table 5.7: Relative contribution of organs to basal metabolic rate

organ	% body weight	% BMR
liver	2.6	21
brain	2.0	20
heart	0.5	9
kidney	0.4	8
skeletal muscle	40.0	22
adipose tissue	21.4	4

Table 5.6: Definitions in energy metabolism

BMR	Basal Metabolic Rate	Energy expenditure in the post-absorptive state; measured under standardized conditions of thermal neutrality (environmental temperature 26-30°C) , awake but completely at rest.
RMR	Resting Metabolic Rate	Energy expenditure at rest, not measured under strictly standardized conditions.
PAR	Physical Activity Ratio	Energy cost of physical activity, on a minute by minute basis, expressed as ratio of BMR.
IEI	Integrated Energy Index	Energy cost of an activity over a period of time, including time spent pausing or resting, expressed as the average (integrated) value over the time, as a ratio of BMR.
PAL	Physical Activity Level	Sum of PAR or IEI × time spent in each activity over 24h, expressed as ratio of BMR.
DIT	Diet-Induced thermogenesis	Increased energy expenditure after a meal.
TEE	Total Energy Expenditure	PAL × BMR (+ DIT).

Table 5.8: Effects of gender, age, and body weight on BMR

	body weight, kg									
	50	60	70	80	90	50	60	70	80	90
			MJ /day					kcal /day		
males										
10-17	6.38	7.11	7.84	8.58	9.31	1524	1699	1874	2049	2224
18-29	6.04	6.68	7.32	7.96	8.60	1443	1596	1749	1902	2054
30-59	6.10	6.58	7.07	7.55	8.04	1456	1572	1688	1804	1919
> 60	4.87	5.43	6.00	6.56	7.13	1162	1297	1432	1567	1702
females										
10-17	5.67	6.18	6.69	7.20	7.71	1355	1476	1598	1720	1842
18-29	5.16	5.77	6.39	7.00	7.62	1231	1378	1525	1672	1819
30-59	5.29	5.65	6.02	6.38	6.75	1264	1351	1438	1525	1612
> 60	4.69	5.12	5.56	6.00	6.44	1119	1224	1329	1434	1539

Source: calculated using the formulae for estimation of BMR from weight in Table 5.10

Table 5.9: Equations for estimating resting metabolic rate from weight, height and age

	MJ /d	kcal /d
males	0.0418w + 0.0261h - 0.0209a - 0.674	9.99w + 6.25h - 5a - 161
females	0.0418w + 0.0261h - 0.0209a - 0.0209	9.99w + 6.25h - 5a + 5

w = body weight (kg); h = height (cm); a = age (years)
Source: from data reported by Mifflin *et al.* 1990, recalculated for estimation of RMR in MJ.

Table 5.10: Equations for estimating basal metabolic rate from weight or weight and height, at different ages

	males		females	
age	MJ /d	kcal /d	MJ /d	kcal /d
0—3	0.2548w - 0.226	60.9w - 54	0.255w - 0.213	61.0w - 51
	0.007w + 6.349h - 2.584	1.673h + 1517h - 617	0.068w + 4.281h - 1.730	16.252w + 1023h - 413
3—10	0.0949w + 2.07	22.7w + 495	0.0941w + 2.09	22.5w + 499
	0.082w + 0.545h + 1.736	19.59w + 130h + 415	0.071w + 0.677h + 1.5453	16.97w + 161h + 531
10—17	0.0732w + 2.72	17.5w + 651	0.0510w + 3.12	12.2w + 746
	0.068w + 0.574h + 2.157	16.25w + 137h + 516	0.035w + 1.948h + 0.837	8.365w + 465h + 200
18—29	0.0640w + 2.84	15.3w + 679	0.0615w + 2.08	14.7w + 496
	0.063w - 0.042h + 2.953	15.06w + 10.04h + 705	0.057w + 1.184h + 0.411	13.62w + 283h + 98
30—59	0.0485w + 3.67	11.6w + 879	0.0364w + 3.47	8.7w + 829
	0.048w - 0.011h + 3.670	11.47w + 2.629h + 877	0.034w + 0.006h + 3.530	8.126w + 4.434h + 843
over 60	0.0565w + 2.04	13.5w + 487	0.0439w + 2.49	10.5w + 596

w = body weight (kg); h = height (m)
Source: from data reported by Schofield *et al.* 1985, recalculated for estimation of BMR in kcal.

Table 5.11: Equations for estimating basal metabolic rate for people living in tropical countries

	males		females	
age	MJ /day	kcal /d	MJ /day	kcal /d
3—10	0.0113w + 1.689	27.00w + 403	0.0163w + 2.466	3.895w + 589
	0.113w + 0.003h + 1.687	27.00w + 0.717h + 403	-0.002w + 3.115h + 0.169	-0478w + 718h + 40
10—17	0.084w + 2.122	20.08w + 507	0.047w + 2.951	11.233w + 705
	0.065w + 1.690h + 0.389	15.535w + 404h + 93	0.037w + 1.095h + 1.744	8.843w + 262h + 417
18—29	0.056w + 2.800	13.38w + 669	0.048w + 2.562	11.472w + 612
	0.057w - 0. 429h + 3.412	13.62w -	0.042w + 1.546h + 0.433	10.04w + 369h + 103
		102h + 815		
30—59	0.046w + 3.160	10.99w + 755	0.048w + 2.448	11.472w + 595
	0.046w - 0.081h + 3.277	10.99w + 19.35h + 783	0.047w + 0.145h + 2.256	11.233w + 34.655h + 539

w = body weight (kg); h = height (m)
Source: from data reported by Henry *et al.* 1991, recalculated for estimation of BMR in kcal.

Table 5.12: Energy cost of activity, by Physical Activity Ratio

PAR

1.0-1.4 Lying, standing or sitting at rest, e.g. watching TV, reading, writing, eating, playing cards and board games

1.5-1.8 *sitting*: sewing, knitting, playing piano, driving
standing: preparing vegetables, washing dishes, ironing, general office and laboratory work

1.9-2.4 *standing*: mixed household chores, cooking, playing snooker or bowls

2.5-3.3 *standing*: dressing, undressing, showering, making beds, vacuum cleaning
walking: 3—4 km/h, playing cricket
occupational: tailoring, shoemaking, electrical and machine tool industry, painting and decorating

3.4-4.4 *standing*: mopping floors, gardening, cleaning windows, table tennis, sailing
walking: 4—6 km/h, playing golf
occupational: motor vehicle repairs, carpentry and joinery, chemical industry, bricklaying

4.5-5.9 *standing*: polishing furniture, chopping wood, heavy gardening, volley ball
walking: 6—7 km/h
exercise: dancing, moderate swimming, gentle cycling, slow jogging
occupational: labouring, hoeing, road construction, digging and shovelling, felling trees

6.0-7.9 *walking*: uphill with load or cross-country, climbing stairs
exercise: jogging, cycling, energetic swimming, skiing, tennis, football

Source: from data reported by Department of Health 1991; FAO/WHO/UNU 1985.

Table 5.13: Energy cost of physical activities, expressed as Physical Activity Ratio

	PAR
sleeping	1.0
lying down	1.2
sitting	
still, reading	1.2
playing cards	1.4
sewing, knitting	1.5
preparing rope	1.5
weaving	1.5–2.1
sharpening axe	1.7
carving	2.1
sharpening machete	2.2
standing	
still	1.4–1.5
washing clothes	2.2
making bows and arrows	2.7
singing and dancing	3.2
chopping firewood	4.1
walking, running	
downhill, slowly	2.3–2.8
strolling around	2.4–2.5
pushing child (pram or stroller)	2.5
slowly	2.8–3.0
downhill at normal pace	3.0–3.1
at normal pace	3.2–3.4
downhill, fast	3.4–3.6
with load	3.5–4.0
using crutches	4.0
uphill, at normal pace	4.6–5.7
hiking, cross-country	6.0
uphill with load	6.0–6.7
race walking	6.5
marching (military)	6.5
uphill, fast	6.6–7.5
jogging	7.0
backpacking	7.0
rock climbing	8.0
running, 6-8 kph	8.0–10.0
running, cross-country	9.0
running, 9-10 kph	11.0–12.5
running, 11-12 kph	13.5–15.0
running upstairs	15.0
running, 13-15 kph	15.0–18.0
household tasks	
spinning cotton	1.4
ironing clothes	1.4–2.3
washing dishes	1.7–2.3
making beds	2.0
cleaning house	2.2
sweeping floors	2.5
sitting playing with children	2.5
child care, general	2.5–3.5
light cleaning	2.7
standing playing with children	2.8
sweeping house	3.0

Table 5.13 (cont'd)

	PAR
washing clothes	3.0
general house cleaning	3.5
sweeping yard	3.5–4.0
polishing, window cleaning	3.7
walking, playing with children	4.0–5.0
fetching water from well	4.1
chopping wood with machete	4.3
heavy cleaning	4.5
scrubbing floors	5.5
moving household furniture	6.0
carrying boxes or furniture upstairs	9.0
domestic repairs	
car repair	3.0
workshop carpentry	3.0
wiring, plumbing	3.0
car body work repair	4.5
carpentry, finishing furniture	4.5
interior decorating	4.5
laying carpet, tiles, linoleum	4.5
wash and polish car, boat, etc	4.5
sanding floors with power sander	4.5
caulking	4.5–5.0
cleaning gutters	5.0
hanging storm windows	5.0
exterior painting	5.0
outdoor carpentry	6.0
roofing	6.0
sawing hardwood	7.5
house building (tropics)	
kneading clay	2.7
roofing house	2.9
weaving bamboo wall	2.9
squatting, making mud bricks	3.0
cutting bamboo	3.2
nailing	3.3
breaking bricks	4.0
cutting palm tree trunks	4.1
laying floor	4.1
shovelling mud	4.4
digging earth to make mud	5.7
digging holes	6.2
earth cutting	6.2
food preparation	
roasting maize	1.3
peeling sweet potato	1.4
removing beans from pod	1.5
peeling taro	1.7
cooking and preparation	1.8–2.5
collecting leaves and herbs	1.9
breaking groundnuts	1.9
making tortillas	2.1
squeezing coconut	2.4
serving food	2.5
putting away groceries	2.5
loading earth oven with food	2.6

Table 5.13 (cont'd)

	PAR
food shopping, supermarket	3.5
stirring porridge	3.7
grinding corn on millstone	3.8
pounding	4.6
carrying groceries upstairs	8.0
hunting and fishing	
fishing with line	2.1
fishing from boat	2.2–2.5
duck hunting, wading	2.5
hunting, bow and arrow	2.5
trap shooting	2.5
fishing with spear	2.6
paddling canoe	3.4
hunting birds	3.4–6.0
fishing from river bank, standing	3.5
hunting pig	3.6
catching fish by hand	3.9
digging worms for bait	4.0
catching crabs	4.5
fishing from river bank, walking	5.0
hunting small game	5.0
fishing in stream, in waders	6.0
hunting large game	6.0
occupational	
sitting at desk	1.3
standing and moving around	1.6–1.7
directing traffic	2.0
electrical industry	2.0
laboratory work	2.0
printing work	2.0–2.3
bookbinding	2.3
chambermaid	2.5
shoemaking / repair	2.5–3.6
bakery work	2.5–4.0
tailoring	2.6
machine tool industry	2.7–3.1
painting and decorating	2.8
brewery work	2.9
chemical industry	2.9–3.5
lathe operation	3.0
welding	3.0
carpentry	3.1
joinery	3.2
bricklaying	3.3
furnishing industry	3.3
laundry work	3.4
carpentry	3.5
electrical work, plumbing	3.5
locksmith	3.5
motor vehicle repairs	3.6
masseur/masseuse	4.0
tapping and drilling	4.0
using power saw	4.2
furriery	4.5
mining, erecting roof supports	4.9–6.5

Table 5.13 (cont'd)

	PAR
planing wood	5.0
punch press operation	5.0
steelmill, fettling	5.0
labouring	5.2
steelmill, tipping moulds	5.5
stelmill, forging	5.5
mining, shovelling	5.7–7.0
grooming horses	6.0
labouring, pneumatic drills, hammers	6.0
mining, working with pick	6.0
road building	6.0
shovelling, light (< 5 kg /min)	6.0
mining, drilling coal, rock	6.5
masonry, concrete work	7.0
shovelling, moderate (5-8 kg /min)	7.0
hand sawing	7.5
carrying boxes upstairs	8.0
carrying heavy loads	8.0
firefighter, hauling hoses on ground	8.0
labouring, shovelling	8.0
steelmill, handrolling	8.0
shovelling, ditch digging	8.5
shovelling, heavy (> 8 kg /min)	9.0
firefighter, climbing ladder with equipment	11.0
steelmill, removing slag	11.0
firefighter, general	12.0
armed services	
cleaning kit	2.4
drill	3.2
jungle patrol	3.5
route marching	4.4
assault course	5.1
jungle march	5.7
transport	
driving car, light truck	1.4–2.0
helicopter pilot, normal flying	1.5
helicopter pilot, hovering	1.6
pilot, preflight checks	1.8
pilot, aeroplane	2.0
police, driving patrol car	2.0
driving forklift, crane	2.5
driving motor cycle	2.5
police, directing traffic	2.5
horseracing, walking	2.6
driving heavy truck, lorry, bus	3.0
cycling, leisure (< 13 kph)	4.0
pulling empty cart	5.3
pulling loaded cart	5.9
cycling, light effort,13-16 kph	6.0
driving lorry, loading and unloading	6.5
horseracing, trotting	6.5
pedaling empty rickshaw	7.2
cycling, moderate effort, 16-18 kph	8.0
horseracing, galloping	8.0

Table 5.13 (cont'd)

	PAR
pedaling rickshaw with passengers	8.5
cycling, vigorous effort, 18-21 kph	10.0
cycling, racing, > 21 kph	12.0–16.0
agriculture	
picking coffee	1.5
preparing tobacco	1.5
kneeling to sort potatoes	1.6
winnowing	1.7–3.9
deseeding cotton	1.8
harvesting sorghum	2.1
driving tractor, harvester	2.1–2.5
beating cotton	2.4
milking by machine	2.5
weeding	2.5–5.0
tying fence posts	2.7
milking by hand	2.9–3.0
planting and sowing	2.9–4.0
clearing ground	2.9–7.9
harvesting root crops	3.1–3.5
cutting fruit from tree	3.4
fence making	3.6
feeding small livestock	3.6–4.0
lifting grain sacks	3.7
planting root crops	3.9
sharpening posts	4.0
binding sheaves	4.2
splitting wood for posts	4.2
digging holes for planting	4.3
hoeing	4.4
feeding cattle	4.5
collecting coconuts (climbing)	4.6
digging ground	4.6
loading sacks	4.7
cutting grass with machete	4.7–5.0
cutting trees (by hand)	4.8
pushing wheelbarrow	4.8
digging holes for posts	5.0
repairing fences	5.0
threshing	5.0
collecting and spreading manure (by hand)	5.2
digging irrigation channels	5.5
shovelling grain	5.5
husking coconuts	6.3
loading manure	6.4
cutting sugarcane	6.5
forking	6.8
loading sacks on lorry	7.4
baling hay	8.0
forking straw bales	8.0
forestry	
in nursery	3.6
weeding	4.0
planting trees	4.0–6.0
using power saw	4.5

Table 5.13 (cont'd)

	PAR
axe chopping, slow	5.0
hoeing	5.0
barking trees	7.0
sawing by hand	7.0
trimming branches off trees	7.3–9.0
felling with axe	7.5–8.0
carrying logs	11.0
axe chopping, fast	17.0
gardening / horticulture	
watering garden with hosepipe	1.5
applying fertilizer, seeding lawn	2.5
mowing lawn, sitting on power mower	2.5
trimming shrubs, trees with power cutter	3.5
planting seedlings, shrubs	4.0
raking lawn	4.0
sacking grass, leaves	4.0
mowing lawn, power mower	4.5
operating snow or leaf blower	4.5
planting trees	4.5
trimming shrubs, trees by hand	4.5
weeding and cultivating	4.5
digging	5.0
laying crushed rock	5.0
laying turf	5.0
gardening with heavy power tools	6.0
mowing lawn, hand mower	6.0
shovelling snow	6.0
recreational activities	
sexual activity	1.0–1.5
sedentary activities	2.1–2.2
light (billiards, golf, cricket, bowls, sailing)	2.2–4.4
moderate (dancing, swimming, tennis)	4.4–6.6
heavy (football, athletics, jogging, rowing)	6.6
conditioning exercise / physical training	
stationary cycle, very light effort (50w)	3.0
stationary rowing, light effort (50w)	3.5
hatha yoga, stretching	4.0
water aerobics, water calisthenics	4.0
calisthenics, light/moderate effort	4.5
stationary cycle, light effort (100w)	5.5
slimnastics	6.0
stair treadmill ergometer	6.0
teaching aerobic class	6.0
weight lifting	6.0
stationary cycle, moderate effort (150w)	7.0
stationary rowing, moderate effort (100w)	7.0
calisthenics, heavy, vigorous effort	8.0
circuit training	8.0
stationary rowing, vigorous effort (150w)	8.5
ski machine	9.5
stationary cycle, vigorous effort (200w)	10.5

Table 5.13 (cont'd)

	PAR
stationary rowing, very vigorous effort (200w)	12.0
stationary cycle, very vigorous effort (250w)	12.5
sport	
billiards	2.5
croquet	2.5
darts	2.5
horse riding	2.5–6.5
bowls	3.0
putting	3.0
quoits	3.0
shuffleboard	3.0
frisbee playing	3.0–3.5
volleyball	3.0–4.0
archery	3.5
hang gliding	3.5
sky diving	3.5
trampolining	3.5
curling	4.0
gymnastics	4.0
juggling	4.0
moto-cross	4.0
table tennis	4.0
tai chi	4.0
golf	4.5–5.5
badminton	4.5–7.0
children's games	5.0
cricket (batting, bowling)	5.0
skateboarding	5.0
softball, baseball	5.0
boxing, punching bag	6.0
drag racing	6.0
fencing	6.0
wrestling	6.0
paddleball	6.0–10.0
basketball	6.0–8.0
tennis	6.0–8.0
kickball	7.0
rollerskating	7.0
football (soccer)	7.0–10.0
racketball	7.0–10.0
beach volleyball	8.0
hockey	8.0
ice hockey	8.0
lacrosse	8.0
polo	8.0
rock climbing	8.0–11.0
handball	8.0–12.0
rope jumping	8.0–12.0
football (American)	8.0–9.0
boxing, sparring	9.0
orienteering	9.0
judo, kick boxing	10.0
rugby football	10.0

Table 5.13 (cont'd)

	PAR
boxing, in ring	12.0
jai alai	12.0
squash	12.0
water sports, recreations	
power boating	2.5
diving	3.0
surfing	3.0
water volleyball	3.0
sailing	3.0–5.0
canoeing, rowing	4.0–12.0
snorkeling	5.0
whitewater rafting	5.0
water skiing	6.0
canoeing, portage	7.0
skimobiling	7.0
skindiving, scuba diving	7.0–12.0
swimming, backstroke	8.0
swimming, slow crawl	8.0
swimming, breaststroke	10.0
swimming laps	8.0–10.0
water polo	10.0
swimming, fast crawl, butterfly stroke	11.0
winter sports	
snowmobiling	3.5
ice skating	5.5–9.0
skiing	5.0–7.0
ski jumping (including climbing up)	7.0
sledding, tobagganing	7.0
skiing, cross-country	8.0–14.0
skiing, uphill	16.5
ice skating, speed racing	15.0
dancing	
ballroom, slow (waltz, foxtrot)	3.0
aerobic, low impact	5.0
ballrooom, fast (disco, square, folk)	5.5
ballet or modern	6.0
aerobic, high impact	7.0
playing musical instruments	
accordion	1.8
cello	2.0
flute, horn, woodwind	2.0
guitar, classical, folk (sitting)	2.0
conducting	2.5
piano, organ	2.5
trumpet	2.5
violin	2.5
guitar, rock (standing)	3.0
trombone	3.5
drums	4.0
marching band	4.0

Source: from data reported by Ainsworth *et al.* 1992; FAO/WHO/UNU/ 1985; James & Schofield 1980; Passmore & Durnin 1955.

Table 5.14: Calculation of Integrated Energy Index of specified activities, allowing for pauses in activity

	PAR	IEE male	IEE female
light activity	1.0-2.5	0.75 × 1.54 + 0.25 × PAR	0.75 × 1.68 + 0.25 × PAR
moderate activity	2.6-3.9	0.25 × 1.54 + 0.75 × PAR	0.25 × 1.68 + 0.75 × PAR
heavy activity	> 4.0	0.40 × 1.54 + 0.60 × PAR	0.40 × 1.68 + 0.60 × PAR

Source: James & Schofield 1980.

Table 5.15: Occupational Physical Activity Levels in developed and less developed countries

	Occupational Physical Activity Level males developed	males less developed	females developed	females less developed
professional and technical workers	1.55	1.61	1.56	1.58
administrative and managerial	1.55	1.61	1.56	1.58
clerical and related workers	1.55	1.61	1.56	1.58
sales workers	1.67	1.78	1.60	1.64
service workers	1.67	1.78	1.60	1.64
agricultural, animal husbandry, forestry, fishing and hunting	1.78	1.86	-	1.69
production and related transport equipment operators and labourers	1.78	1.86	1.64	1.69
housewives	-	-	1.56	1.64
students	1.55	1.61	1.56	1.58
unemployed	1.55	1.61	1.56	1.58
subsistence farmers	1.78	1.86	1.64	1.69
domestic helpers	-	1.78	1.60	1.64
elderly over 65	1.51	1.51	1.56	1.56

Source: James & Schofield 1980.

Table 5.16: Classification of types of occupational work by PAR
(average PAR through 8h working day, excluding leisure activities)

	PAR men	PAR women	
Light	1.7	1.7	professional, clerical and technical workers, administrative and managerial staff, sales representatives, housewives
Moderate	2.7	2.2	sales staff, domestic service, students, transport workers, joiners, roofing workers
Moderately heavy	3.0	2.3	machine operators, labourers, agricultural workers, forestry, hunting and fishing, bricklaying, masonry
Heavy	3.8	2.8	labourers, agricultural workers, bricklaying, masonry where there is little or no mechanization

Source: Department of Health 1991.

Table 5.17: Average Physical Activity Levels for adults in developed and less developed countries

	developed countries males	developed countries females	less developed countries males	less developed countries females
urban areas	1.61	1.58	1.67	1.60
rural areas	1.78	1.64	1.86	1.69

Source: FAO/WHO/UNU 1985.

Table 5.18: Physical Activity Levels for varying levels of occupational work and non-occupational physical activity

| | occupational work (see Table 5.16) | | | | | |
| | males | | | females | | |
non-occupational activity	light	moderate	heavy	light	moderate	heavy
non-active	1.4	1.6	1.7	1.4	1.5	1.5
moderately active	1.5	1.7	1.8	1.5	1.6	1.6
very active	1.6	1.8	1.9	1.6	1.7	1.7

Source: Department of Health 1991.

Table 5.19: Energy requirements for children, without and with desirable physical activity, expressed /kg body weight

| | without desirable physical activity | | | | with desirable physical activity | | | |
| | males | | females | | males | | females | |
age	kJ	kcal	kJ	kcal	kJ	kcal	kJ	kcal
0-1	410	98	410	98	431	103	431	103
1-2	414	99	431	103	435	104	452	108
2-3	414	99	406	97	435	104	427	102
3-4	393	94	377	90	414	99	398	95
4-5	377	90	364	87	398	95	385	92
5-6	364	87	352	84	385	92	368	88
6-7	352	84	331	79	368	88	347	83
7-8	331	79	301	72	347	83	318	76
8-9	306	73	276	66	322	77	289	69
9-10	285	68	247	59	301	72	260	62

Source: James & Schofield 1980.

Table 5.20: Energy requirements for adolescents and adults, without and with desirable physical activity, expressed as PAL

| | without desirable activity | | with desirable activity | |
age	males	females	males	females
10—11	1.74	1.59	1.76	1.65
11—12	1.67	1.55	1.72	1.62
12—13	1.61	1.51	1.69	1.60
13—14	1.56	1.47	1.67	1.58
14—15	1.49	1.46	1.65	1.57
15—16	1.44	1.47	1.62	1.54
16—17	1.40	1.48	1.60	1.52
17—18	1.40	1.50	1.60	1.52
adults, light work	1.41	1.42	1.55	1.56
adults, moderate work	1.70	1.56	1.78	1.64
adults, heavy work	2.01	1.73	2.10	1.82
elderly, over 60	1.40	1.40	1.51	1.56

Source: from data reported by FAO/WHO/UNU 1985; James & Schofield 1980.

Table 5.21: Effects of gender, age, body weight and Physical Activity Level on total energy expenditure

	50	60	70	80	90	50	60	70	80	90
			MJ /day					kcal /day		
males age 10-17										
BMR	6.38	7.11	7.84	8.58	9.31	1524	1699	1874	2049	2224
PAL=1.2	7.66	8.53	9.41	10.29	11.17	1829	2039	2249	2458	2668
PAL=1.4	8.93	9.96	10.98	12.01	13.03	2134	2379	2623	2868	3113
PAL=1.6	10.21	11.38	12.55	13.72	14.89	2439	2718	2998	3278	3558
PAL=1.8	11.48	12.80	14.12	15.44	16.75	2743	3058	3373	3688	4002
PAL=2.0	12.76	14.22	15.69	17.15	18.62	3048	3398	3748	4097	4447
females aged 10-17										
BMR	5.67	6.18	6.69	7.20	7.71	1355	1476	1598	1720	1842
PAL=1.2	6.80	7.42	8.03	8.64	9.25	1625	1772	1918	2064	2210
PAL=1.4	7.94	8.65	9.37	10.08	10.79	1896	2067	2237	2408	2579
PAL=1.6	9.07	9.89	10.70	11.52	12.34	2167	2362	2557	2752	2947
PAL=1.8	10.21	11.12	12.04	12.96	13.88	2438	2657	2877	3096	3315
PAL=2.0	11.34	12.36	13.38	14.40	15.42	2709	2953	3196	3440	3684
males age 18-29										
BMR	6.04	6.68	7.32	7.96	8.60	1443	1596	1749	1902	2054
PAL=1.2	7.25	8.02	8.78	9.55	10.32	1731	1915	2098	2282	2465
PAL=1.4	8.46	9.35	10.25	11.14	12.04	2020	2234	2448	2662	2876
PAL=1.6	9.66	10.69	11.71	12.74	13.76	2309	2553	2798	3043	3287
PAL=1.8	10.87	12.02	13.18	14.33	15.48	2597	2872	3148	3423	3698
PAL=2.0	12.08	13.36	14.64	15.92	17.20	2886	3192	3497	3803	4109
females age 18-29										
BMR	5.16	5.77	6.39	7.00	7.62	1231	1378	1525	1672	1819
PAL=1.2	6.19	6.92	7.66	8.40	9.14	1478	1654	1830	2007	2183
PAL=1.4	7.22	8.08	8.94	9.80	10.66	1724	1930	2135	2341	2547
PAL=1.6	8.25	9.23	10.22	11.20	12.18	1970	2205	2441	2676	2911
PAL=1.8	9.28	10.39	11.49	12.60	13.71	2217	2481	2746	3010	3274
PAL=2.0	10.31	11.54	12.77	14.00	15.23	2463	2757	3051	3344	3638
males age 30-59										
BMR	6.10	6.58	7.07	7.55	8.04	1456	1572	1688	1804	1919
PAL=1.2	7.31	7.90	8.48	9.06	9.64	1747	1886	2025	2164	2303
PAL=1.4	8.53	9.21	9.89	10.57	11.25	2038	2201	2363	2525	2687
PAL=1.6	9.75	10.53	11.30	12.08	12.86	2330	2515	2700	2886	3071
PAL=1.8	10.97	11.84	12.72	13.59	14.46	2621	2829	3038	3247	3455
PAL=2.0	12.19	13.16	14.13	15.10	16.07	2912	3144	3376	3607	3839
females age 30-59										
BMR	5.29	5.65	6.02	6.38	6.75	1264	1351	1438	1525	1612
PAL=1.2	6.35	6.78	7.22	7.66	8.10	1516	1621	1725	1830	1934
PAL=1.4	7.41	7.92	8.43	8.93	9.44	1769	1891	2013	2134	2256
PAL=1.6	8.46	9.05	9.63	10.21	10.79	2022	2161	2300	2439	2578
PAL=1.8	9.52	10.18	10.83	11.49	12.14	2275	2431	2588	2744	2901
PAL=2.0	10.58	11.31	12.04	12.76	13.49	2527	2701	2875	3049	3223

Table 5.21: (Cont'd)

	50	60	70	80	90	50	60	70	80	90
			body weight (kg)							
			MJ /day					kcal /day		
males over 60										
BMR	4.87	5.43	6.00	6.56	7.13	1162	1297	1432	1567	1702
PAL=1.2	5.84	6.52	7.19	7.87	8.55	1395	1557	1719	1881	2043
PAL=1.4	6.81	7.60	8.39	9.18	9.98	1627	1816	2005	2194	2383
PAL=1.6	7.78	8.69	9.59	10.50	11.40	1860	2075	2291	2507	2723
PAL=1.8	8.76	9.77	10.79	11.81	12.83	2092	2335	2578	2821	3064
PAL=2.0	9.73	10.86	11.99	13.12	14.25	2324	2594	2864	3134	3404
females over 60										
BMR	4.69	5.12	5.56	6.00	6.44	1119	1224	1329	1434	1539
PAL=1.2	5.62	6.15	6.68	7.20	7.73	1343	1469	1595	1721	1846
PAL=1.4	6.56	7.17	7.79	8.40	9.02	1567	1714	1861	2007	2154
PAL=1.6	7.50	8.20	8.90	9.60	10.31	1791	1959	2126	2294	2462
PAL=1.8	8.43	9.22	10.01	10.80	11.59	2015	2203	2392	2581	2770
PAL=2.0	9.37	10.25	11.13	12.00	12.88	2238	2448	2658	2868	3077

Source: calculated using the formulae for estimation of BMR from weight in Table 5.10.

Table 5.22: Plasma concentrations of metabolic fuels in the fed and fasting states

mmol /L	fed	40 h fasting	7 d starvation
glucose	5.5	3.6	3.5
free fatty acids	0.3	1.15	1.19
ketones	0.01	2.9	4.5

6

The physiology of feeding and digestion

The gastrointestinal tract (see Fig. 6.1) has two main functions.

1. The digestion of foods by hydrolysis of complex carbohydrates to simple sugars, triacylglycerols and phospholipids to free fatty acids and glycerol, and proteins to small peptides and free amino acids. Digestion of carbohydrates begins in the mouth, and that of proteins and lipids in the stomach, although in all three cases the main site of digestion is the upper small intestine.

2. The absorption of the products of digestion occurs mainly in the lower small intestine. The primary function of the large intestine is the absorption of water and mineral salts, although some absorption also occurs here, and the intestinal flora (see section 6.2.2.1) synthesize significant amounts of some nutrients.

6.1 Structure and secretions of the gastrointestinal tract

Tables 6.1 and 6.2 list the principal digestive secretions of the gastrointestinal tract. For further details of the digestion of carbohydrates see section 7.2, of fats section 8.2 and of proteins section 10.3.

In addition to these secretions, all parts of the gastrointestinal tract also secrete mucus, a solution of glycoproteins and small peptides that serves both to lubricate food (especially important in the mouth and oesophagus) and, more importantly, to protect the gastrointestinal mucosa against the proteolytic and other enzymes secreted into the lumen. As discussed in section 10.8.3, the proteins and peptides of mucus are especially rich in two essential amino acids, threonine and cysteine, and secretion of mucus which is largely lost from the body explains a considerable proportion of the requirement for dietary protein in adults.

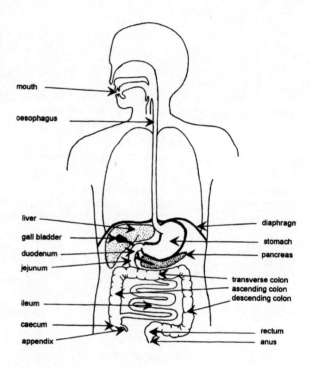

Figure 6.1 The gastrointestinal tract

6.1.1 The mouth

The mouth has three functions in feeding and digestion:

1. appreciation of the flavour and texture of food (its organoleptic properties);

2. secretion of saliva to lubricate food and initiate digestion of carbohydrates;

3. chewing to break up the structure of food, so permitting access to digestive enzymes, and mixing with saliva.

6.1.1.1 The senses of taste and small

There are five types of sensory papillae (taste buds) in the mouth and upper oesophagus which are capable of detecting sweetness, sourness or acidity, bitterness, salt, and 'savouriness'. This last is sometimes called by its Japanese name of *umami*; it is the taste of a number of amino acids and small peptides, most notably monosodium glutamate, which is widely used as a flavour enhancer in savoury foods (E-621). The tongue is also sensitive to the astringency of many plant foods. In general, sweetness, umami, and saltiness are pleasant flavours, while sourness, bitterness and astringency are unpleasant or aversive. These last two may be a protection against the toxic alkaloids in fruits and vegetables, many of which have a bitter flavour or are astringent.

Most of the 2000 taste buds in the mouth are on the tongue, but they also occur on the soft palate, pharynx, larynx, epiglottis, uvula and (especially in infants) on the cheeks and lips. Taste buds at the tip of the tongue (fungiform papillae) respond to salt and sweetness (See Table 7.10), those at the back of the tongue (circumvalate papillae) to bitterness, while those on the sides of the tongue (foliate papillae) respond to sourness. Taste buds on the fungiform papillae, anterior foliate papillae and most on the soft palate are innervated by the seventh (facial) cranial nerve; those on the circumvalate papillae and posterior foliate papillae by the ninth (glossopharyngial), and those in other regions of the mouth by the tenth (vagus) cranial nerve.

Taste buds have a relatively rapid turnover (a life span of some 10 days), and a number of drugs that affect them (including many used in cancer chemotherapy, as antibiotics, antithyroid, antirheumatic, diuretic, and hypoglycaemic agents) can dull or distort the sense of taste. The sense of taste is normally restored within a few days of cessation of medication. Complete loss of sense of taste is termed ageusia, while reduced sensitivity to some or all tastes is hypogeusia (and conversely, increased sensitivity to some or all tastes is hypergeusia). Dysgeusia (or parageusia) is a distortion of the reaction to some or all tastants, so that otherwise pleasant flavours are aversive; it may include perception of taste in the absence of any tastant.

In addition to the basic sense of taste, much of the attractiveness or otherwise of foods is due to the sense of smell. Aroma is detected by sensory cells in the olfactory epithelium of the upper part of the superior turbinate, the nasal septum, and the roof between these regions. These cells are innervated by the first (olfactory) cranial nerve, and have a life-span of some 30 days. The term flavour is used for a combination of taste and aroma.

A number of drugs dull or distort the sense of smell, including antihypertensive, antimicrobial, and antithyroid agents. Complete loss of the sense of smell is anosmia; decreased sensitivity is hyposmia (and enhanced sensitivity hyperosmia). Distortion of the sense of smell for some or all odorants, or sensation of smell when no odorant is present, is dysosmia.

In addition to disturbance of the sense of taste and smell in response to various drugs, and in association with some diseases in the absence of medication, there is a general reduction in sensitivity with increasing age, with the sense of smell being progressively impaired from the age of about 60–70, and the sense of taste later. Not all tastes are equally affected. Schiffman and Gatlin (1993) reported that detection thresholds were approximately 3–fold higher in elderly than young subjects for sweetness, 4–fold for sourness, 5–fold for umami, 7–fold for bitterness, and 12–fold for salt.

6.1.1.2 Saliva

There are two main types of salivary secretion: serous, which contains amylase (see section 7.2); and mucous, which contains mucin. The parotid salivary glands secrete only serous saliva, the sublingual and buccal only mucous, while the submaxillary glands secrete both mucous and serous saliva. As shown in Table 6.3, saliva contains high concentrations of potassium and bicarbonate, but lower concentrations of sodium and chloride ions, than does plasma. The sodium and chloride concentrations vary with the rate of secretion, because there is active resorption from the primary secretion. The concentration of sodium ions in saliva can be estimated from

$$\text{mmol Na}^+ \text{/L} = 7.919 \times \text{secretion rate (mL /min)} + 8.289.$$

Mucous saliva also contains a relatively high concentration of isothiocyanate, which has antibacterial activity, and the proteolytic enzyme lysozyme (EC 3.2.1.17) that also helps to protect against undesirable oral bacteria (see section 6.1.1.4).

Under basal conditions the rate of mucous saliva secretion is 0.5–1.0 mL /min. Both mucous and serous secretions are increased by parasympathetic nervous stimulation, in response to the taste and tactile stimulation of food in the mouth, and reflexes from the stomach and upper small intestine. The appetite centre of the hypothalamus also stimulates secretion of saliva, in response to the sight or smell of food, or in anticipation of food without a direct physical stimulus. Total daily saliva secretion is 1–2 L/day, with a mean density of 1.002–1.008 g/L

6.1.1.3 Teeth

Infants and children have 10 teeth in each of the upper and lower jaws, the first or deciduous teeth. Eruption begins at age about 6 months, and is complete by about 2 years of age (see Table 6.4). The total weight of the deciduous teeth is 9–10 g. From the age of 7–12 the deciduous teeth are shed, and replaced by the adult (permanent) teeth—a total of 16 in each of the upper and lower jaws. Full adult dentition, including the third molars (wisdom teeth) is normally complete by the age of about 21 (see Table 6.5). The total weight of the permanent teeth is about 41 g (in females) to 46 g (in males).

6.1.1.4 Oral bacteria and dental caries

The main bacterial species found in the healthy mouth are shown in Table 6.6; those that are acid forming are associated with the erosion of dental enamel, and hence the development of dental caries. The extent to which caries develops depends on the ability of the acid-forming bacteria to adhere to the tooth surface, forming dental plaque; in turn this is controlled to a considerable extent by the carbohydrates present in the mouth; sucrose enhances adherence, while some sugar alcohols (see section 7.5) reduce adherence and inhibit the growth of cariogenic organisms (Birkhed and Bär 1991). Xylitol is used in the manufacture of 'tooth-friendly' sweets that inhibit dental decay.

Although there may be considerable acid erosion of dental enamel by acidic foods and drinks, and by bacterial action shortly after a meal, when there is an ample supply of substrates, between meals there is considerable recalcification, as the teeth are bathed in alkaline saliva. Fluoride ions both enhance this process and also provide resistance of the dental enamel against acid attack; the fluoride content of saliva (see Table 6.3) varies widely, depending on the intake of fluoride (see also section 25.12). It is noteworthy that in most countries the prevalence of dental caries decreased over the period from 1970–90, largely due to the widespread introduction of fluoride-containing toothpaste and fluoridation of drinking water, despite constant or increased consumption of (extrinsic) sugars (König and Navia 1995).

6.1.2 The stomach

The main functions of the stomach are to mix food to a uniform fluid consistency (chyme), denature and initiate the digestion of proteins (see section 10.3), and protect the gastrointestinal tract against invading micro-organisms. The total capacity of the stomach (as determined at post mortem) ranges from 1.5–4.8 L; the mean physiological capacity, as determined by weighing subjects before and after eating, is 1.3 L, with a range from 1–2.

The total surface area of the gastric mucosa is 500–550 cm^2.

There are three main types of gland in the stomach.

1. Mucus secreting goblet cells. The pH of gastric juice is between 1.0–3.5, and gastric mucus is both alkaline and extremely viscous, providing a protective layer over the gastric mucosa that may be as much as 1 mm thick.

2. Gastric glands, which secrete hydrochloric acid and intrinsic factor (required for the absorption of vitamin B_{12}, see section 21.6.1) from the oxyntic (parietal) cells, and pepsinogen, lipase, and gastric amylase from the peptic (chief) cells, as well as mucus. Gastric acid secretion serves both to denature proteins and also to protect against invading micro-organisms; acid secretion continues between meals (sometimes called basal secretion, but since there is continuing extracellular stimulation to secrete it is better called interdigestive secretion).

3. Pyloric glands, which secrete mucus and pepsinogen. The G cells of the pyloric glands secrete the hormone gastrin, which is a 17 amino acid peptide (there is also a small amount of a dimer, gastrin-34).

6.1.2.1 Control of gastric secretion

The initial increase in gastric secretion from all three types of gland is in response to the sight, smell and taste of food as a result of vagal stimulation (the tenth cranial nerve); this is sometimes called the cephalic phase of gastric secretion.

Gastric secretion is then maintained by the action of gastrin; the gastric phase of secretion. Gastrin is released by the G cells of the pyloric glands in response to vagal stimulation, physical distension of the stomach, or a variety of secretagogues in the lumen of the stomach, including partially digested proteins, and small amounts of alcohol and caffeine. Both the physical distension of the stomach and the response to secretagogues are mediated by local nerve reflexes.

Gastrin is secreted into the lumen of the stomach, and must then be absorbed into the bloodstream before it acts on the G cells. This provides a measure of self-regulation of gastric secretion; as the pH of the stomach contents falls below about 2.0 the absorption of gastrin is considerably impaired, thus reducing the stimulation of further acid secretion.

Gastric secretion continues to be stimulated by the presence of food in the duodenum, which provokes the secretion of enteric gastrin; this is the intestinal phase of gastric secretion.

6.1.2.2 Peptic ulcers

Peptic ulcers may affect the stomach (gastric ulcer) or duodenum (duodenal ulcer). The process of ulceration involves erosion of the gastric or duodenal mucosa by acid and pepsin, as a result of breakdown of the normal protection provided by mucus and, especially in the stomach, the resistant apical surface of the mucosal cells. Stress, non-steroidal anti-inflammatory drugs, and cigarette smoking all increase the risk of development of peptic ulcers.

Symptomatic relief is achieved by use of a variety of antacids, to raise the pH of the gastric (and upper duodenal) contents; magnesium and aluminium carbonates and hydroxides are commonly used. Duodenal ulcers may respond almost as well to antacid treatment as to more specific medication, while gastric ulcers show little healing in response to antacids alone.

Stimulation of mucus secretion also leads to healing of peptic ulcers. Liquorice extract is commonly used, as is the synthetic derivative of glycyrrhizinic acid (the active principle in liquorice), carbenoxolone. In some cases a synthetic 'mucus' can be given, in the form of sucralfate, a basic aluminium salt of sucrose hydrogen sulphate; under acid conditions this forms a sticky polymer that coats the gastric mucosa, and is reported to have especially high affinity for ulcer sites.

Gastric secretion can be reduced by inhibition of vagal stimulation using antagonists of cholinergic receptors. The receptors in the stomach are muscarinic cholinergic receptors (M_1 subclass), and two M_1 inhibitors are used: pirenzepine hydrochloride and telenzepine. Pirenzepine has some degree of selectivity for the gastric M_1 receptors, and at doses that inhibit acid and pepsinogen secretion it has few other anticholinergic effects.

Regardless of whether the gastric glands are being stimulated by the vagus nerve, local nerve reflexes, or gastrin, the final stimulatory transmitter is histamine. Therefore greater reduction in the secretion of gastric acid and pepsinogen can be achieved by inhibition of the histamine H_2 receptors. A number of specific H_2 receptor antagonists are in widespread use, including cimetidine, famotidine, nizatidine, ranitidine, and roxatidine. The introduction of these compounds into clinical practice revolutionized the treatment of peptic ulcers, with a very high rate of cure meaning that few patients now have to undergo surgical repair of ulcers.

A more recent advance in the treatment of ulcers depends on inhibition of the proton pump that is responsible for the secretion of hydrochloric acid by the oxyntic cells. Two compounds are in current use, lansoprazole and omeprazole; they are irreversible (mechanism-dependent) inhibitors of the proton pump, which therefore have a long duration of action, so affording little opportunity to adjust the dose to suit the patient's response.

Although the underlying cause of peptic ulceration is unknown, there is strong evidence that the bacterium *Helicobacter pylori* (*Campylobacter pylori*) may be involved. This organism is found in the antrum of the stomach of more than 95 per cent of patients with gastric ulcers, and accidental exposure to *H. pylori* results in acute symptomatic gastritis. However, the organism is also found in some 20 per cent of apparently healthy, asymptomatic subjects. Colloidal bismuth salts both provide some protection for the mucosa and also eliminate *H. pylori*, leading to rapid cure of ulcers, with a lower rate of recurrence than with other treatments (Soll 1990).

6.1.3 The small intestine

The small intestine can be divided into three regions: the duodenum (so-called because it is 12 fingerbreadths long), the jejunum and the ileum. Table 6.7 shows the size and weight of these regions.

Emptying of the stomach contents into the duodenum is stimulated both by gastrin and also neuronally, as a result of gastric distension. There is also an enterogastric nerve reflex which inhibits gastric emptying, and is activated by distension of the duodenum, irritation of the duodenal mucosa, and high osmolality or acidity of the duodenal chyme.

The entry into the duodenum of chyme from the stomach stimulates the secretion of secretin and cholecystokinin (CCK). Secretin acts on the ductile cells of the exocrine pancreas, stimulating the secretion of bicarbonate into the duodenum, thus neutralizing the acid chyme. CCK stimulates the acinar cells of the exocrine pancreas to secrete enzymes (see Table 6.2). CCK and (to a lesser extent) secretin also stimulate contraction of the gall bladder; the bile duct empties into the duodenum alongside the pancreatic duct.

Pancreatic and bile secretions are also stimulated by the vagus nerve. Table 6.8 shows the inorganic composition of pancreatic juice. The duct cells that secrete bicarbonate compose about 4 per cent of the total weight of the pancreas, and the acinar cells about 82 per cent; the endocrine pancreas (the islets of Langerhans, see section 5.5.1) make up about 1.8 per cent of the total, with the remainder being blood vessels. The role of bile in fat digestion is discussed in section 8.2.3.

The first part of the duodenum has an extensive array of mucus-secreting glands (Brunner's glands), which are stimulated by direct tactile or irritant stimuli, as well as by vagal stimulation and in response to secretin. Mucus is also secreted by goblet cells throughout the intestinal mucosal surface and in the crypts of Lieberkühn, mainly controlled by local nerve reflexes.

The crypts of Lieberkühn (intestinal glands) secrete the succus entericus; this contains pro-aminopeptidases and the enzyme enteropeptidase which is responsible for the action of trypsinogen in the pancreatic juice to active trypsin (see section 10.3.1). The remaining intestinal digestive enzymes (disaccharidases, dipeptidases and tripeptidases) are anchored to the brush border of the intestinal mucosal cells.

There are two types of intestinal motility (in both the small and large intestine): mixing movements, which are local contractions of small segments of gut wall; and propulsive movements which are peristalsis stimulated by distension.

6.2   Absorption of the products of digestion

Compounds that are lipophilic can cross biological membranes by simple diffusion, dissolving in the lipid of the membrane, coming to equilibrium across the membrane. Alcohol and a number of drugs that are lipophilic at low pH are absorbed by diffusion across the gastric mucosa. Otherwise the main site of absorption is the small intestine.

6.2.1 The small intestine

The small intestine has a considerably greater absorptive surface area than would appear from considering it as a simple cylinder (3.3×10^3 cm^2), because of the villi (small finger-like projections of mucosa into the intestinal lumen, some 7500 /cm^2) and the micro-villi (the invaginations of the surface of the mucosal cells

that line the villi. Allowing for the villi the surface area is some 10^5 cm^2, and allowing for the microvilli 2×10^6 cm^2.

As shown in Table 6.9, there is a rapid rate of turnover of mucosal cells; a total of 50–250 g of cells are shed daily into the lumen of the gut; from the rate of DNA loss this amounts to some $20–50 \times 10^6$ cells shed per minute. Most of these cells are lysed in the lumen, and their protein is largely hydrolysed and absorbed.

There are four main mechanisms for intestinal absorption.

1. Simple diffusion for lipophilic substances. This may operate in either direction, depending on concentration gradients across the membrane; there is considerable influx of urea into the intestinal lumen from the bloodstream (see section 10.8.2).

2. Carrier-mediated (passive) uptake. Here there are specific transport proteins in the mucosal cell membrane, but overall the process is not energy requiring, and does not achieve a greater concentration inside the cell than in the intestinal lumen. However, if there are intracellular binding proteins then compounds that have been taken up passively can be sequestered by the binding protein, thus achieving an overall concentration (see, for example, the intestinal transport of iron in section 24.2.3).

3. Active transport, in which there is utilization of ATP to achieve a greater concentration of the compound being transported inside the cell than outside. Active transport is commonly linked to a sodium pump: hydrolysis of ATP to ADP and phosphate in the cell membrane produces a proton gradient across the membrane; protons then re-enter the cell coupled to the efflux of sodium ions. The sodium ions then re-enter the cell together with amino acids (see section 10.3.2) or monosaccharides (see section 7.2).

4. Metabolic trapping is a concentrative process, but the transport of the metabolite across the cell membrane is by (passive) carrier-mediated transport. Once inside the cell it is phosphorylated; in general, phosphorylated metabolites do not cross cell membranes. Such mechanisms are important in the intestinal uptake of vitamins B$_2$ (see section 18.3.1) and B$_6$ (see section 20.3), and also in the uptake of glucose into liver cells.

6.2.2 The colon and rectum

The primary function of the large intestine is the absorption of water (and mineral salts) from the luminal contents. Table 6.10 shows the dimensions of the regions of the large intestine. The absorption of salts and water from the contents of the colon leaves the faeces, the average excretion of which is 110–135 g/day for adults. The principal constituents of faeces are shown in Table 6.11.

6.2.2.1 Intestinal microflora

The normal healthy colon supports a considerable population of bacteria (some 10^{11} organisms /g of luminal contents in the caecum), as well as small numbers of yeasts. The principal intestinal bacteria are shown in Table 6.12; most of these species are normally found only in the colon, rectum, appendix, and most distal segment of the ileum. However, lactobacilli are normally found in the jejunum and ileum, and streptococci in the ileum. This intestinal flora has a number of valuable functions.

1. A considerable amount of resistant starch (see section 7.2.2) and non-starch polysaccharides (see section 7.3) is fermented in the colon; the resulting short chain fatty acids are mainly absorbed, hence adding to available energy. Butyrate formed by colonic fermentation has been suggested to have a role in preventing colo-rectal cancer.

2. Conjugates of the bile acids (see section 8.2.3) are hydrolysed by bacteria, and the resultant free bile acids are absorbed and re-utilized. A number of other conjugates that are excreted in the bile, including those of steroid hormones, may also undergo enterohepatic recycling.

3. As discussed in section 10.8.2, there is considerable entry of urea by passive diffusion from the blood into the colon, where it is hydrolysed by bacterial urease; the resulting ammonia may be absorbed and used for amino acid synthesis in the liver, or may be used for bacterial synthesis of amino acids. Lower down the gut the bacteria are lysed, and significant amounts of essential amino acids may be made available.

4. Intestinal bacteria synthesize significant amounts of biotin (see section 23.1), thiamin (see section 17.1), and vitamin K (see section 16.2).

6.2.2.2 Constipation

The average normal intestinal transit time (the time from ingestion of a food to evacuation in the faeces) is between 20–60 hours. Diets with a low bulk (i.e. a low content of dietary fibre, see section 7.3.2) are generally associated with a considerably longer intestinal transit time, and the eventual passage of hard dry faeces. Failure to evacuate faeces regularly is constipation. Table 6.13 shows the main types of compound used as laxatives (also known as purgatives or cathartics) used in the treatment of severe constipation. Mild constipation can sometimes be relieved by increasing the intake of fibre from foods (i.e. fruits, vegetables, and whole-grain cereals) without recourse to the bulk-forming laxatives, which are pharmaceutical preparations of dietary fibre.

6.2.2.3 Diarrhoea

Diarrhoea, the frequent passage of excessively watery faeces, commonly associated with intestinal pain, may be due to the following.

1. Intestinal infection or parasite infestation (see Table 6.14). Serious intestinal bacterial or protozoal infection will require use of antibiotics, but most common intestinal infections are self-limiting. There are two mechanisms involved in infectious diarrhoea:

   (i) stimulation of intestinal mucosal secretion of water and electrolytes by bacterial enterotoxins (e.g. *Vibrio cholera* and enterotoxicogenic *Escherichia coli*);

   (ii) mucosal damage caused by invasive organisms such as Salmonella spp. and rotaviruses, resulting in reduction in the number of cells available for absorption of fluid and electrolytes. Although diarrhoea caused by invasive organisms commonly resolves within 3–5 days, in some 5–10 per cent of cases (and more in malnourished children) the infection persists for 2 or more weeks. Intestinal mucosal abnormalities, including disaccharide intolerance (see section 7.2.1) may persist for very much longer (Lunn *et al.* 1991).

2. Inflammatory bowel disease, when the long-term remedy is treatment of the underlying condition with sulphasazaline or other 5–aminosalicylic acid derivatives.

3. Disaccharide intolerance (see section 7.2.1), when the long-term remedy is to avoid the offending sugar.

4. Coeliac disease (intolerance of the gliadin fraction of gluten, see section 28.1.4), when the long-term remedy is to avoid wheat, rye and other sources of gluten.

Among children in developing countries, diarrhoea and protein-energy malnutrition (see section 12.2), resulting in impairment of growth, are closely related. Frequent or persistent diarrhoea may be a cause of malnutrition, as a result of impaired absorption, and conversely undernutrition leads to increased susceptibility to diarrhoeal infections (Briend 1990). As well as general undernutrition, deficiencies of zinc (see section 25.26.2) and vitamin A (see section 13.4) are especially associated with susceptibility to diarrhoeal infections (Tomkins *et al.* 1993).

The most important treatment for diarrhoea is replacement of the fluid and salt that are being lost, in order to prevent the development of dehydration; the introduction of oral rehydration solutions containing sugar and salt has been a major advance in paediatric medicine. The intestinal discomfort associated with diarrhoea can be relieved by use of

(1) kaolin, which acts as an absorbent of diarrhoeagenic toxins and also by increasing the bulk of the faeces (cereal bran has a similar action),

(2) diphenoxylate hydrochloride, which inhibits intestinal motility, commonly used together with atropine, to inhibit muscarinic cholinergic receptors,

(3) loperamide, which inhibits gastrointestinal motility and secretion.

6.3　Integration and control of gastrointestinal function

Gastrointestinal motility and secretion are closely regulated by neuronal, endocrine and paracrine mechanisms.

6.3.1 Neuronal control of gastrointestinal function

The nerves that control gastrointestinal function may be divided into two main classes:

(1) enteric neurones with cell bodies within gut wall;

(2) extrinsic neurones with cell bodies outside gut wall.

Further subdivision on the basis of neuroanatomy is shown in Table 6.15, and by the aspects of gut function controlled in Table 6.16. In addition other neurones control or modify secretion of mucus, pepsinogen, gastrin and other gut hormones (see section 6.4.2). There are also primary sensory neurones with cell bodies in dorsal root ganglia and vagal sensory ganglia. Table 6.17 shows the main types of neurotransmitter found in gastrointestinal neurones.

As well as the paracrine and endocrine actions described in section 6.4.2, a number of peptide hormones and neurotransmitters affect gastrointestinal motility and transit time by way of extrinsic neurones; the actions shown in Table 6.18 can all be demonstrated following direct intracerebroventricular injection of the peptides.

6.3.2 Endocrine and paracrine regulation of gastrointestinal function: the gut peptides

A number of peptides are secreted by the gastrointestinal tract, rather than by neurones innervating it, and have either local (paracrine) activity or circulate in the bloodstream (endocrine activity). The sources and actions of the major gut peptides are shown in Table 6.19. The receptors for many of these peptides have now been characterized; known target tissues and the mechanisms of transmembrane signal transduction are shown in Table 6.20.

Ions are transported in both directions across the intestinal mucosa; Table 6.21 shows the principal neurotransmitters and paracrine agents that stimulate ion secretion into the intestinal lumen (secretagogues) and the uptake of ions from the lumen (absorbagogues).

6.4　Hunger and satiety: the control of feeding

There are two hunger centres in the lateral hypothalamus; in experimental animals electrical stimulation of these centres causes the initiation of feeding behaviour, while lesions cause severe anorexia. In addition to simple, but as yet unidentified, changes in blood chemistry and the supply of nutrients, these hunger centres respond to stimulation from higher brain centres. There is increased electrical activity in the lateral hypothalamus in response to the sight or taste of food, and the secretion of saliva and gastric juice increases in anticipation of food intake, with or without visual and olfactory stimulation. At least one of the brain centres involved in the control of the hypothalamic hunger centres is in the temporal lobe of the amygdala; lesions in this region result in inappropriate 'food' responses being made to non-food items.

Cessation of feeding is controlled by the satiety centres in the ventro-medial hypothalamus; electrical stimulation of these centres in experimental animals results in cessation of feeding regardless of whether or not the animal has eaten an adequate amount, and lesions result in hyperphagia. The activities of the satiety centres can also be over-ridden by higher brain centres. After satiety has been reached, the appearance of a new appetizing food will stimulate further feeding, i.e. appetite versus hunger.

The physiological stimuli to the hunger and satiety centres are not known (Blundell 1991; Forbes 1988). Changes in the plasma concentrations of metabolic fuels (especially glucose, non-esterified fatty acids and ketones, see section 5.5) or perhaps the relative concentrations of different amino acids in plasma, and changes in the relative concentrations of insulin and glucagon are obvious candidates for signalling hunger and satiety. The hypoglycaemic rebound following consumption of alcohol together with a small amount of carbohydrate increases hunger, although it is not possible to disentangle the hypoglycaemia from the potentiation of insulin release and action following alcohol intake (O'Keefe and Marks 1977).

Direct neuronal signalling, due to distension of the stomach or small intestine, and indirect (hormonal) signalling from the gastrointestinal tract are also possible mediators of the satiety response (Smith and Gibbs 1992). As shown in Table 6.20, there are central nervous system receptors for several of the gastrointestinal peptides. In addition, there is good evidence that a peptide secreted by adipose tissue may have an effect on longer-term regulation of food intake (Rink 1994; Zhang *et al.* 1994).

A variety of neurotransmitter systems have been implicated in the control of the hypothalamic appetite centres: noradrenergic, dopaminergic, serotoninergic and GABAergic agonists and antagonists all have effects on food intake. It is not possible to determine which provides the ultimate signal. However, while some of the appetite-suppressing drugs (see Table 11.32) affect several different neurotransmitter systems, others (e.g. dexfenfluramine) have purely serotoninergic actions. Together with observations that changes in the uptake of tryptophan into the brain, and consequent changes in serotonin turnover, have predictable effects on food intake, this suggests that the major factor regulating food intake may well be a serotoninergic mechanism (Blundell 1991).

Table 6.1: Secretions of the gastrointestinal tract

	volume secreted (L/day)	pH
saliva (see Table 6.3)	1.2	6.0-7.4
gastric juice	2	1.0-3.5
pancreatic juice (see Table 6.8)	1.2	8.0-8.3
bile (see Table 8.10)	0.7	7.8
Brunner's glands (duodenum)	0.05	8.0-8.9
succus entericus (small intestine)	2	7.8-8.0
large intestinal secretion	0.06	7.5-8.0

Table 6.2: Digestive secretions of the gastrointestinal tract

	carbohydrate digestion see section 7.2	fat digestion see section 8.2	protein digestion see section 10.3	other secretions
salivary glands	α-amylase			
gastric parietal (oxyntic) cells				HCl
				intrinsic factor
gastric chief cells		lipase	pepsinogen	
gall bladder		bile salts		
pancreatic acinar cells	α-amylase	lipase colipase prophospholipase	procarboxypeptidases proelastase trypsinogen chymotrypsinogen ribonuclease	deoxyribonuclease bicarbonate
succus entericus			enteropeptidase pro-aminopeptidases	
mucosal brush border	sucrase-isomaltase maltase lactase		dipeptidases tripeptidases	

Table 6.3: Inorganic constituents of saliva
(Figures show mean and 95% reference ranges)

	mmol /L
sodium	174 (87–240)
nitrogen	64 (25–90)
potassium	19.7 (11.8–27.6)
chloride	11.3–46.5
phosphorus	6.5 (3.9–9.4)
sulphur	2.4
calcium	1.1–2.5
magnesium	0.29 (0.08–0.53)
fluoride	0.005–0.011
copper	0.004
bromide	0.002- 0.088
cobalt	0.001

Source: Snyder *et al.* 1975.

Table 6.4: The deciduous teeth

	age at eruption (months)	age at shedding (years)	mean weight (g /tooth) upper jaw	lower jaw
first (central) incisors	6-12	7	0.3	0.14
second (lateral) incisors	12-14	8	0.22	0.2
cuspid (canine)	14-24	10	0.39	0.40
first molars	18-19	10	0.58	0.57
second molars	20-24	11-12	1.0	1.0

Source: Snyder *et al.* 1975.

Table 6.5: The permanent teeth

	median age of eruption				mean weight (g /tooth)	
	lower jaw		upper jaw			
	males	females	males	females		
first (central) incisors	6.4	6.1	7.1	6.9	1.19	0.55
second (lateral) incisors	7.5	7.0	8.6	7.9	0.82	0.63
cuspid (canine)	10.3	9.6	11.5	10.7	1.28	1.09
first premolar (bicuspid)	10.8	10.1	10.2	9.9	1.23	0.97
second premolar (bicuspid)	11.4	10.8	10.7	10.7	1.13	1.09
first molar	6.4	5.9	6.4	6.1	2.48	2.32
second molar	11.8	11.6	12.8	12.2	2.18	2.27
third molar (wisdom)	17–21	17–21	17–21	17–21	1.73	1.99

Source: Snyder *et al.* 1975.

Table 6.6: Normal oral bacteria

species	intra-oral site	associated oral disease
Actinobacillus actinomycetemcomitans	subgingival plaque	abcesses, juvenile periodontitis
Actinomyces israeli	dental plaque	dental calculus formation
Actinomyces odontolyticus	dental plaque	extension of caries into dentine
Actinomyces naeslundi, A. viscosus	dental plaque	root surface caries, dental calculus formation
Arachnia propionica	dental plaque	carious dentine, necrotic dental pulp, chronic periodontitis
Bacterionema matruchotti	dental plaque	dental calculus formation
Bacteroides endodontalis	dental plaque	root canal and dentoalveolar infection
Bacteroides gingivalis, B. intermedius	gingival crevice, subgingival plaque	chronic periodontitis, dentoalveolar abcesses
Bacteroides melaninogenicus	dental plaque	-
Bacteroides oralis	dental plaque	dentoalveolar infection
Bifidobacterium dentium	dental plaque	-
Branhamella catarrhalis	tongue, saliva, oral mucosa	-
Capnocytophaga sputiga, C. ochhracea, C. gingivalis	dental plaque, oral mucosa	destructive periodontal disease
Eikenella corrodens	dental plaque	dento-alveolar abcesses, chronic periodontitis
Eubacterium suburreum, E. timidum	dental plaque	dental calculus, necrotic dental pulp, carious dentine, chronic periodontitis
Fusobacterium nucleatum	gingival crevice	acute ulcerative gingivitis, dentoalveolar abcesses, chronic periodontitis
Haemophillus parainfluenzae, H. segnis, H. agrophilus	dental plaque, saliva, oral mucosa	dento-alveolar infections
Lactobacillus casei, L. fermentum	dental plaque	extension of caries into dentine
Leptotrichia buccalis	dental plaque	-
Micrococcus mucilangenosus	tongue, gingival crevice	-
Mycoplasma orale, M. salivarium	dental plaque, gingival crevice	-
Neisseria lactamicus, N. pharyngis	tongue, saliva, oral mucosa	-
Peptococcus spp.	sub-gingival plaque	dento-alveolar infections
Peptostreptococcus spp.	sub-gingival plaque	dento-alveolar infections
Propionobacteria acnes	dental plaque	dento-alveolar infections
Rothia dentocariosa	saliva, dental plaque	-
Selenomonas sputagena	gingival crevice	-
Simonsiella spp.	tongue, hard palate	-
Streptococcus milleri	gingival crevice	dento-alveolar and endodontic infections
Streptococcus mitis	dental plaque	-
Streptococcus mutans	tooth surface	caries
Streptococcus oralis	tongue, dental plaque, saliva	-
Streptococcus salivarius	tongue, saliva	-
Streptococcus sanguinis	dental plaque	? caries, apthous ulceration
Treponema denticola, T. macrodentium, T. orale, T. vincenti	gingival crevice	acute ulcerative gingivitis, destructive periodontal disease
Veillonella alcalescens	tongue, saliva, dental plaque	-
Wollinella recta	gingival crevice	destructive periodontal disease
Entamoeba gingivalis (protozoan)	gingival crevice	chronic periodontitis
Trichomonas tenax (protozoan)	gingival crevice	-
Candida albicans, C. glabrata, C. tropicalis (yeasts)	tongue	oral candidiasis

Source: MacFarlane & Samaranayake, 1989.

Table 6.7: Dimensions of the small intestine

	weight (g)	length (cm)	diameter of lumen (cm)
small intestine	640	500	-
duodenum	60	25	3.5-6
jejunum	280	190	2.5-4
ileum	300	285	2-3.8

Source: Snyder *et al.* 1975.

Table 6.8: Inorganic composition of pancreatic juice

	concentration (mmol /L)
sodium	140
potassium	5
calcium	2
bicarbonate	120
chloride	70

Table 6.9: Small intestinal villi and epithelial cell turnover

villus length	700 μm
villus diameter	130 μm
villus volume	9.3×10^6 μm^3
volume of the epithelium of a single villus	8×10^6 μm^3
number of villi	7500 /cm^2 of intestine; total in intestine 9×10^7
total volume of epithelial cells	7.2×10^{14} μm^3 = 720 mL
dimensions of columnar epithelial cells	$5 \times 5 \times 40$ μm = 1000 μm^3
number of epithelial cells	8000 /villus; total in intestine 7.2×10^{11}
total number of mucosal cell turnover	20-50 $\times 10^6$ /min; 2.4×10^{11} /day
number of mitoses /1000 gland cells	6.5 (range 2-11)
duodenal cell turnover time	2-6 days
jejunal cell turnover time	5 days
ileal cell turnover time	3 days
migration from crypt to tip of villus in ileum	80 hours

Source: Snyder *et al.* 1975.

Table 6.10: Dimensions of the large intestine

	weight (g)	length (cm)	diameter of lumen (cm)
large intestine	370	160	7-8 proximally
upper large intestine	210	75	2.5-3 distally
caecum	-	7	5-7
ascending colon	90	18	-
transverse colon	120	50	-
lower large intestine	160	85	-
descending colon	90	30	4
sigmoid colon	70	40	-
rectum	-	15	empty 2.5; extreme distension 7.5

Source: Snyder *et al.* 1975.

Table 6.11: Principal components of faeces

	adult man		adult woman	
	g /day	% of total	g /day	% of total
weight	135	-	110	-
water	105	78	90	82
solids	30	22	20	18
ash	17	12.5	15	13.6
fats	5	3.7	4.5	4.1
other substances	6.5	4.8	5	4.5

Source: Snyder *et al.* 1975

Table 6.12: Major intestinal bacterial flora

Gram-negative anaerobic rods	*Bacteroides* spp.
	Butyrovibrio fibriosolvens
	Desulfomonas pigra
	Fusobacterium spp.
	Leptotrichia buccalis
	Succinomonas amylolytica
	Vibrio succinogenes
Gram-positive anaerobic rods	*Bifidobacterium* spp.
	Clostridium spp.
	Eubacterium spp.
	Lacnospira multiparus
	Propionobacterium spp.
Anaerobic cocci	*Acidaminococcus fermentans*
	Coprococcus spp.
	Gemiger formicilis
	Megasphera elsdenii
	Peptococcus spp.
	Ruminococcus spp.
	Sarcina ventriculi
	Streptococcus spp.
	Veillonella parvula
Facultitive anaerobes	*Citrobacter freundii*
	Escherichia coli
	Enterobacter spp.
	Klebsiella pneumoniae
	Lactobacillus spp.
	Proteus spp.
	Streptococcus spp.
	Staphylococcus epidermidis

See also Table 6.14 for micro-organisms commonly associated with food- and water-borne disease
Source: Drasar & Barrow, 1985.

Table 6.13 Laxative agents

bulk-forming laxatives	cereal bran
	ispaghula–from *Psyllium* spp
	psyllium–from *Psyllium* spp
	sterculia–from *Psyllium* spp
	methylcellulose
stimulant (irritant) laxatives	aloe (extract of leaves of *Aloe vera*)
	bisacodyl
	cascara (bark of *Rhamnus* (*Frangula*) *purshiana*)
	cassia (seed pods of *Cassia fistula*)
	castor oil (ricinoleic acid)
	danthron (1,8-dihydroxyanthroquinone)
	fig extract (*Ficus* spp)
	phenolphthalein
	rhubarb (rhizomes of *Rheum palmatum* or *R. officinale*)
	senna (seed pods of *Cassia senna* (*C. acutifolia*)
osmotic laxatives	magnesium sulphate (Epsom salts), magnesium citrate
	lactulose (see section 7.2.1.1)
emollient laxatives	docusates (Na, K or Ca salts of dioctyl sulphosuccinate)

Table 6.14: Micro-organisms commonly associated with food- and water-borne infection

organism	pathogenic mechanism
Bacillus cereus	ingestion of preformed toxin
Campylobacter jejuni	invasion and enterotoxin
Clostridium botulinum	ingestion of preformed toxin
Clostridium difficile[1]	toxins
Clostridium perfringens	toxin released by ingested bacteria
Entamoeba histolytica	invasion of intestinal mucosa
Escherichia coli	enterotoxins
Listeria monocytogenes	invasion of intestinal mucosa
Salmonella spp.	invasion of intestinal mucosa
Shigella spp[2]	invasion and enterotoxin
Staphylococcus aureus	ingestion of preformed toxin
Vibrio cholera	enterotoxin
Vibrio parahaemolyticus	enterotoxin
Yersinia enterocolitica	invasion and enterotoxin

(1) Infection with *C. difficile* commonly follows the use of antibiotics and the loss of normal intestinal flora. It has been implicated in the aetiology of pseudomembranous colitis.
(2) While infection with most of these pathogens requires a dose of 10^4-10^6 organisms, clinically significant infection with *Shigella* spp. requires only 10–200 organisms.
Source: from data reported by Drasar & Barrow 1985.

Table 6.15 Neurones of the gastrointestinal tract

neurones	location of cell body
enteric	gut wall
extrinsic, vagal	brain stem
extrinsic, pelvic	spinal cord
extrinsic, sympathetic	prevertebral and paravertebral ganglia
extrinsic, primary sensory	dorsal root or vagal sensory ganglion

Table 6.16: Functional categories of gastrointestinal neurones

control of	type	neurones
motility	enteric	excitatory and inhibitory muscle motor neurones
		interneurones of ascending and descending reflex pathways
		enteric primary sensory neurones
		neurones supplying muscularis mucosae and villous smooth muscle
	extrinsic	excitatory and inhibitory vagal neurones
		sympathetic neurones to sphincter muscles
		sympathetic motility inhibiting neurones
		excitatory and inhibitory pelvic preganglionic neurones
fluid movement	enteric	cholinergic and non-cholinergic secretor motor neurones
		neurones of secretomotor reflexes
		primary sensory neurones of secretomotor reflexes
	extrinsic	vagal and pelvic secretomotor excitatory neurones
		sympathetic secretomotor inhibitory neurones
gastric acid secretion	enteric	interneurones for acid secretion reflexes
		primary sensory neurones for acid secretion reflexes
	extrinsic	motor neurones to parietal and gastrin cells
		vagal preganglionic neurones for acid secretion and gastrin release
blood supply	enteric	vasodilator neurones
		interneurones and primary sensory neurones of vasodilator reflexes
	extrinsic	sympathetic vasoconstrictor neurones

Source: McConalogue & Furness (1994).

Table 6.17: Neurotransmitters in gastrointestinal neurones

transmitter	localization and functions
acetylcholine	primary excitatory transmitter to muscle, intestinal epithelium, parietal cells, some gut endocrine cells and neuroneuronal synapses
ATP	contributes to transmission from enteric inhibitory motor neurones
calcitonin-gene related peptide (CGRP)	some secretomotor neurones and axons of extrinsic sensory neurones; role unknown
cholecystokinin (CCK)	some secretomotor neurones and interneurones; generally excites muscle.
enkephalins, dynorphins and endorphins	interneurones and motor neurones; feedback inhibition of transmitter release
GABA	antagonises muscle contraction stimulated by enteric cholinergic neurones; excites cholinergic neurones and enteric inhibitory neurones
galanin	secretomotor cells and descending interneurones; role unknown
gastrin releasing peptide (GRP)	excitatory transmitter to gastrin cells; also present in interneurones and nerve fibres to muscle, where role unknown
histamine	stimulation of gastric acid secretion
5HT	excitatory neuroneuronal transmission
neuropeptide Y	secretomotor neurones; inhibits secretion water and electrolytes
nitric oxide	cotransmitter from enteric inhibitory muscle motor neurones
noradrenaline	extrinsic neurones; inhibition of motility in non-sphincter regions, contraction of sphincter muscle; inhibition of secretomotor reflexes; vasoconstrictor neurones for enteric arterioles
somatostatin	widespread; no clearly defined roles
tachykinins[1]	excitatory transmitters to muscle; cotransmitters with acetyl choline
vasoactive intestinal peptide (VIP)	excitatory transmitter from secretomotor neurones; possibly also transmitter of enteric vasodilator neurones; contributes to transmission from enteric inhibitory motor neurones

(1) tachykinins include: substance P, neurokinin A, neuropeptide K, neuropeptide γ.
Source: from data reported by McConalogue & Furness 1994.

Table 6.18: Effects of central nervous system peptides on gastrointestinal motility and transit.

	stomach	small intestine	colon
stimulation of motility	thyrotropin somatostatin	thyrotropin cholecystokinin	thyrotropin endorphin
stimulation of transit	thyrotropin corticotrophin releasing factor	thyrotropin	thyrotropin corticotrophin releasing factor
inhibition of motility	cholecystokinin oxytocin neurotensin substance P	calcitonin calcitonin-gene related peptide. corticotrophin releasing factor neurotensin endorphin neuropeptide Y substance P	endorphin
inhibition of transit	endorphin calcitonin calcitonin-gene related peptide. corticotrophin releasing factor neurotensin	endorphin calcitonin calcitonin-gene related peptide. corticotrophin releasing factor neurotensin	endorphin enkephalin

Source: from data reported by Taché *et al.* 1990.

Table 6.19: The principal gut peptides

	secreted by	actions
antral chalone	stomach	↓ gastric secretion
bulbogastrone	duodenum	↓ gastric secretion
calcitonin-gene related peptide	throughout gut	↓ gastric acid secretion
cholecystokinin (pancreozymin)	duodenum	↑ gall bladder emptying
		↑ pancreatic secretion of enzymes
		↓ gastric acid secretion
duocrinin	duodenum	↑ intestinal secretion and absorption
enteroglucagon	ileum, colon	↑ gut motility, gut mucosal growth
entero-oxyntin	upper small intestine	↑ gastric secretion
enterocrinin	upper small intestine	↑ intestinal secretion and absorption
enterogastrone	stomach, duodenum	↓ gastric secretion
		↓ gastric motility
gastrin	stomach, ileum	↑ gastric secretion
gastric inhibitory peptide	upper small intestine	↑ insulin secretion
glucagon-like peptide 1	terminal ileum	↑ insulin secretion, ↓ glucagon secretion
motilin	stomach, upper small intestine	↑ intestinal motility
peptide YY	throughout gut	↓ pancreatic secretion of fluid, bicarbonate and enzymes
secretin	duodenum	↑ pancreatic secretion of fluid and bicarbonate;
		↑ choleresis
		↓ gastric secretion and gastrin release
somatostatin	throughout gut	↓ gastric secretion and gastrin release
		↓ pancreatic secretion of bicarbonate and enzymes
		↓ expression and release of gut peptides
		↓ gastric emptying
		↓ intestinal motility
		↓ gall bladder contractility
		↓ absorption of glucose, triacylglycerols, amino acids
		↓ intestinal ion secretion
		↓ splanchnic blood flow

Source: from data reported by Aynsley-Green *et al.* 1990; Davison 1989; Holst 1994; Holst & Schmidt 1994; Lloyd 1994; Schulkes 1994.

Table 6.20: Receptors for gut peptides

peptide	target tissue(s)	signal transduction
cholecystokinin	CCK-A: pancreas, gall bladder, brain	↑ IP3, DAG
	CCK-B: brain	?
galanin	endocrine pancreas, brain	↓ cAMP; ↑ K$^+$ channel
gastric inhibitory peptide	pancreas β-cells	↑ cAMP
gastrin	gastrointestinal smooth muscle, gastric mucosal cells, pancreas	↑ IP3, DAG
gastrin-releasing peptide	exocrine pancreas, brain, gastrointestinal tract	↑ IP3, DAG
glucagon	liver, adipose tissue	↑ cAMP
glucagon-like peptide I	endocrine pancreas, lung	↑ cAMP
neuropeptide Y	Y-1: brain, blood vessels	↓ cAMP; ↑ Ca^{++}
	Y-2: brain, kidney	↓ cAMP
	Y-3: heart	↓ cAMP
neurotensin	brain, stomach, intestine	↓ cAMP; ↑ IP3, DAG
opioid	μ: (β-endorphin) brain, intestinal tract	↓ cAMP; ↑ K$^+$ channel
	δ: (enkephalins) brain, intestinal tract	↓ cAMP; ↑ K$^+$ channel
	κ: (dynorphins) brain, intestinal tract	↓ cAMP; ↑ K$^+$ channel
pancreatic polypeptide	small intestine, nervous tissue, liver	?
peptide YY	small intestine, adipose tissue, brain	↓ cAMP
pituitary adenylate cyclase activating polypeptide	brain, liver	↑ cAMP
secretin	exocrine pancreas, stomach, brain	↑ cAMP
somatostatin	ubiquitous	↓ cAMP; ↑ K$^+$ channel
tachykinins	NK1: (substance P) brain, ileum, carotid artery	↑ IP3, DAG
	NK2: (substance K) brain, duodenum, pulmonary artery	↑ IP3, DAG
	NK3: (neuromedin K) brain, portal vein	↑ IP3, DAG
vasoactive intestinal peptide	ubiquitous	↑ cAMP

Source: from data reported by Laburthe *et al.* (1994).

Table 6.21: Control of intestinal ion transport

	secretagogues	absorbagogues
amines	acetylcholine	adrenaline
	histamine	dopamine
	5-hydroxytryptamine	noradrenaline
peptides	bombesin	angiotensin
	bradykinin	cholecystokinin
	calcitonin	enkephalins
	neurotensin	neuropeptide Y
	substance P	somatostatin
	vasoactive intestinal peptide	vasopressin
other compounds	ATP prostaglandins	

Carbohydrates provide some 35–45 per cent of the energy intake in most developed countries, with a desirable level of intake being 55 per cent of energy, to compensate for the desirable reduction in fat intake (see section 4.2); in less developed countries carbohydrate may provide as much as 75 per cent of energy intake. Average and desirable levels of carbohydrate intake are shown in Table 7.1, and major sources in the average diet in Table 7.2.

7.1 Classification and nomenclature of carbohydrates

Both chemically and nutritionally, carbohydrates can be divided into two groups: sugars (both monosaccharides and small oligosaccharides) and complex carbohydrates, which are linear or branched polymers of monosaccharides. Complex carbohydrates include both starch and non-starch polysaccharides. Non-starch polysaccharides may be simple or mixed polymers, and may include a variety of monosaccharide units other than those shown in Figs 7.5, 7.6 and 7.7, which are the nutritionally important sugars.

7.1.1 Classification of carbohydrates

Carbohydrates can be classified as follows (see Fig. 7.1).

1. Polysaccharides, divided into

    (a) starches, which are the main metabolic fuel, yielding 16 kJ /g;

    (b) non-starch polysaccharides (nsp), the major fraction of dietary fibre (see section 7.3); nsp are precisely defined chemically, and serve as an index of dietary fibre; they have little or no energy value (see section 7.4).

2. Oligosaccharides, divided into

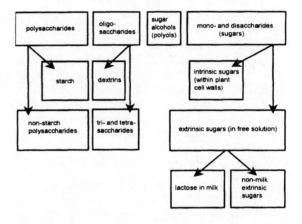

Figure 7.1 Nutritional classification of carbohydrates

    (a) dextrins, derived from starch by partial enzymic hydrolysis, which provide 16 kcal /g;

    (b) indigestible tri- and tetrasaccharides (see section 7.1.3).

3. Sugars, monosaccharides with 3–7 carbon atoms, and disaccharides which are hydrolysed to monosaccharides by digestive enzymes. Sugars are subdivided by their occurrence in foods within plant cells (intrinsic sugars) or in free solution (extrinsic sugars). To distinguish the latter from the lactose of milk, they are termed non-milk extrinsic sugars. Sugars in fresh fruits are considered intrinsic; sugars in fruits that have been canned, stewed or dried are considered half extrinsic, since the cell walls have been partially broken down. So far as dental decay is concerned (see section 6.1.1.4), it is recommended in UK that the intake of non-milk extrinsic sugars should not exceed 60 g /day or 10 per cent of total food energy. This is different from the US recommendation, which differentiates between sugars

that are naturally present (and may be intrinsic or extrinsic) and sugars that are added in food manufacture or preparation.

4. Sugar alcohols (polyols), reduced derivatives of monosaccharides in which the aldehyde or ketone group has been reduced to an alcohol (e.g. sorbitol from glucose, dulcitol from galactose; the trihydric alcohol glycerol (see section 8.1.1) is a sugar alcohol). A number of fruits, especially apples, cherries, pears and plums, are relatively rich in sorbitol, providing between 1–3.5 g /100 g. Sugar alcohols (and especially sorbitol) are widely used as sweeteners in food manufacture (see section 7.5), especially foods suitable for diabetics (see section 7.7.2), and in the manufacture of sugar-free sweets. Unlike sugars, the sugar alcohols do not readily support the growth of plaque-forming oral bacteria (see section 6.1.1.4), and have low cariogenic activity (Birkhed and Bär 1991). Indeed, xylitol has a positive anti-cariogenic action, and is used in the manufacture of 'tooth-friendly' sweets.

A further, chemical, classification of sugars is into those that have an aldehyde group at carbon 1 (aldoses, chemically they are reducing agents, and hence are sometimes known as reducing sugars) and those that have a keto- or oxo- group at carbon-1 (ketoses, which are not chemically reducing agents). Disaccharides and oligosaccharides can also be classified as reducing or non-reducing sugars, depending on whether they have an exposed free aldehyde group on carbon-1 of one of the constituent monosaccharides. This distinction between reducing and non-reducing sugars is not nutritionally relevant, but can be of importance in clinical chemistry; all reducing sugars will give a positive result with the various chemical tests that are sometimes used to detect glucosuria (see section 7.7.2).

7.1.1.1 Monosaccharides

The monosaccharides can be classified by the number of carbon atoms they contain: trioses 3 carbon sugars; tetroses 4 carbon sugars; pentoses 5 carbon sugars; hexoses 6 carbon sugars; heptoses 7 carbon sugars. Of these, hexoses are nutritionally the most important, although the diet provides moderate amounts of pentoses and the triose alcohol glycerol (mainly in triacylglycerols, see section 8.8.1.1). Trioses, tetroses and heptoses occur mainly as metabolic intermediates.

As shown in Fig. 7.2, sugars are capable of undergoing an aldol condensation to yield a ring structure. There are thus three different conventions for show-

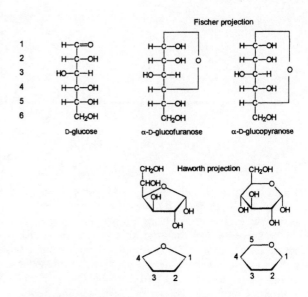

Figure 7.2 The structure of glucose
Glucose can undergo internal condensation to yield the 5-membered furanose or 6-membered pyranose ring, shown above in the Fischer projection, and below in the Haworth projection.

ing the structures of sugars: as a straight-chain formula, as the Fischer projection of the ring and as the Haworth projection of the ring. Glucose is capable of undergoing either 1–4 condensation, forming a 5–membered (furanose) ring or a 1–5 condensation, forming a 6–membered (pyranose) ring.

The assignation of D- or L-conformation to a sugar depends on the orientation of the hydroxyl group on the highest numbered asymmetric carbon, by comparison with Fischer's assigned structures for glyceraldehyde (see Fig. 7.3). (Note that the same comparison with glyceraldehyde, or alanine, (which can be regarded as a glyceraldehyde derivative) is used to assign D- or L-conformation to amino acids; see section 10.2.1.

There are two possible orientations of the hydroxyl group on carbon 1, assigned α- and β-, depending on whether the hydroxyl group is above or below the 'plane' of the ring. In free solution there is interconversion between the α- and β forms, but in oligo- and polysaccharides the orientation at carbon-1 is fixed. This is nutritionally important: starch is an β-1,4-linked glucose polymer and is a major metabolic fuel; cellulose is a α-1,4-linked glucose polymer and has no nutritional value to human beings. In fact, the pyranose ring is not planar, but can adopt either of two possible conformations; these conformations, and the consequent orientations of the hydroxyl

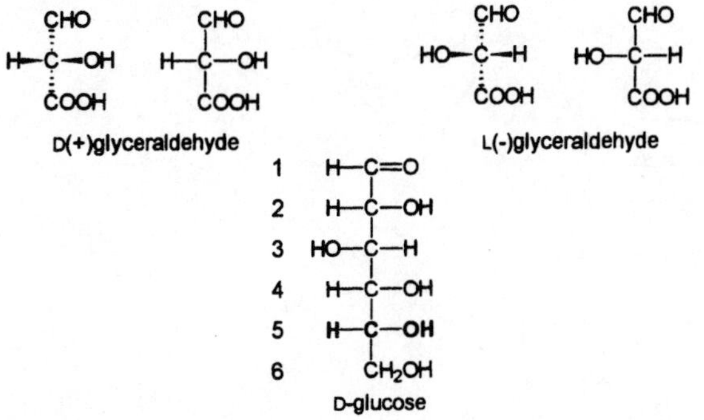

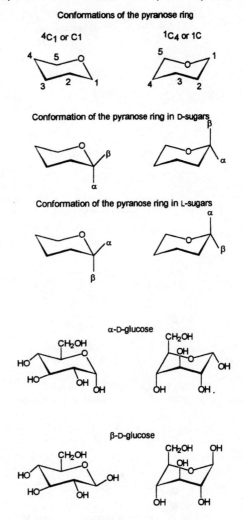

Figure 7.3 Stereochemistry of carbohydrates: D- and L-configurations
The stereochemistry of sugars is determined by the configuration of the asymmetric centre compared with the assigned configurations of glyceraldehyde, shown above.

group at carbon 1 are shown in Fig. 7.4. A further complication to the systematic naming of sugars is that the pyranose ring can take up one of two possible conformations, known as C1 or 1C.

The differences between the other nutritionally important monosaccharides are the result of the orientation of the other hydroxyl groups in the molecule. Nutritionally important hexoses are shown in Figure 7.5 and pentoses in Fig. 7.6.

Some further derivatives of glucose are shown in Fig. 7.7; amino sugars and acetylated amino sugars occur in plant cell walls, and hence in non-starch polysaccharides. Glucuronic acid is not nutritionally important, but is a part of the body's detoxication mechanisms. A number of (potentially) toxic compounds, that may be naturally occurring compounds, drugs or endogenous metabolites such as steroids, are conjugated with glucuronic acid before excretion in the urine or bile. Some of the biliary conjugates may be hydrolysed by intestinal bacterial β-glucuronidase (EC 3.2.1.31), releasing the free steroid metabolite, which is reabsorbed from the colon, leading to a considerable amount of entero-hepatic recycling (see also section 8.2.3).

Figure 7.4 Conformations of the pyranose ring

7.1.1.2 Disaccharides and oligosaccharides
The major disaccharides are shown in Table 7.3; those starred in the Table are also shown in Fig. 7.8. Sucrose (cane or beet sugar, ordinary table sugar) is by far the major dietary disaccharide, accounting for more than 10 per cent of energy intake in average western diets. The only significant source of lactose is milk, although it is also used as a filler in many pharmaceutical preparations. Maltose and isomaltose are formed in the digestion of starch, and in the sprouting (malting) of cereal grains. Trehalose is

found in mushrooms and other fungi, and also in a number of insects. Other disaccharides may occur in small amounts as a result of degradation of various polysaccharides in foods, and small amounts of lactulose are formed when milk is heated.

Trisaccharides and oligosaccharides other than dextrins (see Table 7.4) are not digested by human enzymes, but can serve as substrates for intestinal bacterial fermentation, and so cause flatulence. They include the trisaccharide raffinose and the tetrasaccharides stachyose and verbascose, found in bran, raisins, and legumes, especially soybeans.

7.1.1.3 Starches
Starches are polymers of glucose. Amylose is a linear polymer of glucose linked by α-1,4 links, with about

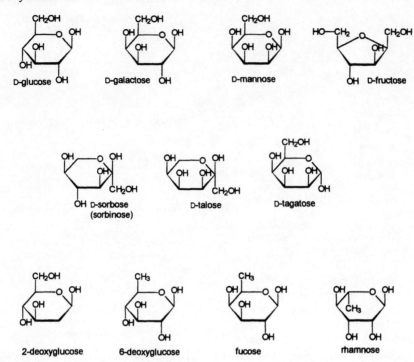

Figure 7.5 The major 6-carbon (hexose) sugars
Relative molecular mass (M_r) of hexose monosaccharides = 180.2

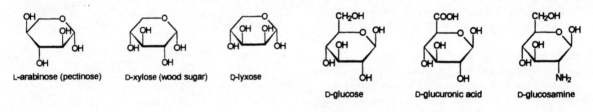

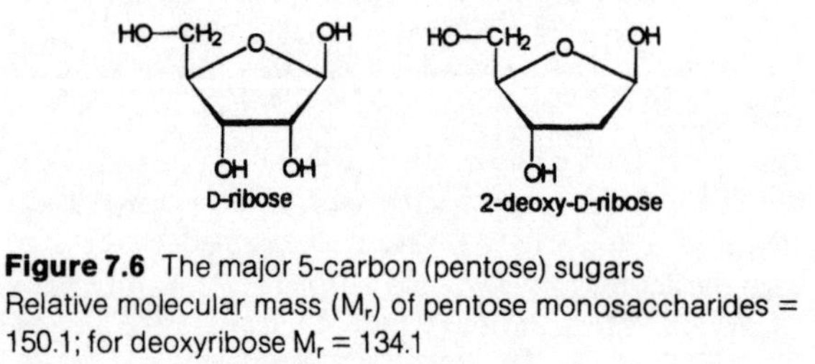

L-arabinose (pectinose) D-xylose (wood sugar) D-lyxose

D-glucose D-glucuronic acid D-glucosamine

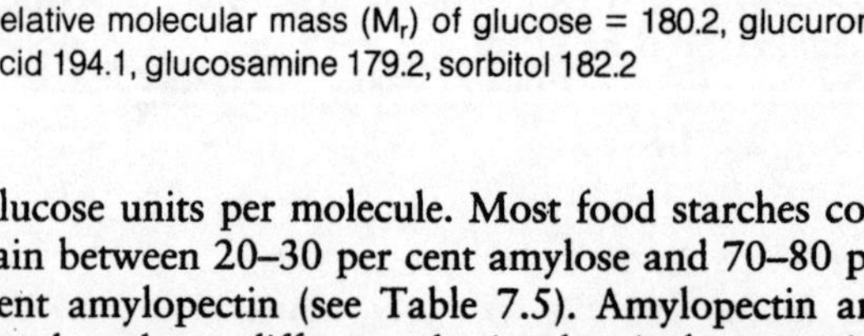

Figure 7.7 Glucose derivatives
Relative molecular mass (M_r) of glucose = 180.2, glucuronic acid 194.1, glucosamine 179.2, sorbitol 182.2

D-ribose 2-deoxy-D-ribose

Figure 7.6 The major 5-carbon (pentose) sugars
Relative molecular mass (M_r) of pentose monosaccharides = 150.1; for deoxyribose M_r = 134.1

250–1,000 glucose units per molecule. Amylopectin is a highly branched polymer, with the chains of 20–25 α-1,4 linked glucose units and branch points provided by α-1,6 links (See Fig. 7.9). Amylopectin is considerably larger than amylose, with 10–100 000 glucose units per molecule. Most food starches contain between 20–30 per cent amylose and 70–80 per cent amylopectin (see Table 7.5). Amylopectin and amylose have different physicochemical properties, which affect their use in food manufacture; the more highly branched the structure, the greater the amount of water that can be taken up in gelatinization. Gelatinized amylose readily undergoes recrystallization (retrogradation, see section 7.2.2), whereas amylopectin gels are stable. Glycogen, the storage carbohydrate in liver and muscle, has a highly branched amylopectin-like structure.

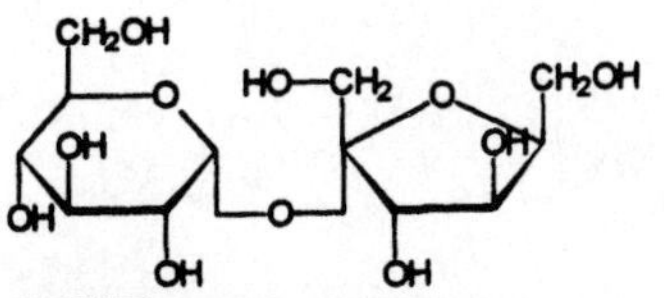

sucrose
(1-α-D-glucopyranosyl-β-fructofuranoside)

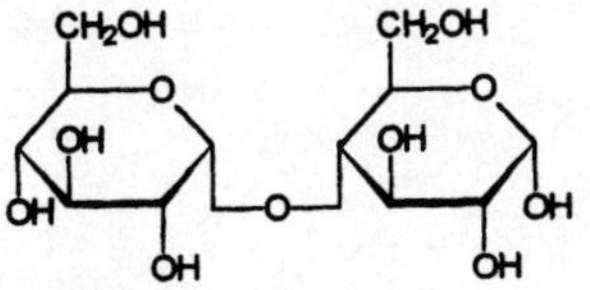

maltose
(4-β-D-glucopyranosyl-D-glucopyranose)

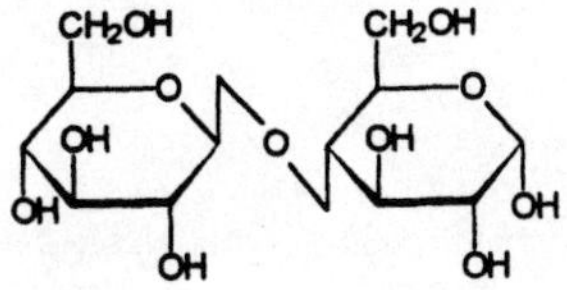

lactose
(4-β-D-galactopyranosyl-D-glucopyranose)

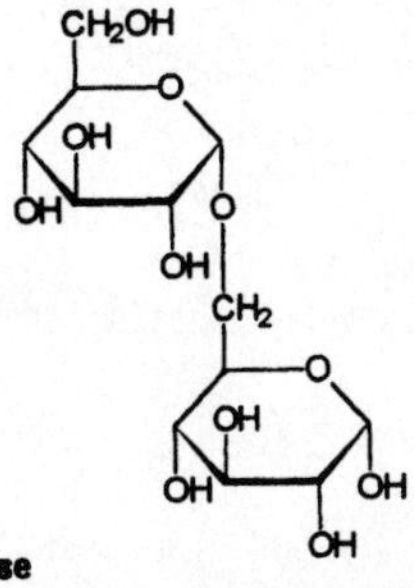

isomaltose
(6-α-D-glucopyranosyl-D-glucopyranose)

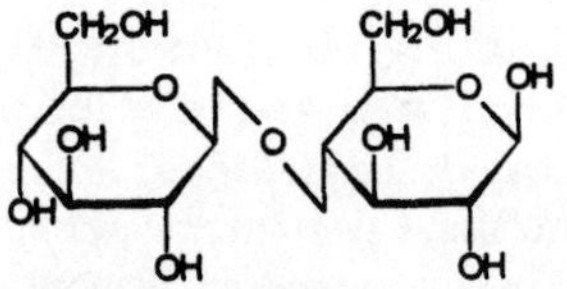

cellobiose (cellose)
(4-β-D-glucopyranosyl-D-glucopyranose)

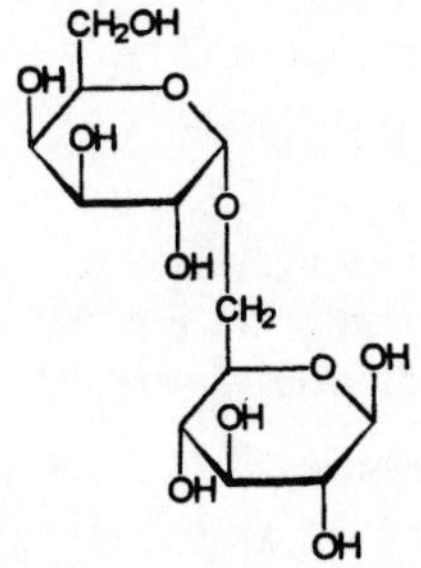

melibiose
(6-α-D-galactopyranosyl-D-glucopyranose)

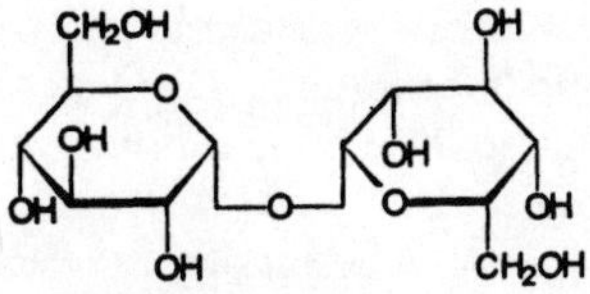

trehalose (mycose)
(1-α-D-glucopyranosyl-α-D-glucopyranoside)

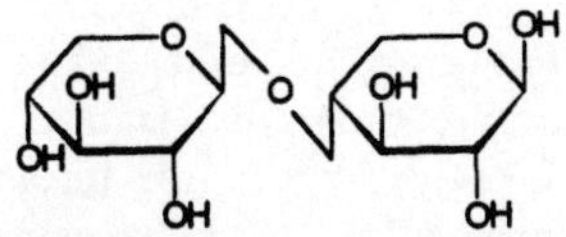

xylobiose
(4-β-D-xylopyranosyl-β-D-xylose)

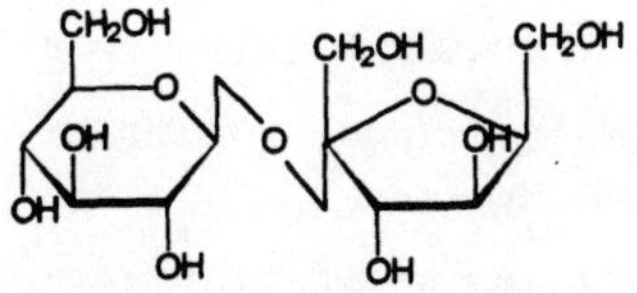

lactulose
(4-β-D-galactopyranosyl-D-fructofuranose)

Figure 7.8 The major disaccharides
Relative molecular mass (M_r) of hexose disaccharides = 342

7.2 Digestion and absorption of carbohydrates

Starch is hydrolysed by amylase, in both saliva (salivary amylase is sometimes called ptyalin) and the pancreatic juice. This is an α-amylase, catalysing random hydrolysis of 1,4-α D-glucosidic bonds internally in oligosaccharides of greater than 3 glucosyl units (EC 3.2.1.1, 1,4-α-D-glucan glucanohydrolase). It thus yields a mixture of glucose, maltose, and dextrins. It does not act on the α-1,6 glucoside links of amylopectin. There is no human (or other mammalian) equivalent of the plant β-amylase, which cat-

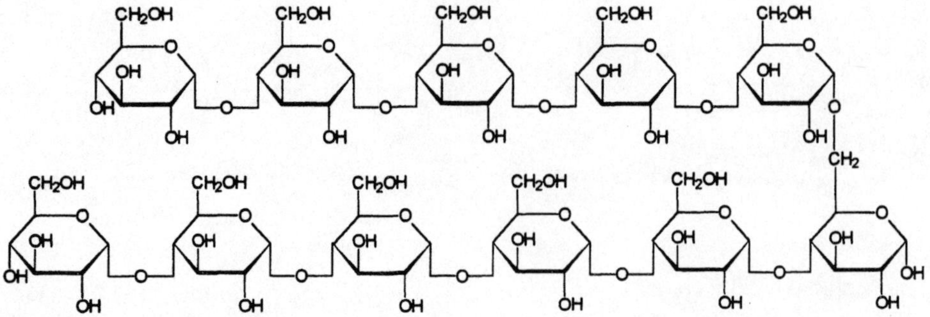

114   *Carbohydrates*

Figure 7.9 The structure of starch and glycogen
Amylose consists entirely of straight chains of glucose units linked α1→4; in amylopectin and glycogen the branch points are provided by α1→6 links.

alyses the exo-hydrolysis of 1,4-α-D-glucosidic bonds, sequentially releasing maltose from the non-reducing end of starch.

In the brush border of the intestinal mucosal cells there are the following disaccharidases.

1. Maltase (α-glucosidase, EC 3.2.1.20, glucoside glucohydrolase) which hydrolyses the non-reducing terminal α-1,4 glycoside links of maltose and small dextrins to liberate free glucose.

2. Isomaltase (limit dextrinase, EC 3.2.1.10, 6-α-D-glucosidase) which hydrolyses isomaltose, maltose, and palatinose. This enzyme occurs as a bifunctional complex together with sucrase.

3. Sucrase (invertase, saccharase, EC 3.2.1.26, β-D-fructofuranoside fructohydrolase) which hydrolyses sucrose, and to a limited extent also maltose. This enzyme occurs as a bifunctional complex together with isomaltase.

4. Trehalase (EC 3.2.1.28, trehalose glucohydrolase) which hydrolyses trehalose.

5. Lactase (EC 3.2.1.108, lactose galactohydrolase) which hydrolyses lactose, and also glucosyl-N-acyl sphingosine, cellobiose and various β-galactosides.

Of the monosaccharides that occur in the diet or are released by hydrolysis of oligosaccharides, only glucose and galactose are absorbed from the small intestine by a process of (sodium dependent) active transport (see section 6.2.1). Fructose is absorbed by a carrier-mediated process, so that it is absorbed considerably more slowly than are glucose and galactose, but faster than sugar alcohols, which are absorbed passively. The presence of glucose increases the rate of fructose absorption; the mechanism is unclear, but may simply reflect the increased uptake of water together with glucose, and a solvent drag effect on the uptake of fructose (Lentze 1995).

A moderately large intake of fructose or sugar alcohols may be greater than can be absorbed during normal intestinal passage, resulting in their accumulation in the large intestine, where their osmotic pressure causes retention of water in the colon, leading to osmotic diarrhoea. The effect of sugar alcohols has been called 'chewing gum diarrhoea', since a significant source of sugar alcohols is sugar-free chewing gum. Foods containing sugar alcohols usually carry a warning to this effect, although an 'excessive intake' is difficult to define. The threshold intake ranges from 20–50 g, not only varying between individuals, but also varying in the same person at different times, with the presence of other foods, etc.

7.2.1 Disaccharidase deficiency

In most ethnic groups, other than northern European (Caucasian) populations, lactase activity is lost in adolescence, leading to an intolerance of lactose. Consumption of even moderate amounts of lactose in milk can lead to severe gastrointestinal discomfort and diarrhoea, as a result of the fermentation of undigested lactose by colon bacteria. This results in formation of lactate (and hence an 8–fold increase in osmotic pressure compared with lactose), as well as significant amounts of hydrogen, methane and other gases—the cause of the abdominal discomfort. For adults who lack lactase the solution is relatively simple—avoidance of milk, since this is the only significant source of lactose in the diet (although it is also used in pharmaceutical preparations). Many alactasic adults can tolerate the relatively small amount of lactose that remains in cheese and yoghurt. Congenital alactasia also occurs, rarely, in infants; here the problem is to provide a lactose-free milk substitute.

Extremely rarely, infants have a congenital lack of sucrase-isomaltase. Their problem is more serious than for alactasic people, since sucrose is widely distributed in many foods. In addition to congenital lack of disaccharidases, and the (normal) loss of lactase in adult life, there can be acquired loss of all five disaccharidase activities from the small intestinal mucosa as a result of intestinal infection with the protozoan parasite *Giardia lambla*, which is a major cause of water-borne disease (giardiasis) when there is faecal contamination of water supplies. Some months after resolution of the infection the activity of the enzymes returns to near normal. Similar temporary loss of disaccharidase activity may also occur as a result of diarrhoeagenic infection with various enteropathogenic bacteria (see section 6.2.2.3).

The old method for diagnosis of alactasia was to give a test dose of 50 g of lactose, and measure the increase in blood glucose—in an alactasic subject there will be no increase. This was a particularly unpleasant experience for the patient, since the test dose of lactose produced a painful, explosive watery diarrhoea. A more recent development is to detect the hydrogen produced by colonic fermentation of lactose by measuring the hydrogen exhaled after a much more modest dose of lactose (Brummer *et al.* 1993; King and Toskes 1983).

7.2.1.1 Lactulose

Lactulose is a synthetic disaccharide, 4-β-galactopyranosyl-fructofuranose (see Fig. 7.8); small amounts are formed when milk is heated. It is not digested by human enzymes, but is fermented by intestinal bacteria to yield lactic acid. For this reason it is used as a mild laxative (see section 6.2.2.2).

Lactulose promotes the growth of *Lactobacillus bifidus*, a desirable intestinal micro-organism, and it has been called the bifidus factor, and for this reason has been added to infant milk formula to mimic the bifidus-promoting effect of human milk (which is not due to the presence of lactulose). Other fructose oligosaccharides, including inulin, also stimulate the growth of *L. bifidus*, and impair the growth of less desirable organisms such as *Clostridium perfringens* (Cummings and Englyst 1995).

Lactulose is also used clinically in the treatment of hyperammonaemia; the increased acidity in the colon resulting from its fermentation to lactic acid leads to trapping of ammonia in the gut lumen as ammonium ions, which cannot cross the gut wall, and hence to increased removal of ammonia from the bloodstream.

7.2.2 Resistant starch

The digestibility of starch in raw foods is very low, both because of the intact cell walls that prevent access of digestive enzymes, and also because of the crystalline nature of the (insoluble) starch granules (the B form of starch crystals is especially resistant to digestion). When a food is cooked, the cell walls are broken down and the starch is solubilized (gelatinized), allowing ready access of amylase. However, digestion is still incomplete. Controlled hydrolysis in vitro provides some information and the availability and absorbability of starches (and other carbohydrates) can be measured in vivo by the glycaemic index—the increase in blood glucose after a test meal relative to that from the same amount of glucose (see Tables 7.6 and 7.7).

The undigested and unabsorbed fraction is termed resistant starch, since it resists amylase digestion in the small intestine; it passes to the colon, where it is a substrate for bacterial fermentation. Resistant starch is formed by the partial recrystallization (retrogradation) of cooked starch as it cools. Depending on the method of analysis, resistant starch may be included with dietary fibre; physiologically it appears to have similar beneficial effects to those of non-starch polysaccharide (see section 7.3).

7.3 Non-starch polysaccharides and dietary fibre

Dietary fibre was originally defined as the remnants of plant cell walls, a definition that was later extended to include all undigested polysaccharides and lignin in foods of vegetable origin (Trowell *et al.* 1976). This definition thus includes not only plant cell wall constituents (including lignin, which is not a carbohydrate, but a polymer of aromatic alcohols), but also storage carbohydrates such as inulin (an indigestible fructose polymer), a variety of gums and mucilages and also that fraction of starch that is resistant to digestion. However, none of the methods described below for analysis of dietary fibre determines inulin, which although it is an unavailable polysaccharide, is soluble in ethanol, and is therefore not recovered from the ethanol precipitation step that is used in all methods to recover water-soluble fibre constituents.

Total dietary fibre may be estimated gravimetrically after enzymic hydrolysis of proteins, sugars and starches; this is the method used for US food composition tables (Prosky *et al.* 1985; 1988). This is a rapid method, but may include non-fibre components of the food. It gives no information on the chemical composition of the material measured, although soluble and insoluble fibre are differentiated by alcohol precipitation of the soluble fibre before gravimetry.

The method for fibre determination as used in UK tables of food composition depends on specific determination of hexoses, pentoses and uronic acids, and thus gives more information on the chemical nature of the material being measured. Full information about the material being measured is obtained by specific determination of the various monosaccharide components of the non-starch polysaccharides (nsp) of the food using gas or high-pressure liquid chromatography (Southgate 1969; Englyst *et al.* 1992; Quigley and Englyst 1992). Lignin and resistant starch are specifically excluded from the determination of nsp; the nsp content of a food is therefore frequently significantly lower than the dietary fibre content determined by other methods—for most foods 1 g of nsp is equivalent to 1.6 g of dietary fibre.

US labelling legislation (see section 4.3.1) includes both dietary fibre and digestible carbohydrates under the heading of carbohydrate—chemically correct but uninformative. By contrast, EU legislation defines carbohydrates as those that are metabolizable (and hence digestible), including sugar alcohols. There is, to date, no EU legislation on the method to be used for determination of fibre or nsp for food labelling.

Table 7.8 shows the principal types of non-starch polysaccharides in foods, and Fig. 7.10 the structures of cellulose, chitin, pectin and inulin; some of the monosaccharide units commonly found in non-starch polysaccharides are shown in Fig. 7.11.

7.3.1 Fructans: inulin and levan

Inulin is a linear polymer of fructose with up to about 50 monosaccharide residues; levan is a branched fructose polymer of up to about 100 monosaccharide units. Together with other smaller fructose-containing oligosaccharides they are known collectively as fructans. The main sources are tubers, including the Jerusalem artichoke (*Helianthus tuberosus*, up to 65 per cent fructans) and salsify (*Scorzonera hispanica*, about 10 per cent fructans). Cereals such as wheat and rye may contain up to about 7 per cent fructans, with considerable seasonal variation, and significant amounts are found in a variety of other vegetables

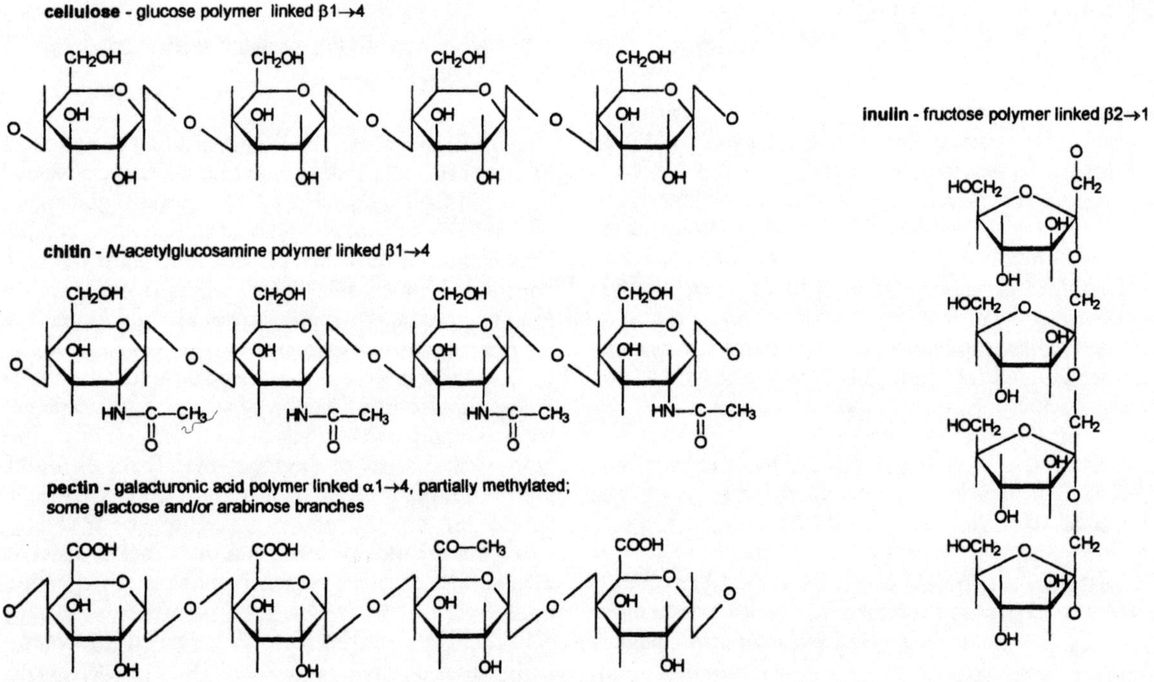

cellulose - glucose polymer linked β1→4

chitin - *N*-acetylglucosamine polymer linked β1→4

pectin - galacturonic acid polymer linked α1→4, partially methylated; some glactose and/or arabinose branches

inulin - fructose polymer linked β2→1

Figure 7.10 Structures of major non-starch polysaccharides

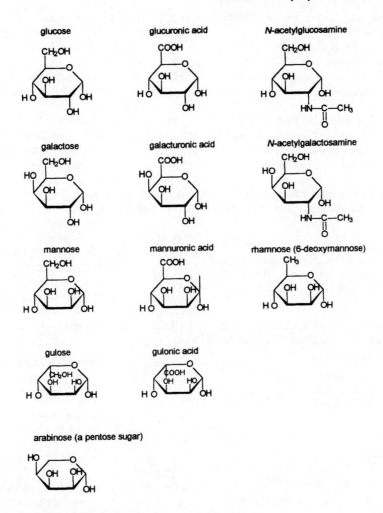

Figure 7.11 Monosaccharides commonly found in non-starch polysaccharides
Relative molecular mass (M_r) of glucose, galactose, mannose, gulose = 180.2, glucuronic acid, galacturonic acid, mannuronic acid = 194.1, rhamnose = 164.2, arabinose = 150.1.

(Rumessen 1992). Fructans are not digested to any significant extent, and as noted above they are not measured as part of either dietary fibre or non-starch polysaccharide. They are readily fermented in the colon.

7.3.2 Beneficial effects of dietary fibre and resistant starch

The main health benefits attributed to a moderately high intake of fibre are due to increased faecal bulk and more uniform intestinal transit time, which results in a reduction in both intra-intestinal pressure and straining on defecation. The average intake of nsp in UK is about 13 g /day (approximately 20 g

dietary fibre), and it is recommended that this should be increased to an average of 18 g nsp (30 g dietary fibre), with an individual range of 12–24 g. Low intakes are associated with constipation, diverticular disease of the colon, haemorrhoids, varicose veins and hiatus hernia, all of which are relieved by increased fibre intake.

Viscous non-starch polysaccharides (the soluble nsp and especially plant gums) are associated with delayed gastric emptying, and hence a greater sense of satiety. They also increase the viscosity of the intestinal contents, and slow the rate of absorption of nutrients. This may be especially valuable in the control of non-insulin-dependent diabetes mellitus, where a slower rate of glucose absorption results in better glycaemic control with less need for dietary restriction and hypoglycaemic agents.

Epidemiological data also suggest a hypocholesterolaemic action of nsp, associated with a reduction in coronary heart disease, and also a reduction in gall bladder disease. It is mainly soluble nsp that has the beneficial effect, which is believed to be due to physical adsorption of the bile salts (see section 8.2.3), thus reducing the extent to which they are available for reabsorption. This leads to increased synthesis of bile salts, and hence a depletion of the body pool of cholesterol.

High intakes of nsp are also associated with lower incidence of colo-rectal cancer. Here there may be three distinct mechanisms.

1. Increased intestinal transit reduces the time in which potential carcinogens can interact with the intestinal mucosa; at the same time the increased faecal bulk dilutes any potential carcinogens.

2. Potential carcinogens are adsorbed onto nsp, and hence are excreted rather than being absorbed or interacting with the intestinal mucosa.

3. The butyrate formed by intestinal fermentation of nsp, resistant starch and fructans may have a protective effect—in vitro butyrate has an antiproliferative action.

7.4   The determination and metabolic energy yield of dietary carbohydrates

Many authoritative tables of food composition quote figures for 'carbohydrate by difference'. This means that they were not analysed, but the protein, fat and ash were subtracted from the total dry weight. This usually introduces only a small error, except for foods relatively rich in non-starch polysaccharides, since these are included in the calculation of carbohydrate by difference. One of the few tables that is based on direct analysis is that of McCance and Widdowson, in which the starch and sugars are hydrolysed to their monosaccharides and the energy calculated by multiplying this figure by 16 kJ /g. 100 g of a disaccharide such as sucrose yields 105 g of glucose + fructose on hydrolysis (the addition of the elements of water); 100 g of starch yields 110 g of glucose. Consequently the quoted 'carbohydrate value' of 100 g of food can exceed 100 g.

The energy yield is measured accurately by this method, since the conversion factor for monosacchar-

ides is 16 kJ (3.75 kcal) /g; for disaccharides it is 16.5 kJ (3.9 kcal) and for starch 17 kJ (4.1 kcal) /g, thus permitting the average value of 4 kcal /g for carbohydrate.

Livesey (1992) has reported that the available energy from (experimental) human diets may vary by as much as 16 per cent of gross energy. This figure is presumably derived from diets that excluded alcohol (see Chapter 9), and he states that much of this variability is the result of variation in the occurrence, availability and metabolism of complex carbohydrates (non-starch polysaccharides and resistant starch) and sugar alcohols. These are carbohydrates that are not digested in the small intestine, but are, or may be, fermented by colonic flora, with availability to the host of a varying amount of metabolizable products of bacterial fermentation—largely short-chain fatty acids such as acetate, propionate, and butyrate.

For the purposes of nutritional labelling, the energy yield of sugar alcohols is taken to be 10 kJ (2.4 kcal) /g. The net energy yield can be calculated from

$$\text{net energy yield} = \text{heat of combustion} \times [(A\text{-}B) + (1\text{--}A) \times f)]$$

where A is the fraction absorbed in the small intestine, B is the fraction not recovered in urine, f is the fraction fermented in the large intestine that is available to the host.

This last term, the fraction of intestinal fermentation products available to the host, is almost impossible to determine with any useful precision, although it can be estimated by measurement of the proportion of carbohydrate energy lost as bacterial mass, and the energy yield of the resultant short chain fatty acids. Conventionally a value of 0.5 is used.

The fraction fermented in the large intestine that is available to the host may be calculated from

$f = (1\text{-}a\text{-}b\text{-}c) \times g$ where *a* is the proportion of carbohydrate energy lost as microbial mass in the faeces; this can be measured with reasonable precision, *b* is the the heat of fermentation, variously estimated as between 0.02–0.05 times the energy value of the carbohydrate. *c* is the efficiency of production of combustible gases such as hydrogen and methane. Livesey (1992) quotes various estimates of the energy loss in hydrogen and methane as between 0.02–0.08 kJ /kJ carbohydrate; the higher values are from animal studies, with lower values for combustible gases in breath and flatus from the few studies that have been performed in human beings. *g* is the efficiency of metabolic utilization of short-chain fatty acids compared with glucose. Livesey (1992) quotes estimates between 0.69–0.85. For mixtures of short-chain fatty acids he proposes that

$$\text{gmix} = 0.848 \times \text{acetate} + 0.865 \times \text{propionate} + 0.920 \times \text{butyrate}.$$

Heats of combustion of carbohydrates are shown in Table 7.9, heats of combustion and metabolic energy of sugar alcohols in Table 7.10, and of complex carbohydrates in Table 7.11.

7.5 Sweetness and sweeteners

Two main types of sweeteners are used in food manufacture and preparation: bulk sweeteners and intense sweeteners.

The major bulk sweeteners are sucrose and glucose syrups. The latter are prepared by the hydrolysis of starch, and some or all of the glucose can be converted into fructose enzymically, using isomerase from *Bacillus megaterium*—so-called iso-syrups, high-fructose syrups or high-fructose corn syrups. Since fructose is sweeter than glucose, these products are as sweet as, or sweeter than, sucrose and cheaper than invert sugar made by hydrolysis of sucrose. High-fructose corn syrups account for almost 50 per cent of total carbohydrate sweeteners in the US food supply. Sucrose, and to a lesser extent glucose syrups, not only contribute to taste but also viscosity and texture in general, serve as preservatives, and also play a role in the structure of some foods (such as biscuits and cakes), as well as the appearance of many foods (Davis 1995).

Intense sweeteners, some of which are synthetic while others occur naturally, are many hundreds or even thousands times as sweet as sucrose and consequently are used in extremely small amounts (see Table 7.12). They thus serve no function other than their prime purpose of reducing the energy content of the food.

Bulk sweeteners include derivatives of the sugars, e.g. hydrogenated glucose, which provide bulk and textural and preservative properties but are slowly absorbed and supply less energy than 16 kJ/g and so are useful in reduced energy foods and products suitable for use by diabetics. Together with the sugar alcohols, they have the special virtue that they do not promote the growth of dental plaque-forming bacteria (see section 6.1.1.4). Xylitol, the alcohol of the pentose sugar xylulose, appears to have a more positive effect in inhibiting the growth of such bacteria (Birkhed and Bär 1991).

Many amino acids (see section 10.2.1) are also sweet; they are not used as sweeteners themselves but in various mixtures, e.g. with saccharine to modify the flavour. D-Tryptophan is about 30–40 times as sweet as sucrose, although L-tryptophan has an intensely bitter taste. Glycerol is also sweet and is used in food manufacture both for its flavour and as a humectant.

In most countries products sweetened with aspartame (β-methylaspartyl-phenylalanine) are specifically labelled because of the possible risk to children with phenylketonuria from ingestion of excessive amounts of phenylalanine (see section 10.10).

Not all of the intense sweeteners shown in Table 7.12 are permitted in all countries, and some are still experimental compounds awaiting approval after toxicological testing. Those that are permitted may be used in 'low calorie' beverages, other foods and/ or as 'table top' sweeteners added to beverages.

7.6 Glucosinolinates and glycosides

A wide variety of alkyl isothiocyanate derivatives of glucose, collectively known as glucosinolates, occur in plants—especially brassicas, but also in other plants. The general structure is shown in Figure 7.12, and the principal glucosinolinates are listed in Table 7.13.

High intakes of glucosinolates are toxic—a problem that has not been encountered in human nutrition, but may occur when animals are fed on large amounts of brassica. One glucosinolinate is of more serious concern; progoitrin is metabolized by the plant enzyme myrosinase to yield goitrin (see Fig. 7.12). Goitrin inhibits the uptake and metabolism of iodine in the thyroid gland, and in cattle with high intakes of brassicas leads to clear signs of hypothyroidism (see section 25.14.4). Although there is no evidence that consumption of modest amounts of cabbage and other brassicas leads to the development of clinical goitre in human beings, changes in thyroid metabolism have been observed after consumption of moderately large amounts, and in areas where iodine and selenium intake are marginal, dietary goitrogens are associated with goitrous cretinism.

There is some evidence that dietary glucosinolates may have beneficial actions, providing protection against chemical carcinogenesis (Nugon-Baudon and Rabot 1994). They induce, and hence increase the activity of, the various enzymes that are involved

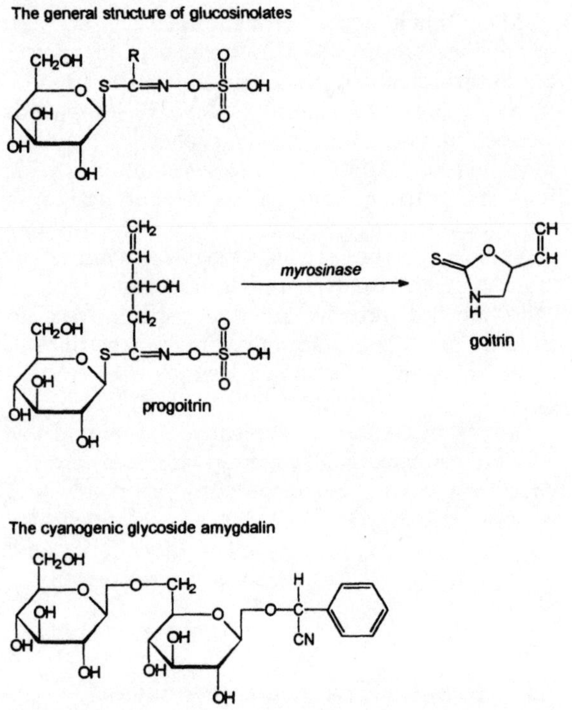

The general structure of glucosinolates

The cyanogenic glycoside amygdalin

Figure 7.12 Structures of glucosinolinates and amygdalin Myrosinase EC 3.2.3.1

in the conjugation of the activated metabolites of xenobiotics, so speeding their clearance from the body.

A number of plants produce the glycoside amygdalin (see Fig. 7.12). Relatively large amounts are found in the kernels of almonds (and especially bitter almonds, *Prunus amygdala*) and apricots (*Prunus armenica*) and, more importantly, in the root of cassava (*Manihot utilissima*), which is the dietary staple in many parts of west Africa and an important food in the Caribbean. When the plant tissue is damaged, the enzymes amygdalase and prunase hydrolyse the glycoside to yield glucose, benzaldehyde (which is partially responsible for the aroma of almonds) and hydrogen cyanide. Traditional methods of preparing cassava involve grating the root in the open air, and allowing the cyanide to evaporate overnight.

Amygdalin has been promoted as a nutrient, under the names of laetrile and 'vitamin B_{17}', although there is no evidence that it has any metabolic function, nor, as was claimed by its proponents, that it has any useful anticancer activity. As a result of a number of fatalities associated with its consumption, the US FDA specifically banned its sale or promotion in

1971. A wide variety of other glycosides occur in plants, including those of the flavonoids (see section 23.3).

7.7 Disorders of carbohydrate metabolism

There are number of rare genetic conditions that affect carbohydrate metabolism, including the following.

1. Disaccharidase deficiencies—either alactasia or, more rarely, lack of sucrase-isomaltase (see section 7.2.1).

2. Deficiency of the glucose–galactose intestinal transport system may also occur, resulting in carbohydrate malabsorption (see section 7.2).

3. Galactosaemia, due to deficiency of galactose-1–phosphate uridyl transferase (EC 2.7.7.10), and hence an inability to metabolize galactose. Since the main source of galactose is the lactose in milk, affected infants require a lactose-free milk substitute.

4. Hereditary fructose intolerance due to deficiency of fructose-bisphosphate aldolase (EC 4.1.2.13); affected infants have to avoid all foods containing sucrose or fructose.

5. Idiopathic pentosuria, a harmless condition characterized by failure to metabolize pentoses, which are therefore excreted in the urine in relatively large amounts. This condition is restricted entirely to people of north European Jewish (Ashkenazi) origin.

6. Glycogen storage diseases, resulting in abnormal accumulation of glycogen in liver and/or muscle; there are seven forms:

   type I (von Gierke's disease) due to deficiency of glucose-6–phosphatase (EC 3.1.3.9) in liver;
   type II (Pompe's disease) due to deficiency of lysosomal acid maltase (EC 3.2.1.3);
   type III (Cori's disease) due to deficiency of the glycogen debranching enzyme, amylo-1,6–glucosidase (EC 3.2.1.3);
   type IV (Andersen's disease) due to deficiency of the branching enzyme (EC 2.4.1.18), so that glycogen is present as linear, rather than branched, polymers;
   type V (McArdle's disease) due to deficiency of muscle glycogen phosphorylase (EC 2.4.1.1);

type VI (Hers' disease) due to deficiency of glycogen phosphorylase (EC 2.4.1.1) or phosphorylase b kinase (EC 2.7.1.37) in liver;
type VII due to deficiency of phosphofructokinase (EC 2.7.1.11).

7.7.1 Favism

Favism is due to partial deficiency of glucose-6–phosphate dehydrogenase (EC 1.1.1.49), and is probably the commonest known enzyme deficiency, with some 200 million people affected world-wide. The enzyme deficiency results in damage to the red blood cell membrane, and affected people suffer acute attacks of haemolytic anaemia and haemoglobinuria. Attacks are precipitated by eating broad beans (*Vicia faba*), or even inhaling the pollen, as well as in response to a number of drugs, including the common antimalarial and antihelminthic drugs, sulphonamides, probenecid, and the synthetic vitamin K analogue menadione (see sections 16.1 and 16.6).

7.7.2 Diabetes mellitus

Diabetes mellitus is an impaired ability to regulate the utilization of blood glucose. Normally an increase in the concentration of glucose in the hepatic portal vein stimulates secretion of insulin from the β-cells of the pancreatic islets of Langerhans. Insulin stimulates the uptake of glucose into muscle and other extra-hepatic tissues, and increases both the utilization of glucose as a metabolic fuel and also the synthesis of glycogen in liver and muscle (see section 5.5.1). In diabetes mellitus there is impaired tolerance to an oral or intravenous load of glucose, and the plasma glucose concentration rises to considerably higher than normal, and remains high for an abnormal period of time. When it rises above the capacity of the kidney to resorb it from the glomerular filtrate (the renal threshold), the result is glucosuria—excretion of glucose in the urine. There are two main types of diabetes mellitus.

1. Type I (insulin dependent) diabetes mellitus (IDDM) is due to a failure to secrete insulin, or, rarely, to secretion of the biologically inactive precursor protein, pro-insulin. It commonly manifests in childhood, and is sometimes known as juvenile-onset diabetes. Treatment is by injection of insulin and strict control of carbohydrate intake; the commonly used preparations of insulin are shown in Table 7.14.

2. Type II (non-insulin-dependent) diabetes mellitus (NIDDM) is due to failure of responsiveness to insulin, as a result of decreased formation or sensitivity of cell surface insulin receptors. Insulin secretion in response to glucose is normal or higher than normal. It usually manifests in middle-age, with a gradual onset, and is sometimes known as maturity-onset diabetes. In mild cases treatment is by control of carbohydrate intake, and possibly use of oral hypoglycaemic agents (see Table 7.15) such as sulphonylureas, which stimulate increased insulin secretion, enhance insulin-receptor function and decrease hepatic gluconeogenesis, or biguanides, which do not stimulate insulin release, but require insulin to be present to exert their hypoglycaemic effect, since they enhance insulin sensitivity and inhibit hepatic gluconeogenesis. See also the discussion on the glucose tolerance factor in section 25.9.1. Increasingly, as biosynthetic human insulin has become widely available, treatment of NIDDM includes insulin injection to maintain better control over blood glucose concentration.

In addition to these two clear diabetic syndromes, impaired glucose tolerance, and sometimes frank diabetes, may develop in pregnancy—so-called gestational diabetes. In many cases glucose tolerance returns to normal on parturition, but in some cases the stress of pregnancy is sufficient to precipitate persistent clinical diabetes. It is likely that the problem in pregnancy is due to formation of a biologically inactive insulin-xanthurenic acid complex, as a result of the changes in tryptophan metabolism in pregnancy (Kotake *et al.* 1975, and see Fig. 19.4).

The immediate result of the failure of glycaemic control in diabetes is excretion of glucose in the urine when the renal threshold is exceeded. Both initial diagnosis of the condition and monitoring of glycaemic control are commonly achieved by determination of urine glucose. Two main methods are used.

1. Determination of total reducing sugars in urine with an alkaline copper reagent. As well as glucose this will give a positive result in cases of pentosuria, and also if there is significant urinary excretion of vitamin C (a reducing compound, see Section 22.4.4).

2. Enzymic determination of glucose using glucose oxidase linked, via the enzyme peroxidase, to the oxidation of a dye-stuff by the hydrogen peroxide produced; this is the basis of urine and blood glucose testing strips. While specific for glucose, this will give a false negative result in the presence of moderately high concentrations of vitamin C.

Persistent failure of glycaemic control results in damage to capillary blood vessels, kidneys, and peripheral nerves, and the development of cataracts in the lens of the eye and abnormal metabolism of plasma lipoproteins (see section 8.3). Three mechanisms have been proposed to explain these effects.

1. At high concentrations, glucose can be reduced to sorbitol by aldose reductase (EC 1.1.1.121). In tissues that cannot metabolize sorbitol, it accumulates, causing osmotic damage. A number of inhibitors of aldose reductase have been developed in order to minimize renal and other damage in diabetes mellitus, including epelrestat, ponelrestat, sorbinol, and tolresat.

2. Glucose can react non-enzymically with exposed lysine residues on proteins, in a reaction akin to the Maillard non-enzymic browning reaction (see section 27.4.1). Such glycated proteins include collagen, serum albumin, apolipoprotein A, α-crystallin in the lens, and haemoglobin A. Glycation of haemoglobin A provides a sensitive means of assessing the adequacy of glycaemic control over the preceding 4–6 weeks, and is commonly measured in diabetes clinics.

3. Glucose may inhibit tissue uptake of inositol (see section 23.7.2).

Table 7.1: Average intakes of carbohydrate in UK, and desirable levels of intake

Figures for intake show mean and (95% range)

	desirable intake % total energy	average intake, men		average intake, women	
		g/d	% total energy	g/d	% total energy
total carbohydrate	53	272 (131—435)	41.6 (29.1—53.8)	193 (83—314)	43.0 (30.5—55.5)
starch	38	156 (69—258)	24.0	106 (42—172)	23.8
sugars	10	115 (37—224)	17.6	86 (25—171)	19.2

Source: Gregory *et al.* 1990.

Table 7.2: Percent of carbohydrate intake from various sources in average UK diets

Figures show the percentage of average total intake of carbohydrate, sugar or fibre, from various sources

	total carbohydrate	sugars	fibre
cereals	**46**	**23**	**47**
white bread	14	-	13
wholemal / brown bread	8	-	17
breakfast cereals	5	-	6
biscuits	-	3	-
cakes and pasries	-	8	-
puddings and ice cream	-	5	-
milk	**6**	**13**	**-**
meat and meat products[1]	**5**	**1**	**5**
fish and fish dishes	**1**	**0**	**1**
vegetables	**16**	**6**	**38**
potatoes	11	-	12
fruit and nuts	**4**	**8**	**8**
sugar and confectionery	13	29	1
beverages	7	17	-

(1) This includes sausages and burgers, which may contain cereal, as well as meat pies
Source: Gregory *et al.* 1990.

Table 7.3 Disaccharides

maltose* (maltobiose)	4-α-D-glucopyranosyl-D-glucose	R, F
isomaltose* (brachyose)	6-α-D-glucopyranosyl-D-glucose	R, NF
kojibiose (sakebiose)	2-α-D-glucopyranosyl-D-glucose	R
sophorose	2-β-D-glucopyranosyl-D-glucose	R
laminaribiose	3-β-D-glucopyranosyl-D-glucose	R
nigerose	3-α-D-glucopyranosyl-D-glucose	R
cellobiose (cellose)	4-β-D-glucopyranosyl-D-glucopyranose	R, NF
gentiobiose (amygdabiose)	6-β-D-glucopyranosyl-D-glucopyranose	R, F[1]
trehalose* (mycose)	1-α-D-glucopyranosyl-α-D-glucopyranoside	NR, F
lactose* (lactobiose)	4-β-D-galactopyranosyl-D-glucopyranose	R, F
melibiose	6-α-D-galactopyranosyl-D-glucopyranose	R, F[1]
sucrose* (saccharose)	1-α-D-glucopyranosyl-β-D-fructofuranose	NR, F
turanose	3-α-D-glucopyranosyl-β-D-fructose	R, NF
xylobiose	4-β-D-xylopyranosyl-β-D-xylose	R

* The structures of these disaccharides are shown in Figure 7.8
R = reducing, N = non-reducing; F= fermented by yeasts; NF=not fermented by yeasts; (1) fermented by bottom fermenting yeasts only.

Table 7.4: Oligosaccharides

cellotriose	β-D-glucopyranosyl-(1,4)-β-D-glucopyranosyl-(1,4)-D-glucose	R
kestose	β-D-fructofuranosyl-(2,6)-β-D-fructofuranosyl(2,1)-α-D-glucopyranoside	NR
isokestose	β-D-fructofuranosyl-(2,6)-β-D-fructofuranosyl(2,1)-α-D-glucopyranoside	NR
neokestose	β-D-fructofuranosyl-(2,1)-β-D-fructofuranosyl(2,1)-α-D-glucopyranoside	NR
laminaritriose	β-D-glucopyranosyl-(1,3-β-D-glucopyranosyl-(1,3-β-D-glucose	R
maltotriose	α-D-glucopyranosyl-(1,4)-α-D-glucopyranosyl-(1,4)-D-glucose	R
isomaltotriose	α-D-glucopyranosyl-(1,6)-α-D-glucopyranosyl-(1,4)-D-glucose	R
melezitose	α-D-glucopyranosyl-(1,3)-β-D-fructofuranosyl-(2,1)-α-D-glucopyranoside	NR
panose	α-D-glucopyranosyl-(1,6)-α-D-glucopyranosyl-(1,4)-D-glucose	R
raffinose	α-D-galactopyranosyl-(1,6)-α-D-glucopyranosyl-(1,2)-β-D-fructofuranoside	NR
stachyose	α-D-galactopyranosyl-(1,6)-α-D-galactopyranosyl-(1,6)-glucopyranosyl-(1,2)-β-D-fructofuranoside	NR
verbascose	α-D-galactopyranosyl-(1,6)-α-D-galactopyranosyl-(1,6)-α-D-galactopyranosyl-(1,6)-α-D-glucopyranosyl-(1,2)-β-D-fructofuranoside	NR

R—reducing, NR = non-reducing.

Table 7.5: Proportions of amylose and amylopectin in different starches

	% amylose	% amylopectin
cassava	17	83
maize	26	74
maize, high amylose	70	30
maize, waxy	1	99
potato	21	79
rice	17	83
wheat	25	75

Table 7.6 Classification of starchy foods based on starch digestibility

type of starch	examples	small intestinal digestion
rapidly digestible	freshly cooked starchy foods	rapid and complete
slowly digestible	raw cereals	slow but complete
resistant—physically inaccessible	partially milled grains and cereals	resistant
resistant granules	raw potato, banana	resistant
retrograded amylose	cooled cooked potato, bread, breakfast cereals	resistant

Source: Cummings & Englyst 1995.

Table 7.7: Percentage of total starch in foods that is rapidly or slowly digestible or resistant

	% of total starch		
	rapid	slow	resistant
white flour	49	48	3
white bread	90	9	1
wholemeal bread	93	7	-
spaghetti, hot	52	41	7
digestive biscuits	77	21	2
cornflakes	94	2	4
shredded wheat	93	6	<1
potato, raw	2	9	81
potato, boiled, hot	96	1	3
potato, boiled, cold	83	11	6

Source: calculated from data reported by Cummings & Englyst 1995.

Table 7.8: The principal types of non-starch polysaccharides in foods

cellulose	linear polymer of up to 10^4 glucose units linked 1 4	insoluble	all plant cell walls
hemicelluloses	heterogeneous branched polymers (50—2000) residues of hexoses, pentoses and uronic acids;	insoluble	most plant cell walls
xylans	xylose polymers, with arabinose and glucuronic acid side-chains	partially soluble	wheat, rye and barley bran
galactomannans	mannose polymers with glucose and galactose side-chains	partially soluble	legumes
xyloglucans	glucose polymers with xylose branches	soluble	associated with cellulose
pectins	polymers of galacturonic acid; partially methylated,; various side chains	soluble	fruit and vegetables (especially under-ripe)
β-glucans	branched polymers of glucose (linked β1→3 and β1→4)	soluble	oats, barley, rye
inulin	polymer of fructose	soluble	artichokes and some other root vegetables
chitin	polymer of amino sugars	insoluble	mushrooms, other fungi, crustacean exoskeletons)
gums	polymers of 1-3 x 10^4 monomer units; various monosaccharides and/or acids; may be methylated or acetylated	soluble	exudates from various plants; some seeds
mucilages	complex polymers; characterised by galacturonic acid; (alginic acid is polymer of mannuronic and galacturonic acid; carageenans are sulphated polymers of galactose)	soluble	seeds, roots, algae

Table 7.9: Heats of combustion of carbohydrates

	kJ /g	kcal /g
pentose monosaccharides	15.6	3.72
hexose monosaccharides	15.6	3.72
dihexose disaccharides	16.5	3.95
trihexoses	16.7	4.00
tetrahexoses	16.9	4.04
pentahexoses	17.0	4.07
polyhexoses (starch)	17.5	4.18
polypentoses	17.6	4.20
polydeoxypentoses	20.6	4.93

Source: Livesey 1992.

Table 7.10: Heats of combustion and net energy yields of sugar alcohols

	heat of combustion		net energy	
	kJ /g	kcal /g	kJ /g	kcal /g
glycerol	18.0	4.30	18	4.3
erythritol	17.2	4.30	0.9	0.2
xylitol	17.0	4.05	>12	>3
sorbitol	16.7	3.99	10—15	2—3.7
mannitol	16.7	3.99	<7	<2
lactitol	17.0	4.06	8.5	2.0
maltitol	17.0	4.06	15.3	3.7
isomalt [1]	17.0	4.06	8.4	2.0

(1) Approximately equimolar mixed disaccharide alcohol, D-glucosyl-α-1,6-D-sorbitol (maltitol, reduced maltose) and D-glucosyl-α-1,6-D-mannitol (reduced palatinose, marketed as Palatinit®).
Source: Livesey 1992.

Table 7.11: Heats of combustion, digestible energy, and net energy of polysaccharides

	heat of combustion		digestible energy		net energy	
	kJ /g	kcal /g	kJ /g	kcal /g	kJ /g	kcal /g
available starch (as starch)	17.5	4.18	17.5	4.2	17.5	4.2
available starch (as monosaccharides)	17.5	4.18	15.7	3.75	15.7	3.75
cellulose	17.5	4.18	0	0	0	0
guar gum	17.5	4.13	12	2.9	8.7	2.1
gum Arabic	17.2	4.11	12	2.9	8.7	2.1
locust bean (carob) gum	17.9	4.28	-	-	-	-
gum karaya	17.2	4.11	2.4	0.6	1.7	0.4
Psyllium gum	-	-	4.0	1.0	2.9	0.7
Beta-fibre®	17.6	4.22	9.1	2.2	6.5	1.6
hydroxypropylmethylcellulose	22.0	5.25	-	-	-	-
polyhexuronic acid	13.1	3.13	-	-	-	-
polymethylhexuronic aid	17.25	4.12	-	-	-	-
pectin (35% methylated)	18.5	3.78	-	-	-	-
soybean oligomers, SOE(1)	16.4	3.91	13	3.1	8.2	2.0
soybean oligomers, SOR(1)	16.8	4.02	13	3.2	8.4	2.0
Polydextrose® (2)	17.0	4.05	-	-	‹10	‹2.5
Neosugar® (3)	16.9	4.03	13	3.2	8.4	2.0
mixed dietary unavailable complex carbohydrates	17.2	4.1	8.4	2.0	6.0	1.5
cereal non-starch polysaccharides	17.5 (16.7—18.5)	4.18 (3.99—4.42)	-	-	-	-
vegetable non-starch polysaccharides	16.8 (16.6—17.9)	4.01 (3.88—4.27)	-	-	-	-
fruit non-starch polysaccharides	16.5 (14.9—17.3)	3.94 (3.56—4.13)	-	-	-	-
wheat bran non-starch polysaccharides	-	-	4.2	1.0	2.9	0.7
apple non-starch polysaccharides	-	-	8.2	2.0	5.8	1.4
carrot non-starch polysaccharides	-	-	8.8	2.1	6.3	1.5
cabbage non-starch polysaccharides	-	-	11	2.6	7.3	1.7

(1) SOE is a water-soluble extract of soya-bean meal, containing more than 95% of the raffinose and stachyose; SOR is a refined product.

(2) Polydextrose® is a synthetic oligosaccharide bulking agent, a random condensation product of glucose and sorbitol in the ratio 9:1

(3) Neosugar® is a mixture of the fructose oligosaccharides (inulin).

Source: Livesey 1992.

Table 7.12: Relative sweetness of sugar, sugar alcohols and other sweeteners

		relative sweetness
sugars	sucrose	1.00
	fructose	1.4
	high-fructose corn syrup[1]	1.0-1.6
	glucose	0.8
	galactose	0.6
	xylose	0.4-0.6
	isomaltulose	0.5
	maltose	0.4
	lactose	0.1-0.3
sugar alcohols	xylitol	1.0
	maltitol	0.6-0.9
	sorbitol	0.5
	mannitol	0.45-0.57
	lactitol	0.3-0.4
intense sweeteners	cyclamate	30-40
	glycyrrhizin	50
	abrusides (saponins from *Abrus precatorius*)	50
	naringin dihydrochalcone	75
	aspartame (β-methylaspartyl-phenylalanine)	180-200
	acesulfame-K	150-200
	dulcin, phyllodulcin	200-300
	stevioside	300
	suosan	350
	sodium saccharin	450
	rebaudioside A	450
	saccharin	300 -550
	sucralose (trichlorosucrose)	600-650
	perillartine	750-2000
	trihalogenated benzamides	1000
	hernandulcin	1000
	neohesperidin dihydrochalcone	1500
	alitame	2000
sweet proteins	miraculin	2500
	monellin	1500-3000
	osladin	3000
	thaumatin	3000-4000

(1) The sweetness of high-fructose syrups depends on the proportion of fructose they contain.

Table 7.13: Glucosinolates in edible plants

trivial name	side chain
glucocapparin	methyl
glucoepidiin	ethyl
glucoputranjivin	isopropyl
glucocochlearin	1-methylpropyl
sinigrin	prop-2-enyl
gluconapin	but-3-enyl
glucobrassicanapin	pent-4-enyl
progoitrin, epiprogoitrin	2-hydroxybut-3-enyl[1]
gluconapoleiferin	2-hydroxypent-4-enyl
glucoiberverin	3-methylthiopropyl
glucoerucin	4-methylthiobutyl
glucoraphasin	4-methylthiobut-3-enyl
glucoberteroin	5-methylthiopentyl
glucoiberin	3-methylsulphinylpropyl
glucoraphanin	4-methylsulphinylbutyl
glucoraphenin	4-methylsulphinylbut-3-enyl
glycoalyssin	5-methylsulphinylpentyl
glucocheirolin	3-methylsulphonylpropyl
glucoerysolin	4-methylsulphonylbutyl
glucotropaeolin	benzyl
gluconasturtiin	2-phenethyl
glucobarbarin, glucosibarin	2-hydroxy-2-phenylethyl[1]
glucolepigramin	3-hydroxybenzyl
sinalbin	4-hydroxybenzyl
glucobrassicin	indolylmethyl
neoglucobrassicin	1-methoxyindolylmethyl
4-hydroxyglucobrassicin	4-hydroxyindolylmethyl
4-methoxyglucobrassicin	4-methoxyindolylmethyl

(1) Two stereoisomers.
Source: from data reported by Nugon-Baudon & Rabot 1994.

Table 7.14: Pharmaceutical preparations of insulin

	time-course of action (h)			
	onset	peak	duration	
short acting	0.5-1	2-5	6-8	soluble insulin
intermediate acting	< 2	4-12	up to 24	biphasic insulin: suspension of crystals of insulin in insulin solution
				biphasic isophane insulin: suspension of insulin complexed with protamine in solution of insulin
				isophane protamine insulin: suspension of insulin-protamine complex
				insulin zinc suspension: suspension of insulin-zinc complex
intermediate / long acting	2-3	6-15	up to 30	insulin zinc suspension, insulin lente: suspension of insulin-zinc complex
long acting	4	10-20	up to 36	crystalline (extended) insulin-zinc suspension, insulin ultralente: crystals of insulin-zinc complex
				insulin protamine zinc: suspension of insulin-zinc-protamine sulphate complex

Table 7.15: Oral hypoglycaemic agents

biguanides	sulphonylureas	other classes
buformin HCl	acetohexamide	glymidine (sulphonamidopyridine)
metformin HCl	carbutamide	glybuzole (benzene sulphonamide)
phenformin HCl	chlorpropamide	midaglizole (benzylpyrimidine)
	glibenclamide	
	gliclazide	
	glipizide	
	glibornuride	
	glipizide	
	gliquidone	
	glisentide	
	glisolamide	
	glisoxepide	
	glyclopyramide	
	glycyclamide	
	metahexamide	
	tolazamide	
	tolbutamide	

Lipids — fats and oils

Fat provides some 40 per cent of the energy intake in developed countries, yielding 37 kJ (9 kcal) per gram. As discussed in section 5.5.2, fat is synthesized in the body as the major reserve of metabolic fuel, either from dietary lipids or from carbohydrates and amino acids surplus to immediate requirements.

Table 8.1 shows the desirable and average intakes of different classes of fat in UK, and Table 8.2 the major sources of fat in the average diet; for reference intakes of mono- and polyunsaturated fatty acids see section 8.1.1.3.

In less developed countries, fat intakes may be considerably lower than 30 per cent of energy. Below about 10 per cent of energy from fat, it is difficult to ingest a sufficient amount of food to meet energy requirements, because of the greater amount of carbohydrate (2.25–fold more) that is required to provide the same energy yield as 1 g of fat, and the absorption of fat-soluble vitamins may be compromized. In addition, dietary fat is important for the following reasons:

(1) it lubricates food in the mouth, assisting chewing and swallowing;

(2) much of the flavour of many foods (especially meats) is in the fat;

(3) two of the fatty acids, linolenic and α-linoleic acids, are dietary essentials, with important functions in cell membranes, and as precursors for the synthesis of prostaglandins and other eicosanoids (see section 8.1.1.3);

(4) the fat-soluble vitamins are present in foods in the fat.

In order to facilitate reduction in total fat intake, and so meet dietary goals (see section 4.2), a number of low-fat bread spreads have been developed as replacements for butter and margarine (see Table 8.3). In most countries the composition of margarine is defined by law, and low-fat spreads may not legally be called margarines. Spreads with fat content down to about 20–25 per cent (compared with 70–82 per cent fat in butter and margarine) are water-in-oil emulsions. Extremely low fat spreads (containing as little as 5 per cent fat) are made using fat substitutes such as Simplesse, a modified protein which has a texture similar to that of fat. A further fat replacer is under development for use in food manufacture: Olestra, a polyacyl sucrose derivative that has properties similar to triacylglycerols, but is not digested, and hence is unabsorbed.

8.1   The chemistry of dietary fats and oils

More than 90 per cent of dietary fat is in the form of triacylglycerols (triglycerides, see section 8.1.1). The remainder is mainly phospholipids (see section 8.1.2), with very much smaller amounts of cholesterol (see section 8.1.3) and other sterols and sterol esters, which are not metabolized as metabolic fuels. Diets also contain small amounts of waxes—esters of fatty acids with higher alcohols; these are not metabolized to any significant extent.

The distinction between oils and fats is based on their melting point; oils are liquids at room temperature (around 20°C), whereas fats are solid. The melting point of a fat depends on the following.

1. The chain length of its constituent fatty acids; the longer the carbon chain, the higher the melting point.

2. The degree of unsaturation of the fatty acids. Unsaturated fatty acids have a lower melting point than saturated fatty acids of the same chain length. In general oils from plants and fish have a higher content of unsaturated fatty acids than fats from animal sources (see Table 8.5).

3. The *cis/trans* isomerism of unsaturated fatty acids (see section 8.1.1.2). *Trans*-isomers have a higher melting point than *cis*-isomers.

8.1.1 Triacylglycerols (triglycerides) and fatty acids

As shown in Fig. 8.1, triacylglycerols (also known as triglycerides) are esters of the trihydric alcohol glycerol with three molecules of fatty acids. The three fatty acids esterified to glycerol may differ; commonly carbon-2 of glycerol is esterified to an unsaturated fatty acid.

Chemically the fatty acids are aliphatic mono-carboxylic acids, with a chain length between 2 and 24 carbon atoms; they may be saturated or unsaturated. Unsaturated fatty acids are divided into mono-unsaturated (only one carbon–carbon double bond in the molecule) and polyunsaturated fatty acids (two or more carbon–carbon double bonds). Figure 8.2 shows the structures of saturated, mono-unsaturated and polyunsaturated C18 fatty acids. The major dietary fatty acids have chain lengths between C12 and C18.

8.1.1.1 Fatty acid nomenclature

Correct chemical nomenclature numbers the carbon atoms of a molecule from the functional group from which the compound is named—i.e. the carboxyl group for fatty acids. However, when considering unsaturated fatty acids this is not a useful convention. Metabolically the unsaturated fatty acids can be classified by the position of the double bond nearest to the methyl group (i.e. furthest from the carboxyl group). This is because, although there are human enzymes that can introduce additional double bonds into fatty acids by dehydrogenation, these desaturase enzymes can only act between the carboxyl group and the most distal double bond; they cannot insert additional double bonds distal to the most distal already present.

Therefore, for nutritional purposes it is usual to name fatty acids by the position of the carbon–carbon double bond most distal from the carboxyl group; in all cases further double bonds are separated from this distal double bond by methylene (–CH$_2$–) bridges, so that in polyunsaturated fatty acids the sequence would be

$$-CH_2-CH=CH-CH_2-CH=CH-CH_2-$$

Three 'families' of unsaturated fatty acids can be distinguished:

(1) with the most distal double bond at carbon-3 from the methyl group, n-3 or ω3 fatty acids;

(2) with the most distal double bond at carbon-6 from the methyl group, n-6 or ω6 fatty acids;

(3) with the most distal double bond at carbon-9 from the methyl group, n-9 or ω9 fatty acids.

Although the trivial names shown in Table 8.4 are widely used, it is common practice to use an abbreviated shorthand notation for the fatty acids, showing the number of carbon atoms, followed by a colon and the number of double bonds, and then the position of the most distal double bond, e.g. n-3, -6 or -9, or ω3, 6, 9. The Greek letter omega (ω) is used to indicate that this is the carbon atom most distal from the α-carbon, to which the carboxyl group is attached. Table 8.5 shows the proportions of saturated, mono- and polyunsaturated fatty acids in a variety of oils and fats.

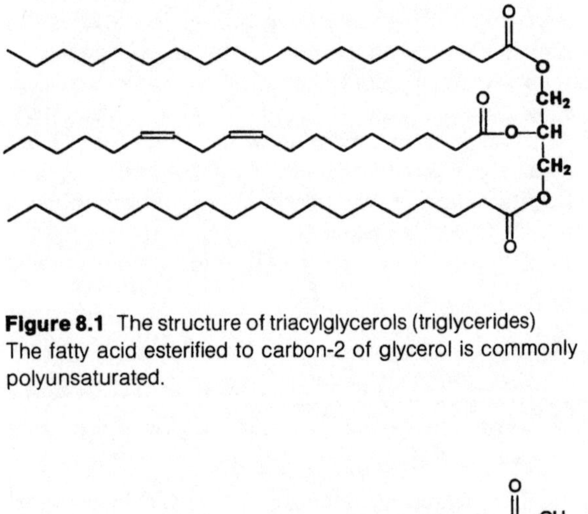

Figure 8.1 The structure of triacylglycerols (triglycerides) The fatty acid esterified to carbon-2 of glycerol is commonly polyunsaturated.

8.1.3 Cis/trans isomerism

Carbon–carbon single bonds permit free rotation within the molecule, whereas double bonds impose rigidity on the structure. Therefore, unsaturated compounds may exist in one of two isomeric forms that are not interconvertible: the *cis*-configuration, in which the carbon chain continues on the same side of the double bond, or the *trans*-configuration, in

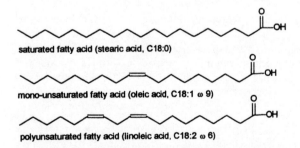

saturated fatty acid (stearic acid, C18:0)

mono-unsaturated fatty acid (oleic acid, C18:1 ω 9)

polyunsaturated fatty acid (linoleic acid, C18:2 ω 6)

Figure 8.2 Saturated and unsaturated fatty acids

which it continues on the opposite side of the double bond (see Fig. 8.3).

The majority of naturally occurring unsaturated fatty acids have the all-*cis* configuration. However, there is significant hydrogenation of unsaturated fatty acids by rumen bacteria in cows and sheep, and during this process there is also isomerization to give rise to *trans* unsaturated fatty acids. These *trans* fatty acids are incorporated into the body and milk fat of ruminants; typically beef, milk and mutton fats contain between 2–9 g of *trans* fatty acids per 100 g fat. The main *trans* fatty acids in these fats are mono-unsaturated, with chain lengths from C14 to C18, especially *trans* ω9, ω10, and ω11 isomers of C18, with *trans*-C18:1 ω11 predominating.

Trans fatty acids also occur as a result of isomerization of fatty acids during catalytic hydrogenation of oils for the manufacture of margarine and cooking fats. Here the mixture of *trans* fatty acids formed depends on both the initial fatty acid composition of the oil being hydrogenated, and also the conditions used for hydrogenation; again the main products are *trans* ω9, ω10 and ω11 isomers of C18:1. However, *trans* isomers of polyunsaturated fatty acids also occur in varying amounts (British Nutrition Foundation 1995).

8.1.1.2.1 Possible hazards of dietary *trans* fatty acids

There are reports in the literature that the consumption of *trans* fatty acids may increase the risk of coronary heart disease—and also contradictory reports. A Task Force of the British Nutrition Foundation examined the evidence of possible hazards of high intakes of *trans* fatty acids. (British Nutrition Foundation 1995). They reported that average intake of *trans* fatty acids in UK is about 4–6 g/day (6 per cent of total dietary fat, or 2 per cent of energy intake), with a 95 per cent range of 2–12 g/day; information from other countries is limited, but in USA such data as are available suggest slightly higher intakes. The main sources of *trans* fatty acids are shown in Tables 8.6.

From such evidence as is available, it can be calculated that for each 1 per cent increase in dietary energy from *trans* fatty acids there will be a 0.9 per cent increase in low density lipoprotein cholesterol and a 1.13 per cent decrease in high density lipoprotein cholesterol—both undesirable effects (see section 8.3.4), but of considerably less importance than the need to reduce saturated fatty acid intake. The main conclusion of the British Nutrition Foundation Report was that intakes of *trans* fatty acids should not increase above the present average of about 2 per cent of energy.

In general the digestion, absorption and metabolism of *trans* fatty acids is comparable to that of the *cis* isomers, although at high levels of intake there is some impairment of the metabolism of essential fatty acids (see section 8.1.1.3). At adequate intakes of essential fatty acids this is unlikely to be significant, and studies in experimental animals show no adverse effects of *trans* fatty acids. Epidemiological studies do not show any clear evidence of hazards of *trans* fatty acid intake.

For labelling purposes, *trans* fatty acids are included with total fat, but since they do not meet the definitions of saturated, mono-unsaturated or polyunsaturated fatty acids, they are not included in the sub-categories that are used in more complete nutritional labelling (see section 4.3).

8.1.1.3 Essential fatty acids: requirements and desirable levels of intake

There is an absolute requirement for a dietary source of ω3 and ω6 pufa, because of their role in membranes, and also as precursors for the prostaglandins and other eicosanoids. The two parent compounds, which are considered to be dietary essentials, are linoleic acid (C18:2 ω6) and α-linolenic acid (C18:3 ω3). These two can undergo chain elongation and further desaturation to yield the precursors of the two families of prostaglandins shown in Figs 8.4 and 8.5: arachidonic acid C20:4 ω6) and docosahexaenoic acid (C22:6 ω3) respectively. The pattern of eicosanoids formed is tissue specific.

The nomenclature of the prostaglandins derives in part from the chemistry of their synthesis (prostaglandins A and B are synthesized using acid and base catalysis respectively), and their solubility in ether (prostaglandin E) or phosphate buffer

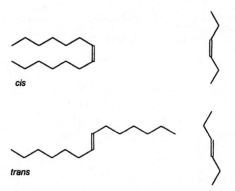

cis

trans

Figure 8.3 *Cis- / trans-isomerism of fatty acids*

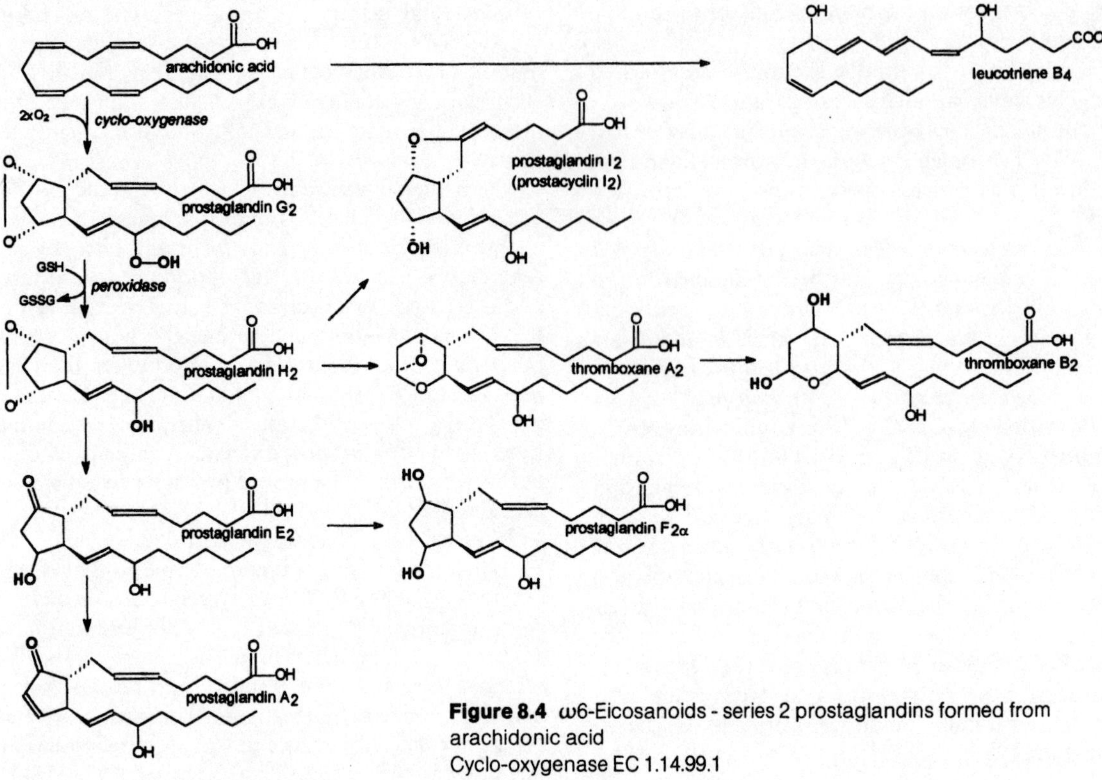

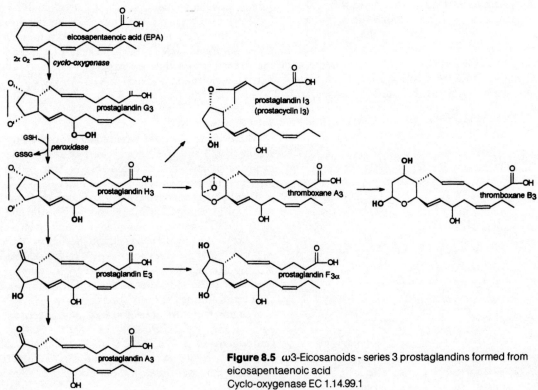

arachidonic acid

2×O₂   cyclo-oxygenase

prostaglandin G₂

GSH
GSSG   peroxidase

prostaglandin H₂

prostaglandin E₂

prostaglandin A₂

leucotriene B₄

prostaglandin I₂ (prostacyclin I₂)

thromboxane A₂

thromboxane B₂

prostaglandin F₂ₐ

Figure 8.4 ω6-Eicosanoids - series 2 prostaglandins formed from arachidonic acid
Cyclo-oxygenase EC 1.14.99.1

eicosapentaenoic acid (EPA)

2× O₂   cyclo-oxygenase

prostaglandin G₃

GSH
GSSG   peroxidase

prostaglandin H₃

prostaglandin E₃

prostaglandin A₃

prostaglandin I₃ (prostacyclin I₃)

thromboxane A₃

thromboxane B₃

prostaglandin F₃ₐ

Figure 8.5 ω3-Eicosanoids - series 3 prostaglandins formed from eicosapentaenoic acid
Cyclo-oxygenase EC 1.14.99.1

(prostaglandin F). The remainder follow in alphabetical order of their discovery after prostaglandin F. The subscript numbers indicate the number of double bonds in the side chain, and where appropriate α or β to indicate the orientation of the ring hydroxyl group.

There is no requirement for a dietary source of the longer chain pufa, but they are potentially desirable in the diet, since their formation from linoleic or linolenic acids is a rate-limiting step. Because the long-chain ω3 and ω6 pufa are mutually competitive for cyclo-oxygenase, increased intakes of ω3 pufa increase the proportions of series 3 prostaglandins and other eicosanoids that are formed, with potentially beneficial effects on blood coagulation; as shown in Table 8.7, the two families of eicosanoids have different effects in different tissues.

Clinical signs of deficiency (growth failure and skin lesions) have been observed in infants fed on diets providing less than 1 per cent of energy as linoleic acid (Hansen *et al.* 1947); there is little evidence on which to base requirements of adults for pufa. In experimental animals maintained on pufa-deficient diets there is an increase in the circulating concentration of ω9 trienoic acids (especially C20:3 ω9), formed by chain elongation and desaturation of oleic acid. It has been suggested that an increase in the ratio of C20:3 ω9 to C20:4 ω6 (the triene:tetraene ratio) may provide an index of inadequate pufa intake in human beings. On this basis the requirement for ω6 pufa is about 1 per cent of energy intake, and a desirable level of intake is 4 per cent of energy (Holman 1971; Sinclair 1982).

The EU estimated average requirement for ω6 pufa is 1 per cent of energy intake (and a population reference intake of 2 per cent of energy), and for ω3 pufa 0.2 per cent of energy (PRI 0.5 per cent of energy). Prudent upper limits of intake are 5 per cent of energy from ω3 pufa or 15 per cent of energy from total pufa (Scientific Committee for Food 1993); the UK Department of Health (1991) report on dietary reference values noted that there was little evidence of undesirable effects of high intakes of pufa, but suggested that the total intake should not exceed 10 per cent of energy.

The UK Reference Nutrient Intakes for fats (Department of Health 1991) are based on effects on serum cholesterol, rather than prevention of deficiency: 10 per cent of energy should be from saturated fats, 6 per cent from pufa (a mixture of ω3 and ω6 pufa) and 12 per cent from mono-unsaturated fatty acids (see Table 8.1). At least 1 per cent of energy should be from linoleic acid and 0.2 per cent from α-linolenic acid.

8.1.2 Phospholipids

The other major class of dietary lipids, comprising about 10 per cent of total fat intake, is the phospholipids. As shown in Fig. 8.6, phospholipids are 2,3–diacylglycerol esters with phosphate esterified at carbon-1 of the glycerol, and a hydrophilic compound esterified to the phosphate. This may be one of a number of compounds, including the amino acid serine, its decarboxylated derivative ethanolamine, and N-trimethylethanolamine (choline), as well as inositol, mannose, glycerol, and aminoacylglycerol derivatives.

The unsubstituted 2,3–diacylglycerol phosphate is known as a phosphatidic acid, and phospholipids are then named as phosphatidyl derivatives of the substituent esterified to the phosphate. Phosphatidylcholine is also known as lecithin, a trivial name that causes some confusion, since a relatively crude mixture of phospholipids extracted from eggs, soybeans, groundnuts, etc., and used as an emulsifying agent in food processing (see section 26.2.6) is also known as lecithin. Phosphatidylcholine is the major, but far from the only, phospholipid present in 'commercial lecithin'.

Phospholipids are amphiphilic, with a hydrophobic 'tail' provided by the two acyl groups, and a

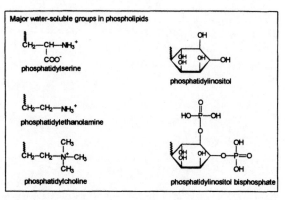

Figure 8.6 The structure of phospholipids

hydrophilic 'head' provided by the phosphate ester. They are thus able to emulsify lipids in aqueous media (hence their use as emulsifying agents), and they form the major part of the lipid bilayer that makes up biological membranes.

Phosphatidylinositol in membranes has a major function in signalling to the intracellular compartment in response to the binding of hormones, etc. to cell membrane receptors—the process of signal transduction. Phosphatidylinositol in the membrane undergoes two phosphorylations to yield phosphatidylinositol bisphosphate. In response to hormone binding to the receptor, an intra-membrane phospholipase is activated which hydrolyses phosphatidylinositol bisphosphate to inositol triphosphate and diacylglycerol. Both of these enter the cell and act as second messengers to the hormone.

The sphingolipids are a group of functionally important phospholipids in membranes; the most abundant is the choline derivative, sphingomyelin. Instead of a diacylglycerol core, as for other phospholipids, the sphingolipids have a single fatty acid and the phosphate esterified to the C-17 dihydroxyamine, sphingosine.

8.1.3 Cholesterol

Cholesterol (see Fig. 8.7) is important both as a component of membrane lipids, and also as the precursor of the steroid hormones. As shown in Table 8.1, average intakes are 280 (women)–390 (men) mg /day; in addition to dietary cholesterol, there is considerable enterohepatic cycling of cholesterol, and as much as 2

g/day is secreted in the bile (see section 8.2.3), almost all of which is reabsorbed in the small intestine.

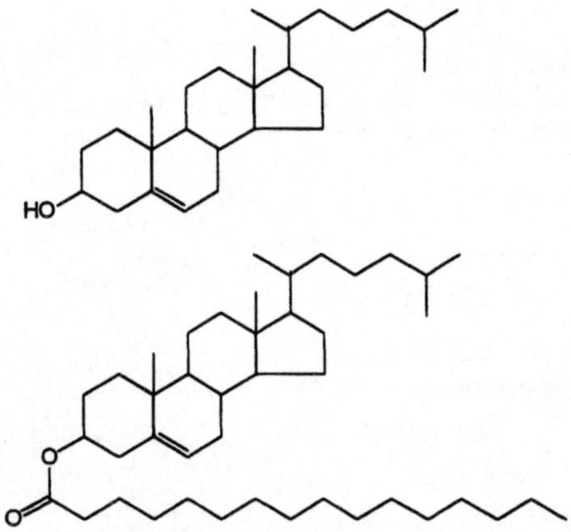

There is no requirement for preformed cholesterol in the diet, since it can readily be synthesized from acetyl CoA. The rate-limiting (controlling) enzyme of cholesterol biosynthesis is hydroxymethylglutaryl CoA (HMG-CoA) reductase (EC 1.1.1.34, 1.1.1.88); as the dietary intake of cholesterol increases, so the activity of this enzyme in the liver is reduced. Normally there is little or no effect of increased dietary cholesterol on plasma cholesterol (see section 8.3.4). Nevertheless, many foods are labelled with their cholesterol content, or make claims of being low in cholesterol. While the cholesterol content of the food is probably unimportant, it does act as a good marker of the presence of saturated fatty acids, since cholesterol is found almost exclusively in animal fats that are also relatively rich in saturated, rather than unsaturated, fatty acids. As discussed in section 8.3.4, inhibitors of HMG-CoA reductase are used clinically to treat hypercholesterolaemia.

8.2   Digestion and absorption of fats

Triacylglycerols are hydrolysed by lipases (see Table 8.8) to yield free fatty acids and, successively, 2,3–diacylglycerol and 2–mono-acylglycerol, which is hydrolysed to glycerol and free fatty acid by esterase activity (see Fig. 8.8). Lipases are secreted by the tongue and in gastric and pancreatic juices; phospholipase is secreted in the pancreatic juice. They act at the oil–water interface of emulsified lipid droplets. In the small intestine both the bile salts (see section 8.2.3) and the products of lipase and phospholipase action (free fatty acids, diacyl- and mono-acylglycerols and lysophospholipids) aid the progressive emulsification of dietary lipids, until the droplets (containing such non-polar lipids as cholesterol, cholesteryl esters, carotenes and the fat-soluble vitamins) are small enough for absorption into the intestinal mucosal cells.

8.2.1 Lingual and gastric lipase

Lipases are secreted both by the serous glands (von Ebner glands) of the tongue (lingual lipase) and also by the gastric parietal (chief) cells. Both of these enzymes act in the stomach; they are especially important in infant nutrition, since they are capable of penetrating into the globules of milk fat. Adults with alcoholic exocrine pancreatic insufficiency, who secrete little or no pancreatic lipase, nevertheless

Figure 8.7 Cholesterol (above) and cholesteryl palmitate (below)

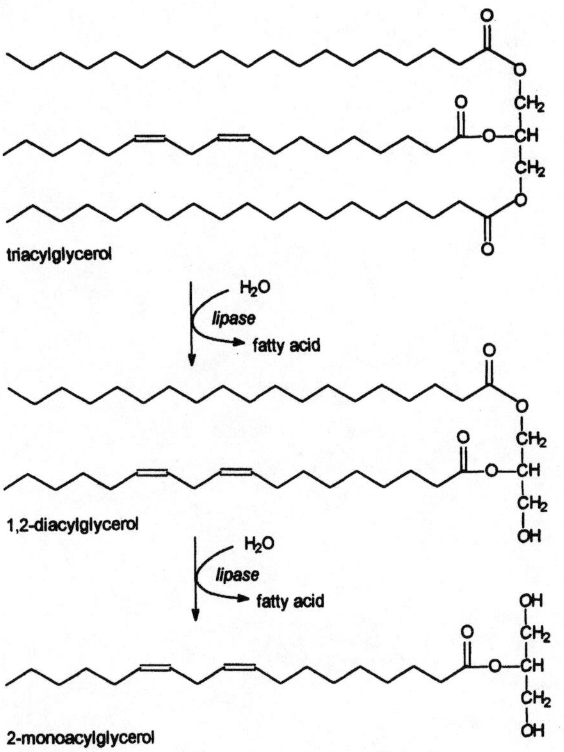

Figure 8.8 Hydrolysis of triacylglycerol by lipase
See Table 8.8 for the classification of intestinal lipases

absorb 50 per cent or more of dietary lipid; both in these patients and in patients with cystic fibrosis, the activity of lingual and gastric lipases continues in the duodenum (Abrams *et al.* 1987; Hamosh 1990).

In response to a test meal containing coarsely emulsified fat, unemulsified lipids (droplets > 100 μm in diameter) represent only a minor proportion of the total gastric fat, and a significant proportion of large droplets (70–100 μm diameter) disappears within the first hour of digestion, leaving finely emulsified droplets (1–10 μm diameter), which are relatively rich in free fatty acids and diacyl- and mono-acylglycerols. As the concentration of free fatty acids in the droplets increases, so the activity of gastric lipase is inhibited (Bernback *et al.* 1989).

8.2.2 Pancreatic lipases

As secreted, pancreatic lipase is catalytically inactive; a region of the polypeptide chain (called the lid) overlies the catalytic site, which is only exposed when the enzyme binds to the oil–water interface of a lipid droplet (Jennens and Lowe 1994). Unlike gastric lipase, which has a hydrophobic lipid-binding tail, pancreatic lipase does not bind to lipid droplets unless it is complexed with a second pancreatic protein, colipase (van Tilbeurgh *et al.* 1992). Colipase is secreted as an inactive precursor protein, procolipase, which is activated in the duodenal lumen by tryptic cleavage (Larsson and Erlanson-Albertsson 1991).

The prior action of lingual and gastric lipases is essential for the activity of pancreatic lipase-colipase; long-chain fatty acids liberated by these two lipases not only aid the emulsification of the lipid droplets, but also permit the binding of lipase-colipase to the droplets (Bernback *et al.* 1989).

Pancreatic lipase is inhibited by the bile salts (see section 8.2.3). However, infants secrete a small amount of a bile salt-stimulated lipase in pancreatic juice, and there is a similar enzyme, in greater amounts, in breast milk. The main activity of this enzyme is to hydrolyse the mono-acylglycerols formed by pancreatic lipase, although it also acts on cholesteryl esters and esters of fat-soluble vitamins. More importantly, bile salt-dependent lipase has considerably greater activity towards long-chain polyunsaturated fatty acyl esters than does pancreatic lipase-colipase (Chen *et al.* 1994; Hernell and Blackberg 1994).

Lipases hydrolyse the esters at carbons-1 and -3 of triacylglycerols; by contrast, phospholipase A2, secreted by the pancreas, hydrolyses the ester at carbon-2 of a phospholipid, yielding a free fatty acid and the corresponding lysophospholipid, with a free hydroxyl group at carbon-2 of the glycerol moiety. Lysophospholipids are potent emulsifying agents; indeed the name derives from their potency in lysing cell membranes *in vitro*.

Pancreatic juice also contains cholesteryl esterase, which hydrolyses cholesteryl esters to cholesterol and free fatty acids.

8.2.3 Bile salts

The bile acids, cholic and chenodeoxycholic acids, are synthesized in the liver by side-chain oxidation and ring hydroxylation of cholesterol, as shown in Fig. 8.9. Before secretion they are conjugated with either glycine or taurine, yielding the bile salts, glycocholic, taurocholic, glycochenodeoxycholic, and taurochenodeoxycholic acids.

Bile salts function to emulsify lipid droplets, and thus increase the surface area for action of lipase-colipase. However, lipase-colipase is significantly inhibited by bile salts. Probably their more important function is in the formation of micelles of fatty acids, mono-acylglycerols and lysophospholipids that dis-

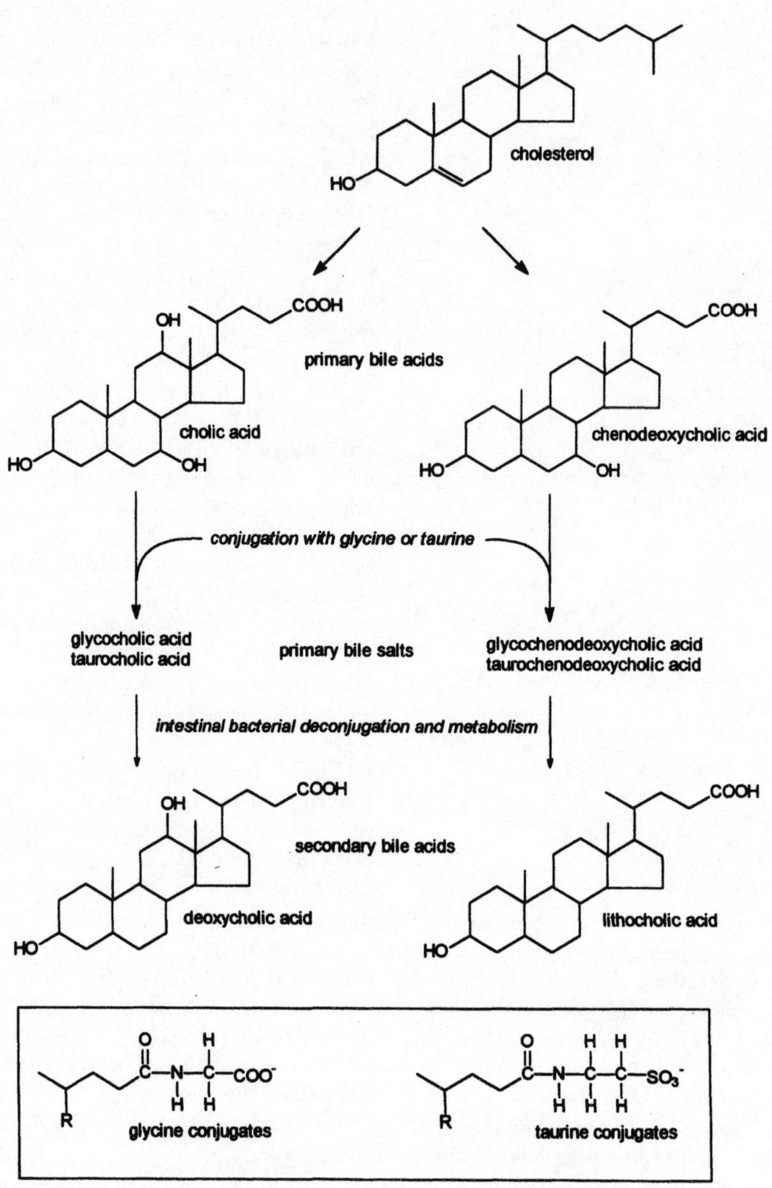

Figure 8.9 The bile salts

solve non-polar lipids (cholesterol and other sterols, carotenoids and vitamins A, D, E, and K), so permitting their absorption.

Bile salts that are not reabsorbed together with lipid micelles in the ileum are susceptible to metabolism by colon bacteria, which hydrolyse the conjugates, and catalyse ring dehydroxylation of cholic acid to deoxycholic acid, and of chenodeoxycholic to lithocholic acid and ursodeoxycholic acid. These secondary bile acids, as well as free cholic and che-

nodoxycholic acids, are reabsorbed together with lipids, and are reconjugated with glycine or taurine, and resecreted. The total secretion of bile salts is some 30 g/day, whereas faecal output of bile salts and steroids is only 0.2–1.0 g/day.

8.2.3.1 Gallstones
More than 80 per cent of all gallstones are composed mainly of cholesterol, and the prevalence of gallstones in industrialized countries is about 10 per

cent, with higher incidence associated with increasing age, a higher incidence in women than men, and a very considerable increase in incidence with obesity (see section 11.2.1).

As shown in Tables 8.9 and 8.10, bile consists mainly of bile salts, phospholipids, and cholesterol. Under normal conditions the concentration of cholesterol relative to the polar bile salts and phospholipids is such that cholesterol is near its limit of solubility. Under conditions where the cholesterol concentration is increased, or that of bile salts and phospholipids is decreased, cholesterol crystallizes in the gall bladder and bile duct—the formation of gallstones (cholelithiasis). The solubility of cholesterol in bile is frequently expressed as the lithogenicity index—the ratio of the cholesterol content of bile to the maximum solubility of cholesterol at the concentration of bile salts and phospholipids present (Metzger *et al.* 1972; Thomas and Hoffman 1973).

Although supersaturation of bile with cholesterol is a necessary condition for the development of gallstones, it is not sufficient; a variety of other factors, including the presence of nucleating compounds that permit crystallization, and the rate of bile secretion, affect the formation of stones (Bouchier 1983; Paumgartner and Sauerbruch 1991).

8.3 Plasma lipoproteins

Lipids are transported in plasma complexed with proteins; there are three major classes of lipoproteins.

1. Chylomicrons, formed in the intestinal mucosa and circulating as a source of triacylglycerol in the fed state.

2. Very low density lipoproteins, formed in the liver and circulating as a source of cholesterol and triacylglycerol for extra-hepatic tissues.

3. High density lipoproteins, synthesized in liver (and also small intestine), which transport cholesterol from tissues to the liver.

In addition, in the fasting state free fatty acids released from adipose tissue circulate bound to serum albumin.

As shown in Table 8.11, the plasma lipoproteins are classified according to their density, which depends on the relative proportions of protein and lipid. They contain different apo-lipoproteins (see Table 8.12), and hence differ in their electrophoretic mobility. This means that quantitation of lipoproteins can be achieved by either centrifugation or electrophoresis of plasma samples.

8.3.1 Chylomicrons

The intestinal micelles of bile salts, free fatty acids, mono-acylglycerols, lysophospholipids and nonpolar lipids enter the intestinal mucosal cells, where acylglycerol lipase and lysophospholipase (see Table 8.8) complete the hydrolysis to yield glycerol and free fatty acids. Medium-chain fatty acids (C10–12) enter the bloodstream directly, bound to serum albumin; long-chain fatty acids are re-esterified to glycerol phosphate to form triacylglycerols with a fatty acid pattern that only partially reflects that of the dietary lipids. This resynthesis of triacylglycerols is an energy-expensive process, making a significant contribution to diet-induced thermogenesis (see section 5.3.3); there is consumption of 2 mol of ATP per mol of fatty acid esterified. Much of the cholesterol that is absorbed in the lipid micelles is esterified to cholesteryl esters, catalysed by acyl CoA : cholesterol acyltransferase in the intestinal mucosa, although chylomicrons also contain some free cholesterol.

The newly synthesized triacylglycerols are then assembled into chylomicrons, which are transported into the lymphatic system of the ileum, entering the bloodstream (subclavian vein) at the thoracic duct. Thus, unlike the products of protein and carbohydrate metabolism, which are absorbed into the hepatic portal vein, and hence are subject to regulation by the liver, the products of fat digestion enter the peripheral circulation unregulated by the liver. The apolipoproteins C-II (which activates lipoprotein lipase, permitting utilization of chylomicron triacylglycerol), C-III (which activates lecithin-cholesterol acyltransferase) and E (which binds to hepatic receptors), are added to the chylomicrons from high density lipoproteins as they enter the bloodstream at the thoracic duct.

In the fed state (the only conditions under which chylomicrons are normally present in the circulation), the major fate of triacylglycerol is uptake into adipose tissue—again the process is ATP expensive, and contributes to diet-induced thermogenesis, since uptake is by hydrolysis to free fatty acids, catalysed by lipoprotein lipase (EC 3.1.1.34), followed by re-esterification intracellularly. Other tissues (especially cardiac and skeletal muscle and lactating mammary gland) also have lipoprotein lipase, phospholipases and cholesteryl esterases, and can therefore take up such lipids as are required, or as are presented to them by the chylomicrons.

The triacylglycerol-depleted chylomicron remnants are taken up by the liver; apo-lipoprotein E binds to a liver cell surface receptor, and the complex undergoes endocytosis, followed by hydrolysis of both the residual lipids and the apo-lipoproteins. The liver receptor for chylomicron remnants is distinct from the low density lipoprotein receptor (see section 8.3.2). Chylomicrons begin to appear in plasma about 60 min after a fatty meal, and are normally completely cleared within 6–8 hours (Sethi *et al.* 1993).

Medium-chain triacylglycerols (with C8–10 fatty acids) can be hydrolysed by limited amounts of lipase, and their fatty acids can be absorbed in the absence of bile salts, directly into the portal blood, and hence the liver. Preparations of medium-chain triacylglycerols (commonly from coconut oil) are used as a dietary source of energy in patients suffering from compromized fat digestion and absorption.

8.3.2 Very low density lipoproteins (VLDL) and low density lipoproteins (LDL)

VLDL are synthesized in the liver, and contain endogenously synthesized triacylglycerol, cholesterol, cholesteryl esters, and phospholipids. Like chylomicrons, VLDL contain apo-lipoprotein C-II which activates cell surface lipoprotein lipase (thus permitting tissue uptake of free fatty acids), as well as apo-lipoproteins C-I and C-III, which activate lecithin-cholesterol acyltransferase.

As the VLDL particles are progressively depleted of lipid in the circulation they transfer their apo-lipoproteins C-I and C-II to circulating high density lipoproteins, forming intermediate density lipoproteins (IDL). IDL take up cholesterol esters from high density lipoproteins (HDL) by means of the HDL cholesterol ester transfer protein, and lose apolipoproteins C-III and E, becoming low density lipoproteins (LDL).

LDL are cleared from the circulation by receptor-mediated uptake into the liver; as with chylomicron remnants, the presence of exposed apo-lipoprotein E on the surface of the LDL particle is required for receptor binding and endocytosis (Brown and Goldstein 1986). The main underlying cause of hypercholesterolaemia (see section 8.3.4) is a failure of this receptor-mediated endocytosis of LDL.

8.3.3 High density lipoproteins (HDL); reverse cholesterol transport

The rate of uptake of cholesterol by peripheral tissues from LDL is considerably greater than normal tissue cholesterol requirements; because most tissues are unable to catalyse oxidation of cholesterol, it must be returned to the liver for catabolism. This is the function of HDL.

HDL are secreted into the circulation from the liver, almost entirely devoid of cholesteryl esters. They take up cholesterol from peripheral tissues by the action of lecithin cholesterol acyltransferase on the HDL surface, forming cholesteryl esters at the expense of HDL phosphatidylcholine. Much of the HDL cholesteryl ester is transferred to chylomicron remnants and LDL for receptor-mediated uptake into the liver; HDL have an active cholesteryl ester transfer protein (Sethi *et al.* 1993).

8.3.4 Hypercholesterolaemia and hyperlipidaemias

One of the main risk factors for the development of atherosclerosis and cardiovascular disease is an elevated plasma cholesterol concentration (see Table 8.13). In fact, the correlation is with low density lipoproteins (LDL cholesterol), and high concentrations of HDL cholesterol are associated with reduced incidence of atherosclerosis and cardiovascular disease. In popular parlance, LDL cholesterol is 'bad' and HDL cholesterol is 'good' or protective.

The main causes of elevated LDL cholesterol are increased synthesis and secretion of LDL, and impaired clearance, as a result of either low activity of the hepatic LDL receptor, or poor affinity of some variants of apo-lipoprotein E for the LDL receptor. Since this latter is genetically determined, this explains at least part of the (important) hereditary element in atherosclerosis and cardiovascular disease.

Whatever the underlying mechanism, the result of increased and prolonged circulation of LDL is that polyunsaturated fatty acids undergo increased non-enzymic oxidation in the circulation; oxidized lipids are taken up by macrophages, and stimulate their transformation into foam cells, which infiltrate the blood vessel endothelium, permitting and stimulating the deposition of atherosclerotic plaque.

The most common cause of hyperlipidaemia is a high intake of saturated fatty acids. Table 8.14 shows the WHO (Fredrickson) classification of hyperlipidaemias, and the conditions in which they occur as secondary problems, while Table 8.15 shows the main types of primary hyperlipidaemia.

Modest elevation of plasma lipoproteins is treated by (fairly severe) restriction of saturated fat intake, and possibly increased intake of mono- and polyunsaturated fats, which lower the levels of LDL cholesterol and triacylglycerol. In addition, a high fibre diet (see section 7.3.2) also lowers LDL cholesterol. The main effect is probably physical adsorption of bile salts and cholesterol in the gut lumen, hence reducing their enterohepatic cycling (see section 8.2.3), and requiring increased utilization of endogenous or dietary cholesterol for bile salt synthesis. The effect of high and low fibre diets on bile composition is shown in Table 8.10.

For more serious hyperlipidaemias, a variety of drug treatments are available (see Table 8.16).

Ion exchange resins function in the same way as high fibre diets, albeit with considerably greater avidity for bile salts, and are thus useful for treatment of hypercholesterolaemia. Relatively large amounts of the granular resins have to be taken to have any significant effect. A more recent development for the treatment of hypercholesterolaemia has been the development of inhibitors of HMG-CoA reductase—the rate-limiting enzyme of endogenous cholesterol synthesis.

Nicotinic acid, at intakes considerably greater than requirement levels (see section 19.7), causes a significant lowering of plasma triacylglycerol. However, at the doses that are effective it causes an unpleasant vasodilatation and flushing, with skin irritation, and may cause liver damage; as shown in Table 8.16, a number of nicotinic acid analogues that have less severe side-effects have been developed. The other treatment for hypertriglyceridaemia is use of clofibrate, or one of the other fibric acid derivatives; two compounds, etofibrate and nicofibrate, are combined nicotinic acid and fibric acid derivatives.

A number of other, miscellaneous, compounds also have useful hypolipidaemic action; dextrothyroxine is a thyroid hormone analogue (see section 25.14.3) which was developed because of the occurrence of secondary hyperlipidaemia in hypothyroidism. Sitosterol is a plant sterol which has some hypocholesterolaemic action, probably acting to down-regulate cholesterol synthesis by inhibiting HMG-CoA reductase.

Further reading

British Nutrition Foundation (1995). *Trans fatty acids*, Report of the British Nutrition Foundation Task Force, British Nutrition Foundation, London.

Lowe, M.E. (1994). Pancreatic triglyceride lipase and colipase: insights into dietary fat digestion. *Gastroenterology* 107, 1524–36.

Sardesai V.M. (1992). Biochemical and nutritional aspects of polyunsaturated fatty acids. *Journal of Nutritional Biochemistry*, 3, 154–67.

Sardesai, V.M. (1992). Biochemical and nutritional aspects of eicosanoids. *Journal of Nutritional Biochemistry*, 3, 562–79.

Simopolous, A.P. (1991). Omega-3 fatty acids in health, and in growth and development. *American Journal of Clinical Nutrition*, 54, 438–63.

Sinclair, H.M. (1982). Essential fatty acids (vitamin F), In *Vitamins in Medicine* (ed. B.M. Barker and D.A. Bender), Vol, II, 4th edn, chapter 5, pp. 168–98. Heinemann Medical, London.

Table 8.1: Fat intake in average UK diets as percentage of food energy (i.e. excluding energy from alcohol)

	average, men		average, women		desirable
	mean	95% range	mean	95% range	
total fat	40.4	30.6-49.5	40.3	27.7-50.1	30
saturated fatty acids	16.5	10.6-22.4	17.0	10.7-23.4	10
mono-unsaturated fatty acids	12.4	8.76-16.6	12.2	8.39-16.4	12
ω-6 pufa	5.44	2.57-10.35	5.27	2.47-10.27	total pufa 6
ω-3 pufa	0.78	0.41-1.46	0.75	0.41-1.45	
trans-fatty acids	2.19	1.06-4.08	2.16	0.92-3.91	no more than 2
P:S ratio	0.40	0.16-0.87	0.38	0.15-0.85	-
cholesterol (mg /d)	390	151-741	280	98-511	300

Source: Gregory *et al.* 1990.

Table 8.2: Percent of intake of fat and fatty acids from various sources in average UK diets

	total fat	saturated	mufa	ω-6 pufa	ω-3 pufa	*trans*
cereal products	19	18	18	22	17	27
biscuits	4	4	3	-	-	7
cakes and pastries	6	6	6	6	4	14
puddings and ice-cream	3	4	-	-	-	3
white bread	-	-	-	4	-	-
pasta, rice, grains	-	-	3	-	4	-
wholemeal /brown bread	-	-	-	4	-	-
milk products	15	23	12	2	6	10
whole milk	7	11	6	-	-	4
cheese	6	9	5	-	-	4
eggs	4	3	5	4	2	2
fat spreads	16	17	11	20	15	30
butter	6	10	4	-	3	5
pufa margarine	4	-	-	13	4	5
low fat spreads	1	-	-	-	-	-
other margarines and spreads	6	-	-	-	-	17
meat	24	23	31	17	19	18
bacon and ham	4	3	5	2	-	-
beef and veal	4	4	5	2	-	-
chicken and turkey	-	-	-	-	4	-
meat pies	5	4	5	3	-	7
fish	3	2	3	4	14	1
oily fish	-	-	-	-	7	-
vegetables	11	6	12	24	22	6
roast and fried potatoes	5	-	6	12	13	-
savoury snacks	2	-	2	5	-	-
fruit and nuts	1	0	1	2	1	0
confectionery	3	4	2	1	1	3

Source: Gregory *et al.* 1990.

Table 8.3: Types of fat spreads

		% fat
butter	traditional churned butter, sometimes called sweetcream butter. may be salted or unsalted	80-82
lactic butter	made from cream with the addition of lactic bacteria to give a sharp taste. unsalted or lightly salted	80-82
hard margarine	hardened marine, animal, and vegetable oils, mainly used for baking	80
soft margarine	mainly vegetable oils, spreads easily	80
pufa margarine	mainly sunflower, corn or soya bean oils, for a high content of poly-unsaturated fatty acids	70-80
dairy spreads	blended cream and vegetable oil, spreads easily	72-75
reduced fat spreads	mainly vegetable oils, may be some animal or dairy fat	60-70
low fat spreads	may contain dairy fat and vegetable oils; not suitable for cooking use	37-40
very low fat spreads	may contain dairy fat and vegetable oils; not suitable for cooking use	20-25
extremely low fat spreads	made with fat substitutes (e.g. Simplesse, a modified protein) to replace almost all of the fat	5

Table 8.4: The fatty acids found in foods

trivial name	systematic name	shorthand code	M_r	mp (°C)	heat of combustion[1] /mmol kJ	/mmol kcal	/g kJ	/g kcal
acetic	ethanoic	C2:0	60.1	16.7	0.885	0.211	53	12.7
propionic	propanoic	C3:0	74.1	-22.0	1.54	0.367	114	27.2
butyric	butanoic	C4:0	88.1	-7.9	2.19	0.523	193	46.1
caproic	hexanoic	C6:0	116.2	-3.4	3.50	0.835	406	97.0
caprylic	octanoic	C8:0	144.2	16.7	4.80	1.147	692	165
capric	decanoic	C10:0	172.3	31.6	6.11	1.459	1052	251
lauric	dodecanoic	C12:0	200.3	44.2	7.42	1.771	1486	355
myristic	tetradecanoic	C14:0	228.4	53.9	8.72	2.083	1992	476
palmitic	hexadecanoic	C16:0	256.4	63.1	10.03	2.395	2752	614
stearic	octadecanoic	C18:0	284.4	69.6	11.33	2.707	3222	769
arachidic	eicosanoic	C20:0	312.5	76.5	12.64	3.019	3950	943
behenic	docosanoic	C22:0	340.6	81.5	13.95	3.331	4751	1135
lignoceric	tetracosanoic	C24:0	368.6	86.0	15.25	3.643	5621	1343
palmitoleic	9-hexadecenoic	C16:1 ω6	254.4	0.0	9.86	2.356	2508	599
oleic	9-octadecenoic	C18:1 ω9	282.5	13.4	11.17	2.668	3155	754
elaidic	*trans*-9-octadecenoic	*trans*-C18:1 ω9	282.5	44.5	11.17	2.668	3155	754
vaccenic	11-octadecenoic	C18:1 ω9	282.5	44.0	11.17	2.668	3155	754
petroselinic	6-octadecenoic	C18:1 ω6	282.5	32-33	11.17	2.668	3155	754
gadoleic	9-eicosaenoic	C20:1 ω9	310.5	24.0-24.5	12.47	2.980	3872	925
erucic	13-docosenoic	C22:1 ω9	338.6	33.5	13.78	3.292	4666	1115
brassidic	*trans*-13-docosenoic	*trans*-C22:1 ω9	338.6	60.0	13.78	3.292	4666	1115
cetoleic	11-docosenoic	C22:1 ω11	338.6	32.5-33.0	13.78	3.292	4666	1115
nervonic	15-tetracosenoic	C24:1 ω9	366.6	39.0	15.09	3.604	5532	1322
α-linolenic	9,12,15-octadecatrienoic	C18:3 ω3	278.4	-16.0	10.84	2.588	3018	721
parinaric	9,11,13,15-octadecatetraenoic	C18:4 ω3	276.4	95-96	10.67	2.549	2949	705
eicosapentaenoic (timnodonic)	5,8,11,14,17-eicosapentaenoic	C20:5 ω3	302.5	-	11.81	2.821	3573	853
docosapentaenoic (clupanodonic)	7,10,13,16,19-docosapentaenoic	C22:5 ω3	334.6	-	13.12	3.133	4390	1048
docosahexaenoic (cervonic)	4,7,10,13,16,19-docosahexaenoic	C22:6 ω3	332.6	-44	12.95	3.093	4307	1029
linoleic	9,12-octadecadienoic	C18:2 ω6	280.4	-4.0	11.00	2.628	3084	737
γ-linolenic	6,9,12-octadecatrienoic	C18:3 ω6	278.6	-	10.84	2.588	3020	721
α-eleostearic	9,11*trans*,13*trans*-octadecatrienoic	*trans*-C18:3 ω6	278.6	48-49	10.84	2.588	3020	721
dihomo-γ-linolenic	8,11,14-eicosatrienoic	C20:3 ω6	306.5	-	12.14	2.900	3721	889
arachidonic	5,8,11,14-eicosatetraenoic	C20:4 ω6	304.5	-49.5	11.98	2.861	3648	871
docosatetraenoic (adrenic)	7,10,13,16-docosatetraenoic	C22:4 ω6	332.6	-	13.28	3.173	4417	1055
docosapentaenoic	4,7,10,13,16-docosapentaenoic	C22:5 ω6	334.6	-	13.12	3.133	4390	1049
mead	5,8,11-eicosatrienoic	C20:3 ω9	306.5	-	12.14	2.900	3721	889

(1) Calculated from heat of combustion (kJ /mmol) = 0.653 x no of carbon atoms - 0.166 x no of double bonds - 0.421 (Livesey 1984).

Table 8.5: Fatty acid composition of oils and fats

		proportion of total fat as			p:s ratio
		saturated	mufa	pufa	
butter	*Bos tauris*	0.71	0.26	0.03	0.05
margarine soft	-	0.32	0.40	0.28	0.87
margarine, hard, veg	-	0.46	0.42	0.12	0.26
margarine, pufa	-	0.21	0.26	0.53	2.54
ghee, butter	*Bos tauris*	0.71	0.26	0.04	0.05
ghee, palm	*Elaies guineensis*	0.52	0.39	0.10	0.19
dripping, beef	*Bos tauris*	0.58	0.39	0.03	0.05
dripping, chicken	*Gallus domesticus*	0.28	0.48	0.24	0.84
dripping, mutton	*Ovis aries*	0.55	0.41	0.04	0.07
lard	*Sus scrofa*	0.43	0.46	0.10	0.24
suet	*Bos tauris*	0.58	0.39	0.03	0.04
almond oil	*Prunus amygdala*	0.09	0.65	0.27	3.02
cocoa butter	*Theobroma cacao*	0.62	0.34	0.04	0.06
coconut oil	*Cocos nucifera*	0.91	0.07	0.02	0.02
corn oil	*Zea mais*	0.13	0.26	0.61	4.55
cottonseed oil	*Gossypium hirsutum*	0.27	0.22	0.51	1.88
groundnut oil	*Arachis hypogea*	0.20	0.50	0.30	1.52
linseed oil	*Linum usitatissum*	0.10	0.18	0.72	7.56
olive oil	*Olea europea sativa*	0.15	0.73	0.12	0.80
palm kernel	*Elaies guineensis*	0.84	0.14	0.02	0.03
palm oil	*Elaies guineensis*	0.48	0.44	0.09	0.18
pecan oil	*Carya illinoensis*	0.07	0.61	0.33	4.71
rapeseed oil, high erucic acid	*Brassica campestris*	0.06	0.68	0.26	4.68
rapeseed oil, low erucic acid	*Brassica campestris*	0.07	0.60	0.33	4.77
safflower oil	*Carthamus tinctorius*	0.11	0.13	0.76	7.07
sesame (til) oil	*Sesamum indicum*	0.15	0.39	0.46	3.09
soybean oil	*Glycine max*	0.15	0.25	0.60	3.90
sunflower oil	*Helianthus annuus*	0.13	0.21	0.66	5.29
walnut oil	*Juglans regia*	0.09	0.19	0.73	8.48
wheatgerm oil	*Triticum aestivum*	0.20	0.17	0.64	3.23
cod liver oil	*Gaddus morrhua*	0.22	0.45	0.33	1.51
menhaden oil	*Brevioorta tyranus*	0.34	0.29	0.37	1.10

Table 8.6: *Trans* fatty acids in spreads and cooking fats

	total fat (g /100 g)	saturated fat (g /100 g)	*trans* fatty acids (g /100 g)	*trans* fatty acids % of total
butter	80	54	4-8	5-10
hard margarine	80	33	9-14	12-18
soft margarine	80	26	7-18	9-23
soft margarine, high in pufa	70-80	16	0.7-6	1-8
reduced / low fat spreads	40-60	11-19	3-11	8-29
reduced / low fat spreads, high in pufa	40-60	8-10	0.4-7	1-18
cooking fats	100	21-52	7-16	7-17

Source: British Nutrition Foundation 1995.

Table 8.7: Major functions of the eicosanoids

leukotrienes B - E₄	thromboxane A₂	formed from arachidonic acid (ω6 series pufa) prostaglandin I₂	prostaglandin D₂	prostaglandin E₂	prostaglandin F₂α
attract phagocytes	↑ platelet aggregation	↓ platelet aggregation	vasodilator; constricts arteries and bronchioles	vasodilator	vasoconstrictor
	↑ smooth muscle contraction (arteries and bronchioles)	vasodilator		↑ kidney diuresis and natriuresis	
	antagonizes PGE₂ in kidney	releases renin in kidney endothelial cells		↑ renal blood flow	

leukotrienes B - E₅	formed from eicosapentaenoic acid (ω3 series pufa) thromboxane A₃	prostaglandin I₃
as leukotrienes B-E₄, but considerably less active	no effect on platelet aggregation	↓ platelet aggregation
	no effect on smooth muscle	vasodilator releases renin in kidney endothelial cells

actions shared by leukotrienes B - E₅, thromboxane A₃, and prostaglandins I₂ and I₃

↓ VLDL synthesis
↑ VLDL clearance from circulation
↑ bile secretion
↑ fibrinolysis
↓ blood pressure and viscosity
↑ red cell deformability
↑ bleeding time (slower clotting)
↓ release of interleukins
↓ acetyl CoA carboxylase (↓ fatty acid synthesis)

Table 8.8: Intestinal lipases

triacylglycerol lipase	EC 3.1.1.3	includes lingual, gastric and pancreatic lipases
acylglycerol lipase	EC 3.1.1.23	mono-acylglycerol lipase
phospholipase A1	EC 3.1.1.32	broad specificity phospholipase 2-acylhydrolase
phospholipase A2	EC 3.1.1.4	phosphatidylcholine 2-acylhydrolase
lysophospholipase	EC 3.1.1.5	phospholipase B, lysophospholipid 1-acylhydrolase
cholesterol esterase	EC 3.1.1.13	-

Table 8.9: The composition of liver and gall bladder bile

	liver bile	gall bladder bile (as secreted)
water (%)	97	86
protein (g/L)	2.73	3.15-5.39
total glucides (g/L)	0.35-0.91	2.4
lipids (g/L)	3	19
inorganic salts (g/L)	7	9
specific gravity	1.088-1.015	1.01-1.032
pH	8.0-8.6	7.0-7.6

Source: Snyder et al 1975

Table 8.10: Lipid composition of bile

Figures show mean ± SD

	no diet data given[1]	diet based on	
		refined carbohydrate[2]	unrefined carbohydrate[2]
cholesterol (molar %)	5.6 ± 0.3	9.1 ± 0.8	6.8 ± 0.6
bile acids (molar %)	73.6 ± 0.6	70.9 ± 2.6	75.8 ± 2.2
phospholipids (molar %)	20.6 ± 0.5	17.8 ± 0.7	18.4 ± 0.9
cholesterol % saturation	0.86 ± 0.03	1.50 ± 0.10	1.20 ± 0.12
bile acids as % of total			
cholate	41.2 ± 1.5	36.9 ± 1.9	42.1 ± 1.9
chenodeoxycholate	34.5 ± 1.2	32.1 ± 2.1	31.0 ± 2.1
deoxycholate	23.4 ± 1.8	28.7 ± 2.8	25.1 ± 2.4
lithocholate	0.7 ± 0.4	2.2 ± 0.3	1.8 ± 0.1
ursodeoxycholate	0.7 ± 0.3	-	-

Source: (1) Einarsson *et al*. 1985; (2) Thornton *et al*. 1983.

Table 8.11: Major classes of plasma lipoproteins

	chylomicrons	VLDL very low density lipoproteins	IDL intermediate density lipoproteins	LDL low density lipoproteins	HDL high density lipoproteins
density (g /mL)	< 0.95	< 1.006	1.006-1.019	1.020-1.063	1.064-1.210
diameter (nm)	75-1200	30-80	25-35	18-25	5-12
M_r (10^3 kDa)	400	10-80	5-10	2.3	0.175-0.36
% protein	1.5-2.5	5-10	15-20	20-25	40-55
% phospholipids	7-9	15-20	22	15-20	20-35
% free cholesterol	1-3	5-10	8	7-10	3-4
% triacylglycerol	84-89	50-65	22	7-10	3-5
% cholesteryl esters	3-5	10-15	30	35-40	12
electrophoretic mobility	at origin	pre-beta	between pre-beta and beta	beta	alpha
major apo-proteins	A-I, A-II, B-48, C-I, C-II, C-III, E	B-100, C-I, C-II, C-III, E	B-100, C-III, E	B-100	A-I, A-II, B-48, C-I, C-II, C-III, D, E
turnover in plasma	4-5 min	1-3 h	1-3 h	45% /day	4 d

Table 8.12: Plasma apo-lipoproteins

	M_r (kDa)	lipoprotein(s)	plasma concentration (mmol/L)	function
A-I	28.3	HDL	31-46	activates lecithin-cholesterol acyltransferase
A-II	17	HDL	18-30	inhibits lecithin-cholesterol acyltransferase, activates hepatic lipase
B-48	264	chylomicrons	< 0.2	unknown
B-100	550	LDL	1.5-1.8	binds to LDL receptor
C-I	6.5	chylomicrons, VLDL	6-11	activates lecithin-cholesterol acyltransferase
C-II	8.8	chylomicrons, VLDL	3-9	activates lipoprotein lipase
C-III	8.75	chylomicrons, VLDL	9-17	inhibits lipoprotein lipase, activates lecithin-cholesterol acyltransferase
D	33	HDL	3	unknown
E	35	chylomicrons, VLDL	0.8-1.7	binds to LDL receptor
cholesterol ester transfer protein	74	HDL	-	transfers cholesterol esters to LDL

Table 8.13: Interpretation of serum cholesterol concentrations

	desirable range	borderline	abnormal	severe elevation
total cholesterol, mmol/L	< 5.2	5.2-6.5	6.5-7.8	> 7.8
LDL cholesterol, mmol/L	< 4.0	4.0-5.0	> 5.0	-
HDL cholesterol, mmol/L	> 1.0	0.9-1.0	< 0.9	-
HDL : total cholesterol ratio	> 0.25	0.20-0.25	< 0.20	-
triacylglycerol	< 2.0	2.0-2.5	> 2.5	-

Table 8.14: WHO (Friedrickson) classification of hyperlipoproteinaemias

type	chylomicrons	VLDL	LDL	cholesterol	triacylglycerol	cholesterol : triacylglycerol ratio	may occur secondary to
I	↑	-	(↓)	-	↑↑	< 0.2	-
IIa	-	-	↑↑	↑↑	-	> 1.5	hypothyroidism, nephrotic syndrome
IIb	-	↑	↑	↑	↑	variable	diabetes mellitus, hypothyroidism, nephrotic syndrome
III	-	broad beta[1]		↑	↑	0.3- > 2.0	hypothyroidism
IV	-	↑	(↓)	(↑)	↑	variable	obesity, diabetes mellitus, excess alcohol consumption, nephrotic syndrome
V	↑	↑	(↓)	(↑)	↑	0.15-0.6	diabetes mellitus, excess alcohol consumption, nephrotic syndrome

↑ = elevated; ↑↑ = markedly elevated; (↓) = may be normal or lower than normal; (↑) = may be normal or elevated
(1) In Type III hyperlipoproteinaemia a broad β-globulin band is seen on electrophoresis, covering the regions occupied by VLDL and LDL.

Table 8.15: Primary hyperlipidaemias

	WHO type	metabolic defect	prevalence	drug therapy
familial hypercholesterolaemia	IIa, IIb	↓ LDL receptor function	1:500 (autosomal dominant)	ion exchange resins, nicotinic acid derivatives
familial hypertriglyceridaemia	IV, V	unknown	1:600 (autosomal dominant)	nicotinic acid and fibric acid derivatives
familial combined hyperlipidaemia	IIa, IIb, IV, V	unknown	1:300 (autosomal dominant)	nicotinic acid and fibric acid derivatives, HMG-CoA reductase inhibitors
polygenic hypercholesterolaemia	IIa, IIb	multiple	very common	rarely required
familial dysbetalipoproteinaemia (broad beta disease)	III	abnormal apolipoprotein E; defective clearance of IDL and chylomicron remnants	1:10,000	nicotinic acid and fibric acid derivatives
abnormal lipoprotein lipase	I	lipoprotein lipase deficiency or inhibition; apolipoprotein CII deficiency	rare	none available

Table 8.16: Major hypolipidaemic drugs

ion exchange resins	HMG CoA reductase inhibitors	fibric acid derivates	nicotinic acid derivatives	miscellaneous
cholestyramine	fluvastatin	benzafibrate	nicotinic acid	dextrothyroxine
colestipol	lovastatin	cipofibrate	acipimox	meglutol
colextran	mevastatin	clinofibrate	glunicate	melinamide
divistyramine	pravastin	clofibrate	homonicotinic acid	pirozadil
polidexide	simvastin	fenofibrate	nicoclonate	probucol
		gemfibrozil	nicomol	sitosterol
		pirifibrate	sorbinicate	tiadenol
		plafibride	tocopheryl nicotinate	xenbucin
		pyridoxine clofibrate		
		ronifibrate	combined fibric and nicotinic acid derivatives	
		simfibrate	etofibrate	
		sitofibrate	nicofibrate	
		theofibrate		
		tocofibrate		

9

Alcohol and alcoholic beverages

Alcoholic beverages, made by fermenting fruit juices, sugars and other fermentable carbohydrates with yeast to form alcohol, have a long history, and are widely consumed in most countries, except where religious observance prohibits their consumption. Moderate consumption of alcohol is associated with lower mortality from cardiovascular disease, but persistent heavy consumption is associated with physiological addiction—alcoholism. In addition to the addiction, there may be damage to the liver (cirrhosis), stomach (gastritis) and pancreas (pancreatitis), as well as behavioural changes and peripheral nerve damage. Both general malnutrition and more specifically deficiency of thiamin (see section 17.5.5), niacin (see section 19.5), and zinc (see section 25.26.2) are associated with alcoholism.

9.1 The energy yield of alcohol

The energy yield of alcohol is 29 kJ (7 kcal) /g. A number of studies have suggested that the true metabolizable energy of alcohol may be considerably lower than this. One factor may be that a relatively large amount can be lost in urine, and on the breath (see Table 9.1); alternative pathways for alcohol oxidation may also account for the observed discrepancy (Lands and Zakhari 1991; Coldlitz *et al*. 1991).

Alcohol is metabolized by oxidation to acetaldehyde, then acetate, which is oxidized by the citric acid cycle (see Fig. 5.2). However, there are two enzymes that can catalyse the oxidation of alcohol to acetaldehyde: alcohol dehydrogenase (EC 1.1.1.1), linked to the reduction of NAD^+ to NADH, and a microsomal cytochrome P_{450}-linked ethanol oxidizing system which oxidizes NADPH to $NADP^+$. The net yield when alcohol is oxidized by way of the dehydrogenase is 16 ATP /mol, but only 10 when it is oxidized by the microsomal system—a difference of 37.5 per cent. The relative activities of alcohol dehydrogenase and the microsomal ethanol oxidizing system are not

known, but there is evidence that the microsomal pathway is induced in heavy drinkers.

The rate of alcohol metabolism in healthy people is such that blood alcohol is cleared by the liver at a rate of about 15 mg/100 mL /hour (3.25 mmol /L / hour); this is increased to some extent by induction of the microsomal ethanol oxidizing system, and then decreases with impaired liver function following prolonged alcohol abuse (see section 9.3.1).

Table 9.2 shows average and extreme ranges of alcohol intake in UK; 21 per cent of men and 35 per cent of women claimed to have consumed no alcohol during the week in which the survey was conducted. In defining dietary goals (see section 4.2), no level of alcohol intake is specified, but it is conventional to assume that on average it provides about 5 per cent of energy. Some tables of dietary goals differentiate between food energy intake, which excludes that from alcohol, and total energy intake.

9.2 Alcoholic beverages

The strength of alcoholic beverages is most often shown as the per centage of alcohol by volume at 20°C (sometimes shown as per cent v/v). Because the density of ethanol is 0.79 g/mL, the percentage of alcohol by weight (per cent w/v) differs markedly from per centage by volume. The old British method of describing the alcohol content of beverages was by reference to proof spirit, originally defined as a solution of alcohol of such strength that it can be ignited when mixed with gunpowder. Proof spirit contains 57.07 per cent alcohol by volume or 49.24 per cent by weight in Great Britain. In the USA it contains 50 per cent alcohol by volume. Pure (absolute) alcohol is 175.25° proof UK or 200° proof USA.

For convenience in calculating intakes of alcohol, a unit of alcohol is defined as 8 g (10 mL) of absolute alcohol; this is the amount in $\frac{1}{2}$ pint (300 mL) of beer, a single measure of spirit (25 mL) or a single glass of wine (100 mL). The Royal College of Physicians (1987) has set upper limits of prudent consumption of alcohol as 21 units (= 168 g alcohol) per week for men and 14 units (= 112 g alcohol) per week for women (see Table 9.3). Table 9.4 shows the alcohol content of the major classes of alcoholic beverages.

9.2.1 Cider, perry and beer

Cider (cyder) is fermented apple juice, perry is fermented pear juice (in UK either may include not more than 25 per cent of the other juice). Sparkling perry is sometimes known as champagne perry. Dry cider contains 2.6 per cent sugars and 3–4 per cent alcohol, sweet cider 4.3 per cent sugars, and vintage cider 7.3 per cent sugars and 10.5 per cent alcohol. In the USA cider or fresh cider is the term used for unfermented apple juice; the fermented product is termed hard or fermented cider.

Beer is made by the fermentation of cereals— traditionally barley, but also maize, rice and sorghum. The first step is the malting of barley—it is allowed to sprout, when the enzyme β-amylase (EC 3.2.1.2) hydrolyses some of the starch to dextrins and maltose. The sprouted (malted) barley is dried, then extracted with hot water (the process of mashing) to produce wort. After the addition of hops for flavour, the wort is allowed to ferment. Two types of yeast are used in brewing: top fermenting yeasts which float on the surface of the wort and bottom or deep fermenters. Most traditional British beers (ale, bitter, stout and porter) are brewed with top fermenting yeasts. Deep fermenting yeasts produce lager, the traditional mainland European type of beer, sometimes called Pilsner lager or Pils, since the original lager was brewed in Pilsen in Bohemia.

Ale is a light-coloured beer, relatively high in alcohol content, and relatively heavily hopped. Bitter beers are darker and contain more hops. Porter and stout are almost black in colour; they are made from wort containing some partly charred malt; milk stout is made from wort containing added lactose.

Lite beer is beer which has been allowed to ferment until virtually all of the carbohydrate has been converted to alcohol and so is lower in carbohydrate and higher in alcohol.

Low alcohol beer may be made either by fermentation of a low carbohydrate wort, or by removal of much of the alcohol after fermentation (de-alcoholized beer).

African sorghum beer, also known by numerous local names such as kaffir beer, bouza, pombé, bantu beer, is a is a thick sour beverage consumed while still fermenting; it may also be made from millet, maize or plantain.

9.2.2 Wines

Wine is the fermented juice of grapes (varieties of *Vitis vinifera*). Red wines are made by fermenting the juice together with the skins at 21–29°C; white wines are made normally from white grapes by fermenting the juice alone at 15–17°C; rosé by removing the skins after 12–36 hours, or by mixing red and white wines. Sulphur dioxide is commonly added to wines to prevent spoilage by bacterial fermentation of alcohol to acetic acid; EU regulations permit no more than 175 mg sulphur dioxide /L in red wines, and no more than 225 mg /L for white wines, with the exception of wines containing less than 5 g /L residual sugar, which may contain up to 275–400 mg /L, depending on type. The principal varieties of grape used in wine making are shown in Table 9.5; those varieties used to make the 'great' wines, the so-called classic grape varieties, are starred in the list.

Beverages made by fermenting other fruit juices and sugar in the presence of vegetables or leaves or roots are also called wines (elderberry, elder flower, parsnip, peapod, rhubarb etc.), although the legal definition is usually restricted to grape juice, fermented in its country of origin. In UK there is a legal distinction between British wine, which is made from imported grape juice concentrate, and English wine, which is made from grapes grown in England.

Sparkling wine contains bubbles of carbon dioxide, and is bottled under pressure. EU regulations require that sparkling wines have a pressure not less than 3 bar at 20°C. There are three methods of production.

1. The méthode champenoise in which the wine undergoes a second fermentation in the bottle. Wine produced outside the Champagne region of France may not be called champagne, even if made by this method.

2. The tank or bulk method, in which the wine is bottled while still fermenting slightly.

3. Wine made with the addition of carbon dioxide gas while bottling.

Lightly sparkling wines are known as pétillante or frizzante; they are often young wines, bottled while still fermenting (e.g. lambrusco, vinho verde). By EU regulations, semi-sparkling wines have a pressure of between 1.1–2.5 bar at 20°C.

Fortified wines are made by adding brandy or other spirit to increase the alcohol content of the wine to 15–18 per cent and so prevent further fermentation (to acids) in warm climates.

1. Madeira wines, from the Island of Madeira: sercial (dry); verdelho (semi-dry), bual (semi-sweet), malmsey (sweet).

2. Port, from the upper Douro valley of north east Portugal. Mostly aged in wood and bottled when ready for drinking; vintage port is aged in wood for 2 years, then in the bottle for at least 10; late bottled vintage is aged less than 6 years. Crusted port is blended from quality vintages, bottled young and develops a sediment (crust) in the bottle. Ruby port is young, old tawny is aged for 10 or more years; fine old tawny is a blend of young and old wines. Tawny port is aged in wood, vintage in the bottle. White port is made from white grapes, generally served chilled as an aperitif. Around 16 per cent alcohol by volume, 12 per cent sugars.

3. Sherry, from the south-west of Spain, around Jerez and Cadiz. Matured by the solera process, rather than by discrete vintages; each year 30 per cent of the wine in the oldest barrel is drawn off for bottling and replaced with wine from the next oldest; this in turn is replaced from the next barrel, and so on. Sherry type wines are also produced in other countries, including South Africa, Cyprus and Britain (made from imported grape juice) and may legally be described as sherry as long as the country of origin is clearly shown. In order of increasing sweetness, sherries are fino (very dry), manzanilla, amontillado, oloroso (may be medium-dry or sweetened and more highly fortified), amoroso or cream. Dry sherry contains 1–2 per cent sugar, medium 3–4 per cent, and sweet 7 per cent sugar.

4. Aperitif wines and vermouths are slightly bitter-tasting fortified wines drunk before meals. They are made from red or white wine fortified with spirit and flavoured with herbs and quinine; usually 15–25 per cent alcohol by volume, and 5–10 per cent sugars.

9.2.2.1 Wine classification

Many of the major wine producing countries have legally enforced systems of classification of wines based on grape varieties used and regions of production. Other countries have a system of denomination of origin for wines grown in defined regions which may or may not reflect quality. The national classifications, in increasing order of quality for each country, are shown in Table 9.6.

The UK Wine Promotion Board classifies white and rosé wines from 1 for very dry wines (0.6 per cent sugars) to 9 (very sweet, 6 per cent sugars). For red wines the classification is from A (light and dry) to E (full-bodied heavy wines). German and Austrian labelling is trocken (dry), halbtrocken (half dry), halbüss or lieben (medium sweet) and süss (very sweet).

9.2.3 Spirits and liqueurs

Spirits are beverages of high alcohol content (usually 40 per cent alcohol by volume, equivalent to 31.7 g per 100 mL) made by distillation of fermented liquors. Liqueurs are prepared by steeping fruit and herbs in spirit, and sweetening; fruit brandies are either distilled from fruit wines (e.g. plum and apple brandies, calvados) or are prepared by soaking fruit in brandy (e.g. cherry and apricot brandies). Eau de vie, sometimes known as white spirit or *alcool blanc* is distilled from fermented grape or other fruit juice, and may be flavoured with fruits, etc.

Brandy is distilled from wine. The name is derived from the German *brandtwein*, meaning burnt wine, corrupted to brandy-wine. Most wine-producing countries also make brandy. The age of brandy is generally designated as follows:

(1) 3-star is 3–5 years old before bottling;

(2) VSOP (very special old pale) is aged 4–10 or more years, the name indicating that it has not been heavily coloured with caramel;

(3) Napoleon brandy is a premium blend aged 6–20 years;

(4) XO (Extraordinary Old) is Extra or Grand Reserve, possibly 50 years old.

Cognac and Armagnac are brandies made in defined regions of France, using defined grape varieties.

Gin is made by distilling fermented maize and rye grains (together with malted barley or rye), flavoured mainly with juniper berries, together with coriander seeds, angelica, cinnamon, orange and lemon peel. The name is derived from French *genièvre* (juniper); originally known as geneva, schiedam or hollands, since it is Dutch in origin.

There are two types of English gin: Plymouth gin with a fuller flavour and London gin. Dutch and German gins are more strongly flavoured than English or American:

(1) Steinhäger and schinkenhäger are distilled from a mash of wheat, barley and juniper berries;

(2) Wacholder is made from neutral spirit flavoured with juniper.

Dutch gin may be *jonge* (young) or *oude* (aged, matured).

Marc is distilled from the fermented residue of grape skins, stalks, and seeds after the grapes have been pressed for wine making. It is often a harsh raw spirit, drunk young, although some varieties are matured and smooth. Equivalent spirits include grappa (Italian), bagaciera (Portugal) and aguardiente (Spain).

Rum is distilled from fermented sugar cane juice or molasses, and may be 35–60 per cent alcohol by volume. It may be colourless and light tasting or dark and with a strong flavour. Traditionally rum is darker and more strongly flavoured the further south in the Caribbean it is made. There are three main categories:

(1) Cuban, Jamaican and Dutch East Indies, several types, aguardiente (Spain, Portugal and S. America);

(2) Bacardi (trade name, originally from Cuba), cachaca (Brazil), cane spirit (S. Africa);

(3) Demerara rum (Guyana), 35–60 per cent alcohol by volume.

Vodka is made from neutral spirit, i.e. alcohol distillate, mainly from potatoes, with little or no acid so that there is no ester formation and hence no flavour. Polish vodka is flavoured with a variety of herbs and fruits.

Whisky (whiskey) is distilled from barley, rye, maize or other cereal which has first been malted and then fermented. Most brands of whisky are a blend of pure malt whisky with spirit distilled from grain. The distilled spirit is diluted to about 62 per cent alcohol and matured in wooden casks, then diluted to 40 per cent alcohol.

1. Irish and Scotch whisky, made from malted barley, is matured for at least 3 years.

2. Bourbon, made from malted maize, is matured for at least one year.

3. Sour mash bourbon is made from mash that has yeast left in it from a previous fermentation.

4. Other American and Canadian whiskies are made from rye.

Both spellings are used, but generally whisky is the Scotch variety and whiskey the Irish and American varieties. The name is derived from the Gaelic *uisge beatha*, water of life.

Arak (arack) is Arabic, an anise and liquorice flavoured spirit (*ouzo* in Greek, *raki* in Turkish). The name is also used generally in the Middle and Far East to mean any one of a variety of spirits, often distilled from fermented dates or palm wine.

9.3 Hazards and benefits of alcohol consumption

9.3.1 Problems of excessive alcohol consumption

Problems associated with excessive alcohol consumption range from those of acute intoxication, with its social consequences and impairment of both judgement and motor coordination, leading to increased risks of accidents, through behavioural and psychosocial problems to physical addition and tissue damage. Table 9.7 shows the effects of acute intoxication, and Table 9.8 the effects of different blood alcohol concentrations on the likelihood of accidents when driving for people with low and high susceptibility to the effects of alcohol.

The Royal College of Physicians (1987) defined four types of drinker.

1. Social drinkers, who consume not more than 2–3 units of alcohol per day (see Table 9.3), do not become intoxicated and are not likely to harm themselves or their families through drinking.

2. Heavy drinkers, who regularly drink more than 6 units of alcohol per day, but with no apparent immediate harm.

3. Problem drinkers, who experience physical, psychological, family, legal, employment, and financial problems attributable to drinking.

4. Dependent drinkers, who are physiologically addicted to alcohol. Initially they have increased alcohol tolerance, but much reduced tolerance at a later stage. They suffer from withdrawal symptoms that are relieved by more alcohol.

Sherlock (1995) has suggested that the prudent upper limits of habitual consumption shown in Table 9.3 are unduly cautious, and indeed overlap the levels of alcohol consumption that are associated with health benefits (see section 9.3.2). She states that consumption of 16 units per day for 5 years is probably the minimum level associated with significant liver damage.

The effects of alcohol withdrawal after prolonged regular intake include the following.

1. Tremor, especially on waking and before the first drink of the day, together with restlessness, agitation and insomnia,

2. Hallucinations, either auditory hallucinations or buzzing and ringing in the ears,

3. Delirium tremens, usually developing 2–5 days after alcohol withdrawal, initially as increasing restlessness, apprehensiveness, nightmares and mental disorientation, leading to trembling, panic, and visual hallucinations,

4. Epileptiform seizures, either isolated or repeated, and sometimes leading to status epilepticus.

The principal adverse effects of heavy alcohol consumption are shown in Table 9.9, and changes in blood chemistry in Table 9.10.

9.3.1.1 Malnutrition and hypoglycaemia in heavy drinkers

Apart from energy, both as alcohol and sugars, most alcoholic beverages provide little in the way of nutrients, although the B vitamin content of beer may make a significant contribution to intake. It is therefore to be expected that people who are obtaining more than about 20–25 per cent of their energy intake from alcohol will be at risk of micronutrient and protein deficiency. Thiamin deficiency is especially prevalent in alcoholics, due to both low intake and also specific inhibition of thiamin absorption by alcohol (see section 17.3.5).

As discussed in section 9.1, the metabolic energy yield of alcohol may be very much lower than 27 kJ / g, and despite their apparently adequate total energy intake, heavy drinkers are at risk of general undernutrition. This is compounded by the fact that heavy alcohol consumption is associated with appetite suppression (again partially attributable to thiamin deficiency). Gastritis and diarrhoea will impair digestion and absorption, and alcoholic pancreatitis results in decreased secretion of digestive enzymes (see section 6.1.3), and hence impaired digestion.

Unfed alcoholics are at risk of profound hypoglycaemia, as a result of inhibition of gluconeogenesis by alcohol (Krebs 1968). Alcohol also potentiates the action of insulin; in response to a modest intake of alcohol together with carbohydrate there is a marked reactive hypoglycaemia among both habituated drinkers and social drinkers (O'Keefe and Marks, 1977). In insulin-treated diabetics heavy alcohol consumption can result in profound, life-threatening, hypoglycaemia (Arky *et al.* 1968).

9.3.1.2 Alcohol in pregnancy

Even moderate consumption of alcohol during pregnancy can have serious effects on foetal development, including the following.

1. Damage to the infant's genetic material during early stages of development, possibly leading to chromosome abnormalities and spontaneous abortion. Spontaneous abortion is twice as common in women who drink heavily.

2. Interference with organ formation (between 16–24 days of gestation, before the mother knows she is pregnant, see Table 3.2).

3. Restriction of the development of tissues, especially the brain, during the period of rapid growth (73–280 days of gestation). Consumption of more than about 6–10 units / day in pregnancy leads to the foetal alcohol syndrome: marked growth retardation, with birth weight 65–70 per cent of that expected; characteristic facial abnormalities and mental handicap, with a mean IQ of the affected child of about 70.

9.3.1.3 Effects of alcohol on drug action

Acute ingestion of alcohol results in decreased metabolism, and hence potentiation of the action of a number of drugs, as shown in column 1 of Table 9.11. By contrast, in chronic alcoholism the induction of the microsomal ethanol oxidizing system leads to increased drug metabolism, and hence diminished action of those drugs listed in column 2 of Table 9.11. As alcoholic liver disease develops, so the metabolism of drugs is impaired, and the actions of those shown in column 3 of Table 9.11 is increased.

9.3.2 Benefits of modest alcohol consumption

Notwithstanding the adverse health effects of excessive alcohol consumption discussed in section 9.3.1, there is a considerable body of evidence that modest consumption confers positive health benefits. Most studies show a J-shaped curve for the relationship between mortality and alcohol consumption (Marmot and Brunner 1991; Veenstra 1991); people who habitually consume a modest amount of alcohol have lower mortality from all causes, and especially cardiovascular disease, than either those who are total abstainers or those whose consumption is excessive.

The effects of moderate alcohol consumption on all-cause mortality for both men and women are shown in Table 9.12, and for death from various causes for men in Table 9.13. As shown in Table 9.12, the beneficial effect is essentially limited to wine, rather than beer or spirits. This has led to suggestions that the protective effect, especially with respect to cardiovascular disease, may be compounds other than alcohol that are present in wine, including polyphenols and flavonoids (see section 23.2). In women the beneficial effect of alcohol consumption on death from cardiovascular disease is countered to a great extent by increased mortality from breast cancer (Fuchs *et al.* 1995).

Table 9.1: Alcohol in breath and urine at various blood concentrations

blood		breath		urine	
mg /100 mL	mmol /L	mg /100 mL	mmol /L	mg /100 mL	mmol /L
50	10.85	22	4.77	67	14.53
80	17.35	35	7.59	107	23.21
150	32.54	66	14.32	200	43.38
250	54.23	110	23.86	333	72.23

Table 9.2: Average consumption of alcohol in UK

	g /day			units /day			% total energy intake		
	mean	median	97.5 centile	mean	median	97.5 centile	mean	median	97.5 centile
all men	25.0	14.4	-	3.1	1.8	-	6.9	4.2	-
excluding abstainers[1]	31.5	23.2	110.7	3.9	2.9	13.8	8.7	6.9	28.4
all women	6.9	2.3	-	0.9	0.3	-	2.8	1.0	-
excluding abstainers[1]	10.6	6.8	39.7	1.3	0.9	5.0	4.3	3.0	15.8

(1) 21% of men and 35% of women claimed to have consumed no alcohol during the survey period.
Source: Gregory *et al.* 1990.

Table 9.3: Health risks of different levels of habitual alcohol consumption and prudent upper limits

		habitual consumption			
		men		women	
		weekly	daily	weekly	daily
low risk	units[1]	< 21	< 3	< 14	< 2
	g alcohol	< 168	< 24	< 112	< 16
	mL alcohol	< 210	< 30	< 140	< 20
prudent upper limit	units	21	3	14	2
	g alcohol	168	24	112	16
	mL alcohol	210	30	140	20
hazardous	units	21-50	3-7	14-35	2-5
	g alcohol	168-400	24-57	112-280	16-40
	mL alcohol	210-500	30-71	140-350	20-50
harmful	units	> 50	> 7	> 35	> 5
	g alcohol	> 400	> 57	> 280	> 40
	mL alcohol	> 500	> 71	> 350	> 50

Source: from data reported by Royal College of Physicians 1987.
(1) 1 unit of alcohol = 8 g (10 mL) absolute alcohol; approximately the amount in ½ pint (300 mL) beer, 100 mL wine, or 25 mL spirits.

Table 9.4: Alcohol content of alcoholic beverages

	% alcohol by volume	% alcohol by weight
beer, cider, perry	4-6	3.2-4.8
table wines	9-13	7.1-10.3
fortified wines, apéritif wines	18-25	14.3-19.8
liqueurs	20-40	15.9-31.7
spirits	38-45	30.1-35.7
proof spirit[1], UK	57.07	49.24
proof spirit, USA	50	39.6

(1) Absolute (100%) alcohol = 175.25° proof (UK) or 200° proof (USA)

Table 9.5: Major grape varieties used for wine making

aleatico	fragrant sweet red wines.
aligoté	Burgundy's second-ranking white grape; the wines need drinking within 3 years.
barbera	the dark fruity and often sharp red wines of northern Italy.
bouchet	also known as cabernet franc
cabernet franc	also known as bouchet.
cabernet sauvignon*	some of the great red wines of Bordeaux, and widely grown throughout the world.
carignan	probably the commonest grape of France, a prolific cropper producing uninspiring wines.
chardonnay*	widely grown throughout the world. Chardonnay wines are among the white wines best adapted to maturing in oak barrels.
chenin blanc*	the great white grape of the middle Loire valley.
cinsaut	the common bulk wine-producing grape of southern France. In South Africa it has been crossed with the pinot noir to produce the pinotage grape.
gamay	the grape of the Beaujolais and Mâcon districts of France, making light fragrant red wines that are best drunk young.
gewürztraminer	the wines have a characteristic spicey flavour and aroma.
grenache	
malvasia	
merlot*	important in some of great fragrant rich red wines; widely grown through the world.
müller-thurgau	the major variety in Rheinhessen and Pfalz in Germany.

Table 9.5: (Cont'd)

muscadet	makes light, very dry wines. also known as melon de bourgogne.
muscat	mostly perfumed sweet white wines.
nebbiolo	
palomino	
pinot noir*	used especially in champagne
pinot blanc	
pinot gris	
pinotage	South African variety, the result of a cross between the cinsaut and pinot noir varieties.
riesling*	the wines have a flowery aroma when young.
sangiovese	the wines are distinctively aromatic and
sauvignon blanc*	sometimes smokey.
sémillon*	especially the great sauternes, graves and white bordeaux. Traditionally called riesling in some parts of Australia.
shiraz*	Australian and Californian name for Syrah.
silvaner	
syrah*	important in the red Rhône wines. Also known as shiraz, especially in Australia and California.
tempranillo	the wine of Rioja.
trebbiano	relatively thin wines of central Italy if not blended with other varieties.
viogner	
welschriesling	also known as Italian riesling; the wines cannot legally be labelled simply riesling.
zinfandel	Californian variety; wines may be blush (rosé) or red. White zinfandel wines are really rosé. The wines have a characteristically fruity flavour.

* Starred varieties are the so-called 9 classic wine grapes.

Table 9.6: Wine classification, in order of increasing quality for each country

Bulgaria	declared variety of brand	
	declared geographical origin (DGO)	
	controliran	specific varieties grown in specific areas
		The best of DGO and controliran wines may be offered as reserve
France	vin de table (or vin ordinaire)	
	vin de pays	vin de pays de zone, wines from a single area
		vin de pays départementaux, wines from one département
		vin de pays régionaux, wines from more than one département
	vin délimité de qualité supérieure (VDQS)	
	appellation contrôlée (AC)	wines from a specified area, from specified grape varieties
	appellation d'origine contrôlée (AOC)	grown under controlled conditions
Germany and Austria	Tafelwein	Deutscher Tafelwein is of German origin; wine labelled simply as tafelwein may be of mixed origin
	Landwein	dry or half-dry wines from one of 15 designated areas
	Qualitätswein bestimmer Anbaugebeite (QbA)	from 11 designated areas and approved grape varieties, sugar may be added to increase sweetness, each bottle carries a batch number (*Amtliche Prüfungsnummer, AP*), *as proof that it complies with QbA status*
	Qualitätswein mit Prädikat (QmP)	six quality gradings based on the level of natural sugar at harvest—extra sugar may not be added:
		Kabinett, light, fruity and delicate, usually dry
		Spätlese, late picked grapes, dry to sweet
		Auslese, selected late picked grapes, rich and sweet
		Ausbruch (in Austria only, intermediate in sweetness between Auslese and Beerenauslese)
		Beerenauslese, late picked grapes affected by 'noble rot', always sweet
		Eiswein, made from grapes that have frozen on the vine, very sweet.
Italy	vini de tavola (Vdt)	
	vini di tavola con indicazione geografica	from a particular area
	vini tipici	equivalent to French vin de pays
	denominazione di origine controllata (DOC)	from specified areas and grape varieties
	denominazione di origine controllata e garantita (DOCG)	as DOC but with more stringent regulations and control
Luxembourg	appellation controlée	must carry a vintage; bottles carry a neck label awarded by the state controlled Marque Nationale, according to the strength of the wine; in order of increasing alcohol content the grades are: non admis, marque nationale, vin classé, premier cru, grand premier cru.
Portugal	vinho de mesa	table wines
	indição de proveniencia regulamentada (IPR)	
	região demarcada (RD)	the same as AC
		wines aged more than 1 year are vinho maduro
South Africa	classification by grape variety and area of production	blue band indicates that origin is certified
		red band guarantees vintage year
		green band certifies grape varieties
		'superior' on gold seal indicates superior quality

Table 9.6: (Cont'd)

Spain	vinos de la tierra	two thirds of the grapes must come from the region named on the label
	denominacion de origen (DO).	the same as AC
USA[1]	American wine or vin de table	blended wine from one or more areas
	multi-State appellation	wine from two or three neighbouring states (the percentage from each must be shown on the label)
	State and County appellation	at least 75% must come from the designated area
	approved viticultural areas	defined boundaries, 85% of the grapes used must come from the defined area
	named vineyard or winery	95% of the grapes must have been grown there

(1) In USA, for tax purposes a table wine must be between 10-14% alcohol—stronger wines are classified as dessert wines, even if dry; dessert wines between 17-21% alcohol are classified by alcoholic strength, not sweetness. US wines may be sold by a generic classification (e.g. Chablis or Loire); such names are prohibited from export to the EU.

Table 9.7: Effects of acute intoxication

units[1] consumed	blood alcohol		effects
	mg /100 mL	mmol /L	
2	30	6.5	increasing likelihood of accident (see Table 9.8)
3	50	10.8	increasing cheerfulness, impaired judgement and loosening of inhibitions
5	80	17.4	legal limit for driving in UK
10	150	32.5	loss of self-control, exuberance, quarrelsomeness, slurred speech
12	200	43.4	stagger, double vision, loss of memory
22	400	86.8	oblivion, sleepiness, coma
30	500	108.5	death possible
> 30	600	130.2	death certain

(1) 1 unit of alcohol = 8 g (10 mL) absolute alcohol; approximately the amount in ½ pint (300 mL) beer, 100 mL wine, or 25 mL spirits.
Source: from data reported by Royal College of Physicians 1987.

Table 9.8: Increased likelihood of accidents when driving, at various blood alcohol concentrations

blood alcohol concentration		increased likelihood of accident	
mg /100 mL	mmol /L	most susceptible	least susceptible
50	10.8	3-fold	negligible
80	17.4	5.5-fold	1.4-fold
100	21.8	10-fold	2.1-fold

Source: from data reported by Transport and Road Research Laboratory 1983.

Table 9.9: Physical health hazards associated with alcohol abuse

central nervous system	psychological	mood and behaviour changes
	brain damage	Wernicke's encephalopathy (cerebellar degeneration)
		Korsakoff's psychosis (dementia)
	cerebrovascular disease	strokes
		subarachnoid haemorrhage
		subdural haematoma after head injury
	withdrawal symptoms	tremor, hallucinations, fits
peripheral nervous system	peripheral neuropathy	weakness
		paralysis
		burning sensation in hands and feet
liver	fasting hypoglycaemia	inhibition of gluconeogenesis (Krebs 1968)
	fatty infiltration	moderate elevation of plasma enzymes
	alcoholic hepatitis	elevated plasma bilirubin and urine urobilinogen
	cirrhosis	eventual liver failure, with hyperammonaemia
	liver cancer	as a late sequel to cirrhosis
gastrointestinal system	oesophageal cancer	
	gastritis	aggravation and impaired healing of peptic ulcers
	diarrhoea	impaired absorption of food
	alcoholic pancreatitis	impaired digestion
		may precipitate diabetes
	thiamin deficiency	inhibition of thiamin absorption (Hoyumpa *et al.* 1977)
cardiovascular system	arrhythmia	
	hypertension	increased risk of stroke and coronary thrombosis
	cardiomegaly and cardiomyopathy	muscle damage leading to heart failure
endocrine system	over-secretion of cortisol	obesity, acne, facial hair
		hypertension
	reproductive system	testicular atrophy and impotence (men)
		menstrual irregularity, shrinkage of breasts and external genitalia (women)
	reactive hypoglycaemia	potentiation of insulin action (O'Keefe & Marks 1977)
skeleton	gout	lactic acidosis impairs uric acid excretion

Source: modified from Royal College of Physicians 1987, and references cited in the Table.

Table 9.10: Blood changes associated with alcohol abuse

	reference range	
γ-glutamyl transpeptidase (EC 2.3.1.1)	< 40 u/L	> 40 indicates mild liver damage, > 100 serious liver damage
plasma aspartate aminotransferase (EC 2.6.1.1)	< 25 u/L	elevation reflects the extent of liver damage
erythrocyte mean cell volume	80-90 fL	> 92 fL in 60% of alcohol abusers
plasma urate	120-360 mol /L	elevated urate results in increased risk of gout and uroliathiasis
fasting triacylglycerol	0.85-2.0 mmol/L	hypertriglyceridaemia (see section 8.3.4) common in alcohol abusers
fasting glucose	3.5-6 mmol/L	fasting hypoglycaemia results from inhibition of gluconeogenesis
		reactive hypoglycaemia results from potentiation of insulin action
serum albumin	35-50 g/L	reduced in cirrhosis because of failure of hepatic synthesis
serum globulins	23-35 g/L	elevated in cirrhosis
prothrombin time	< 2 sec deviation from control	increased in cirrhosis because of failure of prothrombin synthesis
plasma bilirubin	< 7 mol/L	elevated in alcoholic hepatitis, normal in cirrhosis

Table 9.11: Effects of acute and chronic alcohol on drug action

potentiated by acute alcohol	diminished by chronic alcohol	potentiated in alcoholic liver disease
barbiturates	alkylating agents	ampicillin
benzodiazepines	antipyrine	barbiturates
chlormethiazole	barbiturates	benzodiazepines
dextropropoxyphene	benzodiazepines	chlormethiazole
metronidazole	chlormethiazole	frusemide
monoamine oxidase inhibitors	meprobamate	isoniazid
oral hypoglycaemic agents (see Table 7.15)	paracetamol (acetaminophen)	opiates
phenothiazines	phenytoin	phenytoin
tricyclic antidepressants	tolbutamide (oral hypoglycaemic	propanolol
warfarin (see section 16.4)	agent)	rifampicin
	warfarin	theophylline
		tolbutamide

Source: from data reported by Royal College of Physicians 1987.

Table 9.12: The effects of moderate alcohol consumption on mortality (adults aged 40-64)

	all-cause mortality					coronary heart disease		
drinks /day	men	women	wine	beer	spirits	wine	beer	spirits
0	1.0	1.0	1.0	1.0	1.0	1.0	1.0	1.0
0.5	0.8	1.2	-	-	-	-	-	-
0.5-2	0.9	0.9	0.80	0.96	0.81	0.47	0.79	1.16
2 +	1.2	1.9	-	-	-	-	-	-
3-5	-	-	0.50	1.22	1.36	0.44	0.72	1.35

Source: from data reported by Grønbæk *et al.* 1995; Serdula *et al.* 1995.

Table 9.13: The health benefits of moderate alcohol consumption in men

	mortality rate compared with non-drinkers = 1.0				
drinks /day	all causes	cancer	cerebrovascular disease	coronary heart disease	accident / violence
< 1	0.86	0.88	0.94	-	0.95
1	0.84	0.88	0.78	0.78	0.88
2	0.93	0.90	1.00	0.78	0.96
3	1.01	1.06	1.16	0.82	1.32
4	1.08	0.88	1.35	0.75	1.23
5	1.21	1.12	1.29	0.84	1.23
6 +	1.38	1.48	1.50	0.93	1.74

Source: from data reported by Boffetta & Garfinkel 1990.

Protein nutrition

The essentiality of a dietary source of nitrogen was first demonstrated by Magendie in 1816, when he showed that animals fed a nitrogen-free diet were unable to survive. Because of this perceived prime importance of nitrogenous compounds in the diet, the Dutch chemist Johannes Mulder coined the name protein for 'the basic nitrogenous substance present in all nitrogen-rich organic compounds', in 1838, from the Greek προτεοσ meaning *first*. Liebig extended Magendie's original studies, and in 1842 showed that animals maintained on a protein-free diet continued to excrete urea, associated with a loss of muscle tissue. There is thus an obligatory loss of nitrogen from the body; in the adult human being it is between 40–70 mg N /kg body weight /day, equivalent to some 250–440 mg protein /kg body weight /day.

10.1 Nitrogen balance

In 1860 Voit measured the difference between the intake of nitrogenous compounds (mainly protein, but also including nucleic acids) and the urinary excretion of nitrogenous compounds. He showed that dogs fed less than 1.5 kg of meat per day were unable to maintain nitrogen balance, but suffered a net loss of nitrogen from the body, thus establishing the technique of nitrogen balance studies that still provide the basis of estimates of protein requirements.

Nitrogen balance or equilibrium is when the intake and excretion of nitrogenous compounds are equal. Positive balance, when intake is greater than excretion, implies an increase in the total body content of protein (as is normal in growth and recovery from losses). Negative balance, when excretion is greater than intake, implies a loss of body protein and is never a normal state. It implies either an inadequate intake of protein (or total food) or a pathological catabolic state.

In the classical studies that defined amino acid requirements, Rose (1957) regarded the minimum requirement of protein or an individual amino acid as that amount that would permit all of his experimental subjects just to maintain positive N balance. Other studies have considered that a minimum requirement is that amount that will maintain all subjects in an equilibrium zone, with N excretion equal to ±5 per cent of intake.

10.1.1 Crude protein

Total intake and excretion of nitrogenous compounds is generally determined by the Kjeldahl method, first described in 1883: reduction to ammonium sulphate by digestion in concentrated sulphuric acid with a catalyst (commonly a mercury or selenium salt), followed by determination of the ammonium so formed. Based on the average nitrogen content and composition of proteins, crude protein is defined as N × 6.25; for foods whose protein composition differs significantly from the mean, the conversion figures shown in Table 10.1 are used.

10.1.2 Nitrogen losses from the body

Approximately 10–12 per cent of total nitrogen output from the body is in faeces (see Table 6.11). Faecal nitrogen consists of undigested dietary protein, the residue of digestive enzymes, bacterial protein and nucleic acids, protein and nucleic acids from shed intestinal mucosal cells, and mucus secreted into the intestinal lumen to lubricate the passage of faeces and protect the mucosa against damage by digestive enzymes. The major output of nitrogen is in the urine; the principal compounds excreted are shown in Table 10.2.

More precise determination of nitrogen balance requires estimation of losses in sweat, shed skin cells and to a lesser extent the growth of hair and nails. Skin losses (for adult men) are about 5 mg of N /kg body weight /day, falling to 3 mg /kg /d on a protein-free diet. The loss due to hair and nail growth is 30 mg N /day in young men, falling to 15 mg /d in older men (FAO/WHO/UNU 1985).

Sweat loss in temperate climates is about 5 mg N / kg body weight /day for people consuming their accustomed intake of protein, and about 10 mg /kg /d for people acclimatized to tropical climates, falling to 6 mg /kg /d on a low protein diet. Sweating due to strenuous physical activity increases losses by 0.5 mg N /kcal energy expenditure /min (0.13 mg N /kJ /min) (WHO/FAO 1973).

For women, menstrual losses are equivalent to 40–70 mg N /day averaged out over the 28 day cycle; use of hormonal contraceptives reduces this to about 20 mg N /day, while use of intra-uterine devices increases it to 60–100 mg N /day. Other miscellaneous losses are rarely measured, but the following estimates are used: semen and seminal fluid (a mean of 37 mg N /ejaculation), expectorated saliva (1 mg N /g saliva), and toothbrushing (a loss of 14 mg N/ event) (FAO/WHO/UNU 1985).

10.2   Protein composition

Proteins are (mainly linear) polymers of L-amino acids. With the exception of cysteine, all of the L-enantiomers of the protein amino acids have the *S*-configuration. Small amounts of the D-isomers of some amino acids occur in bacterial cell walls and in small peptides in invertebrates; D-serine has a hormonal role in some insects. In addition to this, there is a significant degree of racemization of some amino acids in proteins (especially aspartate), which seems to occur non-enzymically as the proteins age—this has been proposed as one of the mechanisms targeting proteins for intracellular catabolism. Man and Bada (1987) suggest that 10–20 per cent of the aspartate, and a significant proportion of other amino acids in some foods may be present as the D-isomers. There is a D-amino acid oxidase in the kidney, and hence it is possible for D-amino acids to be oxidized to their corresponding oxo-acids, and then undergo transamination to the L-isomers. Although there is evidence that D-amino acids will meet part of the requirement for essential amino acids in experimental animals, there is no information as to whether or not human beings are able to utilize D-amino acids to any significant extent.

10.2.1 Amino acids

The major amino acids are listed in Table 10.3, together with the three-letter abbreviations that are generally used, and the single letter codes that are used in protein sequences, as well as their relative molecular masses (M_r, or molecular weight), the values of pK_a for the ionizable groups and isoelectric point (where such data are reported in the literature) and the codon(s) on mRNA, where appropriate. Table 10.4 shows the genetic code.

Figure 10.1 shows the amino acids that are found in proteins and are incorporated as such in protein synthesis, classified by the chemistry of their side-chains. Figure 10.2 shows additional amino acids that are found in proteins, but are not incorporated as such, being formed by post-synthetic modification of the protein, and Fig.10.3 some amino acids that are not found in proteins, but occur as metabolic intermediates.

10.3   Protein digestion

Protein digestion is by hydrolysis of the α-peptide bonds, initially cleavage of specific bonds by endopeptidases (formerly called proteinases), resulting in a relatively large number of peptide fragments. This is followed by action of exopeptidases (aminopeptidases and carboxypeptidases) which remove single amino acids from the amino and carboxyl terminals respectively, resulting in free amino acids and di- and tripeptides. Tripeptides are hydrolysed by a specific tripeptide exopeptidase, and dipeptides by dipeptidases within the brush border of the intestinal mucosal cells. Peptide bonds from the ε-amino group of lysine, the γ-carboxyl group of glutamate or the β-carboxyl group of aspartate, which are involved in inter- and intra-chain cross-linking, are not hydrolysed by human enzymes, and these amino acids are not biologically available.

10.3.1 Proteolytic enzymes

The digestive proteolytic enzymes are all secreted as inactive precursor proteins (zymogens), and are activated in the intestinal lumen. In each case the zymogen has a terminal peptide region that overlies and blocks the catalytic site of the enzyme; activation is by removal of this blocking peptide by hydrolysis of a specific peptide bond. In the stomach pepsinogen is initially activated to pepsin by gastric acid; thereafter pepsin will catalyse the hydrolysis and activation of pepsinogen. In the small intestine trypsinogen is hydrolysed to active trypsin by enteropeptidase (sometimes incorrectly called enterokinase). Trypsin then catalyses the activation of chymotrypsinogen,

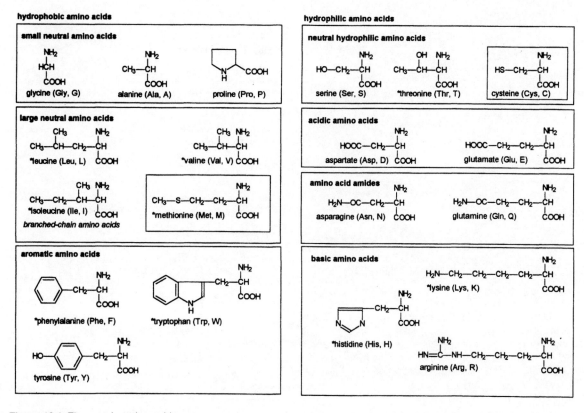

Figure 10.1 The protein amino acids
Hydrophobic amino acids are shown on the left and hydrophilic amino acids on the right; essential amino acids are starred.

proelastase, procarboxypeptidases and pro-amino-peptidases. The major proteolytic enzymes are shown in Table 10.5.

The Enzyme Commission (EC) 1992 classification of proteolytic enzymes (see Table 10.6) recommends that the term 'peptidase' be used for all enzymes that hydrolyse peptide bonds, thus reversing previous nomenclature, which restricted 'peptidase' to exopeptidases, which act only at or near the terminal of a peptide chain, and using the term 'proteinase' for what should now be called endopeptidases, which act in the middle of a peptide chain. Peptidases are in EC class 3.4; further subclassification is on the basis of whether the enzyme is an endo- or exopeptidase, and the reaction mechanism, as shown in Table 10.6.

10.3.2 Absorption of amino acids and peptides

The free amino acids released in the intestinal lumen are absorbed by a variety of group-specific transport mechanisms in the intestinal mucosa; many of the same amino acid transport systems are also found in the renal tubule, blood-brain barrier and other tissues (see Table 10.7). Di- and tripeptides are transported into mucosal cells by separate systems, and undergo hydrolysis to free amino acids within the brush border of the mucosal cell, catalysed by tripeptide aminopeptidase and a variety of dipeptidases.

There is also significant absorption of intact proteins and relatively large peptides from the intestinal lumen; this is especially important in neonates, who can acquire considerable passive immunity from the maternal antibodies in milk, but it continues throughout life. The uptake of intact proteins and peptides may be either paracellular, by diffusion through the tight junctions between epithelial cells, or transcellular, by endocytosis into the intestinal M cells in Peyer's patches, followed by transfer of (potential) antigens to sub-epithelial lymphocytes. Such absorption of proteins is presumably a major factor in food allergy (for a review, see Gardner 1988). In addition, a number of smaller peptides are also absorbed intact; many of these resemble the neuro-active

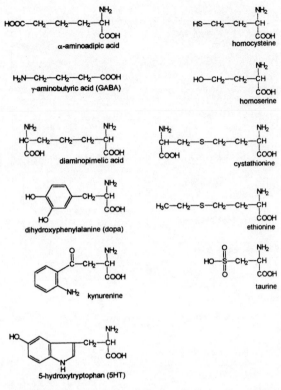

Figure 10.2 Amino acids arising by post-synthetic modification of proteins

See section 16.4 for the synthesis of γ-carboxyglutamate, section 22.4.3 for a discussion of prolyl and lysyl hydroxylases, and section 10.9.2 for a discussion of methylhistidine.

endorphins, and since they have some endorphin-like activity, they have been termed exorphins.

In addition to dietary protein (about 70–100 g/day in an adult), there is a considerable flux of endogenous protein through the gut, composed of

(1) secretion of digestive enzymes, amounting to 15–20 g protein /day;

(2) secretion of serum albumin and other proteins, amounting to about 6 g /day;

(3) shed intestinal mucosal cells and mucus secreted to lubricate the intestinal contents and protect the mucosa against the action of digestive enzymes, which together account for a further 50 g of protein /day.

Most of this protein is also digested and its constituent amino acids absorbed; faecal nitrogen is equivalent to only about 10 g of protein /day.

10.4   The carbon metabolism of amino acids

Despite the importance of amino acids for tissue protein synthesis, the first requirement of the body is for

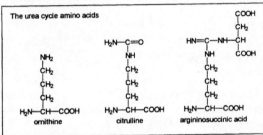

Figure 10.3 Non-protein amino acids that are important metabolic intermediates

a source of metabolic fuel; if total energy intake is inadequate to meet expenditure then amino acids will be oxidized as fuel. The energy yield of protein is 17 kJ /g, about the same as that of carbohydrate (see Table 5.3); this is because the carbon skeletons of most of the amino acids give rise to fragments that are metabolized by the same pathways as are carbohydrates. For an adult in N balance, an amount of protein equal to the dietary intake will be oxidized as metabolic fuel; the energy yields of amino acids are shown in Table 10.8.

Perhaps more importantly, in the fasting state the carbon skeletons of most of the amino acids arising from the continuing breakdown of tissue protein can be used for gluconeogenesis, to maintain a supply of glucose to the nervous system and red blood cells. Other amino acids give rise to acetate or acetoacetate, which cannot be used for gluconeogenesis. It is therefore conventional to divide the amino acids into those that are glucogenic, those that are purely ketogenic, and those that give rise to both glucogenic and ketogenic fragments, as shown in Table 10.9. Figure 10.4 shows the points at which the various amino acids feed into the central metabolic pathways (see also Figure 5.2).

10.5   Estimates of protein requirements

There are two ways in which protein requirements can be estimated: a factorial method of calculation based on replacement of the obligatory N loss that occurs on a protein-free diet and experimental studies of the intakes required to maintain N equilibrium.

10.5.1 Factorial calculation of protein requirements

On a protein-free diet the urinary excretion of N falls sharply for 4–6 days, then more gradually; it never reaches a truly constant level. The obligatory loss is taken as the (reasonably constant) output after 6–10 days on a protein-free diet. When protein was fed in amounts equivalent to the obligatory loss, subjects were still in negative nitrogen balance, and an extra 30 per cent was required to correct this. Allowances are also made for individual variation (20 per cent) and common metabolic stresses (10 per cent). This was the basis of 1973 United Nations Food and Agriculture Organization estimates of protein requirements (WHO/FAO 1973), shown in Table 10.10.

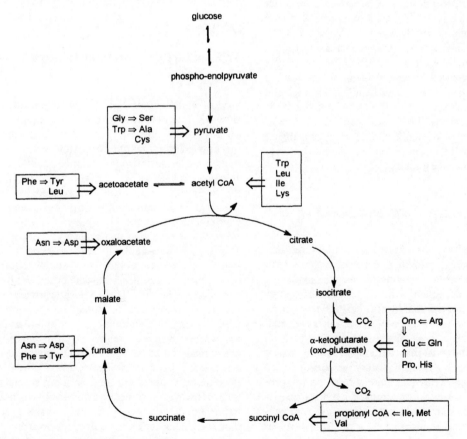

Figure 10.4 Metabolic fates of the amino acids
See also Figure 5.2

10.5.2 Determination of protein requirements by N balance studies

Early studies of N balance used a wide range of intakes, but there is not a linear relationship with intake throughout the sub-maintenance range. More recent studies, which are the basis for the 1985 United Nations estimates of protein requirements (FAO/WHO/UNU 1985) have used intakes around the maintenance requirement. One problem is that nitrogen balance shows some degree of adaptation to changes in intake, so that short-term studies (less than about 3 weeks) suggest higher requirements than do longer-term studies, in which there has been adaptation to the level of protein intake. The 1985 FAO/WHO/UNU report cites data from both short and long-term studies (see Table 10.11); the average requirement for maintenance of N balance was 0.63 g protein /kg body weight in short-term studies and 0.58 g /kg body weight in long-term studies; the mean requirement is therefore taken as 0.6 g protein /kg body weight. The coefficient of variation is 12.5 per cent, so adding $2 \times SD$ gives a reference intake (termed in the UN report a safe level of intake) of 0.75 g protein /kg body weight /day.

The FAO/WHO/UNU (1985) report did not cite a series of short-term studies on 107 subjects who were fed on varying levels of egg protein, which gave a mean requirement of 0.46 g protein /kg body weight, and a 95 per cent range of 0.375–0.59 g /kg body weight (Young *et al.* 1973; Millward *et al.* 1989). This suggests that a significant number of subjects may be able to maintain N balance at intakes very close to the obligatory loss.

10.5.3 Protein requirements as a proportion of energy intake

An alternative way of expressing protein requirements is to express protein as a per centage of total energy intake. Based on average energy expenditure, the average requirement is for 6 per cent of energy from protein, and the safe level is 7.5 per cent. Table 10.12 shows the protein content of a variety of dietary staples expressed as percentage of energy from protein; this suggests that with most of the major dietary staples, if sufficient could be consumed to meet energy requirements, there would be no problem of protein intake for adults. Cassava provides significantly less than 6 per cent of energy from protein, and rice and yam are below the safe level of protein intake. Table 10.13 shows average intakes and major sources of protein in western diets.

10.5.4 Reference intakes of protein

In most countries, Reference Intakes for protein are based on the FAO/WHO/UNU (1985) recommendations. For children, Reference Intakes include allowances for both maintenance and growth; the difference between the WHO/FAO/UNU and European Union figures shown in Table 10.14 is the result of the different basis for estimation of children's requirements used by the EU committee (see section 4.1.3).

Current estimates of infants' requirements include an allowance of 30 per cent, notionally to allow for day-to-day variation in growth rate, but in fact added to match the calculated requirement with the observed intake of breast-fed infants. Since the intake of breast-fed infants is presumably a safe level rather than just meeting requirements, it is possible that estimates of infants' protein requirements will be reduced.

The differences between the various figures for adults shown in Table 10.15 are due to the different average weights of populations in different countries.

10.6   Essential (indispensable) amino acids

Studies in the latter half of the nineteenth century showed that not all proteins were equally capable of supporting nitrogen balance, and that some (notably gelatine) would not permit experimental animals to maintain nitrogen balance at all if fed as the sole protein source. Through the first three decades of the twentieth century this was refined by studies of the amino acid composition of proteins, and the concept emerged that the requirement was not for total protein, but for individual amino acids. Studies of the ability of amino acid mixtures to support nitrogen balance showed that eight are absolute requirements; they cannot be synthesized in the body, but have to be provided in the diet. These are the essential or indispensable amino acids: isoleucine, leucine, lysine, methionine, phenylalanine, threonine, tryptophan, and valine. By contrast, the remaining amino acids are considered to be non-essential, since they can be synthesized from common metabolic intermediates, provided that adequate total amino nitrogen is available. However, it is noteworthy that two non-essential amino acids are only synthesized from precursors that are themselves essential: tyrosine from phenylalanine and cysteine from methionine. It is therefore conventional to consider requirement for (phenylalanine + tyrosine) and for (methionine + cysteine), since an intake of the product amino acid will spare the essential precursor.

A ninth amino acid, histidine, was added to the list of those known to be essential in 1975, following studies of subjects maintained on long-term total parenteral nutrition from which histidine was excluded (Kopple and Swendseid 1975). Early studies had not shown dietary histidine to be essential for the maintenance of nitrogen balance. The simplistic interpretation of this observation is that while there is some ability to synthesize histidine, this is not adequate to meet requirements in the complete absence of a dietary intake. However, it is not known whether or not human tissues are capable of the synthesis of histidine. Irwin and Hegsted (1971) quote Munro, citing unpublished work that demonstrated incorporation of label from [^{14}C]formate into histidine by human liver slices, but there appears to be no further information on this in the literature. One reason why histidine is not required for the maintenance of nitrogen balance in relatively short-term studies may be that it is liberated by hydrolysis of carnosine (β-alanyl-histidine), a muscle dipeptide of unknown function.

10.6.1 Essential amino acid requirements

The requirements for essential amino acids shown in Tables 10.16 and 10.17 have been derived in three different ways. The WHO/FAO (1973) and FAO/WHO/UNU (1985) figures are based on N balance studies, and amino acid scoring patterns have been calculated on the basis of proportion of a safe intake of protein (see Tables 10.14 and 10.15). Studies of the rate of whole body protein turnover and the rates of oxidation of individual amino acids (Young *et al.* 1989; Young 1994) suggest higher apparent requirements for essential amino acids, although the validity of this method of determining amino acid requirements has been challenged (Millward *et al.* 1993). As discussed in section 10.8.3, the rate of whole body protein turnover varies with both protein and energy intake, and therefore reflects the current nutritional status rather than requirements. Similarly, the rate of oxidation of essential amino acids reflects the need to control tissue concentrations rather than requirements to meet the needs for protein synthesis (see section 10.8.3.1).

10.6.2 The need for dispensable amino acids

Visek (1984) noted that apart from threonine and lysine, which do not undergo transamination, all of the amino acids can be replaced, to a greater or lesser extent, by their corresponding oxo-acids. He therefore suggested that only these two amino acids were strictly indispensable, since the others can be synthesized endogenously. This literal interpretation of the definition of an indispensable amino acid has not met with general acceptance, and is not nutritionally relevant, since in the case of the amino acids shown in Table 10.16, the only source of the oxo-acid is the amino acid itself. However, the ability to meet part of the requirement for essential amino acids from oxo-acids (and in some cases the chemically more stable hydroxyl derivatives) has been exploited in the formulation of extremely low protein diets for patients in renal failure (Wrong 1978).

The distinction between essential and non-essential amino acids was based on the assumption that, with the exception of lysine and threonine, all of the amino acids undergo ready transamination, and therefore if there is a pathway for the endogenous synthesis of the carbon skeleton of the amino acid (its oxo-acid), that amino acid is non-essential. Jackson (1983) noted that in fact the distribution of label from many [^{15}N]amino acids is more limited than might be expected. Those amino acids that participate in a large number of transamination reactions (glutamate, aspartate and alanine) readily become labelled, regardless of the source of ^{15}N. Other amino acids, although they can obviously be synthesized in the body, do not readily become labelled, suggesting that there may be only a limited capacity for their synthesis. He proposed a four way classification of amino acids, as shown in Table 10.18, depending on whether or not the carbon skeleton could be synthesized endogenously, and whether or not there was significant labelling of the amino acid from the general ^{15}N pool in tracer studies. Those amino acids whose carbon skeletons can be synthesized, but which are poor substrates for amination (semi-essential amino acids) include glycine and serine.

Laidlaw and Kopple (1987) have proposed two further groups of amino acids, in addition to those defined by Jackson (1983).

1. Conditionally essential amino acids, which may become dietary essentials in the absence of their precursors. This group includes not only tyrosine and cysteine, but also the urea cycle amino acids ornithine and citrulline, since the main source of these is arginine, and there is doubt over the adequacy of the body's capacity for *de novo* synthesis of arginine. Taurine may also be included here, since it is synthesized from cysteine. Although taurine is known to be an absolute diet-

ary essential to cats, it is not known whether or not there is adequate synthesis to meet requirements in human beings in the absence of a dietary intake (see section 23.9).

2. Acquired indispensable amino acids, which can become essential in states of metabolic disorder, immaturity or in severe stress or trauma. This group includes arginine (and possibly citrulline) under conditions of high amino acid intake; glycine when there is a high intake of compounds that are normally excreted as glycine conjugates (hippuric acids); proline in response to severe trauma such as burns (Jaksic *et al.* 1991) and glutamine in response to surgical trauma and sepsis (Souba 1993; Rennie *et al.* 1994).

The only three amino acids that can be regarded as truly dispensable, in that they are formed from common metabolic intermediates that really undergo transamination, are aspartate (formed from oxaloacetate), glutamate (formed from oxoglutarate), and alanine (formed from pyruvate). Nevertheless, in terms of practical nutrition, the amino acids that are most important in terms of the nutritional value of proteins are those listed in Tables 10.16 and 10.17.

10.7   Protein quality (nutritional value)

It is obvious, from the discussion of essential amino acids above, that the body's requirement is for the amino acids that are required for tissue protein synthesis, rather than for total protein. Reduced availability of any amino acid will slow the rate of protein synthesis, and thus, if prolonged, result in negative nitrogen balance, since the catabolism of tissue proteins continues at a more or less constant rate under most conditions (see section 10.8.3). A dietary protein that is relatively deficient in one or more of the essential amino acids will obviously be less useful for tissue protein synthesis than one that provides (more than) enough of all the essential amino acids—i.e. it will be of lower nutritional value or quality.

Protein quality is important in two respects.

1. When the total protein intake is close to the amount that is required, it is obviously a matter of concern if the amino acid composition of the dietary protein does not match requirements. A greater amount of a protein of lower quality will be required to meet requirements than would otherwise be the case.

2. Food labelling legislation in the United States (see section 4.3.1) requires not only that the crude protein content of a food (as determined by the Kjeldahl method) be considered when claims are made, but also that the quality of the protein be taken into account.

10.7.1 The limiting amino acid and complementation between proteins

The limiting amino acid of a protein is that (essential) amino acid present in least amount relative to the requirement for complete utilization of the protein for tissue protein synthesis. Generally cereal proteins are limited by their content of lysine, while legume and animal proteins are limited by their content of the sulphur amino acids (methionine plus cysteine). The result of this is that there is complementation between different proteins eaten in the same meal, and judicious mixtures of proteins may have very much higher nutritional value, as determined experimentally, than would appear likely from the values of the individual proteins. Overall mixed diets, regardless of the major protein sources, have a Biological Value between 0.7–0.8. An example of complementation is shown in Table 10.19.

10.7.2 Biological assays of protein quality

Early methods of assessing the nutritional value of proteins depended on their ability to support nitrogen balance or growth. Studies of N retention may utilize determination of intake and output (classical N balance) or, with experimental animals, carcass analysis, either measuring the increase in total body N after a period on the test diet compared with a control group analysed at the beginning of the experiment, or comparing the test group with a control group fed on a protein-free diet. Methods based on growth are shown in Table 10.20, and the main biological indices of protein quality in Table 10.21.

Such biological assays are time consuming and expensive, and a number of studies have attempted to validate rapid biological assays using insects or micro-organisms (see Table 10.22), specific responses (see Table 10.23) or biochemical indices of nutritional status (see Table 10.24).

It is important to note that, regardless of the method used, all biological methods of protein quality determination are a function solely of the limiting amino acid; unless experimental diets are supplemented with the limiting amino acid, and the experiments repeated, such assays give no information about other amino acids present in the test protein. Furthermore, biological assays give no information about relative surpluses of essential amino acids in the test protein, which are important for complementation (see section 10.7.1).

The Biological Value (BV, Mitchell 1924; Thomas 1909) of a protein is the proportion of the absorbed protein that is retained in the body—i.e. it takes no account of the digestibility of the protein. BV is determined by studies of nitrogen balance; endogenous urinary N loss and metabolic faecal N loss are estimated from a group of control animals fed a protein-free diet. Thomas (1909) estimated endogenous urine N and metabolic faecal N by feeding animals on a protein-free diet; Mitchell's (1924) modification of the method was to feed a low level of a protein of high BV (egg protein) so as to avoid the artefact introduced by the loss of tissue protein that occurs on a protein-free diet. If no correction of N balance data for metabolic and endogenous losses is made, the result is termed apparent BV. Proteins that are completely useable for tissue protein synthesis have BV = 0.95–1.0.

Digestibility is the proportion of food N that is absorbed; it is determined by measurement of faecal N in feeding studies. Apparent digestibility = (intake−faecal N) / intake, while true digestibility includes correction of faecal N for the metabolic faecal N. True digestibility = (intake−(faecal N−metabolic faecal N)) / intake.

Protein Efficiency Ratio (PER, Osborne *et al.* 1919) is the gain in weight of growing animals per gram of dietary protein, and therefore does not require determination of N balance. It therefore has the advantage of simplicity. However, apparent PER varies with the amount of food consumed, the stage of growth of the test animal and the duration of the experiment. Furthermore the weight gain is assumed to be protein tissue, but can include large and variable amounts of fat, which can give erratic and misleading results (Bender 1982). Despite these problems, PER was the basis of expressing protein quality for food labelling in the USA until 1993. The Nitrogen Efficiency Ratio (NER) is the gain in weight per gram of nitrogen consumed; numerically it equals PER × 6.25.

Net Protein Ratio (NPR, Bender and Doell 1957) was developed in order to overcome some of the problems associated with PER; there is a control group of animals fed a protein-free diet and the experiment lasts a standardized 10–14 days. NPR is the weight gain of animals fed on the test protein, plus the weight loss of the protein-free controls, divided by the protein consumed. NPR multiplied by 16 is the Protein Retention Efficiency (PRE) and is numerically equal to NPU.

Net Protein Utilization (NPU, Bender and Miller 1953; Miller and Bender 1955) is the proportion of dietary protein that is retained in the body, and therefore takes account of the digestibility of the protein: NPU = BV × digestibility. By convention NPU is measured at 10 per cent dietary protein (NPU_{10}), a level of intake at which all of the dietary protein can be used for tissue protein synthesis as long as the balance of essential amino acids is appropriate. When fed at 4 per cent of the diet the result is termed NPU standardized. If the food or diet is fed as it is normally eaten the result is NPU operative (NPU_{op}). Determination of NPU may be by N balance or carcass analysis.

Net Dietary Protein is the product of NPU_{op} × crude protein—i.e. it is an index of both the quantity and quality of dietary protein. The Net Dietary Protein:Energy Ratio (NDpE) is the proportion of energy intake provided by protein multiplied by NPU_{op}. When calculated using calories as the unit of energy, it is sometimes called NDpCal%.

10.7.3 Chemical analysis and protein quality

Block and Mitchell (1946) were the first to show that the Biological Value of a protein was related to its amino acid composition. They proposed a Chemical Score, comparing the essential amino acid content of the test protein with that of egg protein, which has a high BV. The lowest ratio reflects the limiting amino acid and is the Chemical Score of the protein.

Oser (1951) proposed a refinement of the Chemical Score procedure, to take into account not only the limiting amino acid but the relative amounts of all of the essential amino acids in the test protein. The Essential Amino Acid Index is the geometric mean of the amounts of all of the essential amino acids as a proportion of their content in the reference protein.

A refinement on the Chemical Score is the Protein Score (FAO 1955), in which the essential amino acid content of the test protein is compared with a reference pattern of essential amino acid requirements rather than the arbitrary comparison with the amino acid content of a protein of high BV. It is obvious from the data shown in Tables 10.16 and 10.17 that choice of the appropriate reference pattern is difficult, since use of the reference pattern for adults would overestimate the value of proteins for children, while use of the patterns for growth would underestimate their value for maintenance in adults. The 1991 FAO/WHO report on protein quality evaluation recommended the WHO/FAO/UNU (1985) reference pattern for children aged between 2–5 years (see Table 10.17), since this is the most demanding pattern of requirements of any age group other than suckling infants.

With the development of relatively rapid and convenient methods of amino acid determination by ion-exchange column chromatography (and more recently by high-pressure liquid chromatography), it would seem that the method of choice for assessing protein quality would be chemical analysis. This would have the added advantage of giving information about all the amino acids present in the food, not just the limiting amino acid as is the case for biological assays.

It is relatively simple to determine the amino acid composition of foods or individual proteins, although the method of hydrolysis of the protein can affect the results: tryptophan is unstable to acid hydrolysis, while cysteine is unstable to alkaline hydrolysis. The method of choice is enzymic hydrolysis with one or a mixture of the broad specificity proteases shown in Table 10.5; however, enzymic hydrolysis may introduce artefacts due to autolysis of the enzyme(s) being used, and consequent determination of their amino acids as well as those of the test protein.

The results of chemical analysis and biological determination can differ widely, especially when lysine is the limiting amino acid. This is because the ε-amino group of lysine can react with reducing sugars and other aldehydes in foods (the Maillard reaction) and can also form cross-links between peptide chains, forming peptide bonds to the γ-carboxyl group of glutamate or the β-carboxyl group of aspartate, as shown in Fig. 10.5. Acid or alkali treatment hydrolyses these ε-amino links, and some bacterial enzymes may also hydrolyse them, so the lysine is shown to be present on chemical analysis. However, ε-amino links to lysine are not substrates for mammalian digestive enzymes, and therefore the lysine is biologically unavailable.

A number of methods have been developed for rapid estimation of the proportion of lysine in a protein that has a free ε-amino group, and therefore is likely to be biologically available; such methods depend on reacting the (denatured) protein with a reagent such as fluorodinitrobenzene (FDNB), which reacts with free amino groups (Carpenter 1960, 1973). The result is termed the available lysine value (ALV); to avoid confusion with biological assays of availability, it is sometimes called FDNB-available or FDNB-reactive lysine. An alternative method involves chemical determination of lysine by ion-exchange chromatography with and without preliminary deamination of exposed ε-amino groups using nitrite. The result is termed chemically available lysine (Allison *et al.* 1973).

Other essential amino acids may also be biologically unavailable in foods; in these cases the chemical nature of the undigested complexes is less well defined than in the case of lysine, and there are no simple methods for correcting chemical analysis for biological availability of other amino acids.

The Protein Digestibility-Corrected Amino Acid Score (PDCAAS) is now the agreed basis for expressing the nutritional quality of proteins (FAO/WHO

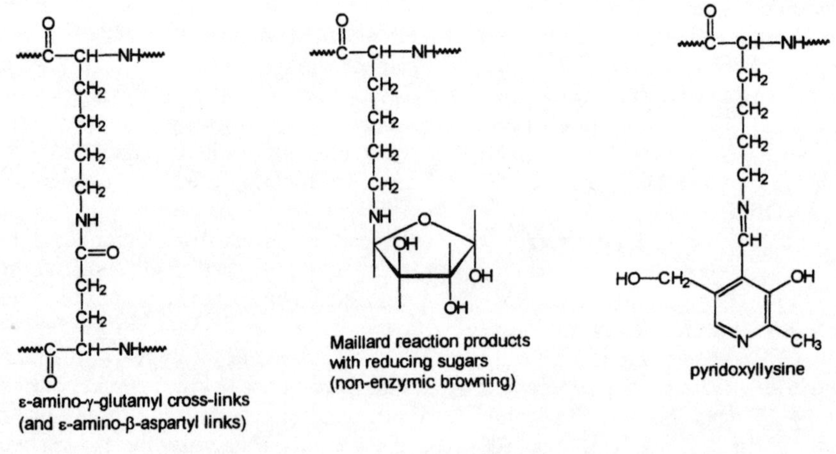

Figure 10.5 Biologically unavailable lysine
See section 20.2.1.2 for a discussion of pyridoxyllysine in vitamin B$_6$ nutrition.

1991; Sarwar and McDonough 1990). This is the Protein Score of the test protein, expressed using the 1985 FAO/WHO/UNU reference pattern for children aged between 2–5 years, corrected for digestibility, as determined by animal feeding studies. US food labelling legislation (see section 4.3.1) requires that the protein content of a food be corrected for the PDCAAS before calculation of the percentage of daily value of protein intake provided by that food.

10.8 Whole body protein turnover

Studies of N balance measure only the difference between intake and excretion, and hence reflect only the net difference between protein synthesis and catabolism. Isotopic studies of whole body protein turnover permit determination of the overall rates of protein synthesis and catabolism, and hence calculation of the energy cost of protein turnover (as discussed below, a significant proportion of BMR), and have permitted elucidation of the mechanisms involved in tissue protein loss in response to trauma, infection and cancer. The physiology of protein turnover has been reviewed by Waterlow (1984).

Early studies of protein turnover used a single dose of a ^{15}N labelled amino acid and estimated the turnover rate and size of the metabolic pool by determination of the isotopic enrichment of urinary urea or the plasma free amino acid during the first few hours. This approach makes three main assumptions, none of which is correct.

1. There is a single homogeneous metabolic amino acid pool—a gross over-simplification.

2. The loss of labelled amino acid from this pool follows first-order kinetics—again a gross over-simplification.

3. Amino acid catabolism is not rate limiting, so that the isotopic enrichment of urea reflects that in the precursor amino acid available for protein synthesis. However, net transamination and deamination of labelled glycine can still be observed 12 hours after a single dose, while the critical measurements are made 3–4 hours after the dose.

10.8.1 The constant infusion, labelled precursor method

If a labelled amino acid is infused at a constant rate over a period of 12–30 hours, rather than being given as a single dose, there will initially be an exponential increase in the isotopic enrichment of the amino acid in plasma, followed by a period over which it will remain constant. The rate of entry of label from the infusion equals the rate of efflux from the free amino acid pool into either protein synthesis or catabolism. Later the isotopic enrichment in plasma will increase again as amino acids enter the pool from protein catabolism. This is the basis of the constant infusion, labelled precursor method developed by Waterlow and Stephen (1967).

This method requires no assumptions about the number of different metabolic pools of the amino acid; a single pool would give a simple exponential increase, whereas multiple pools would give a more complex pattern, but in either case there will be a plateau. At this time

influx (from infusion) = efflux (to protein and metabolites)

hence

rate of infusion × isotopic enrichment of infused amino acid = total efflux from the pool × isotopic enrichment at plateau.

Rearranging gives

total efflux into protein + amino acids = (rate of infusion × isotopic enrichment of infused amino acid) / isotopic enrichment at plateau.

Knowing the amount of amino acid infused, it is possible to calculate the amount entering protein rather than being metabolized.

This method assumes the following

1. When a steady state has been achieved the re-entry of amino acids into the free amino acid pool from protein catabolism is negligible.

2. The amount of amino acid infused is small compared with total flux through the amino acid pool (not justified if stable isotopes are used, because of the relatively large amounts that must be used to enable detection).

3. Isotopic enrichment of the plasma amino acid equals that in the tissues where protein is being synthesized. This is certainly not valid when [^{13}C]leucine is used as the tracer, and a correction is made for the isotopic enrichment of oxo-iso-caproate.

4. The amino acid arising from protein catabolism is treated in the same way as that arising from the diet or infusion.

5. There is no significant isotope effect, and the amino acid chosen is a valid tracer for protein turnover.

10.8.2 The constant infusion, labelled end-product method

Picou and Taylor-Roberts (1969) modified the constant infusion technique by measuring the isotopic enrichment of end-products of metabolism rather than the plasma free amino acid precursor. Such end-products may be exhaled $^{14}CO_2$, or urinary $[^{15}N]$urea and $^{15}NH_4^+$. This has two advantages over the Waterlow and Stephen method: (a) no assumptions are made about the isotopic enrichment in plasma being equal to that in tissues and (b) it is a less invasive procedure, since it does not require plasma samples.

At the plateau of labelling in the end-product, total flux (turnover) of nitrogen

= (measured) dietary intake + entry of amino acid from infusion

= efflux of N to protein synthesis + efflux to metabolites.

Percentage of administered isotope being excreted

= rate of excretion of labelled metabolite / rate of infusion of labelled amino acid

= efflux of N to metabolites / total flux of nitrogen

Hence, protein synthesis = total N flux-excretion.

In addition to the assumptions made in the Waterlow and Stephen method, this method assumes that the recovery of metabolites is complete and constant. This assumption is not wholly valid for measurement of either $^{13}CO_2$ or $[^{15}N]$ urea and ammonia.

1. The recovery of $^{13}CO_2$ in exhaled air after infusion of $H^{13}CO_3^-$ changes from about 90 per cent in the fed state to about 76 per cent in the fasting state, presumably reflecting incorporation of CO_2 into carbohydrates during gluconeogenesis.

2. There is considerable enterohepatic cycling of urea, with hydrolysis by intestinal bacterial urease and re-absorption of much of the ammonia, a considerable proportion of which enters the non-essential amino acid pool by way of formation of glutamate and glutamine. In addition, much of the ammonia may be used for bacterial protein synthesis, releasing a variety of amino acids that can be absorbed into the circulation. Label from $[^{15}N]$urea can be found in all amino acids, including lysine (which does not undergo transamination). Jackson (1993) has reported that at intakes of more than 70 g of protein (160 mg N /kg body weight) /day some 70–75 per cent of the urea synthesized is excreted in the urine, the remainder being salvaged in the colon. At intakes of 35–70 g of protein (80–160 mg N /kg body weight) /day an increasing proportion of the urea synthesized is salvaged rather than being excreted. At an intake of 80 mg N /kg body weight the salvage of urea may account for 115 mg N /kg body weight /day.

Taruvinga *et al.* (1979) compared estimates of whole body protein synthesis by the precursor and end-product methods using a variety of amino acids. They showed that with $[^{15}N]$glycine the two methods give comparable results. However, $[^{15}N]$aspartate resulted in increased labelling of urea (which is predictable, since aspartate is an immediate source of nitrogen for urea synthesis), and hence the end-product method gave a lower apparent rate of protein synthesis than did the labelled precursor method. With $[^{15}N]$leucine, the end-product method gave a higher rate of apparent protein synthesis than did the precursor method, since leucine is mainly transaminated in skeletal muscle rather than the liver, and hence results in less labelling of urea than would otherwise be the case—there is more spread of the label into other amino acids that readily undergo transamination.

10.8.3 Rates of whole body protein turnover

Studies of protein turnover by constant infusion methods have shown that the rate of protein turnover is considerably greater than would be predicted from levels of protein intake required to maintain N balance. Even in growing children there is a considerably greater rate of total protein synthesis than the net increase in body protein shown by positive N balance. Various studies have shown this, even in times of rapid growth; rapidly growing pigs synthesize 2 g of protein for each gram of net synthesis, and in recovery from protein-energy malnutrition children can synthesize 2.5 g protein /g net synthesis. Young and Pellet (1987) have compared rates of protein synthesis and safe levels of protein intake at various ages, as shown in Table 10.25.

Results such as those shown in Table 10.25 imply that there must be considerable re-utilization of the amino acids released by tissue protein catabolism. Indeed, the observation that the total rate of protein synthesis is some 6–fold higher than the dietary intake required to maintain N balance raises the question of why an adult has any need for a dietary intake of protein at all, other than to replace the relatively small amounts lost irreversibly in skin, hair, sweat and mucus.

10.8.3.1 The catabolic drive and amino acid oxidation

Millward and Rivers (1988) have proposed a model of protein turnover that, to a considerable extent, accounts for the continuing need of adults for a dietary source of protein. They proposed that the main controlling factor of protein turnover is a catabolic drive; at any time amino acids released by protein catabolism, or coming from the diet, in excess of immediate requirements for protein synthesis are metabolized, rather than being stored.

Lysine, phenylalanine and the branched-chain amino acids are especially affected; the initial enzymes for the catabolism of these amino acids are normally unsaturated, and hence can respond to increased availability of the substrate by a considerable increase in the rate of amino acid catabolism, whereas the aminoacyl tRNA synthetases involved in protein synthesis are saturated. Withdrawal of these amino acids leaves others that cannot be used for protein synthesis, and therefore will also be catabolized.

The aminoacyl tRNA synthetases have values of K_m such that they are saturated at normal concentrations of substrate, and therefore act at a more or less constant rate to channel amino acids to protein synthesis (Young and Marchini 1990). By contrast, many of the enzymes that channel amino acids towards oxidative metabolism have relatively high values of K_m, and hence show increasing activity as the concentration of substrate rises (see Table 10.26). Furthermore, some, such as phenylalanine hydroxylase and tryptophan dioxygenase, are activated, enhanced or induced by their substrates.

In addition to this catabolic drive, the irreversible losses of amino acids in skin and hair proteins and mucus must be considered. Although these represent minor losses of total body protein (see section 10.1.2), these proteins are unusually rich in cysteine and threonine compared with the amino acid composition of average protein turnover. There is thus an irreversible loss of disproportionate amounts of two essential amino acids. Withdrawal of these from the tissue amino acid pool limits the extent to which other amino acids can be used for replacement protein synthesis. Feeding supplements of threonine and cysteine reduces the obligatory nitrogen loss in subjects maintained on a protein-free diet.

10.8.3.2 The energy cost of protein synthesis

A minimal estimate of the energy cost of protein synthesis can be derived from the biochemistry of protein synthesis. On the ribosome there is utilization of 4 mol of (ATP plus GTP) per peptide bond formed. Robinson *et al.* (1990) therefore calculated the following:

minimum estimate (4 (ATP or GTP) / peptide bond = 2.80 kJ /g protein synthesized

allowing for ATP cost of amino acid transport into tissue = 3.59 kJ /g protein synthesized

allowing for ATP cost of mRNA synthesis = 4.19 kJ /g protein synthesized

On this basis, a 70 kg adult synthesizing 5 g protein /kg body weight /day would expend 1.5 MJ, or almost 20 per cent of BMR, on protein turnover. This is in agreement with the data reported by Waterlow *et al.* (1978) on the rates of whole body protein synthesis and energy cost as a percentage of fasting and total energy expenditure for various species shown in Table 10.27.

Robinson *et al.* (1990) measured energy expenditure using a respiratory chamber and protein synthesis by the end-product methods using [^{13}C]glycine over a 9 hour period in fasting adults and after a high-carbohydrate or high-protein meal. The results are shown in Table 10.28.

It is apparent from the results shown in Table 10.28 that both protein and energy intake affect the rate of whole body protein synthesis. Garza *et al.* (1977) fed six subjects on a diet providing just the safe level of intake (0.57 g /kg body weight) and showed that they were unable to maintain N balance when their diet provided their calculated energy requirement, and were only able to do so when the energy intake was increased to such an extent that they showed a persistent weight gain. The mean change in N balance was 0.355 mg N /kJ additional energy intake.

Motil *et al.* (1981) showed that the daily rate of protein synthesis increased from 2 g /kg body weight at inadequate levels of intake (0.1 g /kg body weight) to 3.15 g /kg body weight at an intake of 0.6 g /kg body weight and to 3.5 g /kg body weight at average levels of protein intake (1.5 g /kg body weight). Chiang and Huang (1988) investigated the effects on N balance of changing energy intake in young men receiving a constant intake of 1.2 g protein /kg body weight. The results are shown in Table 10.29.

The relationship between energy metabolism and protein turnover is seen clearly in studies of different species. As shown in Table 10.30, there is an 11–fold difference in the rate of protein turnover /kg body weight in different species, but a reasonably constant rate between 43–60 mg protein turnover /kJ resting metabolic rate.

10.8.3.3 Diurnal variation in protein turnover

The effect of energy nutrition on protein synthesis is also seen during the normal daily cycle of feeding and fasting. Clugston and Garlick (1982) measured the rates of protein synthesis and catabolism in fed and fasting states. As shown in Table 10.31, the rate of protein catabolism is more or less constant throughout the day, but there is a significant difference in the rate of synthesis between fed and fasting states. There is net positive N balance in the fed state, which is countered by negative N balance in the fasting state. Thus, even for an adult in N equilibrium, there is diurnal cycling between positive and negative balance.

The Millward and Rivers (1988) model (see section 10.8.3.1) predicts that the amplitude of the diurnal cycle of positive and negative N balance will increase with increasing protein intake, and therefore that the requirement for overall maintenance of balance will increase with increasing habitual protein intake—thus providing a biochemical explanation for the difference between short and long-term studies of N balance shown in Table 10.10 (Millward *et al.* 1991). Price *et al.* (1990) have shown that there is indeed such a change in the amplitude of the diurnal cycle of N balance with changing protein intake. In subjects who had been allowed 2 weeks to adapt to the diet, there was a difference between the rates of protein turnover in the fed and fasting states of 55 mg N /kg body weight at an intake of 0.35 g protein /kg body weight, rising to 92 mg N /kg body weight at an intake of 0.75 g protein /kg body weight and to 200 mg N /kg body weight at the average level of protein intake of 1.5 g /kg body weight.

10.8.3.4 Protein turnover in individual organs

Studies in human beings are, of necessity, essentially limited to whole body protein turnover. Studies in experimental animals permit determination of rates of protein turnover in individual organs. As shown in Table 10.32, in the rat some 49 per cent of total body protein turnover is accounted for by the viscera, and 51 per cent by the carcass (skin, bone and skeletal muscle). Half lives for tissue proteins in the rat are shown in Table 10.33.

10.8.3.5 Turnover of individual proteins

Individual proteins show markedly different rates of turnover. In general those enzymes that are key controlling steps of metabolic pathways have very short half-lives, and a range of 2–5–fold variation in activity through the day, while structural proteins have considerably longer half-lives; indeed, for many years it was assumed that collagen does not turn over at all in the adult, because its long half-life (of the order of 150 days) means that its turnover cannot be detected with normal levels of isotopically labelled amino acids. Table 10.34 shows the half-lives and fractional rates of turnover of a range of cytosolic enzymes. It is noteworthy that enzymes inside subcellular organelles (lysosomes, microsomes, mitochondria, etc.) similarly turn over at varying rates, independently of the turnover of the organelles.

10.8.4 The catabolic response to trauma and infection

In response to surgical and other trauma, infection and advanced cancer there is considerable catabolism of tissue protein, and a period of negative N balance; estimates of the amounts of body protein that may be lost over 10 days are shown in Table 10.35.

The early view of this catabolic loss of body protein, cited in many textbooks, was that it represented mobilization of tissue (largely muscle) protein to provide amino acids for repair. This is unlikely, since the amino acids are not used for tissue repair, but are metabolized, resulting in negative N balance for a period up to about 10 days after the trauma. Furthermore, mobilization of amino acids would imply an increase in the rate of protein catabolism, whereas stable isotope studies have shown that under conditions of post-surgical trauma the rate of whole body protein catabolism is unchanged or even reduced. The net loss of protein is the result of a reduced rate of replacement protein synthesis (O'Keefe *et al.* 1974). An alternative explanation that has been advanced is that the loss of tissue protein represents utilization of amino acids as metabolic fuel during the flow phase (the hypermetabolic response to trauma). Again this is unlikely to be the primary mechanism, since the metabolic rate returns to normal within about five days after trauma, whereas negative N balance continues for longer. Furthermore, hypercaloric nutritional supplementation has little effect on N balance under these conditions.

Two related factors may account for the negative N balance associated with trauma: the actions of cortisol, which is secreted in increased amounts under conditions of stress, and the synthesis of acute phase response proteins.

10.8.4.1 Actions of cortisol

At a whole body level, the effect of increased cortisol secretion is to increase the catabolism of muscle protein and to increase the rate of gluconeogenesis from amino acids in the liver. While cortisol does induce the gluconeogenic enzyme phosphoenolpyruvate carboxykinase, its main effect on both physiological processes is indirect, by way of induction of tryptophan dioxygenase and tyrosine aminotransferase. Increased activity of these two enzymes results in depletion of the body pool of two (essential) amino acids. As a result there is a reduced rate of protein synthesis, and accumulation of other amino acids that cannot be used for protein synthesis, and are therefore substrates for deamination and either gluconeogenesis or ketogenesis (see Table 10.9 and Fig. 10.4).

10.8.4.2 Acute phase proteins

In response to a variety of traumatic and other insults, the hepatic synthesis of a number of plasma proteins is changed, mediated by the release of interleukins from the site of injury. The synthesis of albumin, prealbumin and transferrin is considerably reduced, while the synthesis of a variety of other proteins, collectively known as the acute phase proteins, increases (Fleck *et al.* 1985). The major acute phase proteins are shown in Table 10.36. The rates at which the plasma concentrations change in response to injury depend on the half-life, and hence the normal rate of turnover, of the individual proteins. The response reflects the severity of the insult, but not the site or type.

The amounts of acute phase proteins that are synthesized are extremely small compared with the losses of whole body protein shown in Table 10.35. However, the majority of them are disproportionately rich in cysteine and threonine compared with the normal pattern of protein synthesis. Synthesis of acute phase proteins thus represents a disproportionate drain on the body pools of these two essential amino acids, so reducing their availability for the synthesis of other proteins. As a result there is an excess of protein catabolism over replacement synthesis, with those amino acids that cannot be used for protein synthesis (because of the relative lack of threonine and cysteine) undergoing deamination and being used as metabolic fuels.

As discussed in section 12.2, the loss of muscle and other tissue protein in marasmus and kwashiorkor is due to reduced synthesis; the rate of tissue protein catabolism is more or less normal, as it is in response to trauma. However, in patients with cancer cachexia (see section 12.3), and possibly also in patients with AIDS, there is not only a reduction in protein synthesis, as a result of the lack of metabolic fuels associated with hypermetabolism, and increased hepatic synthesis of acute phase proteins, but also an increase in the rate of tissue protein catabolism. This is due to enhancement of protein turnover by tumour necrosis factor-α (cachectin), with greater enhancement of catabolism than of synthesis (Llovera *et al.* 1993).

10.9 Assessment of protein nutritional status

Anthropometric methods such as measurement of arm and leg muscle circumference, and growth, can be used to assess protein nutritional status (see Chapter 3). However, these are insensitive measures, and will only reveal relatively severe protein deficiency; furthermore, as discussed in section 12.2, the effects of energy undernutrition and protein deficiency cannot easily be disentangled, except in the case of stunting with or without wasting in children. A number of laboratory determinations of indices of protein metabolism have been proposed for the assessment of protein nutritional status; none is wholly satisfactory (Gibson 1990).

10.9.1 Plasma protein concentrations

Measurement of total serum protein does not really give any useful information, since this falls to below the reference range only when clear clinical signs of undernutrition are apparent, and anyway does not differentiate between general undernutrition and protein deficiency. A total plasma protein concentration < 60 g /L in young children or pregnant women, and < 64 g /L in children aged over 6 and in adults, is considered to be inadequate, and to indicate risk of malnutrition. Reference ranges for plasma protein concentrations are shown in Table 10.37.

A number of investigators have suggested that a more sensitive indicator of protein nutritional status may be the plasma concentration of one or more specific plasma proteins, such as transferrin, transthyretin (pre-albumin) or retinol binding protein. The problem is that the first two are negative acute phase proteins, whose synthesis will be impaired not only by undernutrition but also by infection, stress and trauma, while retinol binding protein synthesis is especially sensitive to energy nutrition (rather than specifically to protein nutrition) and to zinc status (see sections 13.2.4 and 25.26.2); it is also an early casualty of liver disease.

10.9.2 Plasma amino acid concentrations

Whitehead and Dean (1964) showed that the ratio of total non-essential:essential free amino acids in plasma was high in children with kwashiorkor; about 3.0, compared with a value of 2.0 for children with marasmus or those who were adequately nourished. However, changes in serum amino acids do not provide a sensitive index of protein nutritional status, since there is considerable metabolic control over circulating amino acids. There is less than 30 per cent variation through the day in response to feeding and fasting in the plasma concentrations of most amino acids. The non-essential:essential amino acid index only rises in severely malnourished children with clear signs of kwashiorkor. Reference ranges for plasma amino acids are shown in Table 10.38.

10.9.3 Urine amino acid metabolites

3–Methylhistidine released by catabolism of muscle protein is not re-utilized for protein synthesis but, at least in human beings, is excreted quantitatively (Young and Munro 1978). The majority of the body's 3–methylhistidine is in skeletal muscle, which contains 3.3 μmol /kg, compared with some 2–3 μmol /kg in smooth and cardiac muscle (which are a very much smaller proportion of body protein than is skeletal muscle), and less than 1 μmol /kg in other tissues. However, the rate of 3–methylhistidine turnover in different tissues varies considerably, from less than 1 per cent /day in skeletal muscle to 3.2 per cent /day in skin and 9 per cent /day in intestinal mucosa; Millward and Bates (1983) interpreted these data as indicating that less than 40 per cent of the urinary 3–methylhistidine was the result of muscle protein turnover. Furthermore, there seem to be inadequate published data on 3–methylhistidine excretion to permit reference ranges and hence ranges possibly associated with inadequate protein nutrition, to be constructed.

Like methylhistidine, hydroxyproline is formed by post-synthetic modification of protein, and when released as a result of protein catabolism it is not re-utilized, but is largely excreted unchanged, frequently as small hydroxyproline-containing peptides. While urinary excretion is lower than normal in malnourished children, this occurs in marasmus, kwashiorkor and marasmic kwashiorkor, so reflects general undernutrition rather than protein deficiency. Furthermore, a variety of non-nutritional factors, including hookworm infestation and malaria, as well as collagen ingestion, affect the excretion of hydroxyproline, as does body weight. Whitehead (1965) developed a hydroxyproline index:

$$\frac{mg\ hydroxyproline\ /mL\ urine}{mg\ creatinine/mL\ urine} \times bodyweight(kg).$$

He showed that in adequately nourished children between 1–6 years of age the value of this index was approximately 3.0, falling with increasing severity of malnutrition.

In view of the energy cost of protein synthesis, and the effects of energy nutrition on protein turnover (see section 10.8.3.2), it is perhaps unsurprising that none of these proposed methods of assessing protein nutritional status is capable of differentiating between deficiency of protein and inadequate total food intake. For a discussion of the problems of protein-energy malnutrition see Chapter 12.

10.10   Inborn errors of amino acid metabolism

A number of rare genetic diseases, listed in Table 10.39, affect the metabolism of amino acids; while some cannot (yet) be treated in a satisfactory manner, many can be controlled adequately by more or less severe restriction of the dietary intake of the affected amino acid(s). In some cases the defect is in the coenzyme binding site of the affected enzyme, and patients can be successfully controlled by administration of intakes of vitamin B$_6$ (cystathioninuria, homocystinuria, xanthurenic aciduria, primary hyperoxaluria, see section 20.5.1) or thiamin (maple syrup urine disease, see section 17.4.1) some 50–100 times greater than Reference Intakes. Such conditions have been called vitamin dependency diseases or vitamin responsive inborn errors of metabolism.

Most of these conditions are extremely rare, and indeed for some there are only single case reports in the literature. The frequency per million live births in the north American and European populations of some of the less rare conditions are: phenylketonuria 80; cystinuria 70; Hartnup disease 40; histidinaemia 40; hyperprolinaemia 20; argininosuccinicaciduria 4; maple syrup urine disease 3.

Further reading

Bender, D.A. (1985). *Amino Acid Metabolism*, Wiley, Chichester.

Irwin, M.I. and Hegsted, D.M. (1971). A conspectus of research on amino acid requirements of man. *Journal of Nutrition*, 101, 541–66.

Jackson, A.A. (1983). Amino acids, essential and non-essential. *Lancet*, (i) 1034–7.

Jackson, A.A. (1993). Chronic malnutrition: protein metabolism. *Proceedings of the Nutrition Society*, 52, 1–10.

Millward, D.J. (1994). Can we define indispensable amino acid requirements and assess protein quality in adults? *Journal of Nutrition*, 124, 1509–165.

Millward, D. J., Jackson, A. A., Price, G. and Rivers, J.P. W. (1989). Human amino acid and protein requirements: current dilemmas and uncertainties. *Nutrition Research Reviews*, 2, 109–32.

Waterlow, J.C. (1984). Protein turnover with special reference to man. *Quarterly Journal of Experimental Physiology*, 69, 409–38.

Waterlow, J. C., Garlick, P.J. and Millward, D.J. (1978). *Protein Turnover in Mammalian Tissues and the Whole Body*. North-Holland, Amsterdam.

WHO/FAO (1973). *Energy and protein requirements: Report of a joint FAO/WHO ad hoc expert committee*, WHO Technical Reports Series 522 WHO, Geneva.

WHO/FAO/UNU (1985). *Energy and protein requirements: Report of a joint WHO/FAO/UNU expert comsultation*, WHO Technical Reports Series 724 WHO, Geneva.

Young, V.R. and Pellet, P.L. (1987). Protein intake and requirements with reference to diet and health. *American Journal of Clinical Nutrition*, 45, 1323–43.

Table 10.1: N conversion factors for foods

	factor
wholemeal wheat	5.83
medium/low extraction wheat and pasta	5.70
wheat bran	6.31
rice	5.95
rye, barley, oats	5.83
groundnuts	5.46
soya beans	5.71
almonds	5.18
Brazil nuts	5.46
other nuts and seeds	5.30
milk, cheese, butter	6.38
all other foods	6.25

Source: WHO/FAO 1973.

Table 10.2: Nitrogenous compounds excreted in the urine

	normal range of excretion / 24 h	
urea (varies with protein intake)	10-35 g	150-600 mmol
ammonia (varies with acid-base balance)	340-1200 mg	20-70 mmol
free amino acids, conjugates, small peptides	1.3-3.2 g	20-70 mmol
uric acid	250-750 mg	1.5-4.5 mmol
allantoin	25-30 mg	150-190 µmol
purines	6-40 mg	40-270 µmol
coproporphyrin	5-250 mg	80-380 nmol
uroporphyrin	0-30 mg	< 36 nmol
adrenaline (epinephrine)	< 20 µg	< 109 nmol
noradrenaline (norepinephrine)	< 100 µg	<590 nmol
amino sugars	10-40 mg	50-250 mmol
creatinine[1] (depends on muscle mass)	1.0-2.5 mg	9-22 mmol
creatine[2]	< 100 mg	< 0.75 mmol
proteins	< 150 mg	-
carnitine	80-130 mg	0.5-0.8 mmol
amines	45-100 mg	-

(1) 15-25 mg (0.13-0.22) mmol /kg body weight
(2) Or < 6% of creatinine in adults; < 30% of creatinine in children; < 12% of creatinine in pregnancy.
Source: Bender 1985; Massachussetts General Hospital 1986.

Table 10.3: The amino acids

			M_r	pK_a	iep	codon(s)
Amino acids incorporated in ribosomal protein synthesis						
alanine	Ala	A	89.1	2.35, 9.87	6.11	GCNu[1]
arginine	Arg	R	174.2	1.83, 8.99, 12.48	10.73	CGNu, AGPu[1]
asparagine	Asn[2]	-	132.1	2.1, 8.84	5.41	AAPy[1]
aspartate	Asp	D	133.1	1.99, 3.90, 9.90	2.98	GAPy
cysteine	Cys	C	121.1	1.92, 8.35, 10.46	5.07	UGPy
glutamate	Glu[2]	E	147.1	2.10, 4.07, 9.47	3.21	GAPu
glutamine	Gln	Q	146.1	2.17, 9.13	5.65	CAPu
glycine	Gly	G	75.1	2.35, 9.78	6.20	CGNu
histidine	His	H	155.2	1.80, 6.04, 9.76	7.64	CAPy
isoleucine	Ile	I	131.2	2.32, 9.76	6.04	AUA, AUPu
leucine	Leu	L	131.2	2.33, 9.74	6.04	UUPu, CUNu
lysine	Lys	K	146.2	2.16, 9.18, 10.79	9.47	AAPu
methionine	Met	M	149.2	2.13, 9.28	5.74	AUG
phenylalanine	Phe	F	165.2	2.16, 9.18	5.91	UUPy
proline	Pro	P	115.1	1.95, 10.64	6.30	CCNu
selenocysteine	-	-	168.0	-	5.68	UGA[3]
serine	Ser	S	105.1	2.19, 9.21	5.59	UCNu, AGPy
threonine	Thr	T	119.1	2.09, 9.10	5.88	ACNu
tryptophan	Trp	W	204.2	2.43, 9.44	5.63	UGG
tyrosine	Tyr	Y	181.2	2.20, 9.11, 10.13	6.00	UAPy
valine	Val	V	117.1	2.29, 9.74		GUNu
Amino acids formed by post-synthetic modification of proteins						
γ-carboxyglutamate	Gla	-	199.1	-	-	as Glu
cystine	(Cys)$_2$	-	240.2	< 1.0, 2.1, 8.02, 8.71	5.02	as Cys
hydroxylysine	Hyl	-	162.2	2.13, 8.62, 9.67	9.15	as Lys
hydroxyproline	Hyp	-	131.1	1.82, 9.66	5.82	as Pro
3-methylhistidine	-	-	169.2	-	-	as His
5-oxoproline (pyroglutamate)	-	-	129.1	3.32	-	-
phosphoserine	-	-	185.1	-	-	as Ser
phosphotyrosine	-	-	261.2	-	-	as Tyr
Non-protein amino acids						
α-aminoadipic acid	-	-	161.2	2.14, 4.21, 9.77	-	-
γ-aminobutyric acid)	GABA	-	103.1	4.03, 10.56	-	-
argininosuccinic acid	-	-	290.3	1.62, 2.70, 4.26, 9.58, > 12	-	-
citrulline	-	-	175.2	2.43, 9.41	5.92	-
cystathionine	-	-	223.3	-	-	-
diaminopimelic acid	-	-	190.2	1.8, 2.2, 8.8, 9.9	-	-
dihydroxyphenylalanine	dopa	-	197.2	2.32, 8.72, 9.96, 11.79	-	-
ethionine	-	-	163.2	-	-	-
homocysteine	-	-	117.2	2.22, 8.87, 10.86	-	-
homoserine	-	-	119.1	2.71, 9.62	-	-
5-hydroxytryptophan	5HTP	-	220.2	-	-	-
kynurenine	-	-	208.2	-	-	-
ornithine	Orn	-	132.2	1.71, 8.69, 10.76	9.70	-
taurine	Tau	-	125.2	-0.3, 9.06	-	-

(1) Nu is used to indicate any nucleotide, Pu either purine (A or G), and Py either pyrimidine (C or U)

(2) Where it is not known from protein sequencing whether the amino acid is aspartate or asparagine the abbreviation Asx (and the single letter B) is used; similarly, for either glutamate or glutamine the symbol is Glx and the single letter code is Z.

(3) UGA is normally a stop codon; it is read in a context-sensitive manner as coding for selenocysteine in a very limited number of proteins (see section 15.4.1).

Table 10.4: The Genetic Code

first base	U	C	A	G	third base
		second base of codon			
U	Phe	Ser	Tyr	Cys	U
U	Phe	Ser	Tyr	Cys	C
U	Leu	Ser	STOP	STOP[1]	A
U	Leu	Ser	STOP	Trp	G
C	Leu	Pro	His	Arg	U
C	Leu	Pro	His	Arg	C
C	Leu	Pro	Gln	Arg	A
C	Leu	Pro	Gln	Arg	G
A	Ile	Thr	Asn	Ser	U
A	Ile	Thr	Asn	Ser	C
A	Ile	Thr	Lys	Arg	A
A	Met	Thr	Lys	Arg	G
G	Val	Ala	Asp	Gly	U
G	Val	Ala	Asp	Gly	C
G	Val	Ala	Glu	Gly	A
G	Val	Ala	Glu	Gly	G

(1) UGA is normally a stop codon; it is read in a context-sensitive manner as coding for selenocysteine in a very limited number of proteins (see Section 15.4.1).

Table 10.5: Proteolytic enzymes (peptidases)

	source	EC number[1]	specificity
Digestive endopeptidases			
chymosin (rennin)	neonatal gastric juice	3.4.23.4	hydrophobic, pref aromatic; Phe[105]-Met in κ-casein
chymotrypsin	pancreatic juice	3.4.21.1	Tyr-, Trp-, Phe-, Leu-
elastase	pancreatic juice	3.4.21.36	Ala-
pancreatic elastase II	pancreatic juice	3.4.21.71	Leu-, Met-, Phe-
enteropeptidase	succus entericus	3.4.21.9	Lys[6]-Ile in trypsinogen
pepsin A	gastric juice	3.4.23.1	hydrophobic, pref aromatic
pepsin B (parapepsin)	gastric juice	3.4.23.2	hydrolyses gelatine
gastricsin (pepsin C)	gastric juice	3.4.23.3	Tyr-
trypsin	pancreatic juice	3.4.21.4	Arg-, Lys-
Digestive exopeptidases			
aminopeptidase	succus entericus	3.4.11.1	N terminal except Arg or Lys.
carboxypeptidase A	pancreatic juice	3.4.17.1	C terminal except -Asp, -Glu, -Arg, -Lys, -Pro
carboxypeptidase B	pancreatic juice	3.4.17.2	C-terminal Lys or Arg
dipeptidases	mucosal brush border	3.4.13.3-20	various
tripeptide aminopeptidase	mucosal brush border	3.4.11.4	N terminal of a tripeptide
Tissue proteinases (may be involved in post-mortem changes in meat)			
cathepsin B	lysosomes	3.4.22.1	broad
cathepsin D	lysosomes	3.4.23.5	hydrophobic, pref aromatic
cathepsin L	lysosomes	3.4.22.15	broad, pref hydrophobic
cathepsin H	lysosomes	3.4.22.16	broad endopeptidase, also -Arg aminopeptidase
cathepsin S	lysosomes	3.4.22.27	broad, pref hydrophobic
chymase	skeletal muscle	3.4.21.39	Phe-, Tyr-, Trp-, Leu-
neutrophil collagenase	neutrophil leukocytes	3.4.24.34	interstitial collagen
Plant, bacterial and fungal proteinases			
ananain	pineapple, *Ananas comosus*	3.4.22.31	broad
actinidain	kiwi fruit, *Actinidia chinensis*	3.4.22.14	broad, pref hydrophobic
caricain	pawpaw, *Carica papaya*	3.4.22.30	broad, pref hydrophobic
chymopapain	pawpaw, *Carica papaya*	3.4.22.6	broad, pref hydrophobic
clostripain	*Clostridium histolyticum*	3.4.22.8	Arg-
collagenase	*Clostridium histolyticum*	3.4.24.3	-Gly in collagen
cerevisin	*Saccharomyces cerevisiae*	3.4.21.48	broad
endopeptidase K	*Tritirachium album*	3.4.21.64	broad, hydrolyses keratin
ficin (ficain)	fig, *Ficus glabrata*	3.4.22.3	broad, pref hydrophobic
fruit bromelain	pineapple, *Ananas comosus*	3.4.22.33	broad
mucorpepsin	*Mucor pusillus, M. miehei*		hydrophobic, clots milk
oryzin	*Aspergillus oryzae*	3.4.21.63	broad
papain	pawpaw, *Carica papaya*	3.4.22.2	broad, pref hydrophobic
stem bromelain	pineapple, *Ananas comosus*	3.4.22.32	broad
subtilisin	*Bacillus subtilis*	3.4.21.62	broad
thermolysin	*Bacillus thermoproteolyticus*	3.4.24.27	-Leu, -Phe

(1) See Tables 29.7 and 29.8 for the Enzyme Commission classification of enzymes.

Table 10.6 The Enzyme Commission (EC) classification of peptidases

3.4.11	aminopeptidases
3.4.13	dipeptidases
3.4.14	dipeptidyl peptidases and tripeptidyl peptidases
3.4.15	peptidyl dipeptidases
3.4.16	serine-type carboxypeptidases (Ser in catalytic site)
3.4.17	metallocarboxypeptidases (zinc or another divalent ion in the catalytic site)
3.4.18	cysteine-type carboxypeptidases (Cys in the catalytic site)
3.4.19	omega peptidases (peptide bonds other than α-carboxyl-α-amino)
3.4.21	serine endopeptidases (Ser in the catalytic site)
3.4.22	cysteine endopeptidases (Cys in the catalytic site)
3.4.23	aspartic endopeptidases (Asp in the catalytic site)
3.4.24	metalloendopeptidases (zinc or another divalent ion in the catalytic site)
3.4.99	endopeptidases of (as yet) unknown mechanism

See Tables 29.7 and 29.8 for the Enzyme Commission classification of enzymes.

Table 10.7: Amino acid transport systems in the intestinal mucosa

system A	Na^+-dependent	most neutral amino acids; tolerates N-methyl group
system ASC	Na^+-dependent	most neutral amino acids, but not N-methylated
system $b^{o,+}$	Na^+-independent	lysine, leucine
system Gly	Na^+-dependent	glycine and sarcosine; tolerates N-methyl group
system L	Na^+-independent	branched non-polar side chain or aromatic
system Ly	Na^+-dependent	lysine
system x^-_A	Na^+-dependent	aspartate
system x^-_G	Na^+-dependent	glutamate
system x^-_C	Na^+-independent	acidic amino acids and cystine
system y^+	Na^+-dependent	diamino amino acids and arginine homologues
β-system	Na^+-dependent	taurine, β-alanine, γ-aminobutyrate
imino acid carrier	Na^+-dependent	proline

Source: Bender 1985; Kilberg *et al* 1993.

Table 10.8: Energy yields of amino acids
(Metabolizable energy and RQ quoted for 100% urinary excretion of either ammonia or urea)

	heat of combustion				metabolizable energy								RQ	
	/mmol		/g		/mmol				/g					
	kJ	kcal	kJ	kcal	kJ		kcal		kJ		kcal			
					NH_4^+	urea	NH_4^+	urea	NH_4^+	urea	NH_4^+	urea	NH_4^+	urea
alanine	203.94	48.72	18.17	4.34	166.74	164.15	39.83	39.21	14.86	14.63	3.55	3.49	1.000	0.833
arginine	123.49	29.50	21.51	5.14	84.30	81.61	20.14	19.49	14.68	14.22	3.51	3.40	1.091	0.727
asparagine	110.53	26.40	14.60	3.49	76.65	74.31	18.31	17.75	10.13	9.82	2.42	2.35	1.333	1.000
aspartate	90.42	21.60	12.03	2.88	73.72	72.56	17.61	17.33	9.81	9.66	2.34	2.31	1.333	1.167
cysteine	112.55	26.89	13.63	3.26	152.16	150.78	36.35	36.02	18.43	18.26	4.40	4.36	0.667	0.556
cystine	52.54	12.55	12.62	3.02	72.88	72.20	17.41	17.25	17.51	17.34	4.18	4.14	0.706	0.589
glutamate	103.75	24.79	15.26	3.65	90.09	89.16	21.52	21.30	13.25	13.11	3.17	3.13	1.111	1.000
glutamine	120.54	28.80	17.61	4.21	92.86	90.91	22.18	21.72	13.57	13.28	3.24	3.17	1.111	0.889
glycine	172.62	41.24	12.96	3.10	120.28	116.66	28.74	27.87	9.03	8.76	2.16	2.09	1.143	0.857
histidine	130.84	31.26	20.31	4.85	94.05	91.49	22.47	21.86	14.60	14.20	3.49	3.39	1.200	0.900
isoleucine	208.12	49.72	27.31	6.52	190.99	189.81	45.63	45.34	25.06	24.90	5.99	5.95	0.800	0.733
leucine	208.15	49.73	27.31	6.52	191.05	189.84	45.64	45.35	25.07	24.91	5.99	5.95	0.800	0.733
lysine	172.88	41.30	25.28	6.04	145.22	143.30	34.69	34.23	21.23	20.95	5.07	5.01	0.857	0.714
methionine	125.02	29.87	18.65	4.46	151.08	150.19	36.09	35.88	22.54	22.41	5.39	5.35	0.667	0.601
ornithine	173.93	41.55	22.99	5.49	140.15	137.80	33.48	32.92	18.53	18.22	4.43	4.35	0.909	0.727
phenylalanine	170.35	40.70	28.14	6.72	159.53	158.77	38.11	37.93	26.36	26.23	6.30	6.27	0.900	0.850
proline	206.61	49.36	23.78	5.68	184.24	182.71	44.01	43.65	21.21	21.03	5.07	5.02	0.909	0.818
serine	131.63	31.44	13.85	3.31	104.93	103.06	25.07	24.62	11.04	10.84	2.64	2.59	1.200	1.000
threonine	144.81	34.59	17.25	4.12	123.96	122.52	29.61	29.27	14.76	14.59	3.53	3.49	1.000	0.875
tryptophan	135.05	32.26	27.58	6.59	120.87	119.88	28.87	28.64	24.68	24.48	5.90	5.85	0.957	0.870
tyrosine	135.35	32.33	24.53	5.86	126.37	125.74	30.19	30.04	22.90	22.78	5.47	5.44	0.947	0.895
valine	213.16	50.92	24.96	5.96	191.53	190.03	45.76	45.40	22.43	22.25	5.36	5.32	0.833	0.750
mean	147.56	35.25	20.01	4.78	129.71	128.07	30.99	30.59	17.80	17.59	4.25	4.20	0.976	0.822

Source: recalculated from data reported by May & Hill 1990.

Table 10.9: Metabolic fates of the amino acids

	glucogenic intermediates	ketogenic intermediates
alanine	pyruvate	-
glycine → serine	pyruvate	-
cysteine	pyruvate	-
tryptophan	pyruvate	acetyl CoA
arginine → ornithine	oxoglutarate	-
glutamine → glutamate	oxoglutarate	-
proline → glutamate	oxoglutarate	-
histidine → glutamate	oxoglutarate	-
methionine	propionyl CoA	-
isoleucine	propionyl CoA	acetyl CoA
valine	succinyl CoA	-
asparagine → aspartate	oxaloacetate or fumarate	-
phenylalanine → tyrosine	fumarate	acetoacetate
leucine	-	acetoacetate + acetyl CoA
lysine	-	acetyl CoA

Table 10.10: Factorial calculation of protein requirements

	mg N /kg body weight
obligatory urine loss	37
obligatory faecal loss	12
skin loss (increased in tropics or with heavy work)	3
miscellaneous losses	2
total obligatory N loss	54
increment for maintenance of N balance (+ 30%)	70
+ allowance for individual variation (+ 20%)	84
+ allowance for common stresses (+ 10%)	93
protein requirement	570 mg protein /kg

Source: WHO/FAO 1973.

Table 10.11: N balance studies cited in the FAO/WHO/UNU (1985) report

no of studies	duration	protein source	no of subjects	mean requirement (mg /kg body weight)
9	short-term	single protein sources	93	0.63
8	short-term	typical mixed diets	73	0.63
6	24-98 d	5 egg, 1 milk	34	0.58

Table 10.12: Protein content of dietary staples as percent of energy yield.

	energy kJ/100g	protein g/100g	protein % energy
wheat	1350	13.2	16.6
pasta	1610	13.6	14.3
maize	520	4.1	13.5
oatmeal	1700	12.4	12.4
rye	1430	8.2	9.8
potato	370	2.1	9.6
barley	1540	7.9	8.7
rice	1540	6.5	7.2
yam	560	2.0	6.1
cassava	460	0.9	3.3

Table 10.13: Average intakes and major sources of protein in the average UK diet

Figures show mean intake and (95% range) and the percentage of average total intake of protein from various sources

	g /day	% of energy intake
men	84.7	14.1
	(47-129)	(10-20)
women	62.0	15.2
	(32-92)	(10-23)

major sources of protein	% of total intake
meat and meat products	37(m), 34(f)
milk and milk products	16 (m), 18 (f)
cereal products	23
(bread	14)
vegetables	9
fish	6
eggs	4
fruit and nuts	1
confectionery	1

Source: Gregory *et al.* 1990.

Table 10.14: Reference intakes of protein, g/kg body weight

	FAO/WHO/UNU (1985)	EU (1993)
4-6 m	1.85	1.86
7-9 m	1.65	1.65
10-12 m	1.50	1.48
1-1.5 y	1.20	1.26
1.5-2 y	1.20	1.17
2-3 y	1.15	1.13
3-4 y	1.10	1.09
4-5 y	1.10	1.06
5-6 y	1.00	1.02
6-7 y	1.00	1.01
7-8 y	1.00	1.01
8-9 y	1.00	1.01
9-10 y	1.00	0.99
males		
10 y	1.00	0.99
11 y	1.00	0.98
12 y	1.00	1.0
13 y	1.00	0.97
14 y	0.95	0.96
15 y	0.95	0.92
16 y	0.90	0.90
17 y	0.90	0.86
adult	0.75	0.75
females		
10 y	1.00	1.0
11 y	1.00	0.98
12 y	0.95	0.96
13 y	0.95	0.94
14 y	0.90	0.90
15 y	0.90	0.87
16 y	0.80	0.83
17 y	0.80	0.80
adult	0.75	0.75

Source: Scientific Committee for Food 1993; FAO/WHO/UNU 1985.

Table 10.15: Reference intakes of protein, g/day

	FAO/WHO/UNU (1985)	USA (1989)	UK (1991)	EU (1993)
0-3m	-	13	12.5	-
3-6 m	13	13	12.7	14.5
6-9 m	14	14	13.7	15.0
9-12 m	14	14	13.7	15.0
1-3 y	13.5-17.5 [1]	16	14.5	14.0-15.5[1]
4-6 y	17.5-21[1]	24	19.7	17.0-20.0[1]
7-10 y	27	28	28.3	22.0-29.5[1]
males				
11-14 y	34-43[1]	45	42.1	32.5-51.0[1]
15-18 y	52-56[1]	59	55.2	53.5-55.5[1]
19-24 y	37.5-60[2]	58	55.5	56
25-50 y	37.5-60[2]	63	55.5	56
over 51	37.5-60[2]	63	53.3	56
females				
11-14 y	36-44[1]	46	41.2	34.0-45.5[1]
15-18 y	46-42[1]	44	45.0	45.5-43.5[1]
19-24 y	30-56[2]	46	45.0	47
25-50 y	30-56[2]	50	45.0	47
over 51	30-56[2]	50	46.5	47
pregnant	+6	60	+6	+10
lactating 1-6 m	+17.5	65	+11	+16
lactating over 6 m	+13	62	+8	+12

(1) The range of reference intakes is because the original publication gave values for intermediate age-ranges.
(2) The FAO/WHO/UNU safe levels of protein for adults are calculated on the basis of a range of body weights from 50-80 kg for men and 40-75 for women. The US, UK and EU safe levels are calculated on the basis of average weights in the population for which the figures apply.
Source: FAO/WHO/UNU 1985; National Research Council 1989; Department of Health 1991; Scientific Committee for Food 1993.

Table 10.16: Estimates of essential amino acids requirements and reference pattern for adults

	WHO/FAO (1973)		FAO/WHO/UNU (1985)		protein turnover	amino acid oxidation
	requirement mg /kg bw	pattern mg /g prot	requirement mg /kg bw	pattern mg /g prot	requirement mg /kg bw	requirement mg /kg bw
His	0	0	8-12	16	-	-
Ile	10	18	10	13	38	-
Leu	14	25	14	19	65	66
Lys	12	22	12	16	70	50
Met + Cys	13	24	13	17	27	22
Phe + Tyr	14	25			65	-
Thr	7	13	7	9	35	25
Trp	3.5	6.5	3.5	5	10	-
Val	10	18	10	13	40	33

Source: WHO/FAO 1973; FAO/WHO/UNU 1985, Young *et al. 1989*; Young 1994.

Table 10.17: Essential amino acid requirements and reference pattern for infants and children

	requirement, mg /kg bw /day			pattern, mg /g protein		
	3-4 m	2 years	10-12 years	3-4 m	2 years	10-12 years
His	285	-	-			
Ile	70	31	28-30	46	28	28
Leu	161	73	44-45	93	66	44
Lys	103	64	44-60	66	58	44
Met + Cys	58	27	22-27	42	25	22
Phe + Tyr	125	69	22-27	72	63	22
Thr	87	37	28-35	43	34	28
Trp	17	12.5	3.3-4	17	11	9
Val	93	38	25-33	55	35	25

Source: FAO/WHO/UNU 1985.

Table 10.18: Jackson's classification of amino acids

	synthesis of carbon skeleton	
amination of carbon skeleton	yes	no
yes	non-essential	essential C skeleton
no	semi-essential	essential amino acid

Source: Jackson 1983.

Table 10.19: Complementation between amino acids

	maize meal	yellow pea flour
Biological Value	0.35	0.43
lysine (g/kg protein)	2.6	5.6
methionine + cysteine (g/kg protein)	5.3	2.0

	2 parts maize + 1 part pea protein
Biological value arithmetic mean	0.39
calculated from aminoacids	0.72
determined experimentally	0.70

Source: Bender 1961.

Table 10.20: Evaluation of protein quality by growth assays

Index of quality		Principle of method	Reference
PER	Protein Efficiency Ratio	Weight gain /gram protein consumed	Osborne *et al*.1919
NPR	Net Protein Retention	Weight gain plus weight loss of non-protein group /gram of protein eaten	Bender & Doell 1957
PRE	Protein Retention Efficiency	NPR x protein composition %	Bender & Doell 1957
	Rat repletion	weight gain of protein-depleted adult rat	Cannon 1945
	Weight maintenance	g N required to maintain constant weight in protein-depleted rats	Tomarelli & Barnhart. *1947*
NGI	Nitrogen Growth Index	Gradient of line relating weight gain to N intake	Allison 1959
NU	Nitrogen Utilization Value	Weight change in 14d plus 10% of initial and final weights to allow for maintenance N	McLaughlan 1976
RNU	Relative Nitrogen Utilization value	NU expressed as percentage of that of lactalbumin	McLaughlan 1976
RNPR	Relative Net Protein Ratio	NPR compared with reference protein	McLaughlan *et al.* *1980*
RPV	Relative Protein Value	Gradient of dose response for test protein compared with that of reference protein, omitting zero level	Samonds & Hegsted 1977

Table 10.21 Biological indices of protein quality

index		definition	reference
BV	Biological Value	$\dfrac{\text{retained N}}{\text{absorbed N}}$	Thomas 1909; Mitchell 1924
		$= \dfrac{\text{food N-(faecal N-metabolic N)-(urine N-endogenous N)}}{\text{food N -(faecal N-metabolic N)}}$	
D	true digestibility	$= \dfrac{\text{absorbed N}}{\text{food N}}$	
NPU	Net Protein Utilization	$\dfrac{\text{retained N}}{\text{food N}}$	Bender & Miller 1953; Miller & Bender 1955
		$= \dfrac{\text{food N-(faecal N-metabolic N)}}{\text{food N}}$	
		$= \text{BV} \times \text{D}$	
PER	Protein Efficiency Ratio	$\dfrac{\text{weight increase of experimental animals}}{\text{weight of protein consumed}}$	Osborne *et al.*1919
NPR	Net Protein Retention	$\dfrac{\text{weight gain of experimental animals-weight loss of non-protein group}}{\text{weight of protein consumed}}$	Bender & Doell 1957
NPV	Net Protein Value	BV x D x protein content of foodstuff	
ERV	Egg Replacement Value	$\dfrac{\text{100-N balance on egg-N balance on test protein}}{\text{food N}}$	

Source: Bender 1957; Evans & Whitty 1978.

Table 10.22: Organisms that have been used for rapid evaluation of protein quality

organism	reference
various insects	Loschiavo 1960
mealworm, *Tenebrio molitor*	Davis 1975
red flour beetle, *Tribolium castaneum*	Medrano & Bressani 1977
confused flour beetle, *Tribolium confusum*	Sharma *et al.* 1977
Tetrahymena pyriformis	Rockland & Dunn 1949; Rosen & Fernell 1956; Baker *et al.* 1978
Leuconostoc mesenteroides	Horn *et al.* 1952
Streptococcus faecalis	Halevy & Grosswicz 1953
Escherichia coli	Bell *et al.* 1977
Aspergillus flavus	Moohyuddin *et al.* 1978

Table 10.23: Rapid evaluation of protein quality by specific responses

response	reference
liver protein regeneration	Harrison & Long 1945; Campbell & Kosterlitz 1948
plasma protein regeneration	Robscheitt-Robins & Whipple 1949
plasma protein regeneration after phenylhydrazine-induced anaemia	Moorjani & Subrahmanyan 1950
liver xanthine oxidase activity	Litwack *et al.* 1952
various liver enzymes	Münchow & Bergner 1968
liver protein utilization	Mokady *et al.* 1969

Table 10.24: Biochemical indices used for rapid evaluation of protein quality

index	reference
short-term N retention	Silber & Porter 1950
restitution N	Vardi & Tatar 1955
blood urea nitrogen	Münchow & Bergner 1968
urinary creatinine / total urine N	Münchow & Bergner 1968
plasma amino acid index	Whitakker & Patrick 1971
ribosomal incorporation of amino acids	von der Decken 1975
plasma arginase, ornithine carbamyltransferase and glutamate-pyruvate aminotransferase	Bergner 1977
plasma catalase	Kirchgessner *et al.* 1977

Table 10.25: Protein synthesis and safe levels of intake at various ages

	protein synthesis g /kg bw /day	safe protein intake g /kg bw /d	synthesis rate / safe level of intake
premature infants	11-14	3	4.5
15 m old	6.3	1.3	5
1-8 y old	3.9	1.1	4
13 y old	5	1.0	5
adults	3-6	0.75	6

Source: from data reported by Young & Pellett 1987.

Table 10.26: Kinetic parameters of enzymes involved in amino acid metabolism, compared with liver concentrations of amino acids (on a low-protein diet) of 30-50 µmol/kg and values of K_m for amino acyl tRNA synthetases between 1-50 µmol/L

	EC number	K_m (mmol/L)
glutamate dehydrogenase	1.4.1.2	1.8
glutamine aminotransferase	2.6.1.15	2.0
glycine oxidase	1.4.1.10	0.04
histidine ammonia lyase	4.3.1.3	9-24
isoleucine aminotransferase	2.6.1.32	3.8
leucine aminotransferase	2.6.1.6	3.8
lysine acyltransferase	2.3.1.32	4.2
lysine-oxoglutarate reductase	1.5.1.7	18
methionine aminotransferase	2.6.1.41	1.9
phenylalanine hydroxylase	1.14.16.1	0.66
proline oxido-reductase	1.5.1.1	3.6
serine deaminase	1.4.1.7	52-70
serine hydroxymethyl-transferase (glycine)	2.1.2.1	28
threonine aldolase	4.1.2.5	4.4-20
threonine deaminase	4.2.1.16	29
tryptophan aminotransferase	2.6.1.27	2.7
tryptophan dioxygenase	1.13.11.11	0.3
tyrosine aminotransferase	2.6.1.5	1.5
valine aminotransferase	2.6.1.32	11

Source: from data reported by Barman 1968; Young & Marchini 1990.

Table 10.27: The energy cost of protein synthesis in various species

	protein synthesis g /kg bw /day	% fasting metabolic rate	% total energy expenditure
hooded rat	20.6	19.5	15.3
albino rat	25.7	24.7	19.6
rabbit	13.8	-	17.7
growing pig	9.0	31.0	12.7
adult man	5.7	18.8	12.9

Source: from data reported by Waterlow *et al.* 1978.

Table 10.28: Increased energy expenditure and protein synthesis after feeding

	increased energy expenditure as % of energy intake	protein turnover (g /9 h)	cost of protein synthesis as % of total energy expenditure
fasting	-	17.6 ± 2.2	8.7
high-carbohydrate meal (0.9 g protein /kg bw)	5.7	27.4 ± 1.4	11.7
high-protein meal (4.2 g protein /kg bw)	9.6	58.2 ± 5.3	19.8

Source: from data reported by Robinson *et al.* 1990.

Table 10.29: N balance and changes in energy intake

Energy intake (multiple of initial total energy expenditure)	1.0	1.15	1.3	1.3	1.15	1.0
N balance (mg N /kg bw /day)	7.2	23.8	33.3	27.8	17.6	4.8

Source: from data reported by Chiang & Huang 1988.

Table 10.30: Whole body protein turnover and resting metabolic rate

	protein turnover g /kg bw /day	resting metabolic rate kJ /kg bw / day	protein turnover / RMR g /kJ
mouse	43.5	760	57
rat	22.0	364	60
rabbit	9.2	192	48
sheep	5.6	96	58
human being	4.6	107	43
cow	3.0	60	50

Source: from data reported by Waterlow 1984.

Table 10.31: Protein synthesis and catabolism in the fed and fasting states

	mmol leucine /hour		
	synthesis	catabolism	balance
fed	8.8	8.1	+ 0.7
fasting	6.4	7.85	- 1.45

Source: from data reported by Clugston & Garlick 1982.

Table 10.32: Contribution of different tissues to whole body protein synthesis in the rat

	fractional rate of protein synthesis (% /day)	% of whole body protein synthesis
liver (+ export proteins)	105	24
small intestine	69-143	15
large intestine	62	2.6
stomach	74	1.0
spleen	76	1.8
kidney	48	2.2
lung	33	1.1
heart	17	0.4
brain	17	0.8
skeletal muscle	17	25
skin	64	18
bone	90	8

Source: from data reported by Waterlow 1984.

Table 10.33: Average half-lives of tissue proteins in the rat

	half-life (days)
liver (soluble proteins)	0.9
liver (mitochondrial proteins)	1.8
kidney	1.7
heart (soluble proteins)	4.1
heart (myofibrillar proteins)	5.5
brain	4.6
skeletal muscle (soluble proteins)	10.7
skeletal muscle (myofibrillar proteins)	22.6
skeletal muscle (mitochondrial proteins)	9.0

Source: from data reported by Waterlow *et al. 1978.*

Table 10.34: Turnover rates of liver cytosolic enzymes

	EC number	half life	fractional turnover (% /day)
ornithine decarboxylase	4.1.1.17	11 min	90.7
δ-aminolaevulinate synthase	2.3.1.37	20 min	49.9
tyrosine aminotransferase	2.6.1.5	1.5 h	11.1
tryptophan dioxygenase	1.13.11.11	2 h	8.3
thymidine kinase	2.7.1.21	3 h	5.5
phosphoenolpyruvate carboxylase	4.1.1.31	5 h	3.3
dihydro-orotase	3.5.2.3	12 h	1.39
glucose-6-phosphate dehydrogenase	1.1.1.49	15 h	1.11
phosphoglycerate dehydrogenase	1.1.1.95	15 h	1,11
serine deaminase	1.4.1.7	20 h	0.83
ATP citrate lyase	4.1.3.8	24 h	0.69
glucokinase	2.7.1.1	1.2 d	0.58
ferritin	-	1.3 d	0.53
acetyl CoA carboxylase	6.4.1.2	2.0 d	0.35
aspartate carbamyltransferase	2.1.3.2	2.5 d	0.28
histidine ammonia lyase	4.3.1.3	2.5 d	0.28
aldolase	4.1.2.13	2.8 d	0.25
histidine-pyruvate aminotransferase	2.6.1.38	2.8 d	0.25
aspartate aminotransferase	2.6.1.1	3.0 d	0.23
fatty acid synthetase	2.3.1.85	3.0 d	0.23
alanine aminotransferase	2.6.1.2	3.5 d	0.20
glyceraldehyde-3-phosphate dehydrogenase	1.2.1.12	3.1 d	0.22
pyruvate kinase	2.7.1.40	3.5 d	0.20
urocanase	4.2.1.49	3.5 d	0.20
xanthine oxidase	1.1.3.22	4.0 d	0.173
arginase	3.5.3.1	4-5 d	0.173-0.139

Source: from data reported by Waterlow *et al.* 1978.

Table 10.35: Protein losses (g) over 10 days following trauma and untreated infection.

	tissue loss	blood loss	protein catabolism
fracture of femur	-	up to 200	580-860
muscle wound	500-750	150-400	650
35% burn	500	150-400	600
gastrectomy	up to 60	20-180	525-650
typhoid fever	-	-	675

Source: from data reported by Cuthbertson 1964.

Table 10.36: The major acute phase plasma proteins

	adult reference range (g/L)	half-life (days)	response time
Reduced synthesis			
albumin	0.2-0.4	15-19	-
prealbumin (transthyretin)	35-50	0.5	-
retinol binding protein	0.033-0.096	0.5	-
transferrin	2.0-3.5	7	-
Increased synthesis			
α1-antitrypsin	0.78-2.0	4	-
α1-acidic glycoprotein (orosomucoid)	0.5-1.5	5	24 h
α1-lipoprotein (apolipoprotein A)	1.7-3.25	-	24 h
β1-lipoprotein (apolipoprotein B)	0.6-1.55	-	-
α1-fetoprotein	0.03	-	-
haptoglobin	0.3-2.15	2	24 h
α2-macroglobulin	1.25-4.1	5	-
ceruloplasmin	0.2-0.4	4.5	2-4 d
hemopexin	0.5-1.15	-	-
complement C3	0.7-1.5	-	2-4 d
complement C4	0.1-0.4	-	2-4 d
fibrinogen	2-4	2.5	-
β2-microglobulin	1-2	-	-
immunoglobulin IgA	0.4-3.9	6	-
immunoglobulin IgG	7-15	24	-
immunoglobulin IgM	0.25-3.1	5	-
C-reactive protein	< 8	-	6-10 h

Source: from data reported by Burtis & Ashwood 1994; Fleck *et al.* 1985; Williams & Marks 1983.

Table 10.37: Reference ranges for plasma protein concentrations

	95% reference range g/L
total protein	60-84
albumin	35-50
globulins	23-35
immunoglobulin IgG	7-15
high density lipoprotein[1]	3-8
ceruloplasmin	0.2-0.4
fibrinogen	2-4
plasminogen	0.3
prothrombin	0.1

(1) See also Table 8.11 for plasma lipoproteins
Source: from data reported by Massachussetts General Hospital 1986.

Table 10.38 Reference ranges for plasma amino acids

	mean $\pm$ SD (μmol/L)
alanine	360 $\pm$ 69
arginine	94 $\pm$ 20
asparagine	62 $\pm$ 19
aspartic acid	7 $\pm$ 4
cystine	61 $\pm$ 13
glutamic acid	34 $\pm$ 13
glutamine	656 $\pm$ 146
glycine	232 $\pm$ 44
histidine	94 $\pm$ 14
isoleucine	64 $\pm$ 23
leucine	133 $\pm$ 39
lysine	192 $\pm$ 44
methionine	24 $\pm$ 8
ornithine	66 $\pm$ 17
phenylalanine	58 $\pm$ 14
serine	113 $\pm$ 30
taurine	94 $\pm$ 48
threonine	145 $\pm$ 39
tryptophan	45 $\pm$ 9
tyrosine	64 $\pm$ 19
valine	264 $\pm$ 79

Source: Scriver *et al.* 1985.

Table 10.39: Inborn errors of amino acid metabolism

disease	signs	plasma	urine	intelligence	enzyme defect
alkaptonuria	urine darkens on standing; pigmentation of cartilage; arthritis	-	homogentisic acid	normal	homogentisic acid oxidase (EC 1.13.11.5)
argininaemia	ammonia intoxication	NH_4^+, Arg	Arg, Lys, Orn	normal	arginase (EC 3.5.3.1)
argininosuccinic aciduria	ammonia intoxication	NH_4^+, argininosuccinic acid	argininosuccinic acid	normal	argininosuccinase (EC 4.3.21)
citrullinaemia	ammonia intoxication	NH_4^+, Cit	Cit	retarded	argininosuccinate synthase (EC 6.3.4.5)
cystathioninuria	-	-	cystathionine	normal or retarded	cystathionase (EC 4.4.1.1)
cystinuria	urinary cystine calculi	-	Cys, Lys, Arg, Orn	normal	renal cysteine/basic amino acid transport system
familial goitre	hypothyroid goitre	low thyroxine, tri-iodothyronine	-	normal	thyroid iodide uptake
				normal	thyroglobulin synthesis
			-	cretinous	thyroglobulin tyrosine iodinase (EC 1.11.1.8)
				cretinous	iodotyrosine coupling enzyme
		normal thyroxine, low tri-iodothyronine	-	cretinous	iodotyrosine deiodinase (EC 3.8.1.4)
		high thyrotropin	-	cretinous	thyrotropin receptor
Hartnup disease	pellagra plus neurological signs	low total amino acids	high neutral amino acids, abnormal indoles	normal	intestinal and renal neutral amino acid transport
histidinuria	speech defects	-	histidine, imidazoles	retarded in some cases	histidine ammonia lyase (EC 4.3.1.3)
homocystinuria	fracture of long bones, disolocation of lens, thrombosis	homocysteine, methionine	homocysteine	retarded in 60% of cases	cystathionine synthetase (EC 4.2.1.22)
hydroxykynureninuria	pellagra, growth retardation, bone abnormalities	-	hydroxykynurenine, kynurenine	retarded	kynureninase (EC 3.7.1.3)
hydroxyprolinaemia	-	-	hydroxyproline	severely retarded	hydroxyproline oxidase (EC 1.1.1.104)

Table 10.39: (Cont'd)

disease	signs	plasma	urine	intelligence	enzyme defect
hyperammonaemia	ammonia intoxication	NH_4^+	-	normal	carbamyl phosphate synthase (EC 6.3.4.16)
hyperornithinaemia	ammonia intoxication	NH_4^+, Orn	Orn	normal	ornithine carbamyltransferase (EC 2.1.1.3)
hyperglycinaemia (non-ketotic)	fits, failure to thrive	Gly	Gly	retarded	glycine oxidase (EC 1.4.1.10) or glycine cleavage system (EC 1.4.4.2)
hyperlysinaemia	growth retardation, muscle weakness, abnormal EEG	Lys	Lys, saccharopine	retarded	saccharopine dehydrogenase (EC 1.5.1.10)
hypermethioninaemia	irritability, somnolence	Met	general aminoaciduria	normal	methionine **S**-adenosyltransferase (EC 2.5.1.6)
hyperprolinaemia	renal defects	Pro	Pro, Gly, Hyp	retarded	proline oxidase (EC 1.5.1.1)
hypervalinaemia	failure to thrive, inability to suckle, neurological signs	Val	Val	normal	valine aminotransferase (EC 2.6.1.66)
isovaleric acidaemia	acidosis, coma	isovaleric acid	short-chain fatty acids	retarded	isovaleryl CoA dehydrogenase (EC 1.3.99.10)
kynureninuria	(pellagra)	-	kynurenine	normal	kynurenine hydroxylase (EC 1.14.13.9)
maple syrup urine disease	poor muscle tone, coma	Ile, Leu, Val	Ile, Leu, Val, branched-chain ketones	retarded	branched-chain oxo-acid decarboxylase (EC 4.1.1.72)
oxoprolinuria	-	oxo-proline	oxoproline	slightly retarded	oxoprolinase (EC 3.5.2.9)
phenylketonuria	-	Phe, low Tyr	phenylketones	severely retarded	phenylalanine hydroxylase
primary hyperoxaluria	oxalate renal calculi	oxalate	oxalate	normal	alanine-glyoxylate aminotransferase
tyrosinaemia	failure to thrive	Tyr, low phosphate	**p**-hydroxyphenylketones	normal	**p**-hydroxyphenylpyruvate oxidase

Source: Bender 1985.

11

Overweight and obesity

11.1 Desirable ranges of body weight

Since the 1940s The Metropolitan Life Assurance Company has published tables of desirable ranges of body weight for height, based on actuarial experience of the health risks of overweight. The results of a number of large epidemiological studies show the relationship between body weight and mortality. Data from two such studies are shown in Tables 11.1 and 11.2; more detailed information on causes of excess mortality from these two studies is shown in Tables 11.11, 11.12, and 11.13. The American Cancer Society Study followed 750 000 subjects for 15 years. The 1979 Build and Blood Pressure Study (Stamler *et al.* 1980) collated data from 25 life insurance companies in the USA and Canada—a total of 4.2 million policies issued and 106 000 deaths. This was the basis for the 1983 Metropolitan Life Assurance Company tables of weight for height (Metropolitan Life Assurance Company 1983). In both studies mortality was lowest at weights 10–15 per cent below the population mean, increasing both with overweight and significant underweight. Many studies of overweight and mortality have been reviewed by Kushner (1993).

The most generally accepted method of expressing weight relative to height is the Body Mass Index (Quetelet's Index, the ratio of weight (in kg) / height^2 (in m)). As a general guide, a desirable range of BMI is between 20–25 (World Health Organization 1990). The Minister of National Health and Welfare (1988) of Canada proposed more generously that a 'good range of weight for most people' was BMI = 20–25, while a 'generally acceptable range' was BMI = 20–27. The US National Center for Health Statistics defined overweight for the population aged between 20–74 on the basis of the 85th centile of the BMI for the population aged between 20–29 in the NHANES II study, without regard to health consequences, and proposed a desirable range of BMI for men as 20.7–27.8 and for women as 19.1–27.3 (Najjar and

Rowland 1987). As a practical guide to overweight and obesity, Garrow (1988) has defined the ranges of BMI shown in Table 11.3.

On the basis of the ranges of BMI shown in Table 11.3, 13 per cent of men and 16 per cent of women in UK were classified as obese in 1995—a prevalence of obesity that has doubled since 1983. A further 44 per cent of men and 32 per cent of women are overweight, with BMI between 25–30 (Bennett *et al.* 1995).

11.1.1 The effect of age on desirable body weight

Desirable body weight is not constant with age. Tables 11.4 and 11.5 show more detailed data from the American Cancer Society and Build and Blood Pressure Studies; in both cases significant underweight is associated with higher mortality in older people, while the effect of high body weight is less marked in older people.

From these data, Andres *et al.* (1985) derived the BMI associated with lowest mortality for each decade of life from 20 to 70, shown in Table 11.6, and the National Research Council (1969) of the USA published desirable ranges of BMI with age, shown in Table 11.7. These ranges of desirable BMI have been used to calculate desirable weight for height in metric units (Table 11.8), pounds (Table 11.9) and stones and pounds (Table 11.10). As a more convenient guide to the general public, the US Departments of Agriculture and of Health and Human Services (1990) condensed the data to give two ranges of desirable BMI: age 19–34, BMI 19–25; age over 35, BMI 21–27.

11.2 Causes of excess mortality and morbidity with overweight

Tables 11.11 and 11.12 show the principal causes of excess mortality with under- and overweight in the

American Cancer Society and Build and Blood Pressure Studies, and Table 11.13 the increased risks of hypertension, diabetes, and coronary heart disease in overweight women.

There is a considerably increased incidence of maturity onset diabetes mellitus (see section 7.7.2) in obese people, reflected in the 5–8-fold increase in mortality due to diabetes in severe obesity. This is largely due to impairment of insulin action at cell surface receptors by high concentrations of plasma lipids. In many cases weight reduction to within the desirable range results in a considerable degree of normalization of glucose tolerance (Bierman *et al.* 1968; Felber 1992; Fujioka *et al.* 1987).

Although, as shown in Tables 11.4 and 11.5, excess body weight is less of a risk factor for death in older people, Table 11.14 shows that significant weight gain during adult life significantly increases the risk of ischaemic heart disease.

Additionally, obesity is associated with a higher incidence of gall stones (see Table 11.20), liver disease (see Table 11.21), post-operative complications (see Table 11.24) and mortality during surgery (see Tables 11.23 and 11.24). Morbidity from arthritis, especially of the hip and knee, is increased as a result of the increased stress due to higher body weight, and the incidence of hiatus hernia and haemorrhoids is greater in obesity; this latter may reflect a lower fibre content of the diet (see section 7.3.2).

Overall there is little increase in death from cancer due to overweight. However, as shown in Table 11.15, obesity is associated with increased colorectal and gall bladder cancer, as well as prostate cancer in men, and breast, uterine and ovarian cancer in women. Underweight is associated with increased mortality from lung and bladder cancer.

Cancers of the breast, uterus and ovary are oestrogen-dependent tumours, and the likely explanation of higher incidence in obese women is the formation of oestradiol in adipose tissue, so that they have higher than normal circulating concentrations of oestrogens (Rebuffé-Scrive 1988; Zumoff 1988). Certainly overweight women suffer less from perimenopausal symptoms than do lean women, as a result of the extra-ovarian formation of oestrogens. No such mechanism can be advanced to account for the higher incidence of prostate cancer (an androgen-dependent tumour) in obese men, since the effect of obesity is to reduce rather than increase the circulating concentration of testosterone (Kley *et al.* 1980).

The higher incidence of colorectal and gall bladder cancer in obesity reflects the association of obesity with a high-fat, low-fibre diet, and increased secretion of bile (see also Tables 11.20, 11.21, and section 8.2.3). Bile acids have cocarcinogenic or tumour promoting action. As discussed in section 7.3.2, non-starch polysaccharides have a number of potentially anti-carcinogenic actions, including adsorption of bile acids and potential dietary carcinogens, thus preventing them from interacting with intestinal mucosal cells. Furthermore, a number of potential carcinogens are lipid soluble, and it is likely that a high fat diet will result in a higher intake, and hence increased risk. Fermentation of non-starch polysaccharides by intestinal bacteria results in the production of short-chain fatty acids, some of which (notable butyrate) have anti-proliferative actions *in vitro*, and may thus provide protection *in vivo*. However, such simplistic mechanisms are confounded by the fact that diets that are high in non-starch polysaccharides are also rich in a variety of other protective nutrients and non-nutrients; equally, diets that are rich in non-starch polysaccharides are generally low in fat, and *vice versa*.

The importance of the increased mortality from various causes associated with obesity is shown by the data in Tables 11.16–11.19. Table 11.16 shows the principal causes of premature death in different economic and geographical regions, from WHO data. Table 11.17 shows the five main causes of death at different ages in England; between the ages of 35–54, 37 per cent of male deaths and 49 per cent of female deaths are from conditions in which the risk is significantly increased by excess body weight. Table 11.18 shows the years of potential working life lost as a result of deaths occurring between the ages of 15–64; 22 per cent of the loss due to premature death among men, and 31 per cent of that among women is due to conditions in which obesity is a factor.

11.2.1 Gallstones in obesity

Gallstone formation has long been associated with obesity (Friedman *et al.* 1966; Maclure *et al.* 1989); the medical students' mnemonic is that it is the disease of the 4 Fs: fair, fat, forty and female. Table 11.19 shows data from the Nurses Health Study, in which 90 000 women aged 30–55 were followed for 8 years — there is a considerably increased risk of gallstone formation with overweight.

The cholesterol concentration of normal bile is close to its solubility limit (Mabee *et al.* 1976). Because of this, the composition of bile is conventionally expressed as a lithogenicity index — the ratio of cholesterol : [bile acids + phospholipids]. (For a discussion of bile acid metabolism, see section 8.2.3.) As shown in Table 11.20, two studies have reported the composition of bile in lean and obese subjects; both show an increased lithogenicity index in obese people. Freeman *et al.* (1975), reported on 11 patients weighing 137 ±9 kg; Bennion and Grundy (1975) on 23 patients who weighed 173 ±28 per cent of ideal weight. Freeman *et al.* noted that in all their obese patients the lithogenicity index was above the solubility limit.

11.2.2 Liver disease in obesity

There is widespread liver disease in severely obese people. Bray (1985) cites studies showing that hepatic steatosis occurs in 68–94 per cent of obese patients, and fatty infiltration involving more than half the hepatocytes in 25–35 per cent; inflammatory liver lesions occur less commonly, in under 10 per cent of obese subjects. While excessive alcohol consumption may be a factor in both liver damage and obesity, obesity seems to be a factor independent of alcohol consumption. Unlike alcoholic liver disease (see section 9.3), the results of standard liver function tests (serum aspartate aminotransferase, alkaline phosphatase, serum albumin and bilirubin), are generally normal in obese subjects. Table 11.21 shows the results of lipid analysis in liver biopsy samples; the pattern of lipid accumulation in obesity is different from that seen in alcoholic liver disease

11.2.3 Risks of surgery in obesity

There is a 2–3–fold increased mortality in surgery for conditions such as appendicitis and gallstones in obese patients. Postlethwait and Johnson (1972) quote a mortality rate during duodenal surgery of 2.7 per cent for lean and 6.6 per cent for obese people. Physically, surgery is more difficult, and hence more prolonged, in obese patients, because of the difficulties of operating in the presence of large amounts of subcutaneous and internal adipose tissue.

The induction of anaesthesia is complicated by the difficulty of locating superficial veins under the subcutaneous adipose tissue, and regional anaesthetic techniques are difficult because the usual anatomical landmarks are hidden by adipose tissue. Calculation and control of anaesthetic dose is also more difficult than in lean people, because of both the solubility of most anaesthetic agents in lipid, so that there is a large buffer of the anaesthetic in the body, and the different total body water content /kg body weight (see section 2.2). While obese patients require higher anaesthetic doses than lean people, the dose /kg body weight is lower.

A further problem of anaesthesia in obese patients is the impairment of lung function associated with obesity (see Tables 11.22 and 11.23). The functional residual capacity of the lung is reduced by about 25 per cent in the supine position, and a further 20 per cent by anaesthesia; in severely obese patients functional residual capacity may anyway be only about 75 per cent of expected (Fisher *et al.* 1975; Wilson and Reilly 1993). The reduction in respiratory compliance in obese subjects is almost entirely due to an increase in the elastic resistance of the chest wall—overall nearly a 2–fold increase in workload of respiratory muscles in obesity—and the problem is exacerbated in the supine position because of the additional resistance of the added fat load over the chest. This impaired respiratory function also accounts for an increased mortality from pneumonia and other respiratory diseases in obese people.

In addition to the increased risks during surgery, obese patients are more likely to suffer post-operative complications; Table 11.24 shows the increased incidence of a number of such complications in obese patients undergoing duodenal surgery, with and without pre-existing hypertension or diabetes. The lower incidence of post-operative pneumonia in obese patients presumably reflects more intensive post-operative physiotherapy in this group of patients, known to be at greater risk if they do develop pneumonia.

11.3   The importance of fatness (adiposity) and body fat distribution

Rather than weight for height, the determinant of excess morbidity and mortality in obesity is the excess body fat, and more importantly the distribution of that adipose tissue: as upper body segment (abdominal and chest) fat—the male or android pattern of obesity—or lower body segment (gluteofemoral or hip) fat—the female or gynoid pattern of obesity (Björntorp 1988, 1990; Bouchard *et al.* 1990; Seidell *et al.* 1985). In popular writing these two patterns of fat distribution are sometimes referred to as apple-shaped and pear-shaped obesity.

Table 11.25 shows the results of a 14 year follow-up study of 24 390 adults in whom subcutaneous fat over the trapezius ridge was estimated from chest X-rays. While this presumably reflects upper body segment fat, there is no information on subcutaneous fat in the abdominal region or lower body segment. The association of fatness with excess mortality is more marked for white than black people, and, as for studies of body weight and mortality (see Tables 11.4 and 11.5), there was little effect of fatness on mortality in older subjects. As shown in Table 11.26, the causes of excess mortality in fatter people were the same as those in studies of body weight (see Tables 11.11 and 11.12); it is noteworthy that death from tuberculosis and other respiratory diseases is greater in people with very little subcutaneous fat (< 4 mm would be classified as inadequate body fat reserves, see section 2.2.1.7).

Table 11.27 shows the results of a 12 year study of 8006 men of Japanese extraction in Hawaii (Donahue *et al.* 1987). The upper part of the table shows the expected increase in coronary heart disease with increasing BMI; classification by subscapular skinfold thickness, as an index of upper body segment obesity, shows the same distribution. The importance of fat distribution rather than total excess weight is shown in the lower part of the table. Within each tertile of BMI there is an increasing incidence of coronary heart disease with increasing subscapular skinfold thickness, but within any tertile of skinfold thickness there is considerably less effect of BMI.

Table 11.28 again shows the importance of fat distribution rather than total excess weight in coronary heart disease. Larsson *et al.* (1992) reported a 12 year follow-up study of 1462 women and 792 men aged 54. There was the expected higher incidence of coronary heart disease in men (9.6 per cent) than women (3.4 per cent). Correcting the data for blood pressure, plasma cholesterol, smoking and BMI did not affect the gender difference. However, correcting for waist:hip ratio (mean for men = 0.927, for women 0.754) more or less completely abolished the gender difference.

The effect of fat distribution, rather than BMI, as a risk factor for women is shown in Tables 11.29–11.31. Table 11.29 shows the results of a 5 year study of 41 837 women aged 55–69, who were grouped by quintile of BMI or waist:hip ratio (median values for the quintiles are not given in the paper). There was a lower risk of death with increasing BMI, but increasing waist:hip ratio, reflecting upper rather than lower body segment obesity, was associated with increased mortality.

Table 11.30 shows that excess body weight and waist:hip ratio are independent risk factors for both hypertension and diabetes, in a group of overweight women aged 40–59 attending slimming clubs (Hartz *et al.* 1984).

Table 11.31 shows the results of glucose tolerance tests in healthy lean and obese premenopausal women (Evans *et al.* 1984). A higher waist:hip ratio was associated with higher fasting insulin and greater insulin secretion after oral glucose, but impaired glucose tolerance. There was no significant difference in the degree of overweight of the three groups classified by waist:hip ratio.

11.4 Weight reduction and slimming regimes

The total amount of food that anyone eats is his or her diet but the terms 'diet' and 'dieting' are popularly associated with a reduced energy intake, that is they are weight-losing regimes or 'slimming diets'. Since overweight is the result of an energy intake greater than output, surplus weight can be removed by reversing this state of affairs.

Weight loss is, of necessity, a slow process. Adipose tissue consists of 80 per cent triacylglycerol (37 kJ (9 kcal) /g, yielding 29.6 kJ (7.1 kcal) /g of tissue), and 5 per cent protein (17 kJ (4 kcal) /g, yielding 0.85 kJ (0.2 kcal) /g of tissue); the total energy yield of adipose tissue is therefore 30.45 kJ (7.3 kcal) /g. Loss of 1 kg of adipose tissue requires some 30 MJ energy deficit—therefore per MJ energy deficit there is a loss of 33 g of body weight. For a person with energy expenditure of 10 MJ /day, total starvation would result in a maximum possible loss of 330 g /day or 2.3 kg /week.

During the first 7–10 days of a moderately severe restriction of energy intake there is a considerably greater rate of weight loss than can possibly be accounted for by utilization of adipose tissue. This is the result of depletion of liver and muscle reserves of glycogen—the highly branched structure of glycogen (see Fig. 7.9) means that it contains a considerable amount of interstitial water. As glycogen is utilized, so this water is lost from tissues, leading to a rapid rate of weight loss which, of course, cannot be sustained.

'Slimming diets' by their very name indicate a dietary modification continued for a limited period of time, too often followed by reversion to the original pattern of intake and so a return of the problem. What is required is a modification of one's eating pattern *for life*. A temporary weight loss followed by a return to overweight is not only useless but can be harmful if repeated frequently since it involves some loss of essential tissues, as a result of both utilization of tissue protein for gluconeogenesis and also the lower rate of protein synthesis in negative energy balance (see section 12.2).

Exercise, while beneficial to health in several ways, has relatively little effect in losing excess adipose tissue (see section 5.4). Nevertheless, as discussed in section 5.3.2, a low level of physical activity is one of the major factors associated with the high level of obesity in western countries. The mean Physical Activity Level in Britain is 1.4 times BMR, compared with a desirable PAL for fitness of 1.7—this desirable level of physical activity is achieved by only 22 per cent of men and 13 per cent of women in UK.

11.4.1 Useless diets and slimming aids

Since many people find that control of appetite is difficult, large numbers of slimming diets, devices and diet books have been and still are being introduced. A consumer guide in the USA listed over 100 diets that were common in the United States in the 1980s and new ones appear almost weekly in UK. Many tend to suffer from short-termism, reliance on gimmicks, or are unusual or outlandish.

New, 'Revolutionary', and 'Magic' Diets are introduced as fast as the courts remove them from sale for making misleading and unsubstantiated claims. These diets are often promoted with sensational titles—'The Amazing Secret Diet', 'Calories don't Count', 'The Carvers Diet', 'The Drinkers Diet', etc. They are often promoted with the aid of fashionable figures or named after specific foods or geographical locations. They include foods claimed, without evidence, to assist weight loss — so there have been grapefruit, potato, liquid protein, peanut, rice diets, and almost every food that strikes the imagination of the promoter. Certainly if only potato or bread or grapefruit is permitted or predominates in the diet the monotony would severely restrict the energy intake (and the intake of nutrients).

There are so-called fat-burners on the market which are simply a collection of vitamins of dubious value, and there has been a vogue for starch-blockers which are claimed to inhibit the digestion of starch. These compounds inhibit amylase (see section 7.2), but since resistant starch is a metabolic energy source as a result of intestinal bacterial fermentation (see section 7.2.2), their value as slimming aids *in vivo* is doubtful. Claims have even been made that certain foods supply 'negative calories'—a nonsensical notion.

Devices range from skin patches said to be impregnated with seaweed (which has no effect anyway) and bath salts of various types to ear pinching and ingesting insignificant amounts of substances that swell in the stomach and are supposed therefore to limit the amount of food eaten. Some are simply vitamin preparations.

A dietetic theory originally proposed by Hay in the 1930s, and recently revived as 'food combining' or the Hay diet, is that weight loss can be achieved by consumption of carbohydrates and proteins at separate meals. There is no physiological rationale for such a suggestion, nor any evidence that it is effective. Furthermore, the underlying concept of separating dietary carbohydrates and proteins is impossible; as shown in Table 10.12, the major starchy foods provide between 7–15 per cent of energy from protein.

11.4.2 Sensible diets

The basis of a practical, useful and sensible weight-reducing regime is one that supplies less energy than is used (around 5 MJ (1200 kcal) per day), is palatable, composed of ordinary foods that are generally available, suits the individual's likes and dislikes, fits in with life style and family life, allows the individual to eat away from home, and supplies adequate amounts of all the nutrients. Such diets are relatively low in fat, since fats are energy dense, and rich in fruits and vegetables since many of these are bulky foods which help to provide satiation.

An intake of 5 MJ would allow a steady slow weight loss of between 1–2 kg per week depending on physical activity. Diets providing less than about 5 MJ/day are unlikely to provide adequate nutrient intakes unless specially formulated supplements or enriched foods are included.

Motivation and perseverance are important in weight reduction regimes; most people would balk at a diet that bans a favourite food completely, and it is important to allow (modest) consumption of all foods, both while weight is being lost and later, when the aim is to maintain the lower body weight and not return to positive energy balance. Essentially, a well-planned weight reducing diet follows the same guidelines for a healthy diet as those discussed in section 4.2, with a more severe restriction of fat and sugars than would be appropriate for a person within the desirable range of weight.

Despite the widespread labelling of foods with nutritional information (see section 4.3), it is no simple matter to formulate a palatable and nutritionally balanced diet that is sufficiently low in energy to permit an adequate rate of weight loss, without recourse to food composition tables, advice from a dietitian and weighing foods. Two relatively simple approaches are restriction of carbohydrate or fat intake.

11.4.2.1 Carbohydrate-restricted diets
The aim of restriction of carbohydrate intake is that it is unlikely that the energy intake that has been lost would be replaced by increased fat or protein intake, especially since high fat and high protein foods have a

high satiety value (Yudkin 1971). It is relatively easy to identify the main sources of dietary carbohydrate, as shown in Table 7.2. The most extreme variants of this approach involve so severe a restriction of carbohydrate intake that the subject becomes ketotic, which is undesirable.

While restriction of carbohydrate intake does indeed result in reduced energy intake, and hence weight loss, it is contrary to the dietary goals for health (see section 4.2); it is considered desirable to increase the percentage of energy intake from carbohydrates, rather than to reduce it.

11.4.2.2 Fat-restricted diets

Average diets in developed countries provide 40 per cent of energy from fat, and it is considered desirable that this should be reduced to 30 per cent, to minimize risks of cardiovascular disease and some forms of cancer (see section 4.2). Therefore restriction of fat intake not only permits a relatively simple way of reducing energy intake, and so achieving weight reduction, but also trains the overweight person into what is a more desirable pattern of eating for maintenance of body weight once the target weight has been reached. Again it is relatively easy to identify the major sources of dietary fat, as shown in Table 8.2. As an aid to reducing fat intake, both for overweight people and those of normal weight, a number of low-fat spreads (see Table 8.3) and low-fat alternatives to traditional foods are widely available.

11.4.2.3 High-fibre diets

A diet that is rich in fruits, vegetables and wholegrain cereal products (i.e. a high fibre diet, Eyton 1982) will be both filling and also low in energy, and especially low in fat. Such a diet for weight reduction is really no more than a modest exaggeration of the advice that is anyway proffered to meet dietary goals to people of acceptable weight. An extension of this is the use of dietary fibre preparations as bulking agents to reduce food intake, either as tablets or suspensions taken before meals, or incorporated into foods (see section 7.3.2).

11.4.3 Aids to weight reduction

A number of foods are available with substantially lower energy content than their normal counterparts. This is achieved by reducing the amount of fat, substituting low-energy ingredients for fats and sugars, and diluting the overall energy content with bulking agents. One example is that of breadspreads, which traditionally contain the same amount of fat as butter—80 per cent. Products have been developed ranging from 60 per cent fat to 40 per cent and even 25 per cent, with fat substitutes permitting breadspreads with as little as 5 per cent fat (see Table 8.3).

So far as sugar is concerned it can be replaced by intense sweeteners (synthetic sweeteners) which do not supply any energy but neither do they provide the various textural properties of sucrose. These can be provided by bulk sweeteners, which are sugar derivatives with varying degrees of sweetness, and providing only 25–75 per cent of the energy yield of sugar (see Table 7.12).

However, since it is the total diet that must be considered, these special products can be useful in controlling energy intake only if they are part of an energy-controlled total diet.

11.4.4 Drug treatment

There are two approaches to drug treatment for obesity, either decreasing the appetite (see section 6.5) or increasing the metabolic rate (see section 5.3). At one time, thyroid extract was used to increase the metabolic rate but this could be continued for only a short time, and the effective dose has side effects. It is used only in the rare cases where obesity is associated with hypothyroidism (see section 25.14.4).

Amphetamine has been used both to suppress appetite and increase metabolic rate; it is, however, highly addictive, and its use is strictly controlled in most countries. A number of amphetamine derivatives with similar effects on appetite and metabolic rate, but little potential for abuse, have been developed. These, and the other anorectic drugs shown in Table 11.32, are usefully prescribed for a few weeks, to encourage the patient, but their effect diminishes after some weeks and some patients suffer a variety of side effects. Nor, of course, do they help to instil the new eating habits that are essential for the maintenance of lower body weight (Bray 1993).

11.4.5 Very low energy diets

Very low energy diets are those that involve a severe restriction of energy intake, to one-third or even one-sixth of energy expenditure; obviously such a regime will result in a faster rate of weight loss, but there is concern that there may be greater loss of lean tissue than with more modest energy restriction. Although it is possible to formulate a diet providing only 2.5 MJ (600 kcal) /day from ordinary foods, in general very low energy diets are based on nutrient mixtures used to replace foods more or less completely.

The early commercial very low energy diets, called liquid protein diets, were marketed in the USA in the

1970s. They were generally prepared from hydrolysed cattle hide, a protein source that is markedly deficient in the essential amino acids tryptophan and lysine (see section 10.6), enriched with varying levels of vitamins and minerals. They were withdrawn from sale in 1977, following a number of deaths from cardiac arrest. Subsequent studies showed the development of cardiac arrhythmias within two weeks of taking these preparations as the source of nourishment; while essential amino acid deficiency may have been responsible, it is more likely that the problem was due to the very high sodium content (the result of neutralizing an acid hydrolysate with sodium hydroxide) and a very low potassium content.

More recent very low energy diets have been based on a patent granted to A.N. Howard in 1972, for a diet formulated from at least 15 g of an amino acid mixture or protein of high quality (see section 10.7), with 15–17 g of carbohydrate, providing a total of 1–2.5 MJ (200–600 kcal). Such diets have been reported to be both effective and safe when used for a period of no more than 3–4 weeks (Wadden *et al.* 1983; Department of Health and Social Security 1987).

The UK Department of Health and Social Security (1987) recommended that very low energy diets should not be regarded as the first means of weight reduction, and should not be used by those whose BMI was less than 30. The report also recommended that the following groups of people should not use very low energy diets:

(1) those with serious cardiac disorders, cerebrovascular disease, severe hepatic or renal disease, gout;

(2) pregnant women and breast-feeding mothers;

(3) those with diabetes mellitus treated with insulin or oral hypoglycaemic agents (see section 7.7.2), unless under close medical supervision to adjust their therapy to avoid hypoglycaemia;

(4) those being treated for hypertension, without modification of medication to prevent the development of hypotension;

(5) those with porphyria, in whom attacks may be precipitated by severe restriction of food intake;

(6) infants, children, adolescents and the elderly.

11.4.6 Surgical intervention

When the degree of obesity is sufficient to pose a major hazard to health, and other means have failed, surgery is sometimes the last resort. Apart from simple physical removal of adipose tissue, two groups of surgical techniques have been used to treat obesity, those that result in impaired absorption of food from the small intestine, and those that reduce the physical capacity of the stomach, so reducing the amount that can be eaten at any one meal.

In intestinal bypass surgery, about 30 cm of the proximal jejunum is anastomized with about 10 cm of the distal ileum, so reducing very considerably the length of intestine available for digestion and the surface area available for absorption of the products of digestion. Such techniques give very impressive initial rates of weight loss, albeit at the cost of persistent foul-smelling diarrhoea and flatulence. In longer term follow-up, the results are less impressive; deficiency of a number of micronutrients has been reported, as has the failure of much oral medication, as a simple result of malabsorption. Overall the mortality attributed to intestinal bypass surgery is about 10 per cent, with about 50 per cent of patients suffering severe and persistent morbidity; the technique has been more or less completely abandoned for the treatment of obesity (Anderson *et al.* 1980; Gries 1987; Griffen *et al.* 1983).

Gastric bypass and gastric stapling (gastroplasty) to reduce the volume of the stomach, and hence the amount of food consumed, seem to result in considerably fewer adverse side-effects, but a good rate of weight reduction; digestion and absorption of the reduced food intake are normal (Cohn *et al.* 1981; Griffen 1979). Although gastroplasty and gastric bypass have been considered effective on the basis of acceptable post-operative morbidity and mortality, there have been few, if any, follow-up studies to determine whether or not the procedure confers any long-term benefit, or indeed whether or not the life expectancy of the patients is increased by the surgical intervention.

11.4.7 Conclusion

It is difficult to achieve the discipline needed to lose weight. Slimming clubs, in which professional counsellors advise, and members help one another, are valuable here, and in some cases behaviour modification therapy is also helpful. However, the numbers who regain surplus fat after successful weight reduction indicate that the maintenance of target weight is even more difficult than losing it, so emphasizing the need for soundly based diets and changes in eating habits, rather than dramatic methods of weight reduction.

Further reading

Yudkin, J. (1971). *This Slimming Business*. MacGibbon & Kee, London.

Bray, G. A.. (1985). Complications of obesity. *Annals of Internal Medicine.*, **103**, 1052–62.

Garrow, J.S. (1988). *Obesity and Related Disorders*, 2nd edn. Churchill-Livingstone, Edinburgh.

Pi-Sunyer, F.X. (1991). Health implications of obesity. *American Journal of Clinical Nutrition*, **53**, 1595–1603s.

Kushner, R.F. (1993). Body weight and mortality. *Nutrition Reviews*, **51**, 127–36.

Lardy, H. and Shrago, E. (1990). Biochemical aspects of obesity. *Annual Review of Biochemistry*, **59**, 689–710.

Royal College of Physicians (1983). Report on obesity. *Journal of the Royal College of Physicians*, **17**, 5–65.

Table 11.1: Relative mortality and body weight: American Cancer Society Study

	< 80	80-89	90-109	110-119	120-129	130-139	> 140
			Body weight as % of mean of study population				
men	1.25	1.05	1.00	1.15	1.27	1.46	1.87
women	1.19	0.96	1.00	1.17	1.29	1.46	1.89

Source: from data reported by Lew & Garfinkel 1979.

Table 11.2: Relative mortality and body weight: Build and Blood Pressure Study

	80	90	100	110	120	130	140	150	160
				Body weight as % of mean of study population					
men	1.05	0.94	1.00	1.11	1.20	1.35	1.53	1.77	2.10
women	1.10	0.97	1.00	1.07	1.10	1.25	1.36	1.49	1.67

Source: from data reported by Pi-Sunyer 1991.

Table 11.3: Ranges of Body Mass Index and grades of obesity

		BMI	% desirable weight
Grade 0	normal weight	20-25	100
Grade I	overweight	25-30	110-120
Grade II	obese	30-40	120-160
Grade III	severely obese	> 40	> 160

Table 11.4: Mortality ratio by % of average weight and age, all causes of death, American Cancer Society Study

% mean weight	age			
	40-49	50-59	60-69	70-79
men				
< 80	1.09	1.24	1.24	1.32
80-90	1.01	1.02	1.06	1.12
90-109	1.00	1.00	1.00	1.00
110-119	1.24	1.18	1.12	1.06
120-129	1.63	1.34	1.23	1.08
130-139	1.81	1.64	1.38	1.30
> 140	2.19	2.09	1.85	1.41
women				
< 80	1.20	1.19	1.19	1.20
80-90	0.94	0.92	0.96	0.97
90-109	1.00	1.00	1.00	1.00
110-119	1.09	1.29	1.27	1.08
120-129	1.38	1.46	1.37	1.15
130-139	1.51	1.62	1.59	1.34
> 140	2.02	2.31	1.85	1.65

Source: from data reported by Garfinkel 1986.

Table 11.5: Mortality as percentage of contemporaneous death rates of insured lives by age and body weight relative to desirable range, Build and Blood Pressure Study 1979.

% desirable weight	20-29	30-39	age 40-49	50-59	60-69
men					
< 75	102	105	112	128	135
75-85	94	93	98	113	120
85-95	95	92	93	100	100
95-105	98	95	96	94	95
105-115	103	112	109	100	99
115-125	125	128	118	109	101
women					
< 75	-	-	117	146	134
75-85	118	124	110	105	106
85-95	88	101	92	93	90
95-105	112	86	96	97	101
105-115	90	99	103	99	102
115-125	118	110	115	103	103

Source: from data reported by Lew 1985.

Table 11.6: BMI associated with minimum mortality at different ages

age range	men	women
20-29	21.4	19.5
30-39	21.6	23.4
40-49	22.9	23.2
50-59	25.8	25.2
60-69	26.6	27.3

Source: from data reported by Andres *et al.* 1985.

Table 11.7: Desirable ranges of BMI at different ages

age	BMI
19-24	19-24
25-34	20-25
35-44	21-26
45-54	22-27
55-64	23-28
> 65	24-29

Source: from data reported by National Research Council / National Academy of Science 1989.

Table 11.8: Body weight (kg) for height at different values of Body Mass Index

height (cm)	Body Mass Index										
	19	**20**	21	22	23	24	**25**	26	27	28	29
150	42.8	**45.0**	47.3	49.5	51.8	54.0	**56.3**	58.5	60.8	63.0	65.3
152	43.9	**46.2**	48.5	50.8	53.1	55.4	**57.8**	60.1	62.4	64.7	67.0
154	45.1	**47.4**	49.8	52.2	54.5	56.9	**59.3**	61.7	64.0	66.4	68.8
156	46.2	**48.7**	51.1	53.5	56.0	58.4	**60.8**	63.3	65.7	68.1	70.6
158	47.4	**49.9**	52.4	54.9	57.4	59.9	**62.4**	64.9	67.4	69.9	72.4
160	48.6	**51.2**	53.8	56.3	58.9	61.4	**64.0**	66.6	69.1	71.7	74.2
162	49.9	**52.5**	55.1	57.7	60.4	63.0	**65.6**	68.2	70.9	73.5	76.1
164	51.1	**53.8**	56.5	59.2	61.9	64.6	**67.2**	69.9	72.6	75.3	78.0
166	52.4	**55.1**	57.9	60.6	63.4	66.1	**68.9**	71.6	74.4	77.2	79.9
168	53.6	**56.4**	59.3	62.1	64.9	67.7	**70.6**	73.4	76.2	79.0	81.8
170	54.9	**57.8**	60.7	63.6	66.5	69.4	**72.3**	75.1	78.0	80.9	83.8
172	56.2	**59.2**	62.1	65.1	68.0	71.0	**74.0**	76.9	79.9	82.8	85.8
174	57.5	**60.6**	63.6	66.6	69.6	72.7	**75.7**	78.7	81.7	84.8	87.8
176	58.9	**62.0**	65.0	68.1	71.2	74.3	**77.4**	80.5	83.6	86.7	89.8
178	60.2	**63.4**	66.5	69.7	72.9	76.0	**79.2**	82.4	85.5	88.7	91.9
180	61.6	**64.8**	68.0	71.3	74.5	77.8	**81.0**	84.2	87.5	90.7	94.0
182	62.9	**66.2**	69.6	72.9	76.2	79.5	**82.8**	86.1	89.4	92.7	96.1
184	64.3	**67.7**	71.1	74.5	77.9	81.3	**84.6**	88.0	91.4	94.8	98.2
186	65.7	**69.2**	72.7	76.1	79.6	83.0	**86.5**	89.9	93.4	96.9	111.3
188	67.2	**70.7**	74.2	77.8	81.3	84.8	**88.4**	91.9	95.4	99.0	102.5
190	68.6	**72.2**	75.8	79.4	83.0	86.6	**90.3**	93.9	97.5	101.1	104.7
192	70.0	**73.7**	77.4	81.1	84.8	88.5	**92.2**	95.8	99.5	103.2	106.9
194	71.5	**75.3**	79.0	82.8	86.6	90.3	**94.1**	97.9	101.6	105.4	109.1
196	73.0	**76.8**	80.7	84.5	88.4	92.2	**96.0**	99.9	103.7	107.6	111.4
198	74.5	**78.4**	82.3	86.2	90.2	94.1	**98.0**	101.9	105.9	109.8	113.7

Table 11.9: Body weight (lb) for height at different values of Body Mass Index

height		Body Mass Index (kg /m^2)										
ft	in	19	**20**	21	22	23	24	**25**	26	27	28	29
4	11	94	**99**	104	109	114	119	**124**	129	134	139	143
5	0	97	**102**	107	113	118	123	**128**	133	138	143	148
5	1	100	**106**	111	116	122	127	**132**	137	143	148	153
5	2	104	**109**	115	120	126	131	**137**	142	147	153	158
5	3	107	**113**	118	124	130	135	**141**	147	152	158	164
5	4	111	**116**	122	128	134	140	**146**	151	157	163	169
5	5	114	**120**	126	132	138	144	**150**	156	162	168	174
5	6	118	**124**	130	136	142	149	**155**	161	167	173	180
5	7	121	**128**	134	140	147	153	**159**	166	172	179	185
5	8	125	**131**	138	145	151	158	**164**	171	177	184	191
5	9	129	**135**	142	149	156	162	**169**	176	183	189	196
5	10	132	**139**	146	153	160	167	**174**	181	188	195	202
5	11	136	**143**	150	158	165	172	**179**	186	193	201	208
6	0	140	**147**	155	162	169	177	**184**	192	199	206	214
6	1	144	**151**	159	167	174	182	**189**	197	204	212	220
6	2	148	**156**	163	171	179	187	**195**	202	210	218	226
6	3	152	**160**	168	176	184	192	**200**	208	216	224	232
6	4	156	**164**	172	181	189	197	**205**	213	222	230	238
6	5	160	**169**	177	185	194	202	**211**	219	227	236	244
6	6	164	**173**	182	190	199	207	**216**	225	233	242	251

Table 11.10: Body weight (stones and pounds) for height at different values of Body Mass Index

height		19		20		21		22		23		24		25		26		27		28		29	
ft	in	st	lb	st	lb	st	lb	st	lb	st	lb	st	lb	st	lb	st	lb	st	lb	st	lb	st	lb
4	11	6	10	7	1	7	6	7	11	8	2	8	7	8	12	9	3	9	8	9	13	10	3
5	0	6	13	7	4	7	9	8	1	8	6	8	11	9	2	9	7	9	12	10	3	10	8
5	1	7	2	7	8	7	13	8	4	8	10	9	1	9	6	9	11	10	3	10	8	10	13
5	2	7	6	7	11	8	3	8	8	9	0	9	5	9	11	10	2	10	7	10	13	11	4
5	3	7	9	8	1	8	6	8	12	9	4	9	9	10	1	10	7	10	12	11	4	11	10
5	4	7	13	8	4	8	10	9	2	9	8	10	0	10	6	10	11	11	3	11	9	12	1
5	5	8	2	8	8	9	0	9	6	9	12	10	4	10	10	11	2	11	8	12	0	12	6
5	6	8	6	8	12	9	4	9	10	10	2	10	9	11	1	11	7	11	13	12	5	12	12
5	7	8	9	9	2	9	8	10	0	10	7	10	13	11	5	11	12	12	4	12	11	13	3
5	8	8	13	9	5	9	12	10	5	10	11	11	4	11	10	12	3	12	9	13	2	13	9
5	9	9	3	9	9	10	2	10	9	11	2	11	8	12	1	12	8	13	1	13	7	14	0
5	10	9	6	9	13	10	6	10	13	11	6	11	13	12	6	12	13	13	6	13	13	14	6
5	11	9	10	10	3	10	10	11	4	11	11	12	4	12	11	13	4	13	11	14	5	14	12
6	0	10	0	10	7	11	1	11	8	12	1	12	9	13	2	13	10	14	3	14	10	15	4
6	1	10	4	10	11	11	5	11	13	12	6	13	0	13	7	14	1	14	8	15	2	15	10
6	2	10	8	11	2	11	9	12	3	12	11	13	5	13	13	14	6	15	0	15	8	16	2
6	3	10	12	11	6	12	0	12	8	13	2	13	10	14	4	14	12	15	6	16	0	16	8
6	4	11	2	11	10	12	4	12	13	13	7	14	1	14	9	15	3	15	12	16	6	17	0
6	5	11	6	12	1	12	9	13	3	13	12	14	6	15	1	15	9	16	3	16	12	17	6
6	6	11	10	12	5	13	0	13	8	14	3	14	11	15	6	16	1	16	9	17	4	17 · 13	

Table 11.11: Cause-specific mortality ratios and body weight, American Cancer Society Study

	Body weight as % of mean						
	< 80%	80-89	90-109	110-119	120-129	130-139	> 140
men							
all causes	1.25	1.05	1.00	1.15	1.27	1.46	1.87
CHD	0.88	0.90	1.00	1.23	1.32	1.55	1.95
cancer	1.33	1.13	1.00	1.02	1.09	1.14	1.33
diabetes	0.88	0.84	1.00	1.65	2.56	3.51	5.19
digestive diseases	1.39	1.28	1.00	1.45	1.88	2.89	3.99
cerebro-vascular disease	1.21	1.09	1.00	1.15	1.17	1.54	2.27
women							
all causes	1.19	0.96	1.00	1.17	1.29	1.46	1.89
CHD	1.01	0.89	1.00	1.23	1.39	1.54	2.07
cancer	0.96	0.92	1.00	1.10	1.19	1.23	1.55
diabetes	0.65	0.61	1.00	1.92	3.34	3.78	7.90
digestive diseases	1.58	0.92	1.00	1.66	1.61	2.19	2.29
cerebro-vascular disease	1.33	0.98	1.00	1.09	1.16	1.40	1.52

Source: from data reported by Lew & Garfinkel 1979.

Table 11.12: Relative mortality compared with population as a whole, by weight relative to desirable weight; 1979 Build and Blood Pressure Study

	\< 75	75-85	85-95	95-105	105-115	115-125	125-135	135-145	145-155	155-165
				Body weight as % of population mean						
men										
all causes	1.17	1.02	0.95	0.95	1.06	1.17	1.30	1.39	1.68	1.86
cancer	1.30	1.09	0.89	0.84	0.85	0.93	0.94	0.93	-	-
diabetes mellitus	-	-	0.75	1.12	1.24	1.93	-	-	-	-
cerebrovascular disease	1.13	1.13	1.02	0.94	1.08	1.06	1.27	1.38	-	-
coronary artery disease	0.80	0.84	0.90	0.96	1.16	1.30	1.56	1.55	1.62	1.83
hypertensive heart disease	-	1.27	1.29	1.32	1.71	2.61	2.02	-	-	-
women										
all causes	1.28	1.11	0.93	0.97	1.00	1.09	1.03	1.09	1.31	1.40
cancer	1.12	1.02	0.90	0.91	0.93	0.91	0.88	0.91	1.33	-
diabetes mellitus										
cerebrovascular disease	1.47	1.22	1.05	0.90	0.88	1.20	-	-	-	-
coronary artery disease	-	0.98	0.78	0.97	1.13	1.38	1.39	1.13	1.60	-

Source: from data reported by Sankey 1984.

Table 11.13: Morbidity and mortality with obesity in women

% with:	\< 21	21-22.9	23-24.9	25-28.9	\> 29
			BMI		
hypertension	6.4	7.9	9.4	13.8	26.5
diabetes mellitus	1.0	1.0	1.2	1.7	5.1
elevated serum cholesterol	2.3	2.5	3.1	3.5	4.8
relative risk, corrected for age and smoking					
non-fatal myocardial infarction	1.0	1.2	1.3	1.6	3.2
fatal coronary heart disease	1.0	1.6	1.4	2.4	3.5
angina pectoris	1.0	1.2	1.7	1.7	1.8

Source: from data reported by Manson *et al.* 1990.

Table 11.14: Relative risk of non-fatal myocardiac infarction or fatal coronary heart disease with weight gain since age 18, corrected for age and initial BMI

weight gain (kg)	no of cases	relative risk
\< 3	44	1.0
3-4.9	16	0.6
5-9.9	52	1.0
10-19.9	97	1.7
20-34.9	59	2.5

Source: from data reported by Manson *et al.* 1990.

Table 11.15: Mortality ratios for cancer deaths, American Cancer Society Study

Significant weight effects are shown in bold type; dash (-) indicates too few deaths from this cause for reliable interpretation.

	< 80%	80-89	weight as % of mean 90-109	110-119	120-129	130-139	> 140
men							
stomach	1.34	0.61	1.00	1.22	0.97	0.73	1.88
colon-rectum	0.90	0.86	1.00	**1.26**	**1.23**	**1.53**	**1.73**
gall bladder	-	0.81	1.00	0.90	1.19	-	-
pancreas	1.20	0.82	1.00	0.91	0.88	0.76	1.62
lung	**1.78**	**1.38**	1.00	0.85	1.04	1.00	1.27
prostate	1.02	0.92	1.00	0.90	**1.37**	**1.33**	**1.29**
kidney	1.06	0.96	1.00	1.63	1.39	1.51	-
bladder	**1.47**	**1.27**	1.00	0.95	0.95	0.97	-
brain	0.87	1.19	1.00	0.91	1.02	-	3.20
leukemia	1.09	1.06	1.00	1.00	1.02	1.17	-
lymphomas	0.87	1.03	1.00	1.11	0.99	1.54	-
women							
stomach	0.74	0.95	1.00	1.07	1.28	1.26	1.03
colon-rectum	0.93	0.84	1.00	0.96	1.10	1.30	1.22
gall bladder	0.68	0.74	1.00	**1.59**	**1.74**	**1.80**	**3.58**
pancreas	1.17	1.06	1.00	1.36	1.43	1.18	0.61
lung	**1.49**	**1.20**	1.00	1.10	1.06	1.06	1.22
breast	0.82	0.86	1.00	**1.19**	**1.16**	**1.22**	**1.53**
cervix	0.76	0.77	1.00	**1.24**	**1.51**	**1.42**	**2.39**
endometrium	0.89	1.04	1.00	**1.36**	**1.85**	**2.30**	**5.42**
uterus (unspecified)	1.00	0.64	1.00	**1.22**	**1.81**	**1.40**	**4.65**
ovary	0.86	0.98	1.00	1.15	0.99	0.88	**1.63**
kidney	1.12	0.70	1.00	1.09	1.30	1.85	2.03
bladder	0.92	0.99	1.00	1.04	0.85	-	-
brain	0.86	0.89	1.00	0.95	1.52	0.69	1.01
leukemia	0.73	1.00	1.00	1.01	0.88	0.85	1.24
lymphomas	0.83	1.00	1.00	1.06	1.00	0.92	1.13

Source: from data reported by Lew & Garfinkel 1979.

Table 11.16: Percentage probability of dying between ages 15-60 years from selected causes, by region 1990

	Established market economies		Formerly Socialist economies of Eastern Europe		China		India		Other Asia and Islands		Middle Eastern Crescent		Latin America and Caribbean		Sub-Saharan Africa	
	M	F	M	F	M	F	M	F	M	F	M	F	M	F	M	F
all causes	14.67	7.35	28.09	11.24	20.11	14.97	27.21	22.88	24.28	17.71	22.09	16.64	22.82	16.35	38.04	32.16
tuberculosis	-	-	0.54	-	1.45	0.98	4.37	2.33	4.18	2.31	2.75	1.64	2.02	1.15	7.98	5.10
HIV infection	0.57	0.10	-	-	-	-	-	-	-	-	-	-	0.67	0.13	2.04	2.30
diarrhoeal diseases	-	-	-	-	-	-	0.45	0.44	0.25	0.28	0.26	0.32	0.16	0.28	0.29	0.34
malaria	-	-	-	-	-	-	0.14	0.14	0.38	0.42	-	-	0.11	0.12	0.97	1.14
respiratory infection	0.19	0.10	0.33	0.11	0.11	-	0.79	0.80	0.45	0.49	0.27	0.33	0.50	0.62	0.71	0.84
maternal conditions	-	-	-	-	-	0.31	-	2.03	-	1.30	-	1.11	-	0.68	-	3.64
stomach cancer	0.33	0.18	0.95	0.43	1.06	0.58	0.37	0.21	0.39	0.22	0.36	0.23	0.35	0.18	0.30	0.31
colorectal cancer	0.37	0.28	0.39	0.35	0.25	0.23	0.12	-	0.12	0.14	0.11	0.11	0.16	0.17	-	0.35
liver cancer	0.16	-	-	-	1.81	0.59	0.14	-	0.66	0.20	0.15	0.10	-	-	0.79	0.10
lung cancer	1.14	0.40	2.14	0.25	0.65	0.34	0.38	-	0.59	0.20	0.72	0.17	0.35	0.10	0.24	0.24
diabetes mellitus	0.20	0.14	0.15	0.15	0.14	0.17	0.49	0.65	0.37	0.57	0.60	0.83	0.54	0.72	0.13	0.94
rheumatic heart disease	-	-	0.30	0.33	0.39	0.64	0.35	0.86	0.11	0.32	0.15	0.39	-	0.14	0.33	0.40
ischaemic heart disease	2.19	0.56	5.34	1.33	0.87	0.45	2.61	1.09	2.68	1.33	1.95	0.82	2.04	1.06	0.81	2.16
cerebrovascular disease	0.63	0.42	1.93	1.29	2.06	1.75	1.08	1.32	0.96	1.23	1.41	1.50	1.52	1.46	1.73	1.60
inflammatory cardiac disease	0.22	0.08	0.29	0.11	0.20	0.17	2.31	1.48	0.75	0.58	1.03	0.69	1.09	0.77	2.21	0.33
chronic obstructive lung disease	0.18	0.10	0.52	0.15	1.22	0.98	0.36	0.36	0.23	0.24	0.30	0.25	0.31	0.23	0.26	0.16
asthma	-	-	0.12	-	-	-	0.11	0.18	-	0.12	-	0.12	0.10	0.12	-	0.64
liver cirrhosis	0.71	0.26	0.45	0.16	1.00	0.47	1.42	0.58	1.17	0.50	0.70	0.36	1.38	0.43	1.30	0.27
road traffic accident	1.196	0.39	2.25	0.45	0.85	0.32	1.05	0.22	1.61	0.29	1.14	0.26	1.60	0.37	2.06	0.34
suicide	1.00	0.35	1.89	0.42	1.27	1.65	0.58	0.50	1.21	0.35	0.88	0.32	0.37	0.12	1.52	0.10
homicide / violence	0.34	0.10	0.75	0.23	0.23	0.10	0.20	-	0.66	0.10	0.46	-	1.47	0.13	0.87	1.23

dash (-) indicates less than 0.1 %
Source: from data reported by Murray & Lopez 1994.

Table 11.17: Five main causes of death at different ages, England 1992

age 15-34		age 35-54		age 55-74		age over 75	
males							
road accidents	21%	ischaemic heart disease	28%	ischaemic heart disease	34%	ischaemic heart disease	27%
other injury and poisoning	20%	cancer of digestive organs and peritoneum	9%	cancer of respiratory and intrathoracic organs	13%	cerebrovascular disease	12%
suicide and self-inflicted injury	17%	cancer of respiratory and intrathoracic organs	8%	cancer of digestive organs and peritoneum	10%	chronic obstructive pulmonary disease	8%
diseases of nervous system and sense organs	5%	other injury and poisoning	6%	cerebrovascular disease	7%	cancer of respiratory and intrathoracic organs	7%
cancer of lymphatic and haematopoetic system	4%	suicide	6%	chronic obstructive pulmonary disease	6%	cancer of digestive organs and peritoneum	7%
females							
road accidents	14%	cancer of bone, connective tissue, skin and breast	22%	ischaemic heart disease	24%	ischaemic heart disease	25%
other injury and poisoning	12%	cancer of genitourinary organs	10%	cancer of digestive organs and peritoneum	10%	cerebrovascular disease	17%
suicide and self-inflicted injury	9%	cancer of digestive organs and peritoneum	9%	cerebrovascular disease	9%	pneumonia	8%
diseases of nervous system and sense organs	8%	ischaemic heart disease	8%	cancer of respiratory and intrathoracic organs	8%	cancer of digestive organs and peritoneum	6%
cancer of bone, connective tissue, skin and breast	7%	cancer of respiratory and intrathoracic organs	7%	cancer of bone, connective tissue, skin and breast	8%	mental disorders	4%

Source: from data reported by Department of Health 1994.

Table 11.18: Years of working life lost (thousands) by death between ages 15-64, England and Wales 1992

		men	women
all causes		832	480
all cancer		183	195
	lung cancer	39	20
	breast cancer	-	59
	genito-urinary cancer	16	35
	leukemia	14	16
circulatory disease		201	74
	ischaemic heart disease	144	32
	cerebrovascular disease	26	23
respiratory disease		36	21
	pneumonia	14	6
	bronchitis, emphysema and asthma	9	7
all accidental deaths		131	29
	traffic accidents	77	23
suicide		67	15

Source: from data reported by Department of Health 1994.

Table 11.19: Relative risk of cholecystectomy and / or symptomatic gallstones

BMI	< 24	24.5	25.5	26.5	28	29.5	32.5	37.5	42.5	> 45
relative risk	1.0	1.43	1.74	2.11	2.53	2.67	3.69	4.72	5.11	7.36

Source: from data reported by Stampfer *et al.* 1992.

Table 11.20: Composition of gall bladder bile in lean and obese subjects

	Freeman *et al.* mol /L		Bennion & Grundy molar percent	
	lean	obese	lean	obese
cholesterol	15	26	6.5	9.7
bile acids	40	52	74	67.2
phospholipids	169	131	19.5	23.1
lithogenicity index	0.068	0.158	0.088	0.144

Source: from data reported by Bennion & Grundy 1975;
Freeman *et al.* 1975.

Table 11.21: Liver lipids in biopsy samples from control and obese subjects and patients with alcoholic liver disease.

	control		obesity		alcoholic liver disease	
	µmol /g	molar %	µmol /g	molar %	µmol /g	molar %
free fatty acids	1.6 ± 0.7	9.6	13.7 ± 1.6	5.4	19.9 ± 2.4	9.6
monoacylglycerols	0.3 ± 1.2	1.8	3.1 ± 1.0	1.2	6.0 ± 1.4	2.9
diacylglycerols	0.6 ± 0.2	3.6	5.9 ± 1.1	2.3	15.5 ± 3.6	7.5
triacylglycerols	14.1 ± 2.4	84.9	228.4 ± 43.2	90.9	164.5 ± 24.6	79.8
cholesterol	5.0 ± 1.3	-	5.3 ± 0.2	-	7.5 ± 0.6	-

See also section 9.3.1
Source: from data reported by Mavrelis *et al.* 1983.

Table 11.22: Respiratory function in lean and obese subjects

	lean	obese
vital capacity (mL)	5333 ± 1083	3073 ± 766
% of expected	131 ± 17.3	98 ± 15.8
maximum breathing capacity (L/min)	162 ± 42.2	65 ± 24.7
% of expected	133 ± 25.8	73 ± 29.8
total lung capacity, mL	6824 ± 1352	4606 ± 855
respiratory compliance, L/cm H_2O		
total, seated	0.119 ± 0.045	0.052 ± 0.025
total, supine	0.122 ± 0.029	0.043 ± 0.011
lung, seated	0.283 ± 0.088	0.200 ± 0.113
lung, supine	0.263 ± 0.089	0.181 ± 0.098
chest wall, seated	0.224 ± 0.110	0.077 ± 0.041
chest wall, supine	0.260 ± 0.102	0.059 ± 0.014
mechanical work of respiratory muscles (kg-m /L)	0.227	0.540

Source: from data reported by Naimark & Cherniak 1960.

Table 11.23: Respiratory function with weight for height as % of predicted values

	weight (kg) / height (cm)							
	0.4-0.49	0.5-0.59	0.6-0.69	0.7-0.79	0.8-0.89	0.9-0.99	1.0-1.09	1.1-1.19
vital capacity	116	107	108	100	100	105	82	69
inspiratory capacity	116	109	112	119	120	125	105	87
expiratory reserve volume	114	103	100	63	60	64	35	32
total lung capacity	109	93	95	93	90	100	95	79
functional residual capacity	102	78	80	70	80	79	87	75
residual volume	91	59	63	77	103	97	156	141
max voluntary ventilation	110	98	102	92	93	93	77	61

Source: from data reported by Ray *et al.* 1983.

Table 11.24: Post-operative complications and mortality in lean and overweight patients with and without hypertension and diabetes

	post-operative complications (% of each group)				
pre-existing	thrombophlebitis	pneumonia	atelectasis	wound infection	death
hypertension					
overweight	7.1	0	7.1	14.3	7.1
not overweight	0	2.5	2.5	3.7	4.9
no hypertension					
overweight	3.6	3.6	9.1	15.5	6.4
not overweight	0.7	6.2	4.8	8.3	2.6
diabetes					
overweight	0	0	0	28.6	0
not overweight	1.7	6.9	6.9	10.3	5.2
no diabetes					
overweight	4.3	3.4	9.4	14.5	6.8
not overweight	0.7	6.0	4.7	8.2	2.6

Source: from data reported by Postlethwait & Johnson 1972.

Table 11.25: Mortality ratio for all causes of death, by gender and ethnicity, with subcutaneous fat over the trapezius ridge, relative to mortality in the study population as a whole = 1.0.

	age	subcutaneous fat, mm		
		0-4	5-9	> 10
white males	15-34	0.61	1.32	1.88
	35-54	0.98	0.97	1.21
	> 55	1.08	0.96	0.96
white females	15-34	1.35	0.64	1.52
	35-54	0.89	1.01	1.04
	> 55	0.94	0.96	1.06
black males	15-34	0.91	1.17	0.98
	35-54	1.13	0.83	1.12
	> 55	0.88	1.09	1.16
black females	15-34	0.85	0.79	1.21
	35-54	1.24	0.83	1.06
	> 55	0.95	1.02	1.00

Source: from data reported by Comstock *et al.* 1966.

Table 11.26: Mortality ratio for different causes of death, regardless of gender and ethnicity, by subcutaneous adipose tissue over the trapezius ridge.

	subcutaneous fat, mm		
	0-4	5-9	> 10
all causes of death	0.98	0.96	1.12
coronary heart disease	0.91	0.89	1.37
strokes	0.94	0.97	1.14
hypertension	0.98	0.95	1.13
other cardio-vascular / renal disease	0.83	1.13	0.98
diabetes	0.55	0.92	1.62
cancer	1.06	0.93	1.08
tuberculosis	1.74	0.70	0.28
other respiratory disease	1.17	1.04	0.64
accidents	0.82	1.06	1.26

Source: from data reported by Comstock *et al.* 1966.

Table 11.27: Incidence of coronary heart disease with subscapular skinfold thickness and body mass index

	CHD rate / 1000
BMI 14.3-22.4	39.7
BMI 22.5-25.1	58.2
BMI 25.2-39.9	77.0
subscapular skinfold 2-12 mm	35.8
subscapular skinfold 13-19 mm	59.8
subscapular skinfold 20-51 mm	80.0

BMI	subscapular skinfold	CHD rate / 1000
14.3-22.4	2-12 mm	33.0
	13-19 mm	52.7
	20-51 mm	72.2
22.5-25.1	2-12 mm	40.1
	13-19 mm	54.6
	20-51 mm	72.8
25.2-39.9	2-12 mm	45.9
	13-19 mm	72.3
	20-51 mm	85.2

subscapular skinfold	BMI	CHD rate / 1000
2-12 mm	14.3-22.4	33.0
	22.5-25.1	40.1
	25.2-39.9	45.9
13-19 mm	14.3-22.4	52.7
	22.5-25.1	54.6
	25.2-39.9	72.3
20-51 mm	14.3-22.4	72.2
	22.5-25.1	72.8
	25.2-39.9	85.2

Source: from data reported by Donahue *et al.* 1987.

Table 11.28: The effect of waist : hip ratio on the gender difference in coronary heart disease

	odds ratio men : women
raw data	3.2
corrected for blood pressure, cholesterol, BMI and smoking	3.1
corrected for waist : hip ratio	1.4
corrected for blood pressure, cholesterol, BMI, smoking and waist:hip ratio	1.1

Source: from data reported by Larsson *et al.* 1992.

Table 11.29: Relative risk of death from all causes or specific causes, by BMI

	quintile of BMI					quintile of waist : hip ratio				
	1	2	3	4	5	1	2	3	4	5
all causes of death										
all subjects	1.0	0.75	0.68	0.64	0.74	1.0	1.51	1.63	2.09	2.56
never smokers	1.0	0.83	0.64	0.65	0.80	1.0	1.44	1.56	2.11	2.39
ever smokers	1.0	0.68	0.74	0.66	0.69	1.0	1.50	1.60	1.87	2.42
never smokers										
cardiovascular disease	1.0	0.76	0.65	0.76	1.03	1.0	1.67	1.86	2.77	3.39
cancer	1.0	0.87	0.64	0.64	0.76	1.0	1.35	1.57	1.88	1.87
injury and poisoning	1.0	0.85	0.57	0.51	0.82	1.0	1.89	0.74	2.30	2.65
other	1.0	0.79	0.63	0.48	0.45	1.0	1.47	1.35	2.12	2.99

Source: from data reported by Folsom *et al.* 1993.

Table 11.30: Hypertension and diabetes with excess weight and waist : hip ratio, women

	% over ideal weight		
	< 21%	21-50%	> 50%
percent with hypertension			
waist : hip ratio			
< 0.73	20.6	28.8	52.2
0.73-0.76	23.9	35.0	56.1
0.77-0.80	30.2	41.2	58.9
> 0.80	32.1	46.0	64.7
Percent with diabetes			
waist : hip ratio			
< 0.73	2.0	3.2	6.1
0.73-0.76	2.8	4.2	6.6
0.77-0.80	3.4	4.4	10.8
> 0.80	5.5	10.8	16.9

Source: from data reported by Hartz *et al.* 1984.

Table 11.31: Waist : hip ratio and glucose tolerance.

	non-obese	Obese subjects, waist : hip ratio		
		< 0.76	0.76-0.85	> 0.85
% ideal body weight	111 ± 3	175 ± 8	184 ± 9	177 ± 9
fasting plasma triacylglycerol (mg/dl)	60 ± 5	110 ± 13	129 ± 10	152 ± 16
fasting plasma cholesterol (mg/dl)	162 ± 5	181 ± 11	184 ± 7	188 ± 7
fasting plasma insulin (μU/ml)	19 ± 1	28 ± 3	30 ± 2	40 ± 3
glucose area under curve (arbitrary units)	453 ± 17	538 ± 23	584 ± 17	593 ± 21
insulin area under curve (arbitrary units)	304 ± 32	508 ± 65	538 ± 40	718 ± 77

Source: from data reported by Evans *et al.* 1984.

Table 11.32: Anorectic drugs

benzphetamine hydrochloride
dexamphetamine sulphate
dexfenfluramine hydrochloride
diethylpropion hydrochloride
fenfluramine hydrochloride
mazindol
mefenorex hydrochloride
phendimetrazine tartrate
phenmetrazine hydrochloride
phentermine hydrochloride

World food supplies and protein-energy malnutrition

The term protein-energy malnutrition (pem or pcm, protein-calorie malnutrition) is used to mean an inadequate intake of total food to meet energy and protein requirements. In fact the problem is one of energy shortage, not protein deficiency. As shown in Table 10.12, most dietary staples provide at least enough protein to meet requirements if enough can be eaten to meet energy needs. Three distinct types of protein-energy malnutrition can be defined.

1. Marasmus, which is the predictable physiological response to an inadequate intake of energy to meet expenditure (see section 12.2).

2. Cachexia, which is seen in patients with advanced cancer, AIDS, and other chronic diseases, where an apparently adequate intake of food is insufficient to meet requirements because of an increased metabolic rate (see section 12.3).

3. Kwashiorkor; oedematous malnutrition seen only in young children. The factors that precipitate kwashiorkor in undernourished children are not well understood (see section 12.4).

At its simplest, the problem of protein-energy malnutrition is one of matching food production and population. From the publication of Malthus' *Essay on the Principles of Population* in 1798 until the 1970s, it was widely believed that there never had been, nor ever could be, adequate food produced world-wide to feed the people of the world. Malthus' thesis was that population tends to increase faster than the supply of food, and when there is a relative gain of food production over population growth, a higher rate of population growth follows. As discussed below, despite the continuing increase in world population, from the 1960s to 1990s world food production has increased more, so as to permit an increase in food available per head of population in most countries.

12.1 Population and food availability

The world population is estimated to be 5.7 billion in 1995, having grown from 300 million in AD 0, and only passing 1 billion in AD 1805. It is forecast to reach 6 billion in 1998, and to continue to increase, before stabilizing at around 11.6 billion by the year 2200 (see Fig. 12.1 and Table 12.1). The projected population by the year 2025 ranges from a low of 7.6 billion to a high of 8.98 billion, with a median of 8.29 billion. The average annual rate of increase from 1960 to 1990 was 2.2 per cent, peaking in the late 1960s and falling to 1.6 per cent annually by 1994—an increase of 86 million people in 1994. Table 12.2 shows global and regional population changes; figures for individual countries are shown in Table 12.8. Table 12.3 shows the total population and proportion of elderly people, and Table 12.4 birth, death and fertility rates, in developed, less developed and least developed countries. Table 12.5 shows birth and age-specific fertility rates by geographical region, and Table 12.6 estimated numbers of deaths in developed and less developed countries. More detailed mortality statistics are shown in Table 11.16.

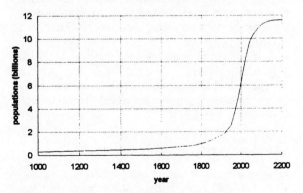

Figure 12.1 World population growth from AD 1000 to predicted stabilization in AD 2200
Plotted from data reported by United Nations 1995a

12.1.1 The impact of AIDS on population growth

The estimate of the effects of AIDS on population growth is that by 2005 the population of the 15 African countries most affected (Benin, Burkina Faso, Burundi, Central African Republic, Congo, Côte d'Ivoire, Kenya, Malawi, Mozambique, Rwanda, Tanzania, Uganda, Zaire, Zambia and Zimbabwe) will be 3.8 per cent lower than would otherwise have been expected (United Nations 1995a). The effect will be most severe in Zambia and Zimbabwe, with 6.9 per cent lower population than would otherwise be expected, and Uganda (6.1 per cent lower).

For these 15 countries, the crude death rate in 1990–95 was 15.4 deaths per thousand, compared with 13.7 /1000 excluding AIDS. Despite this, the population of these 15 countries is forecast to reach 291.8 million by 2005, more than double that in 1980.

12.1.2 Loss of land and water resources

United Nations data estimate that annually 6–7 million hectares of agricultural land are lost to erosion, and a further 1.5 million hectares are lost due to waterlogging, salinization or alkalinization; in recent decades poor land and water management practices have led to the degradation of 1.2 billion hectares—11 per cent of the earth's total fertile soil, an area equal to that of China and India combined. Additionally 16–20 million hectares of tropical forests and woodlands are lost annually.

Water scarcity (defined as less than 1000 m^3 of water /person /year) affects more than 130 million people, in 20 countries, and water shortage may impede industrial development, since industrialization increases water demand; currently almost 80 per cent of the fresh water used world-wide goes to agriculture. An estimated 1.3 billion people were without access to clean drinking water in 1990, and 1.8 billion lacked access to sanitation services. World-wide 2 billion people are at risk from water-borne diseases, leading to 4 million deaths annually (United Nations 1995b).

12.1.3 World food supplies

Despite a 64.8 per cent increase in world population from 1960–90, and the loss of agricultural land, total food available per person increased by 16.5 per cent; regional increases of food availability per head of population from 1960–90 are shown in Table 12.7, and national figures in Table 12.8. Such figures show

total food (theoretically) available per head of population, and make no allowance for losses in storage and distribution, nor for the, sometimes considerable, differences in food distribution to different regions of any one country. It is striking from the data in Table 12.7 that of those countries where food available per head of population in 1960 was marginal or inadequate, most have achieved a significant increase in food availability. The exceptions are those countries with very high rates of population growth, and those that have been severely affected by drought and/or wars.

Table 12.9 shows the food available per head of population, the proportion of food energy consumption that is imported, and the proportion of food energy production that is exported, globally and regionally. Table 12.10 shows the same data for individual countries.

12.2   Marasmus

Marasmus is the predictable physiological response to an inadequate intake to meet energy expenditure. Affected people are obviously emaciated and wasted. Reserves of adipose tissue are extremely low; the normal proportion of adipose tissue is 28 ± 6 per cent of body weight in men and 35 ± 9 per cent in women (see section 2.2). Table 12.11 shows the classification of protein-energy malnutrition by body mass index (the ratio of weight / height^2). More precise evaluation of nutritional status can be made using measurements of skinfold thickness (see section 2.2.1.7) and arm anthropometry (see section 3.3.4).

For children, the severity of malnutrition can be assessed by the percentage of their expected weight for age—the basis of the Gomez classification, shown in Table 12.12.

In a child, low body weight for age may be a result of short stature, with normal weight for height. Waterlow (1972, 1973) proposed a two-way classification of undernutrition in children, based on both wasting (lower than expected weight for height) and stunting (lower than expected height for age). See section 3.3 for a discussion of reference standards of weight and height. Stunting of linear growth reflects past undernutrition; growth once achieved cannot be reversed. Stunting is also likely to reflect past protein deficiency, since if protein intake is inadequate then growth will be reduced. However, energy deficiency with adequate protein intake will also lead to stunting, because of the high energy cost of protein synthesis (see section 10.8.3.2) and growth. By contrast, wasting reflects current under-nutrition, and especially energy deficiency; it may occur relatively suddenly. The original Waterlow classification used four grades of each of wasting and stunting, to produce a 16–way classification; this was later simplified to give a four-way classification, shown in Table 12.13. The most seriously affected children are those who are both stunted and wasted; they are the priority group for nutritional rehabilitation. Those who are only mildly stunted or wasted are not seriously undernourished, and they have a low priority for intervention.

Because of the high energy cost of protein synthesis (see section 10.8.3.2), synthesis of protein is greatly reduced in pem, although body protein catabolism continues at the normal rate. Initially this affects mainly muscle, increasing the obvious wasting of affected people. As the condition worsens, so there is impaired replacement of other tissues as well; when essential organ protein is lost, death is inevitable.

The reduced protein synthesis also leads to impaired immunoglobulin synthesis, and hence greater susceptibility to infection. The normal increase in metabolic rate in response to infection leads to increased energy expenditure, and so worsens the condition. Infections that might be mild in adequately fed people can prove fatal in undernourished adults or children.

A further consequence of impaired tissue protein synthesis is a considerable slowing in the proliferation of intestinal mucosal cells (see Table 6.9). This leads to a loss of intestinal mucosa, with severe flattening of the villi, and considerable impairment of the absorption of such food as is available. Intestinal parasites and infections will exacerbate the problem.

12.3 Cachexia

Cachexia is the severe emaciation and wasting seen in patients with advanced cancer, AIDS and other chronic diseases. Superficially it resembles marasmus, and inadequate food intake is certainly a factor. Severe illness impairs appetite, and many of the drugs used in chemotherapy both induce nausea and distort the senses of taste and smell, so reducing food intake further. In addition, both radiotherapy and chemotherapy reduce cell division (the aim of therapy in cancer), with the undesired effect of reducing the turnover of intestinal mucosal cells, leading to flattening of the villi and loss of absorptive surface. However, cachexia is also associated with hypermetabolism (a considerable increase in resting metabolic

rate), and an increase in the rate of tissue protein catabolism. Unlike marasmus, where protein catabolism is unchanged, and the net loss of tissue protein is the result of reduced replacement, in cachexia there is an increase in the rate of both protein synthesis and catabolism, leading not only to a net increase in protein breakdown, but also an increased energy requirement for the increased rate of turnover (Pisters and Brennan 1990).

12.3.1 Gastrointestinal tract manifestations of AIDS

Infection with human immuno-deficiency virus has a major impact on the function of the gastrointestinal tract, quite apart from the effects of opportunistic infections resulting from impaired immune status. The result is both decreased food intake and also malabsorption, both of which contribute to cachexia—AIDS was originally called 'slim disease' in East Africa, because of the severe emaciation it causes.

One of the causes of decreased food intake is the oral pathology that is commonly associated with AIDS. Oral and oesophageal infection with *Candida* spp. (candidiasis or thrush) is common, and leads to loss of the sense of taste, and pain and difficulty in swallowing. Aphthous ulceration is a common problem in patients with AIDS; the aetiology is unknown. Peptic ulcers (see section 6.1.2.2) are common, probably as a result of infection with cytomegalovirus, leading to dyspepsia, and again decreasing appetite.

The most serious nutritional problem is the diarrhoea, and consequent malabsorption, that is commonly associated with AIDS as a result of infection by a wide range of pathogens, as shown in Table 12.14. In many patients no infective organisms can be found to explain the diarrhoea and malabsorption. However, HIV has been isolated from small and large intestinal mucosal cells, suggesting that it has an adverse effect on the gut mucosa even in the absence of opportunistic infections, causing partial villus atrophy. The mechanism is unclear (Keutsch and Farthing 1990).

12.3.2 Hypermetabolism and responses to cytokines

The key feature which distinguishes cachexia from marasmus is the positive wasting that occurs; in marasmus wasting is a consequence of inadequate energy intake, and the metabolic rate is either unchanged or falls, while in cachexia there is an increase in metabolic rate, leading to an increased energy demand, regardless of whether or not intake is reduced. There is also an increased rate of tissue protein catabolism.

The increase in metabolic rate and protein catabolism is believed to be due to cytokines—especially tumour necrosis factor-α (also known as cachectin), interleukin-1 and interleukin-6, potentiated by interferon-γ. The cytokines are small proteins secreted by macrophages, monocytes and other cells in response to a variety of stimuli. Virtually all cells of the body have receptors for the various cytokines, which normally function as signals to immune cells, growth factors in wound healing, and cellular cytotoxins against pathogens and tumour cells.

Excessive production of cytokines occurs acutely in septic shock, and chronically in persistent infection, AIDS, and metastatic cancer. In experimental animals, administration of cachectin (the best-studied of the cytokines) leads to dehydration, anorexia, and a variety of metabolic responses shown in Table 12.15, the end result of which is severe emaciation and wasting (Langstein and Norton 1991; Tracey and Cerami 1990).

At least part of the increased resting metabolic rate in patients with advanced cancer can be accounted for by anaerobic glycolysis in the tumour, leading to the production of lactate, which is used for gluconeogenesis in the liver. Additionally, as shown in Table 12.13, one of the actions of cachectin is to increase the rate of glycogenolysis and anaerobic glycolysis in muscle, thus increasing the amount of lactate to be converted back to glucose in the liver. Anaerobic glycolysis has a net yield of 2 mol of ATP per mol of glucose metabolized; gluconeogenesis from lactate in the liver incurs a net cost of 4 ATP / mol of glucose formed. Significant cycling between anaerobic glycolysis and gluconeogenesis (the Cori cycle) thus has a considerable energy cost. Holroyd *et al.* (1975) have reported the rates of such glucose cycling in patients with cancer cachexia shown in Table 12.16, and have suggested that this alone would account for 50 per cent of the increased metabolic rate, and a loss of 0.5–1 kg body weight per month.

12.4   Kwashiorkor

Kwashiorkor is a protein-energy deficiency disease that occurs only in young children. It was originally described in west Africa by Cicely Williams in 1935; kwashiorkor is the Ga name for the disease. The key feature that distinguishes kwashiorkor from marasmus is the presence of oedema; in addition there is a sooty dermatitis, resembling sunburn, fatty infiltration of the liver, leading to hepatomegaly and a pot-bellied appearance, and the hair is sparse, wispy and poorly pigmented.

McLaren *et al.* (1967) devised a system of scoring clinical signs to differentiate between kwashiorkor and marasmus in children. As shown in Table 12.17, this relies on measurement of serum albumin or total protein, which is not practicable in field studies. It also creates an apparently intermediate classification of marasmic-kwashiorkor.

A simpler classification is that devised by the Wellcome Trust Working Party (1970), based on just two criteria: the degree of underweight and the presence or absence of oedema (see Table 12.18). This classification, which is the most widely used, shows that marasmic-kwashiorkor is not an intermediate stage in the development of kwashiorkor, but is the most serious form of undernutrition, with both a severe degree of underweight and also oedema (and presumably therefore also the other clinical signs of kwashiorkor).

12.4.1 The aetiology of kwashiorkor

The original hypothesis to explain the aetiology of kwashiorkor was that it was the result of an inadequate intake of protein with adequate energy intake. Comparison of the diets of children with kwashiorkor with those of children with marasmus provides no evidence for this. Neither group of children has an adequate intake of energy, and the protein intakes of children with kwashiorkor are not lower than those of children with marasmus. Furthermore, protein deficiency would be expected to lead to stunting, whereas the data in Table 12.17 show that children with kwashiorkor are not significantly stunted, while those with marasmus or marasmic kwashiorkor are severely stunted.

Further evidence against the role of simple protein deficiency in the aetiology of kwashiorkor comes from the observation that during rehabilitation of severely undernourished children, resolution of the oedema is correlated with energy intake, not protein intake. An intake of only 2.5 per cent of energy from protein (well below the normal maintenance requirement) leads to resolution of the oedema as fast as an intake of 12.5 per cent of energy from protein, provided that energy intake is greater than 245–270 kJ / kg body weight /day (Golden 1982).

The most likely explanation of the development of kwashiorkor is that it is the result of an acute increase in the oxygen radical burden in children whose intake of antioxidant nutrients, as well as total food, is inadequate (Golden and Ramdath 1987). Unsuppressed radical damage to membrane lipids will result in leakiness of capillaries and impairment of the normal renal handling of sodium (see section 24.1), leading to sodium and fluid retention, and hence oedema.

Similarly, peroxidative damage to mitochondrial membranes may account for the fatty infiltration of the liver that is characteristic of kwashiorkor. Jackson (1991) has suggested that the extent of fatty infiltration of the liver is related to the availability of cysteine for synthesis of glutathione—a major antioxidant involved in reduction of lipid peroxides (see section 15.5.1). Plasma glutathione is significantly lower in children with kwashiorkor than in those with marasmus, is lowest in the sickest children, and rises on recovery.

A number of toxins, and especially mycotoxins such as aflatoxin (see section 27.5.1), which are commonly found in foods in developing countries, have been associated with the onset of kwashiorkor. Many of these toxins are metabolized by epoxide formation, a process that results in the formation of reactive oxygen species.

More commonly, kwashiorkor is precipitated by an infection; the macrophage response to infection is production of oxygen radicals. There is commonly an increase in the incidence of kwashiorkor some 6 months after an outbreak of measles and other childhood illnesses.

A further factor increasing oxygen radical stress may be the moderate degree of iron overload that is seen in many children with kwashiorkor; the synthesis of iron binding proteins (see section 24.3) is depressed in protein-energy malnutrition, and free iron ions catalyse non-enzymic production of oxygen radicals.

Further reading

Keutsch, G.T. and Farthing, M.J.G. (1990). Nutritional aspects of AIDS. *Annual Review of Nutrition*, 10, 475–501.

Langstein, H.N. and Norton, J.A. (1991). Mechanisms of cancer cachexia. *Haematology and Oncology Clinics of North America*, 5, 103–23.

Tomkins, A. and Watson, F. (1989). *Malnutrition and Infection: a review*. United Nations Administrative Committee on Coordination / Sub-Committee on Nutrition, Geneva.

Waterlow, J.C. (1992). *Protein-Energy Malnutrition*. Edward Arnold, London.

Table 12.1: World population milestones

billions achieved	year	years elapsed
1	1804	-
2	1927	123
3	1960	33
4	1974	14
5	1987	13
billions estimated		
6	1998	11
7	2009	11
8	2021	12
9	2035	14
10	2054	19
11	2093	39

Source: United Nations 1995b.

Table 12.2: Changes in population 1960-1990

	% change mean	1960-90 annual %
world average	64.8	2.2
Africa	80.7	2.7
Asia	66.8	2.2
Europe	21.5	0.7
Latin America / Caribbean	56.8	2.2
Middle East	111.8	3.8
Oceania	64.1	2.6
North America	34.5	1.5

Table 12.3: World population 1950-2025

	1950	1990	predicted 2000	2025
total, millions	2516	5292	6261	8504
developed countries	832	1207	1264	1354
less developed	1684	4085	4997	7150
least developed	169	444	595	1039
elderly (> 64 y), % of population				
total	5.1	6.2	6.8	9.7
developed countries	7.6	12.1	13.7	19.0
less developed	3.8	4.5	5.0	8.0
least developed	3.4	3.0	3.0	4.0

Source: WHO 1995.

Table 12.4: Birth, death and fertility rates and life expectancy, 1990

	birth rate /1000	death rate /1000	fertility rate[1]	life expectancy (years)
developed countries	14.2	9.7	1.9	74.5
developing countries	30.5	9.5	3.8	62.4
least developed countries	44.3	15.8	6.1	50.6

(1) Number of children a women can expect to bear in her reproductive life
Source: WHO 1995.

Table 12.5: Births and age-specific fertility rates 1990-1995

	births millions	fertility /woman	fertility rate /1000 women by age						
			15-19	20-24	25-29	30-34	35-39	40-45	45-49
World	687.422	3.1	60	181	177	112	59	24	8
More developed regions	72.484	1.7	32	96	111	71	26	5	0
Less developed regions	614.938	3.5	65	200	194	124	71	31	11
Least developed countries	114.735	5.8	140	275	273	218	149	79	27
Africa	142.412	5.8	136	267	272	219	149	82	35
Eastern Africa	48.686	6.5	151	305	299	242	166	97	34
Middle Africa	17.611	6.5	207	305	271	230	163	89	26
Northern Africa	23.732	4.2	60	187	236	179	112	50	14
Southern Africa	7.154	4.2	75	198	217	165	98	63	28
Western Africa	45.228	6.5	164	290	289	240	171	99	56
Asia	417.929	3.0	45	186	183	108	56	22	7
Eastern Asia	123.218	1.9	14	160	134	55	15	4	1
South-central Asia	206.320	4.1	73	223	237	152	89	38	12
South-east Asia	63.091	3.3	47	162	181	139	87	33	9
Western Asia	25.299	4.4	65	206	240	173	121	58	21
Europe	42.056	1.6	27	98	102	62	23	5	0
Eastern Europe	17.818	1.6	38	132	89	44	18	4	0
Northern Europe	6.252	1.8	27	92	125	87	32	6	0
Southern Europe	7.762	1.4	17	73	99	64	25	6	0
Western Europe	10.224	1.5	11	66	113	79	29	5	0
Latin America and Caribbean	59.806	3.1	79	173	156	111	66	28	5
Caribbean	·4.069	2.8	78	153	138	95	57	24	8
Central America	17.762	3.5	89	194	181	126	75	31	8
South America	37.975	3.0	75	167	149	108	65	27	4
Northern America	22.578	2.1	60	113	120	81	32	5	0
Oceania	2.642	2.5	28	111	163	119	53	20	8
Australia and New Zealand	594	1.9	24	83	141	98	33	5	0

Source: United Nations 1995a.

Table 12.6: Estimated number of deaths 1990

	world	developed countries	less developed countries
millions			
total	50.225	11.712	38.514
0-4 y	13.148	0.284	12.864
5-14 y	2.792	0.071	2.721
15-44 y	5.737	0.663	5.074
45-59 y	5.393	1.348	4.045
60-64 y	2.989	0.884	2.106
> 65 y	20.166	8.462	11.704
percent			
0-4 y	26.2	2.4	33.4
5-14 y	5.6	0.6	7.1
15-44 y	11.4	5.7	13.2
45-59 y	10.7	11.5	10.5
60-64 y	6.0	7.5	5.5
> 65 y	40.2	72.3	30.4

Table 12.7: Changes in food availability and population 1960-1990, regional averages

	kcal /head /day			population change annual %
	1961-3	1988-90	% change	
Global average	2300	2648	16.5	2.2
Africa	2068	2278	11.2	2.7
Asia	2084	2473	19.8	2.2
Europe	3076	3397	11.0	0.7
Latin America / Caribbean	2108	2564	18.5	2.2
Middle East	2217	2920	34.3	3.8
Oceania	2486	2831	15.4	2.6
North America	2995	3440	14.8	1.5

Source: FAO 1995.

Table 12.8: Population 1994 and changes in food availability and population 1960-1990, arranged by % change in food availability 1960-90

	1994	Population change 1960-90	annual change	1961-3	1988-90	change 1960-90
	millions	%	%	kcal	kcal	%
Chad	6.183	63	2.1	2300	1740	-24.3
Afghanistan	18.79	36	1.2	2350	1890	-19.6
Central African Republic	3.235	67	2.2	2170	1850	-14.7
Nigeria	108.467	94	3.1	2470	2200	-10.9
Madagascar	14.303	81	2.7	2360	2160	-8.5
Peru	23.331	77	2.6	2220	2040	-8.1
Bangladesh	117.787	80	2.7	2110	1950	-7.6
Mozambique	15.527	74	2.5	1950	1810	-7.2
Cambodia	90968	42	1.4	2520	2340	-7.1
Comoros	0.630	94	3.1	1880	1760	-6.4
Ethiopia	53.435	72	2.4	1800	1700	-5.6
Finland	5.083	12	0.4	3210	3050	-5.0
Burundi	6.209	62	2.1	2050	1950	-4.9
Uganda	20.621	105	3.5	2290	2180	-4.8
Kenya	27.343	106	3.5	2160	2060	-4.6
Togo	4.010	93	3.1	2380	2270	-4.6
Zaire	42.552	84	2.8	2220	2130	-4.1
Iceland	0.266	35	1.2	3230	3100	-4.0
Uruguay	3.167	19	0.6	2790	2690	-3.6
Senegal	8.102	83	2.8	2400	2320	-3.3
Zambia	9.196	99	3.3	2090	2020	-3.3
Chile	14.044	55	1.8	2530	2480	-2.0
Angola	10.674	72	2.4	1910	1880	-1.6
São Tome and Principé	0.130	63	2.1	2180	2150	-1.4
Switzerland	7.131	20	0.7	3510	3460	-1.4
Malawi	10.843	91	3.0	2070	2050	-1.0
Solomon Islands	0.366	100	3.3	2270	2250	-0.9
Nicaragua	4.275	95	3.2	2250	2240	-0.4
Argentina	34.182	45	1.5	3070	3070	0.0
United Kingdom	58.091	8	0.3	3270	3270	0.0
Australia	17.853	51	1.7	3140	3150	0.3
New Caledonia	0.178	81	2.7	2780	2790	0.4
Guinea	6.501	61	2.0	2210	2240	1.4
Haiti	7.035	54	1.8	1970	2010	2.0
Gambia	1.081	89	3.0	2240	2290	2.2
The Netherlands	15.397	25	0.8	3060	3150	2.9
Cameroon	12.781	81	2.7	2140	2210	3.3
Sweden	8.738	14	0.5	2870	2970	3.5
Sierra Leone	4.402	62	2.1	1830	1900	3.8
Mali	10.462	73	2.4	2170	2260	4.1
Panama	2.585	74	2.5	2170	2270	4.6
Poland	38.341	25	0.8	3320	3480	4.8
Rwanda	7.750	97	3.2	1820	1910	4.9
Ghana	16.944	78	2.6	2030	2140	5.4
Congo	2.516	84	2.8	2180	2300	5.5
Sri Lanka	18.125	57	1.9	2100	2220	5.7
Vietnam	72.931	66	2.2	2060	2180	5.8
Lesotho	1.996	71	2.4	2000	2120	6.0
Namibia	1.500	78	2.6	1850	1970	6.5
former USSR	280.703	29	1.0	3110	3320	6.8
Austria	7.918	8	0.3	3260	3490	7.1

Table 12.8: (Cont'd)

	1994 millions	Population change 1960-90 %	annual change %	food available/head /day 1961-3 kcal	1988-90 kcal	change 1960-90 %
Liberia	2.941	86	2.9	2110	2260	7.1
Malta	0.364	13	0.4	2960	3180	7.4
Macau	0.398	91	3.0	2080	2240	7.7
former Czechoslovakia	15.628	14	0.5	3350	3610	7.8
Somalia	9.077	93	3.1	1720	1870	8.7
Ireland	3.539	23	0.8	3360	3660	8.9
Antigua and Barbuda	0.65	33	1.1	2120	2310	9.0
Niger	8.846	90	3.0	2050	2240	9.3
French Polynesia	0.215	92	3.1	2540	2780	9.4
France	57.747	21	0.7	3300	3620	9.7
Guyana	0.825	33	1.1	2270	2500	10.1
Zimbabwe	11.002	94	3.1	2050	2260	10.2
New Zealand	3.531	33	1.1	3160	3490	10.4
Vanuatu	0.165	85	2.8	2470	2730	10.5
United Arab Emirates	1.861	289	9.6	2990	3310	10.7
Sudan	27.361	82	2.7	1840	2040	10.9
Canada	29.141	38	1.3	2920	3240	11.0
Denmark	5.173	11	0.4	3260	3620	11.0
Mongolia	2.363	82	2.7	2040	2270	11.3
Venezuela	21.378	97	3.2	2190	2440	11.4
Bolivia	7.237	75	2.5	1800	2010	11.7
Paraguay	4.830	88	2.9	2400	2680	11.7
India	918.570	66	2.2	2050	2310	12.7
Romania	22.922	24	0.8	2870	3250	13.2
Colombia	34.545	72	2.4	2160	2450	13.4
Kuwait	1.633	187	6.2	2590	2940	13.5
former Yugoslavia	10.763	26	0.9	3120	3550	13.8
Israel	5.458	76	2.5	2830	3220	13.8
Thailand	58.183	72	2.4	2040	2330	14.2
Honduras	5.493	97	3.2	1930	2210	14.5
Japan	124.815	28	0.9	2510	2890	15.1
Trinidad and Tobago	1.292	43	1.4	2400	2770	15.4
Malaysia	19.695	78	2.6	2340	2710	15.8
Belgium	10.080	9	0.3	3120	3630	16.3
Bermuda	0.063	27	0.9	2540	2960	16.5
Guatemala	10.322	85	2.8	1930	2250	16.6
Benin	5.246	73	2.4	2040	2380	16.7
Italy	57.157	14	0.5	2980	3480	16.8
South Africa	40.555	70	2.3	2680	3130	16.8
Laos	4.742	66	2.2	1880	2200	17.0
Nepal	21.360	74	2.5	1920	2250	17.2
Côte d'Ivoire	13.780	117	3.9	2190	2570	17.4
Brazil	159.143	72	2.4	2320	2730	17.7
Tonga	0.098	38	1.3	2480	2920	17.7
Germany	81.278	8	0.3	2980	3510	17.8
Hungary	10.161	3	0.1	3120	3680	17.9
Ecuador	11.220	88	2.9	2030	2400	18.2
USA	260.631	31	1.0	3070	3640	18.6
Guinea Bissau	1.050	57	1.9	1880	2240	19.1
Albania	3.414	70	2.3	2370	2830	19.4
Burkina Faso	10.046	71	2.4	1860	2220	19.4
Belize	0.210	69	2.3	2150	2580	20.0

Table 12.8: (Cont'd)

	1994	Population change 1960-90	annual change	food available/head /day 1961-3	1988-90	change 1960-90
	millions	%	%	kcal	kcal	%
Fiji	0.771	62	2.1	2440	2930	20.1
Swaziland	0.832	89	3.0	2160	2630	21.8
Tanzania	28.846	100	3.3	1800	2200	22.2
St Kitts	0.041	-14	-0.5	1990	2440	22.6
Mexico	91.858	85	2.8	2490	3060	22.9
Costa Rica	3.347	89	3.0	2200	2710	23.2
Yemen	13.873	79	2.6	1730	2140	23.7
Jordan	5.198	54	1.8	2230	2760	23.8
Surinam	0.418	37	1.2	1970	2440	23.9
Mauritania	2.217	71	2.4	1970	2450	24.4
Dominican Republic	7.684	80	2.7	1850	2310	24.9
Gabon	1.283	87	2.9	1950	2440	25.1
Jamaica	2.429	42	1.4	2040	2560	25.5
Kiribati	0.077	57	1.9	2110	2650	25.6
Turkey	60.771	71	2.4	2820	3550	25.9
Bahamas	0.272	77	2.6	2200	2780	26.4
St Vincent / Grenadines	0.111	40	1.3	1940	2460	26.8
Seychelles	0.073	49	1.6	1850	2360	27.6
Barbados	0.261	10	0.3	2520	3220	27.8
Réunion	0.644	55	1.8	2400	3080	28.3
Korea, Dem Peoples Rep	23.483	69	2.3	2430	3120	28.4
Pakistan	136.645	87	2.9	1800	2340	30.0
Spain	39.568	25	0.8	2740	3580	30.7
Papua New Guinea	4.205	70	2.3	1970	2590	31.5
El Salvador	5.641	71	2.4	1770	2330	31.6
Lebanon	2.915	38	1.3	2400	3160	31.7
French Guiana	0.141	112	3.7	2120	2800	32.1
Portugal	9.830	9	0.3	2640	3490	32.2
Syria	14.171	100	3.3	2370	3180	34.2
Philippines	66.188	82	2.7	1700	2290	34.7
Martinique	0.375	16	0.5	2050	2770	35.1
Grenada	0.092	-10	-0.3	1770	2400	35.6
Cuba	10.960	42	1.4	2300	3130	36.1
Guadeloupe	0.421	21	0.7	1990	2780	39.7
Brunei Darussalam	0.280	115	3.8	2040	2860	40.2
Myanmar (Burma)	45.555	65	2.2	1810	2570	42.0
Indonesia	194.615	66	2.2	1840	2630	42.9
Cyprus	0.734	21	0.7	2420	3460	43.0
Samoa	0.169	36	1.2	1990	2870	44.2
Egypt	61.636	70	2.3	2290	3310	44.5
Iran	65.758	100	3.3	1830	2700	47.5
Korea, Republic of	44.563	55	1.8	2220	3280	47.7
Tunisia	8.733	67	2.2	2070	3120	50.7
Cape Verde	0.381	63	2.1	1830	2780	51.9
Djibouti	0.566	166	5.5	1520	2360	55.3
Saudi Arabia	17.451	131	4.4	1730	2690	55.5
Dominica	0.071	30	1.0	1850	2910	57.3
China, Peoples Republic	1208.841	64	2.1	1660	2620	57.8
Iraq	19.925	101	3.4	1960	3120	59.2
Maldives	0.246	77	2.6	1490	2520	69.1
Algeria	27.325	87	2.9	1720	2940	70.9
Libya	5.225	124	4.1	1640	3290	100.6

Source: FAO 1995; United Nations 1995a.

Table 12.9: World food supplies, imports, and exports 1960-90

	Food available, kcal /person /day				% of food energy consumption imported				% of food energy production exported			
	1961-3	1969-71	1979-81	1988-90	1961-3	1969-71	1979-81	1988-90	1961-3	1969-71	1979-81	1988-90
Global average	2300	2413	2705	2648	19.6	25.6	28.1	29.7	18.1	17.0	16.0	15.2
Africa	2068	2119	2701	2278	11.3	15.6	22.3	24.6	13.9	12.3	7.5	6.6
Asia	2084	2242	2359	2473	17.1	18.3	20.7	22.9	10.2	7.7	9.9	9.8
Europe	3076	3175	3302	3397	22.9	23.7	25.5	24.4	9.9	12.1	16.5	19.4
Latin America / Caribbean	2181	2319	2509	2564	21.5	23.5	30.7	33.3	28.8	27.5	23.9	21.9
Middle East	2217	2407	2708	2920	49.3	95.8	68.2	67.8	8..5	6.5	7.6	7.2
Oceania	2486	2624	2721	2832	14.4	19.4	22.9	27.2	47.0	43.9	44.9	38.7
North America	2995	3165	3230	3440	6.5	6.0	5.5	5.5	27.0	26.5	39.0	37.0

Source: FAO 1995.

Table 12.10: World food supplies, imports, and exports 1960-90, arranged by availability per head of population in 1988-90

	Food available, kcal /person /day				% of food energy consumption imported				% of food energy production exported			
	1961-3	1969-71	1979-81	1988-90	1961-3	1969-71	1979-81	1988-90	1961-3	1969-71	1979-81	1988-90
Ethiopia	1800	1720	1800	1700	0	1	4	9	3	3	1	1
Chad	2300	2150	1710	1740	2	4	3	5	2	2	2	0
Comoros	1880	1880	1780	1760	17	24	33	37	11	10	4	1
Mozambique	1950	1920	1950	1810	4	6	14	22	15	17	6	2
Central African Republic	2170	2300	2140	1850	3	6	4	10	2	1	0	0
Somalia	1720	1740	1940	1870	10	12	28	17	2	2	1	1
Angola	1910	2120	2120	1880	5	8	32	36	24	21	1	0
Afghanistan	2350	2200	2210	1890	2	7	6	13	1	1	2	1
Sierra Leone	1830	2100	2310	1900	10	14	18	19	14	10	4	2
Rwanda	1820	2050	2060	1910	0	2	4	7	0	0	0	1
Burundi	2050	2100	2060	1950	1	2	4	3	0	1	0	1
Bangladesh	2110	2120	1910	1950	7	8	8	12	0	0	0	0
Namibia	1850	1970	1950	1970	24	33	29	29	8	9	6	6
Haiti	1970	1940	2070	2010	7	7	20	27	4	2	1	1
Bolivia	1800	1970	2120	2010	22	20	22	11	0	1	5	8
Zambia	2090	2190	2190	2020	9	22	24	7	1	1	0	0
Sudan	1840	2170	2220	2040	8	9	9	14	14	9	8	7
Peru	2220	2270	2100	2040	10	12	27	23	35	36	10	15
Malawi	2070	2370	2270	2050	2	4	4	5	6	7	8	5
Kenya	2160	2230	2150	2060	9	7	11	9	7	6	4	4
Lesotho	2000	2010	2350	2120	14	30	49	57	2	2	0	4
Zaire	2220	2210	2130	2130	3	4	6	5	11	8	1	1
Yemen	1730	1770	1940	2140	20	30	48	64	8	2	0	0
Ghana	2030	2230	1970	2140	11	11	10	11	23	10	3	4
São Tomé and Principé	2180	2170	2060	2150	23	29	42	37	48	43	21	8
Madagascar	2360	2460	2470	2160	2	4	9	5	8	7	2	3
Vietnam	2060	2190	2100	2180	5	19	9	2	2	0	1	8
Uganda	2290	2280	2110	2180	2	2	2	1	5	2	0	0
Tanzania	1800	1800	2240	2200	7	4	6	3	8	8	3	2
Nigeria	2470	2340	2130	2200	1	2	16	4	11	6	2	1
Laos	1880	2150	2360	2200	22	10	11	4	0	0	0	0
Honduras	1930	2160	2130	2210	7	9	12	12	17	22	21	16
Cameroon	2140	2310	2340	2210	3	6	9	16	8	7	4	7
Sri Lanka	2100	2270	2320	2220	32	34	24	29	16	9	4	5
Burkina Faso	1860	1780	1820	2220	2	4	9	9	2	4	3	1
Niger	2050	1990	2220	2240	1	2	7	10	12	16	3	1
Nicaragua	2250	2380	2280	2240	8	9	22	25	17	20	15	9
Macau	2080	2130	2230	2240	94	62	64	95	6	4	5	8
Guinea Bissau	1880	2070	2060	2240	5	21	19	23	28	14	10	14
Guinea	2210	2170	2270	2240	6	5	11	17	4	2	1	0
Solomon Islands	2270	2280	2270	2250	7	9	8	14	48	42	59	58
Nepal	1920	1910	1870	2250	0	0	2	3	13	9	1	1
Guatemala	1930	208	2150	2250	10	10	12	16	7	9	15	17
Zimbabwe	2050	2140	2180	2260	7	4	4	4	20	18	15	18
Mali	2170	2000	1900	2260	3	6	10	8	6	4	4	3
Liberia	2110	2220	2400	2260	16	18	24	24	5	5	4	4
Togo	2380	2380	2270	2270	4	5	12	19	7	9	4	8
Panama	2170	2370	2320	2270	14	15	18	20	12	21	28	20

Table 12.10: (Cont'd)

	Food available, kcal /person /day				% of food energy consumption imported				% of food energy production exported			
	1961-3	1969-71	1979-81	1988-90	1961-3	1969-71	1979-81	1988-90	1961-3	1969-71	1979-81	1988-90
Mongolia	2040	2250	2400	2270	10	20	25	12	19	8	6	6
Philippines	1700	1770	2200	2290	6	6	5	10	31	25	25	15
Gambia	2240	2200	2100	2290	9	11	30	48	40	42	30	26
Congo	2180	2090	2240	2300	8	10	21	24	15	23	2	4
India	2050	2040	2080	2310	4	3	3	2	1	0	1	1
Dominican Republic	1850	2020	2270	2310	6	9	20	30	52	42	36	21
Antigua and Barbuda	2120	2250	2090	2310	27	59	81	82	63	30	3	3
Senegal	2400	2470	2420	2320	18	24	32	32	38	22	12	17
Thailand	2040	2190	2220	2330	0	1	2	2	22	25	43	51
El Salvador	1770	1850	2320	2330	-	14	18	23	-	15	11	6
Pakistan	1800	2180	2150	2340	8	3	9	13	4	3	6	4
Cambodia	2520	2490	1770	2340	2	2	16	3	19	7	0	0
Seychelles	1850	1940	2280	2360	40	49	66	79	53	41	22	8
Djibouti	1520	1690	1740	2360	88	90	88	88	0	0	0	0
Benin	2040	2120	2140	2380	3	5	7	11	14	17	6	8
Grenada	1770	2210	2240	2400	44	47	51	63	22	24	22	20
Ecuador	2030	2150	2290	2400	4	6	14	12	13	13	14	12
Venezuela	2190	2380	2720	2440	30	32	53	43	1	2	0	1
Suriname	1970	2240	2440	2440	25	26	22	27	26	21	44	33
St Kitts	1990	2140	2160	2440	15	20	17	33	78	64	68	62
Gabon	1950	2190	2380	2440	13	19	27	32	1	2	1	4
Mauritania	1970	1940	2080	2450	27	32	55	58	3	4	2	3
Colombia	2160	2060	2410	2450	6	8	11	10	3	6	6	6
St Vincent / Grenadines	1940	2190	2450	2460	27	41	57	59	40	29	27	48
Chile	2530	2630	2640	2480	22	22	32	9	4	4	11	20
Guyana	2270	2270	2500	2500	9	10	11	14	71	65	54	39
Maldives	1490	1670	2120	2520	56	49	66	60	13	20	11	12
Jamaica	2040	2520	2630	2560	25	39	50	53	52	36	18	18
Myanmar (Burma)	1810	2060	2320	2570	2	1	1	1	28	10	7	2
Côte d'Ivoire	2190	2420	2840	2570	10	13	17	15	14	13	19	17
Belize	2150	2320	2680	2580	30	20	16	17	54	58	65	59
Papua New Guinea	1970	2160	2390	2590	8	14	18	19	29	28	31	34
China, Peoples' Republic	1660	2000	2340	2620	4	2	4	5	1	1	1	2
Swaziland	2160	2270	2460	2630	17	12	14	14	42	53	58	55
Indonesia	1840	2050	2450	2630	5	4	8	5	3	5	4	9
Kiribati	2110	2420	2650	2650	11	16	21	22	62	58	50	48
Paraguay	2400	2670	2660	2680	10	5	4	1	8	10	11	30
Uruguay	2790	2970	2810	2690	7	7	10	5	14	20	29	40
Saudi Arabia	1730	1880	2850	2690	54	58	88	61	0	0	1	14
Iran	1830	2080	2650	2700	12	10	31	32	1	1	0	0
Malaysia	2340	2470	2690	2710	41	32	19	18	21	31	59	69
Costa Rica	2200	2410	2580	2710	13	17	16	23	19	29	28	25
Vanuatu	2470	2540	2590	2730	6	10	10	9	68	63	57	44
Brazil	2320	2500	2710	2730	5	4	8	3	5	8	11	9
Jordan	2230	2440	2660	2760	53	57	82	83	4	6	12	4

Table 12.10: (Cont'd)

	Food available, kcal /person /day				% of food energy consumption imported				% of food energy production exported			
	1961-3	1969-71	1979-81	1988-90	1961-3	1969-71	1979-81	1988-90	1961-3	1969-71	1979-81	1988-90
Trinidad and Tobago	2400	2500	2930	2770	35	43	65	69	47	40	18	16
Martinique	2050	2290	2600	2770	25	44	64	61	62	33	20	24
Guadeloupe	1990	2260	2430	2780	18	24	47	54	73	64	53	46
French Polynesia	2540	2840	2750	2780	27	43	55	68	59	31	32	18
Cape Verde	1830	1930	2590	2780	30	74	76	71	3	3	2	1
Bahamas	2200	2570	2450	2780	77	61	60	67	3	19	7	6
New Caledonia	2780	2780	2820	2790	52	66	72	80	6	2	2	0
French Guiana	2120	2440	2490	2800	49	72	74	55	0	3	4	16
Albania	2370	2450	2740	2830	28	14	7	18	0	1	2	2
Brunei Darussalam	2040	2360	2540	2860	73	81	89	93	1	1	1	2
Samoa	1990	2250	2500	2870	16	19	24	26	47	42	42	31
Japan	2510	2680	2750	2890	27	45	55	58	1	3	2	1
Dominica	1850	2090	2360	2910	38	40	48	57	25	22	10	14
Tonga	2480	2640	2860	2920	7	12	15	25	42	35	33	10
Fiji	2440	2500	2680	2930	11	14	19	20	65	73	69	68
Kuwait	2590	2640	3000	2940	96	96	95	93	30	13	13	5
Algeria	1720	1820	2610	2940	29	31	63	77	14	10	1	0
China, Republic of	2470	2630	2780	2950	9	22	45	58	17	11	9	4
Bermuda	2540	2780	3020	2960	92	48	36	94	0	48	62	0
Sweden	2870	2900	3010	2970	16	16	14	16	11	15	17	16
Finland	3210	3140	3050	3050	17	13	18	12	5	9	9	12
Mexico	2490	2630	3000	3060	3	3	20	24	5	6	1	3
Argentina	3070	3270	3200	3070	0	1	0	0	31	38	50	48
Réunion	2400	2560	2820	3080	26	32	38	50	63	64	48	42
Iceland	3230	2930	3240	3100	19	22	13	17	65	65	75	71
Tunisia	2070	2290	2800	3120	28	36	43	58	14	8	8	4
Korea, N	2430	2380	3020	3120	5	9	8	10	1	2	4	2
Iraq	1960	2260	2760	3120	22	30	63	64	7	3	0	1
South Africa	2680	2820	2980	3130	4	5	5	8	27	17	24	17
Cuba	2300	2650	2950	3130	15	18	21	21	71	62	60	56
Netherlands	3060	3020	3050	3150	50	57	62	69	22	33	44	52
Australia	3140	3200	3080	3150	1	2	2	3	50	56	62	60
Lebanon	2400	2330	2700	3160	64	73	79	69	10	10	16	6
Syria	2370	2340	2970	3180	13	29	22	31	18	8	2	3
Malta	2960	3230	3220	3180	83	85	83	83	4	5	3	1
Israel	2830	3050	3010	3220	65	68	69	73	10	9	9	6
Barbados	2520	2830	3070	3220	21	27	37	50	72	62	44	33
Canada	2920	3080	3110	3240	9	8	8	7	36	36	45	43
Romania	2870	3060	3380	3250	1	3	10	5	12	9	7	2
United Kingdom	3270	3290	3180	3270	51	47	35	30	4	4	12	20
Korea, S	2220	2820	3120	3280	11	25	42	51	1	0	3	2
Libya	1640	2440	3470	3290	47	69	70	78	4	0	0	0
United Arab Emirates	2990	3140	3300	3310	72	82	94	93	0	8	23	33
Egypt	2290	2440	3090	3310	21	18	41	42	5	9	1	1
former USSR	3110	3280	3300	3320	3	3	15	14	5	5	1	1
Switzerland	3510	3510	3540	3460	49	53	48	38	3	5	5	6

Table 12.10: (Cont'd)

	Food available, kcal /person /day				% of food energy consumption imported				% of food energy production exported			
	1961-3	1969-71	1979-81	1988-90	1961-3	1969-71	1979-81	1988-90	1961-3	1969-71	1979-81	1988-90
Cyprus	2420	3270	2920	3460	33	36	59	62	14	18	15	14
Poland	3320	3470	3580	3480	9	8	18	7	4	3	2	5
Italy	2980	3380	3560	3480	22	29	29	31	4	6	10	15
Portugal	2640	2990	2900	3490	19	31	60	51	4	4	4	5
New Zealand	3160	3250	3340	3490	12	8	8	13	41	53	57	55
Austria	3260	3250	3370	3490	18	13	13	13	2	3	9	17
Germany	2980	3200	3370	3510	26	29	29	29	4	8	15	22
former Yugoslavia	3120	3340	3570	3550	10	6	9	8	3	3	3	5
Turkey	2820	2990	3270	3550	5	3	2	10	2	2	4	8
Spain	2740	2810	3250	3580	14	17	24	18	4	8	9	14
former Czechoslovakia	3350	3360	3350	3610	20	19	15	8	9	6	6	6
France	3300	3350	3470	3620	11	10	12	10	15	26	37	46
Denmark	3260	3220	3460	3620	14	13	12	12	22	22	31	40
Belgium	3120	3260	3300	3630	40	51	62	63	12	23	45	42
USA	3070	3250	3350	3640	4	4	3	4	18	17	33	31
Ireland	3360	3440	3620	3660	15	18	20	20	14	17	32	39
Hungary	3120	3350	3480	3680	10	8	3	4	7	9	13	19

Source: FAO 1995.

Table 12.11: Body mass index in protein-energy malnutrition in adults

body mass index	classification
20-25	acceptable / desirable range
18.4-20	underweight
17-18.4	moderate protein-energy malnutrition
16-17	moderately severe protein-energy malnutrition
< 16	severe protein-energy malnutrition

Table 12.12: The Gomez classification of protein-energy malnutrition in children

		% of expected weight for age
normal		> 90
mild	1st degree malnutrition	76-90
moderate	2nd degree malnutrition	61-75
severe	3rd degree malnutrition	< 60

Source: Modified from Gomez *et al.* 1956.

Table 12.13: The Waterlow classification of protein-energy malnutrition in children

			stunting % of expected height for age			
wasting % of expected weight for height			>95 grade 0 normal	90-95 grade 1 mild	85-90 grade 2 moderate	<85 grade 3 severe
> 90	grade 0	normal	no action		action	
80-90	grade 1	mild	no action		action	
70-80	grade 2	moderate	action		priority	
< 70	grade 3	severe	action		priority	

Source: Modified from Waterlow 1972; 1973.

Table 12.14: Prevalence of gastrointestinal infections in patients with HIV infection and diarrhoea

	prevalence %
Campylobacter spp.	9-11
Chlamydia trachomatis	11
Clostridium difficile	7
Cryptosporidium spp.	15-16
Cytomegalovirus	7-45
Entamoeba histolytica	11-25
Giardia lamblia	4-15
Herpes simplex virus	4-18
Isospora bella	2
Mycobacterium avium intracellulare	5-12
Salmonella spp.	5-25
Shigella spp.	1-5
Vibrio parahaemolyticus	4

See also Table 6.14
Source: from data reported by Keutsch & Farthing 1990.

Table 12.16: Increased glucose turnover in cancer cachexia

	glucose turnover mmol / m^2 body surface area /24h		
	total	oxidation	Cori cycle
normal, overnight fast	850	700	154
normal, 7 d fast	615	460	154
cancer, stable weight	800	660	141
cancer, weight loss	1145	654	491
cancer, hypermetabolic	1580	675	905

Source: from data reported by Holroyd *et al.* 1975.

Table 12.15: Metabolic responses to cachectin (tumour necrosis factor-α)

↑ synthesis of acute phase proteins
↑ hepatic lipogenesis→hepatomegaly
↑synthesis of muscle protein
↑↑ catabolism of muscle protein
↑ glucagon-stimulated amino acid uptake in hepatocytes
↑ whole body lipolysis
↓ of lipoprotein lipase→hypertriglyceridaemia and insulin resistance
↑ muscle glycogenolysis and anaerobic glycolysis
↓ adipose tissue lipogenesis

Table 12.17: The McLaren scoring system for classification of protein-energy malnutrition

serum albumin (g/L)	serum total protein (g/L)	score
> 4.0	> 7.75	0
3.5-3.99	7.0-7.74	1
3.0-3.49	6.25-6.99	2
2.5-2.99	5.5-6.24	3
2.0-2.49	4.75-5.49	4
1.5-1.99	4.0-4.74	5
1.0-1.49	3.25-3.99	6
< 1.0	< 3.25	7
hepatomegaly		1
hair changes		1
dermatosis		2
oedema		3
oedema and dermatosis		6

final score	classification
0-3	marasmus
4-8	marasmic-kwashiorkor
9-15	kwashiorkor

Source: Modified from McLaren *et al.* 1967.

Table 12.18: The Wellcome classification of protein-energy malnutrition

% of expected weight for age	no oedema	oedema
60-80	underweight	kwashiorkor
<60	marasmus	marasmic-kwashiorkor

Source: modified from Wellcome Trust Working Party 1970.

Table 12.19: Wasting and stunting in severely malnourished children

	kwashiorkor	marasmus	marasmic kwashiorkor
% of expected weight for age	67.0 ± 7.5	45.3 ± 7.8	47.0 ± 6.3
% of expected height for age	91.8 ± 3.6	86.1 ± 4.8	84.6 ± 4.5
stunting	mild	moderate	severe
% of expected weight for height	80.3 ± 11.0	65.7 ± 8.9	69.5 ± 8.6
wasting	moderate	severe	severe

Source: from data reported by Waterlow 1972.

13

Vitamin A and carotenes

Historically, the best defined role of vitamin A is in the visual process, as the prosthetic group of the opsins, the proteins that sense light in the retina and initiate the nervous impulse. It also functions as a carrier of mannosyl residues in the synthesis of some glycoproteins and, most importantly, it is a regulator and modulator of growth and tissue differentiation.

Vitamin A deficiency is a serious problem of public health nutrition, and is probably the most important cause of preventable blindness in children in developing countries. Deficiency of vitamin A is second in scale only to protein-energy malnutrition among nutritional problems world-wide, and even in developed countries vitamin A (along with iron) is the nutrient most likely to be supplied in marginal amounts. In addition to primary deficiency of the vitamin, secondary (functional) vitamin A deficiency can be caused by zinc deficiency (see section 25.26.2) or, more importantly, protein-energy malnutrition (see section 12.2) as a result of impaired synthesis of the plasma retinol-binding protein which is required for transport of the vitamin from liver reserves to its sites of action.

Vitamin A may be provided in the diet either as preformed retinol (from animal foods), or as carotenoids that can be cleaved to yield retinol—the provitamin A carotenoids. Carotenoids are radical trapping antioxidants, and may be nutritionally important in their own right, in addition to their role as vitamin A precursors.

13.1 Vitamin A vitamers and units of activity

The term vitamin A applies correctly only to retinol, its aldehyde retinaldehyde, and retinoic acid (see Fig. 13.1). However, the term vitamin A intake is generally used to mean the dietary intake of both the preformed vitamin and provitamin A carotenoids—those carotenes and carotene derivatives that have a β-ionone ring, and a polyene side-chain with at least 11 carbons, and can therefore be cleaved to yield at least one molecule of retinaldehyde. Some 50 or more dietary carotenoids are potential sources of vitamin A; α-, β- and γ-carotenes and cryptoxanthin are quantitatively the most important.

Retinoic acid is a metabolite of retinol; it has important biological activities in its own right, and will support growth in vitamin A deficient animals. The oxidation of retinaldehyde to retinoic acid is irreversible, and retinoic acid cannot be converted *in vivo* to retinol, and does not support either vision or fertility in deficient animals.

Retinol is found only in foods of animal origin, and a small number of bacteria. Free retinol is chemically unstable, and does not occur to any significant extent in foods or tissues, but is present as esters, mainly retinyl palmitate. Retinyl acetate is generally used as an analytical standard and in pharmaceutical preparations. Small amounts of retinaldehyde and retinoic acid may occur in foods; in almost all cases these will be in the all-*trans* conformation. Dehydroretinol (vitamin A_2) is found in freshwater fishes and amphibians; it can be reduced to retinol *in vivo*, and has about half the biological activity of retinol.

Carotenoids that have an unsubstituted β-ionone ring are known collectively as provitamin A carotenoids; they can be cleaved oxidatively to yield retinaldehyde, which is then reduced to retinol. They may also give rise to retinoic acid directly (see section 13.2.1).

The obsolete international unit of vitamin A activity was based on biological assay of the ability of the test compound to support growth in deficient animals; 1 iu = 10.47 nmol of retinol = 0.3 µg free retinol or 0.344 µg retinyl acetate.

13.1.1 Retinol equivalents

Correctly, the vitamin A content of foods is expressed in terms of retinol equivalents—the sum of the vitamin provided by preformed retinol and carotenoids.

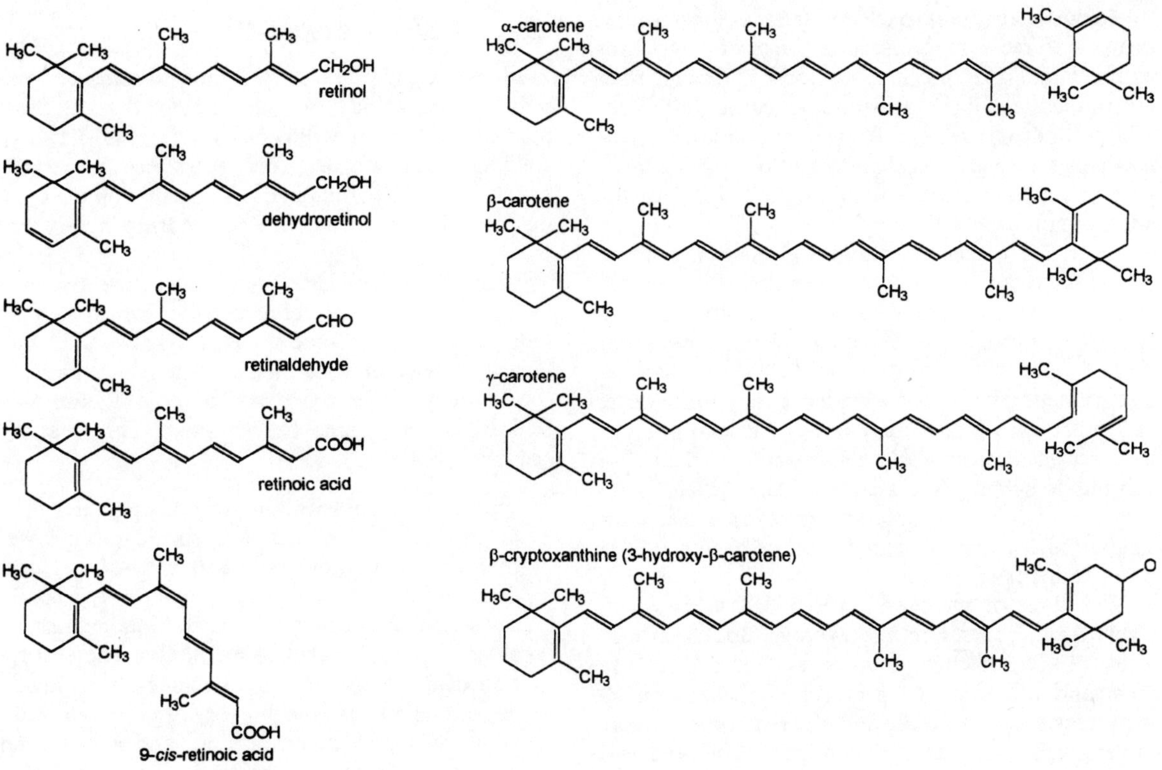

Figure 13.1 Vitamin A and pro-vitamin A carotenoids (9-, 13-, and 15-*cis*-isomers of carotenes also occur in foods)

Because of both the relatively low absorption of carotenes and incomplete cleavage to yield retinol, it is generally accepted that 6 µg β-carotene is 1µg retinol equivalent—a molar ratio of 3.2 mol of β-carotene equivalent to 1 mol of retinol, far from the theoretical yield of 2 mol of retinol per mol of β-carotene (see section 13.2.1)

The absorption and oxidation of carotene vary with intake. It is suggested that the amount of carotene equivalent to 1 µg retinol increases from 4 µg at intakes below 1000 µg, to 6 µg at intakes between 1–4000 µg, and 10 µg at intakes above 4000 µg (FAO/WHO 1988). β-Carotene is very much better absorbed from milk than from other foods, and in milk 2 µg β-carotene is 1 µg retinol equivalent (1.07 mol equivalent to 1 mol of retinol). Other pro-vitamin A carotenoids yield at most half the retinol of β-carotene—i.e. 12µg of these compounds = 1µg retinol equivalent.

13.2 Intake, absorption and metabolism of vitamin A

Very few direct studies have been performed to determine human vitamin A requirements. In the Sheffield study (Hume and Krebs 1949), 16 subjects were depleted of vitamin A for 2 years; only three showed clear signs of impaired dark adaptation (see section 13.4). One was repleted with 390 µg retinol /day, which resulted in a gradual restoration of dark adaptation; the other two received β-carotene. Since then a further 8 subjects have been studied (Sauberlich *et al.* 1974*b*; Hodges *et al.* 1978). On the basis of these studies RDA for adult men was set at 1000 µg retinol equivalent, with a minimum physiological requirement of 600 µg /day. Because the signs of deficiency resolve only slowly, it is likely that such depletion / repletion studies overestimate requirements.

An alternative approach to determining requirements is to measure the fractional rate of catabolism
of the vitamin by use of a radioactive tracer, then
determine the intake that would be required to maintain an appropriate level of liver reserves. Such studies suggest a mean requirement of 6.7 µg /kg body
weight, and a reference intake of 650–700 µg for
adult men (Olson 1987*b*).

Reference intakes of vitamin A are shown in Table
13.1; because of the cumulative toxicity of retinol (see
section 13.7), it is recommended that habitual intakes
should not exceed those shown in the final column of
Table 13.1.

Although there is some evidence that β-carotene,
and other carotenoids, may have beneficial antioxidant actions in their own right, apart from their pro-
vitamin A activity (see section 13.6.2), there is no
evidence on which to base any recommendations or
suggestions of requirements for carotene other than
as a precursor of retinol.

The range of average intakes in UK is shown in
Table 13.2, sources in the average British diet in
Table 13.3 and rich sources in Table 13.4. In
meat and fish some 10 per cent of the vitamin A
is present as carotenoids, and the remainder largely
as retinol, with traces of retinaldehyde, retinoic acid
and glycosides of retinol and retinoic acid; in poultry, eggs, and milk 30 per cent is present as carotenoids.

About 70–90 per cent of the dietary retinol is
absorbed, and even at high intakes this falls only
slightly. However, because it is absorbed dissolved
in lipid micelles, absorption is reduced on very
low fat diets (see section 8.2). Retinyl esters are
hydrolysed at the outer surface of the intestinal
mucosal cell, and the resultant free retinol is re-
esterified intracellularly to the palmitate, by a
microsomal acyltransferase, before entering the
lymphatic system in chylomicrons (Norum *et al.*
1986).

Retinyl palmitate in chylomicron remnants is
taken up by the liver parenchymal cells, where it is
hydrolysed to retinol, which is then transferred to
apo-retinol binding protein (Chen *et al.* 1981).
When liver reserves of the vitamin are adequate,
recently ingested retinol is transferred to storage in
the stellate cells, as retinyl esters, otherwise it is
mainly released into the circulation bound to retinol-binding protein (see section 13.2.4). The predominant ester in the stellate cells is retinyl palmitate
(76–82 per cent), with smaller amounts of stearate
(9–12 per cent), oleate (5–7 per cent) and linoleate
(3–4 per cent), reflecting the pattern of fatty acids in
the diet.

13.2.1 Carotene dioxygenase

As shown in Fig. 13.2, β-carotene and other provitamin A carotenoids are cleaved in the intestinal
mucosa by carotene dioxygenase (EC 1.13.11.21),
yielding retinaldehyde. This is reduced to retinol,
which is esterified and enters the circulation in chylomicrons together with esters formed from dietary retinol.

Central oxidative cleavage of β-carotene gives rise
to two molecules of retinaldehyde, which can be
reduced to retinol. However, as noted above, the biological activity of β-carotene, on a molar basis, is
considerably lower than that of retinol, not two-
fold higher as might be expected. Three factors
account for this:

1. The limited absorption of carotenoids. The
   absorption of β-carotene is considerably lower
   than that of retinol—only about 20–50 per cent
   of a test dose is absorbed under normal conditions, falling considerably as the intake rises, to
   as little as 10 per cent of the intake. The absorption of carotene from foods may be even lower,
   depending on both the integrity of plant cell walls,
   which will prevent absorption, and also the fat
   content of the diet or test meal.

2. The limited activity of carotene dioxygenase.
   While the activity of carotene dioxygenase is adequate to meet vitamin A requirements solely from
   dietary carotene, it is low enough to ensure that
   even very high intakes of carotene will not result
   in the formation of potentially toxic amounts of
   retinol; a relatively large proportion of ingested β-
   carotene appears in the circulation unchanged.

3. The reaction specificity of the enzyme. The principal site of carotene dioxygenase attack is the 15–
   15′ central bond of β-carotene, but asymmetric
   cleavage also occurs, leading to the formation of
   8′-, 10′- and 12′-apo-carotenals, as shown in Fig
   13.2. Apo-carotenals are oxidized to retinoic acid,
   but cannot give rise to retinaldehyde. (Sharma *et
   al.* 1976, 1977*a*).

13.2.2 Liver reserves of retinol

The concentration of retinol in most tissues is
between 1–5 µmol /kg; in liver the mean concentration is 500 µmol /kg, with a very wide range of individual variation. Appropriate levels of liver reserves
are between 70–140 µmol /kg; when the concentration rises above 70 µmol /kg the rate of catabolism

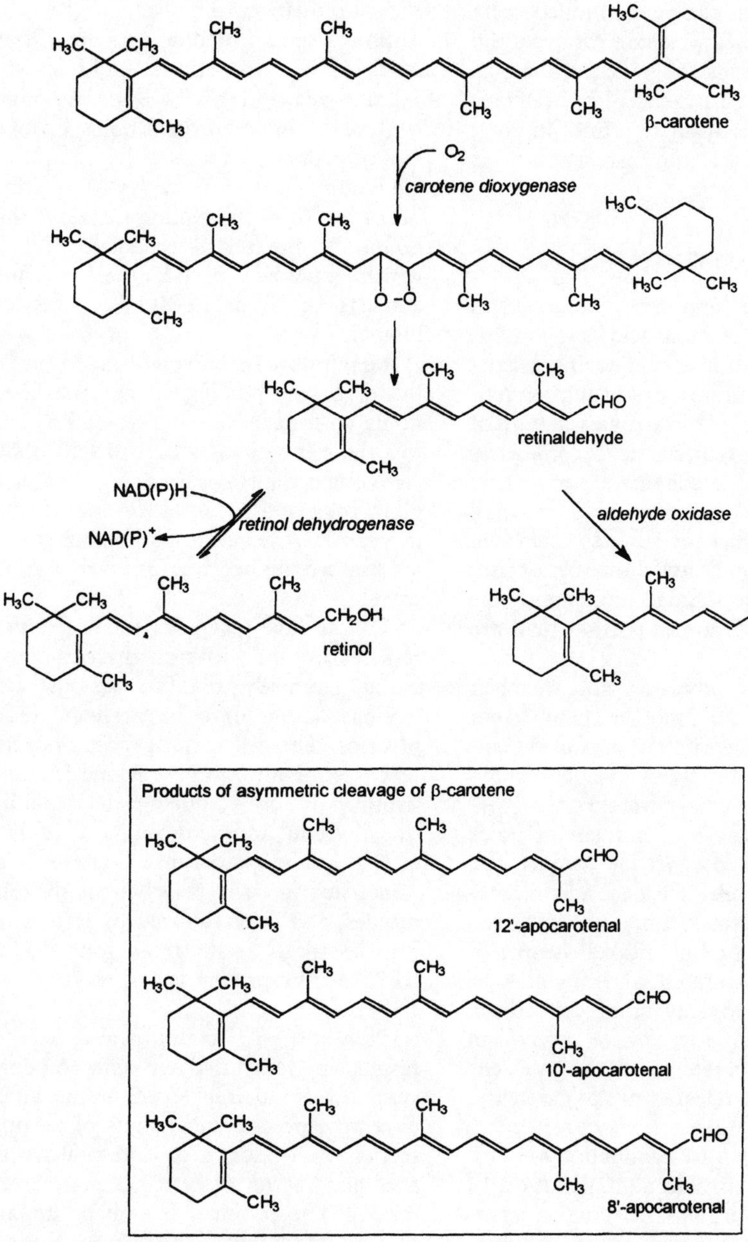

Figure 13.2 The reaction of carotene dioxygenase
Carotene dioxygenase EC 1.13.11.21, retinol dehydrogenase EC 1.1.1.105, retinaldehyde oxidase EC 1.2.3.11

increases (Hodges *et al.* 1978; Olson 1987*b*; Sauberlich *et al* 1974*b*).

In a number of studies of *post mortem* tissue, between 10–30 per cent of the population of the United States had liver retinol below 140 μmol /kg and about 5 per cent had reserves in excess of 1700

μmol /kg. Some 5–10 per cent of samples analysed in Canada showed undetectably low liver reserves of retinol, although similar studies in Britain did not show any significant proportion of the population with extremely low liver reserves (Huque 1982; Sauberlich *et al.* 1974*b*).

Abnormally low liver reserves may be due not only to prolonged low intake, but also to the induction by barbiturates of cytochrome P_{450}, which catalyses the catabolism of retinol. Chlorinated hydrocarbons, as in many agricultural pesticides, also deplete liver retinol, by effects on the metabolism of retinol binding protein (see section 13.2.4), and urinary loss is increased in fever.

13.2.3 Catabolism and excretion of retinol

At modest levels of intake, and with liver reserves below about 70 μmol /kg, retinoic acid is the major metabolite of retinol in both liver and peripheral tissues. After tracer doses of radioactive retinol or retinoic acid there are similar patterns of excretion of metabolites, with mainly retinoic acid conjugates (glucuronides and the taurine conjugate, see section 23.9.2.1) excreted in the bile, but there also are small amounts of a number of other metabolites, including epoxy-retinoic acid glucuronide and a number of products of side-chain oxidation. Small amounts of the products of side-chain oxidation of retinoic acid are also excreted in the urine.

As the intake of retinol increases, and the liver concentration rises above 70 μmol /kg, a different pathway becomes increasingly important for the catabolism of newly ingested retinol in liver parenchymal cells. This is microsomal cytochrome P_{450}-dependent oxidation, leading to a number of polar metabolites, including 4–hydroxyretinol, which are excreted in the urine and bile. Thus there is a catabolic mechanism which allows excretion of excess retinol to a certain extent. At high intakes the microsomal pathway becomes saturated, and this may be one of the factors in the toxicity of excess retinol, since there is no further capacity for its catabolism and excretion. Stored retinyl esters in the stellate cells of the liver are only slowly released to the parenchymal cells for catabolism, so retinol has considerable chronic toxicity (see section 13.7). Induction of cytochrome P_{450} enzymes by chronic administration of barbiturates can result in depletion of liver reserves of retinol, and may be a factor in drug-induced vitamin A deficiency (Leo *et al.* 1989; Leo and Lieber 1985; Olson 1986).

13.2.4   Plasma retinol binding protein (RBP)

Retinol is released from the liver bound to an α-globulin, retinol binding protein (RBP); this serves to maintain the vitamin in aqueous solution, protect it against oxidation, and also deliver it to target tissues. Although retinol binding protein will also bind retinoic acid *in vitro*, retinoic acid released into the circulation by the liver is transported bound to albumin.

Retinol binding protein binds 1 mol of retinol per mol of protein. It forms a 1:1 complex with thyroxine-binding pre-albumin (transthyretin, see section 25.14.2), thus preventing urinary loss of retinol bound to the relatively small RBP (M_r 21 000), which would be filtered by the glomerulus; transthyretin has an M_r of 54 000, and the complex is not filtered.

Metabolites of polychlorinated biphenyls bind to the thyroxine binding site of transthyretin, and in doing so impair the binding of RBP. As a result of this there is retinol bound to RBP that is not associated with transthyretin and so can be filtered at the glomerulus and lost in the urine. This may be a factor in vitamin A deficiency following exposure to polychlorinated biphenyls (Brouwer and van den Berg 1986).

Cell surface receptors on target tissues take up retinol from the RBP-transthyretin complex, esterifying it externally, then transferring free retinol by esterase action onto intracellular retinoid binding proteins. The cell surface receptors remove the carboxyl terminal arginine residue from RBP, so inactivating it by reducing its affinity for both transthyretin and retinol. As a result, apo-RBP is filtered at the glomerulus. Some may be lost in the urine, but most is resorbed in the proximal renal tubules, and is catabolized by lysosomal hydrolases. This seems to be the main route for catabolism of RBP; the apo-protein is not recycled (Peterson *et al.* 1974).

Protein-energy malnutrition (see section 12.2) results in functional vitamin A deficiency, with very low circulating levels of the vitamin, and the development of clinical signs of xerophthalmia (see section 13.4), which is unresponsive to vitamin A, and may occur despite adequate liver reserves of retinol. The problem is one of impaired synthesis of RBP in the liver, and hence a seriously impaired ability to release retinol from liver stores. The synthesis of RBP is very considerably depressed in protein-energy malnutrition in experimental animals, although not markedly more so than that of other serum proteins. Zinc deficiency (see section 25.26.2) similarly impairs the synthesis of RBP and can be a cause of secondary functional vitamin A deficiency unresponsive to vitamin A but responsive to zinc supplementation (Smith *et al.* 1973; Solomons and Russell 1980).

13.2.5 Cellular retinoid binding proteins

Retinol taken up by the cell surface receptors for retinol binding protein is bound by an intracellular retinol binding protein. This is found in most tissues other than muscle. Within tissues (other than the retina, see section 13.3.1), retinol is oxidized to retinaldehyde, then retinoic acid. Retinoic acid is also taken up from the plasma, by an intracellular retinoic acid binding protein, which is found in many tissues, but not in muscle, kidney, small intestine, liver, lung, or spleen. Reversible isomerization of all-*trans*-retinoic acid to 9–*cis*-retinoic acid occurs to a varying degree in different tissues.

13.3 Metabolic functions of vitamin A

Vitamin A has three metabolic roles: as the prosthetic group of the visual pigments; as a carrier of mannosyl units in the synthesis of hydrophobic glycoproteins; and as a nuclear-acting hormone in the control of cell proliferation and differentiation.

Retinoic acid has specific functions in its own right, distinct from those of retinol. Testis and uterus contain both cellular retinol and retinoic acid binding proteins, and both retinol and retinoic acid are essential in the functions of these organs. Although retinoic acid will support testosterone synthesis, it will not support spermatogenesis, nor will it support placental development in female vitamin A deficient animals (Appling and Chytil 1981). Similarly, retinol and retinoic acid have different actions on bone cells in culture, so that both are required for normal bone development. Retinol inhibits collagen synthesis, while retinoic acid stimulates the synthesis of non-collagen bone proteins (Dickson *et al.* 1989).

13.3.1 Retinol and retinaldehyde in the visual cycle

Binding of retinaldehyde to the opsin proteins in the rods and cones of the retina gives rise to rhodopsin (in rods) and iodopsin (in cones). These are highly photosensitive proteins; a single photon results in a measurable change in the current across the outer membrane of the retina, and the propagation of a nerve impulse.

In the pigment epithelium of the retina, all-*trans*-retinol is isomerized to 11–*cis*-retinol and then undergoes oxidation to 11–*cis*-retinaldehyde. This reacts with a lysine residue in opsin, forming the holo-protein rhodopsin. Opsins are cell-type specific; they serve to shift the absorption of 11–*cis*-retinaldehyde from the UV into what we call, in consequence, the visible range—either a relatively broad spectrum of sensitivity for vision in dim light (in the rods, with an absorbance peak at 500 nm) or more defined spectral peaks for differentiation of colours in stronger light (in the cones), with absorption maxima at 419, 531 or 559 nm, depending on the cell type.

Any one cone cell contains only one type of opsin, and hence is sensitive to only one colour of light. Colour blindness results from loss or mutation of one or other of the cone opsins. The combination of 11–*cis*-retinaldehyde with cone opsin is sometimes called iodopsin, with rhodopsin meaning more specifically the holo-protein of rod opsin. Most studies of the mechanisms of vision have been performed using rods; by extrapolation it is assumed that the same mechanisms are involved in cone vision.

As shown in Fig. 13.3, the absorption of light by rhodopsin causes a change in the configuration of the retinaldehyde from the 11–*cis* to the all-*trans* isomer, and a conformational change in opsin. This results in the release of retinaldehyde from the protein, and the initiation of a nerve impulse. The overall process is known as bleaching, since it results in the loss of the colour of rhodopsin.

The all-*trans*-retinaldehyde released from rhodopsin is reduced to all-*trans*-retinol, and joins the pool of retinol in the pigment epithelium for isomerization to 11–*cis*-retinol and regeneration of rhodopsin. The key to initiation of the visual cycle is the availability of 11–*cis*-retinaldehyde, and hence vitamin A. In deficiency both the time taken to adapt to darkness and the ability to see in poor light will be impaired.

The formation of the initial excited form of rhodopsin, bathorhodopsin, depends on the isomerization of 11–*cis*-retinaldehyde to a strained form of all-*trans*-retinaldehyde. This occurs within picoseconds of illumination and is the only light-dependent step in the visual cycle. Thereafter there is a series of conformational changes, shown in Fig. 13.4, leading to the formation of metarhodopsin II. The conversion of metarhodopsin II to metarhodopsin III is relatively slow, with a time-course of minutes, and is the result of multiple phosphorylation of serine and threonine residues on the protein, catalysed by rhodopsin kinase. The final step is hydrolysis to release all-*trans*-retinaldehyde and opsin.

Metarhodopsin II is the excited form of rhodopsin which initiates a guanine nucleotide amplification cascade leading to a nerve impulse. The final event is a hyperpolarization of the outer section membrane of the rod or cone, caused by the closure of sodium channels through the membrane—excitation of a sin-

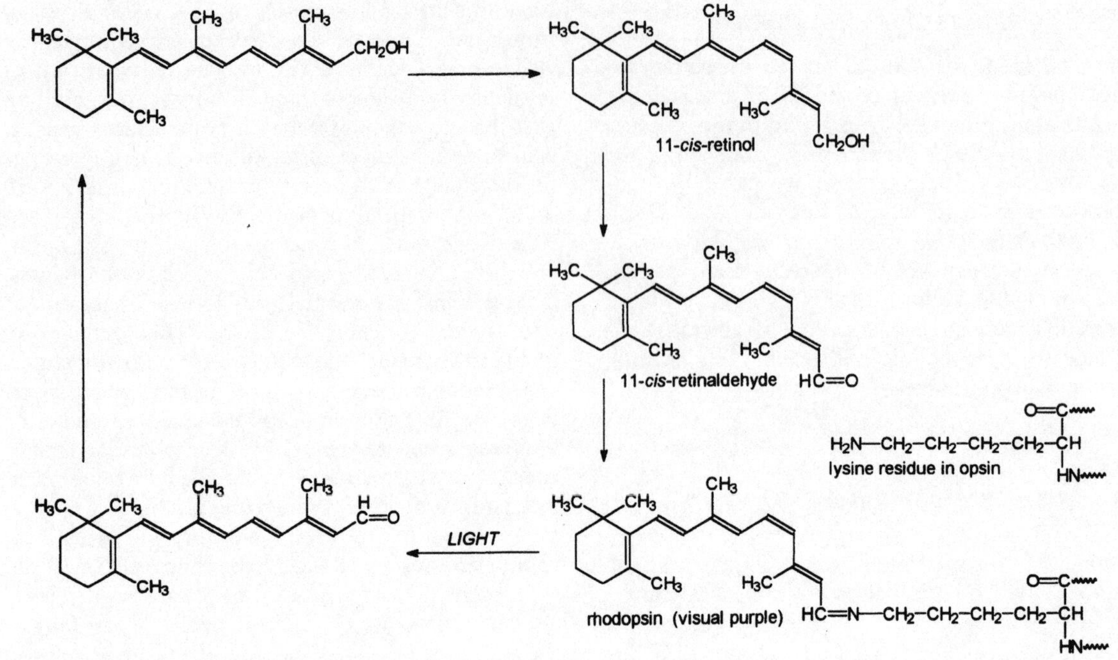

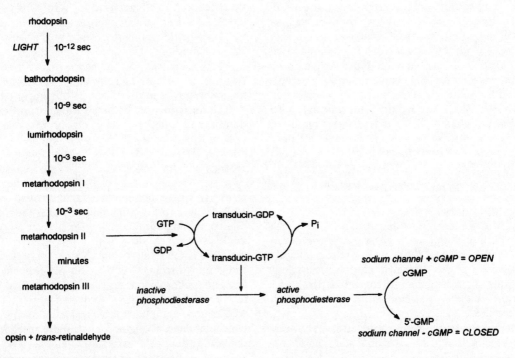

Figure 13.3 The role of retinaldehyde in vision
retinol isomerase EC 5.2.1.3

Figure 13.4 The cyclic GMP cascade in vision
phosphodiesterase EC 3.1.4.35

gle molecule of rhodopsin, the action of a single photon, causes a drop of 1 pA in the normal dark current across this membrane.

13.3.2 Retinyl phosphate as a mannosyl carrier

In the synthesis of most glycoproteins containing mannose, the intermediate carrier of the mannosyl moiety is the polyene dolichol phosphate. However, in some systems retinyl phosphate can act as the intermediate carrier between UDP-mannose and the acceptor glycoprotein. Retinyl phosphate mannose seems be involved especially in the synthesis of hydrophobic regions of glycoproteins (DeLuca 1977; Frot-Coutaz *et al.* 1985).

13.3.3 Retinol and retinoic acid in cell proliferation and differentiation

Apart from effects on vision, most of the effects of vitamin A deficiency (see section 13.4) involve derangements of cell proliferation and differentiation—squamous metaplasia and keratinization of epithelia, dedifferentiation, and loss of ciliated epithelia. Retinoic acid has both a general role in growth and a specific morphogenic role in development, while retinol is essential for fertility in both male and female animals. These functions are the result of nuclear effects of the vitamin, mediated by nuclear receptors in target tissues. Like other nuclear acting hormone receptors, these are zinc-finger proteins (see section 25.26.1).

The expression of a bewildering variety of genes is modulated by vitamin A. Ul-Haq and Chytil (1988) reported that the administration of retinol to deficient animals resulted in decreased synthesis of 286 proteins, and increased synthesis of 101; retinoic acid had similar effects, but on a different spectrum of proteins as isolated by two-dimensional electrophoresis. Among genes regulated by vitamin A are those for keratins, collagen, collagenase and lamanin, all of which are important in the cytoskeleton and extra-cellular matrix, and alkaline phosphatase, plasminogen activator and epidermal growth factor.

There are two families of nuclear retinoid receptors. The first to be characterized were shown to bind retinoic acid, and were called the retinoic acid receptors (RAR); there are three types, α-, β-, γ- RAR proteins. The physiological ligand for the second family of retinoid receptors was not known when they were first discovered, and they were called the RXR (unknown retinoid) receptors; again there are α-, β- and γ-RXR proteins. It is now known that the RXR bind only 9-*cis*-retinoic acid, while the RAR bind either all-*trans*- or 9-*cis*-retinoic acid.

On binding retinoic acid, the receptors undergo dimerization and activation, then bind to hormone-response elements on DNA. The receptors form not only RAR and RXR homodimers, but also RAR-RXR heterodimers, and the RXR can form heterodimers with calcitriol (see section 14.3.3.1) and thyroid hormone (see section 25.14.3) receptors, as well as heterodimers with at least two other zinc finger proteins whose physiological ligands have not yet been identified—the COUP and PPAR receptors (Roe and Brickell 1993).

The different tissue responses to vitamin A thus depend on

(1) the presence of cellular retinol and/or retinoic acid binding proteins,

(2) the extent to which all-*trans*-retinoic acid is isomerized to 9-*cis*-retinoic acid,

(3) the relative amounts of the α-, β- and γ-RAR and RXR proteins;

(4) the presence of thyroxine, calcitriol, COUP and PPAR receptor proteins;

as well as the presence of hormone response elements for the various receptor dimers on genes that are expressed in that tissue.

Retinoic acid has a specific morphogenic role in limb development. There is a small concentration gradient of retinoic acid across the developing limb bud, and a gradient of retinoic acid binding protein in the opposite direction, suggesting that the resultant relatively steep gradient of free retinoic acid may be the important factor determining the pattern of development (Thaller and Eichele 1987). It may also be important in the development of the central nervous system—retinoic acid binding protein has a strictly delimited anatomical localization in the developing mouse brain, and is only expressed transiently, between days 11–14 of gestation (Momoi *et al.* 1990). See section 13.6 for a discussion of the therapeutic uses of retinol and retinoic acid.

13.4 Vitamin A deficiency (xerophthalmia)

Vitamin A deficient experimental animals fail to grow; adults are blind and sterile, with testicular degeneration in males and keratinization of the uterine epithelium in females. Although deficient female animals will conceive, and the foetuses will implant, formation of the placenta is impaired, and the foetuses are resorbed. Epithelia in general are hyperplastic and keratinized, and there is impaired cellular immunity with increased susceptibility to infection.

Vitamin A deficiency is a major problem of public health nutrition in many countries. Table 13.5 shows the numbers of people at risk of deficiency in different regions—a total of 190 million people world-wide. Globally at least 40 million preschool children are vitamin A deficient, and, as shown in Table 13.5, some 13.8 million show signs of eye damage (xerophthalmia) as a result of vitamin A deficiency. WHO estimates that annually some 250 000–500 000 preschool children lose their sight, either partially or totally, as a result of vitamin A deficiency, and two-thirds of them die within a few months of becoming blind. Vitamin A deficiency is the single most common preventable cause of blindness. Table 13.6 shows those countries in which vitamin A deficiency is a significant public health problem, affecting more than 10 per cent of the population—in some regions deficiency may affect 75 per cent of the population.

In addition to dietary deficiency of vitamin A, functional vitamin A deficiency may occur despite adequate liver reserves of retinol, as a result of impaired synthesis of retinol binding protein in protein-energy malnutrition, and possibly also in zinc deficiency, as discussed in section 13.2.4 (Smith *et al* 1973; Solomons and Russell 1980).

Mild deficiency results in impaired dark adaptation; as the deficiency progresses there is inability to see in dim light (nyctalopia or night blindness), followed by conjunctival xerosis—squamous metaplasia and keratinization of the epithelial cells of the conjunctiva, leading to dryness, wrinkling and thickening of the cornea (xerophthalmia). As the deficiency progresses, so there is keratinization of the cornea. At this stage the condition is still reversible, although there may be residual scarring of the cornea. The next stage is ulceration of the cornea due to increased proteolytic action, causing irreversible blindness (Pirie *et al.* 1975). Table 13.7 shows the WHO classification of xerophthalmia.

13.4.1 Control of vitamin A deficiency

There are four types of regional and local programme aimed at preventing blindness and death of children aged under 5 from vitamin A deficiency.

1. As a temporary measure, the provision of a single massive dose of 60 000 μg of retinol acetate or palmitate, either in oil or as water-dispersible beadlets. The dose is given either orally or by injection, and is repeated at 4–6 monthly intervals. Half this dose is given to infants under 1 year of age, and one-quarter to neonates. About half the dose is absorbed and retained in the body (Reddy and Sivakumar 1972). Such massive doses of retinol may lead to transient signs of intoxication, variously reported as affecting between 0.7–2.5 per cent of children; inclusion of 40 mg tocopherol (see Chapter 15) reduces the acute toxicity of retinol.

2. As a long-term measure, an educational approach to encourage the consumption of green leafy vegetables and orange-yellow fruits and vegetables. These are sources of the carotenoids, which are less well absorbed than is preformed retinol, but animal foods are not readily available in areas where xerophthalmia is common. Relatively small amounts of the fruits and vegetables shown in Table 13.8 will meet a child's vitamin A requirement, but these locally available foods are often shunned for cultural or superstitious reasons. However, the absorption and utilization of carotene from green leafy vegetables is relatively poor; de Pee *et al.* (1995) reported that a daily portion of green vegetables had no significant effect on the vitamin A status of breast-feeding women in Indonesia, although the equivalent amount of β-carotene in an enriched biscuit did increase vitamin A status.

3. Food enrichment. Vitamin A can be added to a variety of foods (and carotenoids are useful colouring agents), but from the public health point of view enriched foods must be carefully targeted at the vulnerable groups of the population. Food enrichment is difficult in less developed countries because of the cost, and the availability of appropriate technology, and means of enforcement and prevention of potentially toxic overdosage. Since the target group for vitamin A enrichment is children, the food chosen as the vehicle must be one that they consume in such quantities as to provide an adequate yet safe intake of vitamin A; such foods vary from one region to another. Successful projects are in operation for the enrichment of sugar (in south America), salt (in Indonesia) and monosodium glutamate (in the Philippines). For powdered foods such as these water-dispersible beadlets of retinol palmitate are used.

4. A public health and horticultural approach involves encouragement of, and guidance on, home production of carotene rich fruits and vege-

tables. This will also increase the intakes of other nutrients.

13.5 Assessment of vitamin A nutritional status

The only direct assessment of vitamin A status is by liver biopsy and measurement of retinyl ester reserves (see Table 13.9)—an invasive procedure that cannot be considered for routine investigations and population surveys. Status can also be assessed by clinical and functional tests, the plasma concentrations of retinol and retinol binding protein, and the response to a test dose of vitamin A, the relative dose response.

13.5.1 Clinical and functional tests of status

In field surveys, clinical signs of vitamin A deficiency, including Bitot's spots, corneal xerosis, corneal ulceration and keratomalacia can be used to identify those suffering from vitamin A deficiency. The earliest signs of corneal damage are detected by conjunctival impression cytology (CIC); however, abnormalities only develop when liver reserves are seriously depleted.

The ability to adapt to dim light is impaired early in deficiency, and dark adaptation time is sometimes used to assess vitamin A status. However, the test is not suitable for use on children (the group most at risk of deficiency), and the apparatus is not suited to use in field studies.

In adults maintained on vitamin A-deficient diets for a period of months, there are a number of early signs, apparent before the impairment of dark adaptation: impairment of the senses of taste, smell and balance and distortion of colour vision, with impaired sensitivity to green light. With the exception of the effects on colour vision, these can all be attributed to dedifferentiation of ciliated epithelia (Sauberlich *et al.* 1974*b*; Hodges *et al.* 1978). There seems to be no correlation between impairment of taste, smell, colour vision, and balance and plasma concentrations of vitamin A or retinol binding protein in the few field studies that have been reported.

13.5.2 Plasma concentrations of retinol and carotene

Because retinol binding protein is released from liver only as the holo-protein, and apo-RBP is cleared from the circulation rapidly after tissue uptake of retinol, the fasting plasma concentration of retinol remains constant over a wide range of intakes. It is only when liver reserves are nearly depleted that it falls significantly, and it rises significantly only at the onset of toxic signs. Therefore while less sensitive to subtle changes within the normal range than some methods of assessing nutritional status, measurement of plasma retinol does provide a convenient and sensitive means of detecting people whose intake of vitamin A is inadequate to permit normal liver reserves to be maintained.

Carotene in plasma is mainly in lipoproteins, so, as with vitamin E (see section 15.7), measurements of plasma concentrations of carotene should be related to either cholesterol or total plasma lipids. Only 10–20 per cent of total plasma carotenoids is β-carotene, with a very wide range of individual variation. There are no reliable determinations of β-carotene or total provitamin A carotenoids in appropriate populations to permit plasma concentrations of carotene to be related to vitamin A nutritional status. Plasma concentrations of β-carotene below 0.25 μmol /L are associated with increased risk of cancer; the other carotenoids in plasma, whether or not they have pro-vitamin A activity, have significant free radical trapping and antioxidant activity.

13.5.3 Plasma retinol binding-protein

Measurement of plasma concentrations of retinol binding-protein may give some additional information, and indeed it has been suggested that because retinol is susceptible to oxidation on storage of blood samples, measurement of the more stable RBP may be a better indication of the state of vitamin A nutritional status. In adequately nourished subjects about 13 per cent of immunologically reactive RBP in plasma is present as the apo-protein, while in vitamin A-deficient children the proportion of apo-protein may rise to 50–90 per cent of circulating RBP.

The problem of trying to interpret plasma concentrations of retinol or RBP is that the synthesis and secretion of RBP are severely impaired in both protein-energy malnutrition and zinc deficiency; while this may result in functional vitamin A deficiency, and even night blindness or xerophthalmia, it will be unresponsive to vitamin A supplements, and the liver concentration of retinyl esters may be within the normal range. Improving general nutritional status for children suffering from protein-energy malnutrition, and giving zinc supplements to those who are zinc deficient, improve vitamin A status by increasing the synthesis and release of holo-RBP, with no change in vitamin A intake.

13.5.4 The relative dose response (RDR) test

During the development of vitamin A deficiency in experimental animals, the plasma concentration of RBP falls, while the liver content rises. The administration of retinol to deficient animals results in a considerable release of holo-RBP from the liver. This is a rapid effect on the release of pre-formed apo-RBP in response to the availability of retinol, rather than an increase in the synthesis of the protein, and there is no evidence that retinol controls the synthesis of RBP (Muto *et al.* 1972; Soprano *et al.* 1982).

The relative dose response test is a test of the ability of a dose of retinol to raise the plasma concentration several hours later, after chylomicrons have been cleared from the circulation. The relative dose response is the ratio of the rise in plasma retinol 5 hours after the dose:the plasma concentration of retinol at the time. A relative dose response greater than 20 per cent indicates depletion of liver reserves of retinol to under 70 µmol /kg (Loerch *et al.* 1979; Underwood 1990).

The modified RDR test involves giving a test dose of dehydroretinol, then determining the ratio of dehydroretinol:retinol in a single plasma sample taken 3–8 hours later. Again because of the accumulation of retinol binding protein in the liver in deficiency, and because in deficiency there is less dilution of the dehydroretinol with liver pools of retinyl esters, the ratio is inversely proportional to the liver stores of retinol in the deficient or marginal range—when reserves are < 0.07 µmol /g liver (Tanumihardjo *et al.* 1987).

13.6 Vitamin A and carotene in cancer prevention and therapy

Since the discovery of vitamin A, the observation that the main effects of deficiency are hyperplasia and loss of differentiation of squamous epithelium has raised speculation that the vitamin may be involved with carcinogenesis—either that deficiency may be a risk factor for cancer, or that increased intake may be protective. Deficient animals develop more spontaneous tumours, and are more sensitive to chemical carcinogens, while liver reserves of vitamin A are lower in patients with cancer than in controls. It is now known that one of the genes repressed by retinoic acid is the *myc*-oncogene.

The addition of relatively high concentrations of retinol to organ culture media produces changes that are apparently the opposite of those seen in deficiency; chick epidermis, which is normally kerati-

nized, becomes mucus-producing and in some cases ciliated. Studies of experimentally induced and transplanted tumours in experimental animals given very high intakes of retinol or retinoic acid, and of tumours in tissue culture with very high concentrations of retinol and retinoic acid, suggest that there is a potentially beneficial effect of very high intakes in inhibiting the initiation and growth of epithelial tumours.

13.6.1 Antiproliferative retinoids

The doses that are protective in animals are in the toxic range (see section 13.7) and therefore unlikely to be useful in cancer therapy or prevention in man. A considerable number of synthetic analogues (collectively called retinoids) have been developed, in a search for compounds that show anti-cancer activity, but are metabolized, stored and transported differently, and so are less toxic. Table 13.10 lists some of these retinoids, together with the dose needed to cause 50 per cent regression of established chemically induced tumours in mice (ED_{50}), the lowest daily dose at which toxic signs are observed in mice, and hence the therapeutic index—the ratio of ED_{50}:toxic threshold dose. It is apparent that even those with the lowest toxicity relative to effective dose have only a very small margin of safety.

In addition to the regression of established tumours, a number of retinoids show apparent inhibition of the chemical induction of bladder and other epithelial tumours in experimental animals. The effect is not in fact inhibition of carcinogenesis, but rather a lengthening of the latent period between the initiation step of carcinogenesis and the development of tumours. While perhaps not as exciting as compounds which prevent the development of cancers, such a delaying action may be useful. If the results can be scaled from experimental animals to man then it seems that the recurrence of bladder tumours after initial surgery or chemotherapy might be delayed by 5–10 years—a clinically useful effect (Hicks 1983; Hicks and Turton 1986).

13.6.2 Dietary carotene

Epidemiological and case–control studies show a negative association between vitamin A intake and a number of cancers, an association which is stronger for dietary carotene than for preformed retinol (Peto *et al.* 1981). This has given rise to the suggestion that β-carotene may have a protective effect against some forms of cancer, and hence a function in its own right, not simply as a precursor of retinol. At least under conditions of low oxygen tension, carotenes can act as antioxidants, trapping singlet oxygen generated by photochemical reactions or lipid peroxidation of membranes to form stable delocalized carotene radicals (Krinsky and Deneke 1982; Burton and Ingold 1984).

What the studies which suggest a protective effect of β-carotene have actually shown is a negative association between various types of cancer and the consumption of fruits and vegetables which are rich in β-carotene, other carotenoids, and a great many other potentially protective compounds (see sections 7.6 and 23.3). It may be that β-carotene is simply a marker for some other protective factor; the results of a major intervention study in smokers showed an increase in deaths from lung cancer in those receiving β-carotene (alpha-Tocopherol, beta-Carotene Cancer Prevention Study Group 1994).

13.7 Toxicity of vitamin A

Retinol is both acutely and chronically toxic. Acutely, large doses of retinol (in excess of 300 mg in a single dose to adults) cause nausea, vomiting and headache, with increased pressure in the cerebrospinal fluid; signs that disappear within a few days. After very large doses there may also be drowsiness and malaise, with itching and exfoliation of the skin, and extremely high doses can prove fatal. Single doses of 60 mg of retinol are given to children in developing countries as a prophylactic against vitamin A deficiency—an amount adequate to meet the child's needs for 4–6 months. About 1 per cent of children so treated show transient signs of toxicity.

The chronic toxicity of vitamin A is a more general cause for concern; prolonged and habitual intake of more than about 7.5–9 mg /day by adults (and proportionately reduced for children, see Table 13.1) causes signs and symptoms of toxicity affecting the following.

1. The central nervous system: headache, nausea, ataxia and anorexia, all associated with increased cerebrospinal fluid pressure.

2. The liver: hepatomegaly, hyperlipidaemia and histological changes in the liver, including increased collagen formation.

3. Bones: joint pains, thickening of the long bones, hypercalcaemia and calcification of soft tissues.

4. The skin: excessive dryness, scaling and chapping of the skin, desquamation and alopecia.

As the intake of vitamin A increases, once adequate liver reserves have been established there is an increase in the excretion of metabolites in bile. However, the biliary excretion of retinol metabolites reaches a plateau at relatively low levels, and it seems likely that this explains the relatively low toxic threshold (Olson 1986). Vitamin A intoxication is associated with the appearance of both retinol and retinyl esters associated with albumin and plasma lipoproteins; the amount of circulating retinol bound to retinol binding protein does not increase. This excess plasma retinol is not subject to the normal regulation of RBP binding, and has a membrane lytic action; one of the functions of RBP binding seems to be to protect tissues against retinol, as well as to protect retinol against oxidation (Meeks *et al.* 1981).

Retinoic acid and some of the synthetic retinoids which are used in dermatology are highly teratogenic. There is less evidence of a teratogenic effect of retinol, but there is the possibility of foetal intoxication, and intakes of above 3300 µg /day during pregnancy have been associated with birth defects. The critical period is the first month of pregnancy, before the placental and foetal retinol binding protein systems are fully developed, so that there is unspecific and uncontrolled uptake of retinol by the foetus. After the RBP systems have developed, foetal uptake is tightly controlled (Underwood 1989). The Teratology Society (1987) has recommended that vitamin A supplements in pregnancy should not exceed 2400 µg / day, while in UK the Chief Medical Officer has advised against any vitamin A supplements in pregnancy except on medical advice.

As discussed in section 13.2.1, the conversion of carotenoids to retinol is very limited, so vitamin A intoxication is unlikely to occur. Accumulation of even abnormally high amounts of carotenoids seems to have no adverse effects, although plasma, body fat and skin can have a strong orange-yellow colour (hypercarotinaemia) following prolonged high intakes of carotenoids. A small number of people lack carotene dioxygenase, and suffer from (asymptomatic) carotinaemia with normal modest intakes.

Further reading

14th Maribou Symposium (1994). Vitamin A: from molecular biology to public health. *Nutrition Reviews*, 52, 1s–90s.

Anon (1984). Vitamin A and cancer prevention. *Journal of the National Cancer Institute*, 73, 1365–89.

Bauernfeind, J.C. (1986). *Vitamin A Deficiency and its Control*. Academic Press, New York.

Bender, D.A. (1992). Vitamin A: retinol and β-carotene. In *Nutritional Biochemistry of the Vitamins*, Chapter 2, pp. 19–50. Cambridge University Press.

Chabre, M. and Deterre, P. (1989). Molecular mechanisms of visual transduction. *European Journal of Biochemistry*, 179, 255–66.

Friedrich, W. (1988). Vitamin A and its provitamins. In *Vitamins*, Chapter 2, pp. 63–140. Walter de Gruyter, Berlin.

Gerstler, H. (1993). Anticarcinogenic effect of common carotenoids. *International Journal of Vitamin and Nutrition Research*, 63, 93–121.

Giguère, V. (1994). Retinoic acid receptors. In *Vitamin Receptors: Vitamins as Ligands in Cell Communication*, (ed. K. Dakshinamurti), Chapter 2, pp. 28–58. Cambridge University Press.

Goodman, D.S. (1984). Vitamin A and retinoids in health and disease. *New England Journal of Medicine*, 310, 1023–31.

Hill, D.L. and Grubbs, C.J. (1992). Retinoids and cancer prevention. *Annual Review of Nutrition*, 12, 161–81.

Petkovich, M. (1992). Regulation of gene expression by vitamin A: the role of nuclear retinoic acid receptors. *Annual Review of Nutrition*, 12, 443–72.

Pitt, G. A.J. (1985). Vitamin A. In *Fat-soluble Vitamins: their Biochemistry and Applications*, (ed. A.T. Diplock), Chapter 1, pp. 1–75. Heinemann, London.

Soprano, D.R. (1994). Serum and cellular retinoid-binding proteins. In *Vitamin Receptors: Vitamins and Ligands in Cell Communication*, (ed. K. Dakshinamurti), Chapter 1, pp. 1–27. Cambridge University Press.

Stryer, L. (1986). Cyclic GMP cascade of vision. *Annual Review of Neuroscience*, 9, 87–119.

Wald, G. (1968). The molecular basis of visual excitation. *Nature*, 219, 800–7.

West, K. P., Howard, G.R. and Sommer, A. (1989). Vitamin A and infection: public health implications. *Annual Review of Nutrition*, 9, 63–86.

Table 13.1: Reference Intakes for vitamin A

age (years)	US RDA (1989)	UK RNI (1991)	EU PRI (1993)	upper limit of safe habitual intake
	μg	μg	μg	μg
birth - 1	375	350	350	900
1 - 3	400	400	400	1800
4 - 6	500	500	400	3000
7 - 10	700	500	500	4500
males				
11 - 18	1000	600	600	6000
adult	1000	700	700	9000
females				
11 - 18	800	600	600	6000
adult	800	600	600	7500
pregnant	800	+100	700	3300
lactating	1300	+350	950	-

Source: National Research Council 1989; Department of Health 1991; Scientific Committee for Food 1993.

Table 13.2: Average intakes of vitamin A

(Apart from the SENECA study of the elderly, which involved 17 centres throughout Europe, all the studies quoted were in UK)

age	mean	males median	range[1]	mean	females median	range[1]	reference
total (µg retinol equivalents /day)							
16-24	1164	786	224-5962	1051	633	221-6159	Gregory et al. 1990
25-34	1552	965	269-7257	1234	719	177-6700	Gregory et al. 1990
35-49	1759	1084	389-8024	1531	884	309-6116	Gregory et al. 1990
50-64	1897	1132	369-7335	1655	951	330-5875	Gregory et al. 1990
62-74	1158	-	-	1014	-	-	Lonergan et al. 1975
73-78[2]	-	794 (252-1583)	70-2956	-	709 (229-1505)	56-3090	Euronut SENECA Investigators 1991
75-90	1004	-		825	-	-	Lonergan et al. 1975
preformed retinol (µg /day)							
1.5-2.5	456	317	77-997	456	317	77-997	Gregory et al. 1995
2.5-3.5	433	277	79-1056	433	277	79-1056	Gregory et al. 1995
3.5-4.5	396	277	90-1144	414	269	67-1388	Gregory et al. 1995
16-24	848	487	163-5788	788	389	114-5896	Gregory et al. 1990
25-34	1184	584	188-6671	906	438	106-6056	Gregory et al. 1990
35-49	1333	633	232-7427	1140	481	136-5654	Gregory et al. 1990
50-64	1425	670	212-6793	1263	516	192-5487	Gregory et al. 1990
58-65	1256	-	111-5340	1287	-	117-7506	Davies & Holdsworth 1985
total carotene (µg β-carotene equivalents /day)							
1.5-2.5	796	659	133-2324	796	659	133-2324	Gregory et al. 1995
2.5-3.5	874	640	164-2997	874	640	164-2997	Gregory et al. 1995
3.5-4.5	1029	700	144-3881	884	621	162-3382	Gregory et al. 1995
16-24	1893	1229	175-6488	1576	1179	166-5671	Gregory et al. 1990
25-34	2211	1676	212-7971	1965	1567	173-6449	Gregory et al. 1990
35-49	2555	1999	332-7563	2344	1934	353-6746	Gregory et al. 1990
50-64	2833	2360	421-8361	2353	1848	214-7121	Gregory et al. 1990
58-65	2096	-	425-4392	1726	-	186-4837	Davies & Holdsworth 1985
73-78[2]	-	2057 (379-5382)	157-8088	-	1929 (501-4860)	248-7037	Euronut SENECA Investigators 1991

(1) The range shown is the 2.5-97.5 centile for the studies of Gregory *et al.*, the 10-90 centile for the SENECA study, and the observed extreme range for the study of Davies & Holdsworth.
(2) Data were reported for 17 separate centres; the mean and extreme values of the published median values are shown, with the lowest 10th centile and highest 90th centile of those reported.

Table 13.3: Sources of vitamin A in the average British diet

	% of average intake	
	preformed retinol	carotene
meat[1]	61	12
milk and milk poroducts	14	3
fat spreads	13	2
cereal products	6	2
eggs	4	0
fish	1	0
vegetables	1	70
fruit and nuts	0	3

(1) 60% of total intake of preformed retinol is from liver.
Source: Gregory *et al.* 1990.

Table 13.4: Rich sources of vitamin A

	portion (g)	μg retinol equivalents/ portion
mainly as preformed retinol		
kidney	150	375
milk, full cream	560	280
liver [1]	150	250
cheese [2]	40	100-180
cod roe, hard	100	150
salmon, canned	150	150
cream, double	30	120
butter	10	100
margarine	10	100
egg	70	98
cream, whipping	30	90
bloater	150	75
cream, single	30	75
herring or kipper	150	75
as carotene		
spring greens	75	750
nectarines	110	550
broccoli	75	375
spinach	130	300
banana	135	270
pumpkin	90	270
carrots	35	200
chickpeas	150	135
oranges	250	125
endive	30	120
apricots	40	100
orange juice	200	100
French beans	100	80
tomato juice	100	80
watercress	15	75

(1) The vitamin A content of liver may be considerably higher than this (literature) value.
(2) The vitamin A content of cheese depends on its fat content.

Table 13.5: Millions of people at risk of vitamin A deficiency

	at risk	preschool children with xerophthalmia
south-east Asia	138	10.0
western Pacific	19	1.4
Africa	18	1.3
eastern Mediterranean	13	1.0
Americas	2	0.1
Europe	-	-

Source: WHO 1995.

Table 13.6: Countries classified by the public health significance of vitamin A deficiency

	class 1 significant public health problem in part or whole of country	class 2 insufficient information, but high probability of significant public health problem in part or whole of country	class 3 sporadic cases, but prevalence not such that it constitutes a significant public health problem
south-east Asia	Bangladesh, India, Indonesia, Nepal, Sri Lanka	Burma, Bhutan	Thailand
western Pacific	Philippines, Vietnam	Kampuchea, Fiji, Laos	China, Malaysia
Africa	Benin, Burkina Faso, Chad, Ethiopia, Ghana, Malawi, Mali, Mauritania, Niger, Nigeria, Tanzania, Zambia	Angola, Kenya, Mozambique, Uganda, Rwanda	Algeria, Botswana, Burundi, Lesotho, Madagascar, Senegal, Zimbabwe
eastern Mediterranean	Oman, Somalia, Sudan	Afghanistan, Iran, Pakistan	Egypt, Iraq, Jordan, Syria, Yemen
Americas	Brazil, El Salvador, Haiti, Mexico	-	Bolivia, Ecuador, Jamaica, Peru
Europe	-	-	Morocco, Turkey

Source: Xerophthalmia Club 1990.

Table 13.7: The WHO classification of xerophthalmia

classification code	clinical description	prevalence among preschool children to indicate significant public health problem
XN	night blindness	> 1%
X1A	conjunctival xerosis	-
X1B	Bitot's spots	> 0.5 %
X2	corneal xerosis	
X3A	corneal ulceration / keratomalacia involving < 1/3 of corneal surface	> 0.01 %
X3B	corneal ulceration / keratomalacia involving > 1/3 of corneal surface	> 0.01 %
XS	corneal scar	> 0.05 %
XF	xerophthalmic fundus	
biochemical	plasma retinol < 0.35 µmol /L	> 5%

Table 13.8: Quantities of leafy vegetables needed to supply the vitamin A needs of a preschool child

	English name	g containing 750 µg carotene
Morinda citrofolia	Indian mulberry	2
Carica papaya	pawpaw	4
Leucaena glauca	wild tamarind	4
Manihot utilissima	cassava	4
Colacasia spp.	taro	7
Gnetum gnemon	jointfir	7
Moringa oleifera	drumstick	7
Sauropus androgynous	katuk	7
Hibiscus manihot	-	10
Brassica rugosa	radish	11
Centella asiatica	-	11
Sesbania grandiflora	agati	12
Amaranthus spp.	spinach	13
Ipomea aquatica	water cabbage	13
Ipomea reptans	sweet potato	13
Murraya koenigi	curry leaves	13
Nothopanax scutellaris	-	14
Psophocarpus tetragono	winged bean	14
Vigna sinensis	string bean	14
Momordica charantia	bitter gourd	15
Nasturtium officinale	watercress	15
Ocimum basilicum	basil	15
Basella rubra	Ceylon spinach	18
Talinum triangulare	perslane	19

Source: Xerophthalmia Club 1990.

Table 13.9: Biochemical indices of vitamin A nutritional status

liver retinyl esters (as retinol)	µmol/kg	mg/kg
adequate	> 70	> 20
marginal	35-70	10-20
poor	17.5-35	5-10
deficient	< 17.5	< 5
plasma retinol	µmol/L	µg/L
elevated	> 1.75	>500
normal	0.7-1.75	200-500
unsatisfactory	0.35-0.7	100-200
liver stores depleted / deficient	< 0.35	< 100
plasma total carotenoids[1]	µmol/L	µg/L
adult reference range	0.4-4.0	240-2200
acceptable	> 0.75	> 400
hypercarotinaemia	> 5.6	> 3000
plasma retinoic acid	nmol/L	g/L
adults	10-13	3-4
plasma retinol binding protein	µmol/L	µg/L
adults	1.9-4.28	40-90
preschool children	1.19-1.67	25-35
relative dose response		
normal	< 20%	
marginal deficiency	> 20%	
modified dose response	dehydroretinol / retinol	
normal	< 0.03	
marginal deficiency	> 0.03	

(1) β-carotene is 10-20% of total plasma carotenoids.
Source: from data reported by International Vitamin A Consultative Group 1983; Underwood 1990.

Table 13.10: Efficacy and toxicity of retinoids.

Figures show ED_{50} (the daily dose required to cause 50% regression of established chemically induced tumours in mice), the toxic threshold (the lowest daily dose at which toxic signs are observed in mice) and the therapeutic ratio = ED_{50} / toxic threshold.

	ED_{50} mg/kg body weight	toxic threshold mg/kg body weight	therapeutic ratio
all-*trans* retinoic acid [tretinoin]	400	80	5
13-*cis* retinoic acid [isotretinoin]	800	400	2
Trimethyl-methoxy-phenyl analogue of retinoic acid ethylamide	50	100	0.5
Trimethyl-methoxy-phenyl analogue of ethyl retinoate [etretinate]	25	50	0.5
Arotinoid ethyl ester	0.05	0.1	0.5
4-Fluoro trimethyl-methoxy-phenyl analogue of ethyl retinoate	11.5	25	0.46
Trimethyl-3-thienyl analogue of retinoic acid	75	200	0.375

Source: from data reported by Bollag & Matter 1981.

Vitamin D, calcium and phosphorus

Vitamin D is not strictly a vitamin; it is a hormone which is synthesized in the skin non-enzymatically in UV light. Nevertheless, where sunlight exposure is inadequate a dietary source of preformed vitamin is essential, and deficiency (rickets in children, osteomalacia in adults, see section 14.4) is, or has been, a major problem of public health in northern latitudes.

The function of the active metabolite of vitamin D (see section 14.3.2) is in the regulation of calcium homeostasis and the uptake of calcium into tissues. It is therefore appropriate to consider vitamin D and calcium nutrition together; since the major body pool of phosphate is as calcium phosphates in the skeleton, requirements for phosphorus are closely related to those for calcium.

14.1   Intakes and dietary sources

Tables 14.1-3 show average intakes of calcium, phosphorus (almost entirely as phosphates), and vitamin D, compared with reference intakes and estimates of requirements.

The total body contents of calcium and phosphate are equal; about 25 mol of each. Almost all of this (99 per cent) is present in bones and teeth as calcium phosphates, and therefore it is assumed that requirements for replacement of metabolic turnover are equal on a molar basis. The UK and EU estimated average requirements and reference intakes for calcium and phosphate are calculated on this basis. The UK DRV report notes that phosphorus intake should be equimolar with the actual intake of calcium rather than the reference intake. By contrast the United States RDA are calculated on the basis of equal weights of calcium and phosphate; therefore on a molar basis the RDA for phosphorus is greater than that for calcium (see Table 14.1).

The reference intake for vitamin D is for the housebound elderly, and is a level of intake that will maintain plasma concentrations of calcidiol equal to those seen in late winter in younger people with adequate sunlight exposure.

As shown in Table 14.1, average intakes of phosphate (on a molar basis) are approximately twice as great as those of calcium. There is a considerable body of evidence that significant imbalance between calcium and phosphate in infant formula results in impaired calcium absorption, bone development and calcium homeostasis, and it has been suggested that a persistently low calcium intake with a significant excess of phosphate (as is common in many diets) is a factor in the aetiology of osteoporosis (see section 14.5), since it results in the development of a lower peak bone mass than would otherwise be the case (Calvo 1993). The main sources of this excess phosphate intake are phosphates used as food additives (see section 26.2) and especially the relatively large amounts of phosphate in carbonated beverages.

Much of the dietary phosphate is as phosphoproteins, in which the hydroxyl groups of serine or tyrosine are phosphorylated; casein in milk is especially highly phosphorylated.

Table 14.4 shows the main sources of calcium in the diet; milk and dairy products account for some 58 per cent of average intakes. The significant contribution made by white bread is because white flour is enriched with calcium.

Table 14.5 shows the sources of vitamin D in average diets; the contribution of baked goods is mainly due to the butter or (enriched) margarine used in their preparation. Table 14.6 shows the vitamin D content of those relatively few foods that are significant sources of the vitamin. The vitamin D content of milk and milk products shows a 2-fold seasonal variation, with a maximum in summer; margarine is fortified with vitamin D to the level found in summer butter.

14.1.1 Desirable levels of calcium intake

The Consensus Development Panel of the American Medical Association (NIH Consensus Development

Panel 1994) recommended a considerable increase in calcium intakes over those of the reference intakes in order to promote attainment of high peak bone mass, and attempt to overcome the negative calcium balance seen post-menopausally, in order to reduce the development of osteoporosis (see Table 14.7). As discussed in section 14.5, negative calcium balance in the elderly is a result of osteoporosis rather than a cause, and there is little evidence that higher intakes of calcium after the age of about 40 will have any significant effect on bone mineral loss.

At such levels of calcium intake with meals, it is likely that there would be a considerable and undesirable impairment of the absorption of both haem and non-haem iron consumed in the same meal (Whiting 1995; Hallberg *et al.* 1991, and see section 24.2.3.1).

14.2   Metabolic functions of calcium and phosphate

Almost all of the body's 25 mol of calcium and phosphate is present in bones, mainly as hydroxyapatite ($Ca_{10}(PO_4)_6(OH)_2$), although bone mineral also contains magnesium (see section 25.16), traces of strontium (see section 25.22), carbonate, citrate and fluoride (see section 25.12) ions.

As well as its role in bone structure, bone mineral acts as a reservoir of calcium and phosphate to maintain normal concentrations in plasma and extracellular fluid. The total plasma ionized calcium content of the body is 7 mmol (280 mg), and calcium in body fluids plus exchangeable bone calcium is 50 mmol (2 g); bone mineral turnover amounts to some 10 mmol (400 mg) calcium per day, while the daily exchange between plasma and bone calcium amounts to some 150 mmol (6 g). The maintenance of calcium homeostasis is discussed in section 14.3.3.

In addition to its role in bone, phosphate is important in the following.

1. The nucleic acids, DNA and RNA.

2. Other nucleotides and coenzymes. Although the turnover of ATP is considerable (a total of some 100 mol is synthesized daily), the total body content is only 325 mmol.

3. Phosphorylation of serine and tyrosine residues in enzymes is a major mechanism of metabolic regulation in response to hormone action.

4. The metabolism of carbohydrates involves the intermediate formation of phosphates (see section 5.5.3).

5. Phosphorylated proteins and free phosphate ions in plasma and intracellular provide a significant proportion of total buffering for the maintenance of normal pH and acid–base balance.

About 0.6 per cent of the total body calcium is in soft tissues; muscle contains 15 mmol /kg calcium, other tissues somewhat less. Table 14.8 lists the main calcium-binding proteins in various tissues.

A number of metallo-enzymes, such as α-amylase and phospholipases, contain calcium as an essential part of the catalytic site. Osteocalcin is a bone protein that is important in the normal crystallization of bone mineral (see sections 14.3.3.3 and 16.4.2). Calbindin D is essential for the intestinal absorption of calcium (see section 14.3.3.2), the uptake of calcium into cells and the resorption of calcium from the glomerular filtrate in the kidney. Several of the blood clotting proteins (see section 16.4.1) require to bind calcium for activity; many of the anticoagulants used to prevent clotting of blood samples *in vitro* act by chelating calcium (e.g. EDTA, citrate).

The major functional role of calcium is in metabolic regulation. The protein kinases that modulate the activity of key enzymes in response to the binding of hormones at the cell surface are activated by calcium, either directly or bound to the high affinity calcium binding protein calmodulin. The intracellular cytoplasmic pool of free calcium is normally about 0.1 μmol /L, and is closely regulated by both binding of calcium to proteins and also the active pumping of calcium into various intracellullar compartments.

Calcium is also important in the regulation of muscle contraction; the protein troponin regulates the contractility of actin and myosin, and is calcium dependent; both hypo- and hypercalcaemia lead to disturbance of the control of muscle contraction and tetany.

Calcium binding proteins are also essential for the following.

1. The secretion of hormones and neurotransmitters. The annexins are proteins that require to bind calcium before they can bind to membrane phospholipids to initiate the fusion of intracellular secretory vesicles with the cell surface membrane for exocytosis.

2. Cell adhesion. The cadherins are calcium-dependent proteins that regulate cell adhesion and the normal contact inhibition of cell replication;

defects in cadherin function have been associated with the development of malignancy.

3. The function of the cytoskeletal proteins.

The concentration of calcium in plasma and extracellular fluids is closely regulated, so as to maintain a total concentration between 2.0–2.5 mmol /L, representing some 0.06 per cent of total body calcium. Of this, 10 per cent is chelated by citrate and other ions, 45 per cent is bound to albumin and other proteins, and 45 per cent (0.9–1.125 mmol /L) is free ionized calcium—the functionally active, available, pool in extracellular fluids.

14.3 Vitamin D

Two compounds have vitamin D activity: cholecalciferol (vitamin D_3), which is the naturally occurring vitamin, and ergocalciferol (vitamin D_2), which is formed by UV irradiation of the yeast sterol, ergosterol, and is used in food enrichment and fortification—see Fig. 14.1. The name vitamin D_1 was given to the crude product of the irradiation of ergosterol, which contained a mixture of compounds. When ergocalciferol was identified as the active component of this mixture, it was called vitamin D_2; the phy-

siological compound, cholecalciferol, was identified later, and was called vitamin D_3.

14.3.1 Endogenous synthesis of cholecalciferol

As shown in Fig. 14.2, cholecalciferol is formed nonenzymically in the skin by UV irradiation of 7-dehydrocholesterol.

7-Dehydrocholesterol is an intermediate in the synthesis of cholesterol which accumulates in skin, but not other tissues. It is synthesized in the sebaceous glands, secreted onto the surface of the skin, and then absorbed into the epidermis. It is found throughout the epidermis and dermis, with the highest concentra-

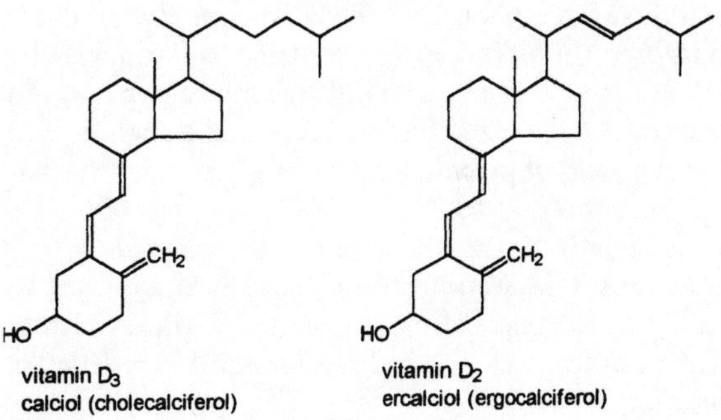

vitamin D_3
calciol (cholecalciferol)

vitamin D_2
ercalciol (ergocalciferol)

Figure 14.1 Vitamin D vitamers

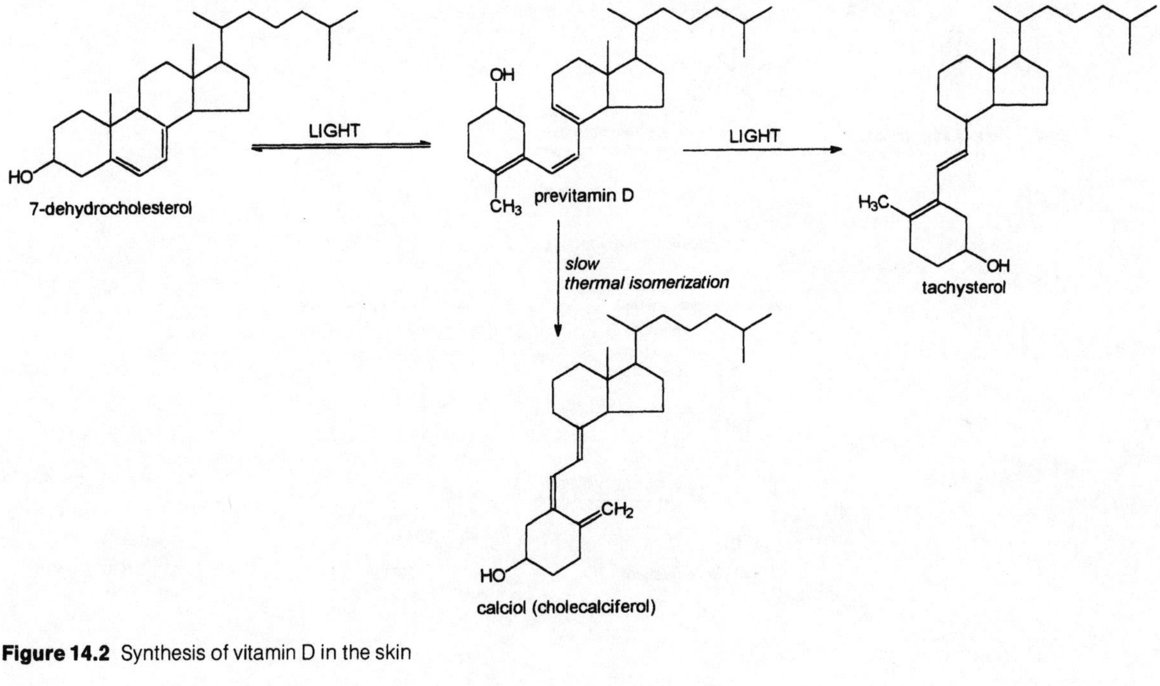

Figure 14.2 Synthesis of vitamin D in the skin

tion per unit surface area in the stratum basale and stratum spinosum, which therefore have the highest capacity for cholecalciferol synthesis. One of the possible causes of vitamin D deficiency in the elderly is the age-dependent decrease in the concentration of 7-dehydrocholesterol in the epidermis, and hence a reduction in the capacity for endogenous cholecalciferol synthesis, quite apart from reduced sunlight exposure compared with younger people (Webb and Holick 1988).

On exposure to UV light, 7-dehydrocholesterol undergoes photolysis, with cleavage of the B-ring and inversion of the A-ring, to yield precalciferol (previtamin D or tacalciol). Precalciferol undergoes slow thermal isomerization to cholecalciferol, which is absorbed into the bloodstream. The peak wavelength for the photolysis is 296.5 nm; for practical purposes the useful range of solar radiation is the UV-B range, between 290 nm (the lowest wavelength transmitted by ozone) and 310 nm, although at 310 nm the yield of precalciferol is only 1 per cent of that at 296.5 nm.

Although excess oral vitamin D results in hypercalcaemia (see section 14.6), excessive exposure to sunlight does not result in vitamin D intoxication. The photolysis of 7-dehydrocholesterol is reversible; light-catalysed closure of the B-ring can result in formation of either 7-dehydrocholesterol or lumisterol. In addition, precalciferol undergoes photo-isomeriza-

tion to tachysterol, which is biologically inactive, and cholecalciferol is also sensitive to photodegradation, yielding 5,6-*trans*-cholecalciferol and biologically inactive suprasterols.

Sunlight is not strictly essential for cutaneous synthesis of cholecalciferol, since UV-B penetrates cloud reasonably well—complete cloud cover reduces the available intensity by about 50 per cent. It also penetrates light clothing. However, low intensity irradiation does not result in significant formation of previtamin D, and whole body exposure to UV-B irradiation below 18 MJ /cm^2 does not result in any detectable increase in plasma cholecalciferol. In temperate regions (beyond about 40° N or S), the intensity of UV-B is below this threshold in winter, so there is unlikely to be any significant cutaneous synthesis of the vitamin in winter.

14.3.2 Metabolism of vitamin D

Both cholecalciferol (formed in the skin or arising from the diet) and ergocalciferol undergo further metabolism to the final active hormones, calcitriol, formed from cholecalciferol and ercalcitriol formed from ergocalciferol. Fig. 14.2 shows the sequence of reactions for cholecalciferol; ergocalciferol undergoes the same reactions. Table 14.9 shows the trivial and systematic names for the vitamin D metabolites.

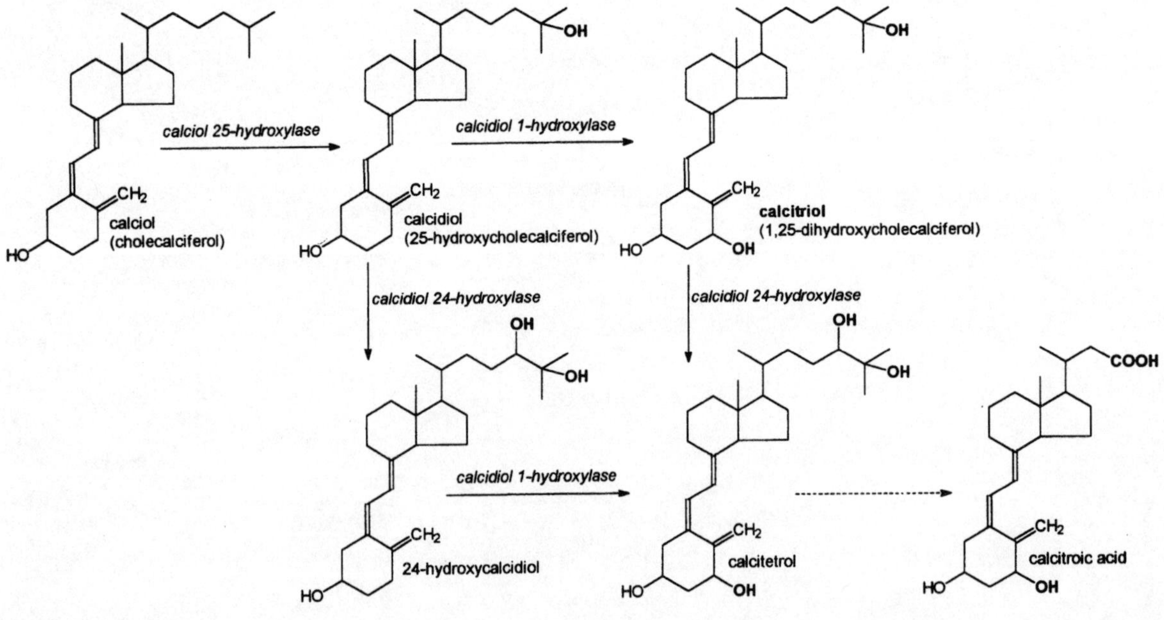

Figure 14.3 Metabolism of cholecalciferol

The first step in vitamin D metabolism is 25–hydroxylation to yield calcidiol (25–hydroxycholecalciferol), which is both the main circulating form of the vitamin and also the main storage form in the body. There is negligible storage of vitamin D in the liver in human beings, and although significant amounts may be present in adipose tissue, this cannot really be regarded as a storage form of the vitamin, since it is released as adipose tissue is catabolized, rather than in response to vitamin D requirements. The half-life of calcidiol in plasma is about 3 weeks (Holick 1990), and there is considerable seasonal variation in the plasma concentration in temperate climates (see Table 14.10).

Calcidiol undergoes 1-hydroxylation in the kidney to yield the active hormone, calcitriol (1,25–dihydroxycholecalciferol), or 24-hydroxylation in the kidney and other tissues to yield 24-hydroxycalcidiol (24,25–dihydroxycholecalciferol), which has no known metabolic function in human beings (see section 14.3.2.3).

The concentration of calcitriol in plasma remains relatively constant, varying with the state of calcium balance (see section 14.3.2.4), but not varying significantly with vitamin D status until deficiency is extreme. By contrast, as shown in Tables 14.10 and 14.15, plasma concentrations of calcidiol fall sharply in deficiency.

Calcitriol is inactivated by 24-hydroxylation, to yield calcitetrol; the same product is formed by 1-hydroxylation of 24-hydroxycalcidiol. Calcitetrol then undergoes side-chain oxidation to calcitroic acid, which is the main excretory product of the vitamin, excreted in the bile. A number of other hydroxylated and oxidized derivatives are also excreted in the bile; less than 5 per cent of total vitamin D is excreted in the urine in the form of a variety of conjugates.

14.3.2.1 Cholecalciferol 25–hydroxylase

There are two separate enzymes in the liver that catalyse the 25–hydroxylation of cholecalciferol. Both are cytochrome P_{450}-dependent mixed function oxidases; one is microsomal and the other is mitochondrial. The mitochondrial enzyme hydroxylates cholecalciferol twice as fast as it does ergocalciferol; the microsomal enzyme does not act on ergocalciferol to any significant extent. The activities of both enzymes are higher in liver from vitamin D-deficient animals, and there is some evidence that both are inhibited or repressed by calcitriol. However, this is unlikely to be a physiologically important control over vitamin D metabolism, which is regulated mainly by the activities of the 1- and 24-hydroxylation of calcidiol.

14.3.2.2 Calcidiol 1-hydroxylase

The active metabolite of vitamin D, calcitriol, is formed in the proximal tubules of the kidney by 1-hydroxylation of calcidiol. The enzyme is a mitochondrial cytochrome P_{450}-dependent mixed function oxidase. As well as the kidney, calcidiol 1-hydroxylase is found in the placenta, bone cells (in culture), mammary gland and keratinocytes. The placental enzyme makes a significant contribution to foetal calcitriol, but it is not known whether or not the enzyme in other tissues is physiologically important.

Renal failure is associated with the development of vitamin D-resistant rickets or osteomalacia (renal osteodystrophy), because the active metabolite cannot be formed. The condition can be treated by administration of the synthetic compound, 1α-hydroxycholecalciferol (hydroxycalciol), which is hydroxylated by the liver 25–hydroxylase to yield calcitriol.

Calcidiol 1-hydroxylase is inhibited or repressed by strontium ions; the result of strontium intoxication is the development of vitamin D-resistant rickets or osteomalacia which responds to the administration of calcitriol or 1α-hydroxycholecalciferol, but not cholecaliciferol or calcidiol (Omdahl and DeLuca 1971).

14.3.2.3 Calcidiol 24-hydroxylase

Both calcidiol and calcitriol are substrates for 24-hydroxylation, again catalysed by a cytochrome P_{450}-dependent enzyme. This enzyme is found in kidney, intestinal mucosa, cartilage and a variety of other tissues that contain calcitriol receptors (see section 14.3.3.1).

Calcidiol 1- and 24-hydroxylases in the kidney are regulated in opposite directions, so that decreased requirement for, and formation of, calcitriol results in increased formation of 24-hydroxycalcidiol (see section 14.3.2.4)

In tissues that have calcitriol receptors, calcidiol 24-hydroxylase is induced and activated by calcitriol, as a mechanism for inactivation of the hormone (Reichel et al. 1989; Yamamoto et al. 1989). Most of the evidence suggests that 24-hydroxylation of calcidiol represents a pathway for inactivation of vitamin D, and regulation of the formation of the active product of 1-hydroxylation. Like calcidiol, plasma concentrations of 24-hydroxycalcidiol show seasonal fluctuation, whereas plasma concentrations of calcitriol do not.

There is some evidence that 24-hydroxycalcidiol may have a function; calcitriol alone will not reverse the hypertrophy of the parathyroid gland that is seen in vitamin D deficient chicks, nor will it support normal hatchability of eggs. Both can be normalized by feeding 24-hydroxycalcidiol together with calcitriol, although it has no effect alone.

14.3.2.4 Regulation of vitamin D metabolism

The main function of vitamin D is in the control of calcium homeostasis, and in turn vitamin D metabolism is regulated, at the level of 1- or 24-hydroxylation, by factors that respond to plasma concentrations of calcium and phosphate.

1. Calcitriol acts to reduce its own synthesis. It induces calcidiol 24-hydroxylase and represses the synthesis of 1-hydroxylase in the kidney, acting on gene expression by way of calcitriol receptors (see section 14.3.3.1).

2. Parathyroid hormone is secreted in response to a fall in plasma calcium. In the kidney it acts to increase the activity of calcidiol 1-hydroxylase and decrease that of the 24-hydroxylase. This is not an effect on protein synthesis, but the result of changes in the activity of existing enzyme protein, mediated by cAMP. In turn, both calcitriol and high concentrations of calcium repress the synthesis of parathyroid hormone; calcium also inhibits the secretion of the hormone from the parathyroid gland, whereas calcitriol does not (Sherwood and Russell 1989).

3. Calcitonin stimulates the 1-hydroxylation of calcidiol in the kidney, acting both to increase the activity of existing enzyme (a cAMP-dependent effect) and also to increase enzyme synthesis. Neither effect is seen when calcitonin is given to thyro-parathyroidectomized animals, nor with isolated kidney cells in culture, suggesting that the action of calcitonin may be mediated indirectly, by way of stimulation of secretion of parathyroid hormone.

4. Calcium exerts its main effect on the synthesis and secretion of parathyroid hormone. However, calcium ions also have a direct effect on the kidney, reducing the activity of calcidiol 1-hydroxylase (but with no effect on the activity of 24-hydroxylase).

5. Phosphate also affects calcidiol metabolism; throughout the day there is an inverse fluctuation of plasma phosphate and calcitriol, and feeding subjects on a low phosphate diet results in increased circulating concentrations of calcitriol (Portale *et al.* 1989).

14.3.3 Metabolic functions of vitamin D

The principal function of vitamin D is to maintain the plasma concentration of calcium; calcitriol achieves this in three ways:

(1) increased intestinal absorption of calcium;

(2) reduced excretion of calcium by increased resorption in the distal renal tubules (due to increased calbindin D synthesis);

(3) mobilization of bone mineral.

In addition, calcitriol has a variety of permissive or modulatory effects, in which it is a necessary, but not sufficient, regulatory factor, in the following:

(1) secretion of insulin;

(2) synthesis and secretion of parathyroid and thyroid hormones;

(3) inhibition of production of interleukin by activated T-lymphocytes and of immunoglobin by activated B-lymphocytes;

(4) differentiation of monocyte precursor cells;

(5) modulation of cell proliferation (at least in culture).

In all of these actions, the role of calcitriol seems to be in the induction or maintenance of synthesis of calbindin D (and other calcium binding proteins), and the effects are secondary to increased calcium uptake into the target cells. Several of these actions are also modulated by vitamin A; as discussed in section 13.3.3, vitamin A receptors form hetero-dimers with calcitriol receptors, so that both vitamins are required together for some actions.

14.3.3.1 Calcitriol receptors

With the exception of the short-term effects on intestinal calcium absorption, all of the actions of calcitriol are due to modulation of gene expression in target cells that have calcitriol receptors. Calcitriol receptors have been identified in a wide range of tissues, as shown in Table 14.11.

The calcitriol receptor is a member of the 'zinc finger' steroid hormone receptor family (see section 25.26). On binding calcitriol (or ercalcitriol) the receptor undergoes activation and dimerization, then binds to hormone response elements on DNA, stimulating the transcription of the associated genes.

Type II (familial) vitamin D resistant rickets is due to either lack of functional calcitriol receptors, or to the presence of receptors with abnormally low affinity for calcitriol (Anon 1989; Griffin and Zerwekh

1983). Two major allelic variants of the calcitriol receptor are known, and peak bone mineral mass, and the subsequent risk of developing osteoporosis (see section 14.5), is predicted by the calcitriol receptor subtype (Morrison *et al.* 1994).

The principal response to calcitriol is induction of the calcium binding protein calbindin D. In bone, the vitamin K-dependent γ-carboxyglutamate-containing protein osteocalcin is also induced by vitamin D. A considerable number of other genes are also regulated by calcitriol, as shown in Table 14.12.

14.3.3.2 Intestinal absorption of calcium and phosphate

Calcitriol has two effects in the small intestine: a rapid increase in the uptake of calcium and phosphate, and a slower response associated with new synthesis of calbindin D.

In duodenal tissue from vitamin D replete animals (but not from deficient animals), calcitriol causes an increase in the uptake of calcium within a few minutes. This is due to an increase in the permeability of the intestinal mucosal brush border to calcium ions, associated with changes in the membrane topology. There is also increased activity of alkaline phosphatase, which will hydrolyse organic phosphates, and in the activity of the sodium-dependent phosphate transport system.

The slower and more prolonged effect of calcitriol on calcium absorption is due to the induction of the calcium-binding protein calbindin D, which permits intracellular accumulation and transport of calcium. It is almost undetectable in intestinal mucosal cells from vitamin D deficient animals, and represents as much as 1-3 per cent of cytosolic protein in duodenal columnar epithelial cells.

Transfer of calcium from the mucosal cell across the baso-lateral membrane is by means of a calcium-magnesium ATPase; magnesium (see section 25.16) thus has a role in the normal absorption of calcium.

A number of substances present in the intestinal lumen affect the absorption, and hence availability, of dietary calcium, as shown in Table 14.13. The absorption of radioactive calcium added to foods is between 20–46 per cent in adults, with some decrease with increasing age; young children may absorb as much as 75 per cent of dietary calcium (National Research Council / National Academy of Sciences 1989; Department of Health 1991).

14.3.3.3 The role of calcitriol in bone metabolism

The maintenance of bone structure is due to balanced activity of osteoclasts, which erode existing bone mineral and organic matrix, and osteoblasts, which both synthesize and secrete the proteins of bone matrix and also have resorptive activity. Mineralization of the organic matrix is largely controlled by the availability of adequate concentrations of calcium and phosphate. The mineral has a very fine crystal structure, and hence a large surface area; one of the main functions of osteocalcin, the γ-carboxyglutamate-containing calcium binding protein in bone matrix, is to modify the crystallization of bone mineral. The rates of turnover of bones in adults are shown in Table 14.14; bone turnover in young children is considerably more rapid, as a result of the continual remodelling of bone that accompanies growth.

Osteoblasts also synthesize and secrete into the bone matrix a variety of compounds which modify the responsiveness of osteoclasts to inhibition by calcitonin and prostaglandins, and also have some direct role in bone resorption. Osteoclasts are not directly affected by calcitriol or parathyroid hormone.

By contrast, osteoblasts have receptors for parathyroid hormone, calcitriol, glucocorticoids, epidermal growth factor, prostaglandins, oestrogens, and androgens, and so are susceptible to multiple hormonal modulation of activity. In response to calcitriol and parathyroid hormone, they show decreased synthesis of collagen and alkaline phosphatase, while in response to calcitriol they show increased synthesis of osteocalcin and increased secretion of resorptive enzymes.

Physiologically, the response of bone to calcitriol is resorption of bone mineral and matrix protein. Both calcitriol and parathyroid hormone increase bone resorption *in vivo* and in bone organ culture, but have no effect on the activity of isolated osteoblasts. In addition to direct stimulation of the resorptive activity of osteoblasts, calcitriol increases osteoclastic activity. This is not due to a direct effect of calcitriol on osteoclasts, which lack calcitriol receptors, but rather to an increase in the differentiation of osteoclast precursor cells into mature osteoclasts, so increasing the number of osteoclasts. It is not known whether osteoclast precursors respond directly to calcitriol, or whether the effect is indirect, mediated by calcitriol-responsive leukocytes or osteoblasts. Osteoblasts stimulated by calcitriol or parathyroid hormone secrete one or more small proteins which increase the activity of osteoclasts.

Osteoclastic activity is inhibited by calcitonin and prostaglandins I_2, E_1 and E_2, all of which act directly on the osteoclast; there is some evidence that osteoblasts may synthesize and secrete some of the osteoclast inhibitory prostaglandins.

Calcitriol and parathyroid hormone stimulation of osteoblast resorptive activity also causes the synthesis and release of a variety of growth factors from the osteoblasts. These accumulate in the bone and act as delayed activators of osteoblast proliferation and activation.

Although the immediate response of osteoblasts to calcitriol is repression of the synthesis of collagen and alkaline phosphatase, between 24-48 hours after calcitriol administration there is increased collagen synthesis, with both new mRNA synthesis and an increased rate of translation of the existing mRNA, and induction of alkaline phosphatase and osteocalcin. Alkaline phosphatase may have an important role in mineralization, by hydrolysing pyrophosphate and ATP in the bone matrix, both of which are inhibitors of mineralization; inhibition of alkaline phosphatase inhibits calcification of cartilage in culture.

The combined effect of the delayed autocrine activators of osteoblast proliferation released by parathyroid hormone or calcitriol-stimulated osteoblasts, and the delayed induction of collagen, osteocalcin and alkaline phosphatase synthesis is thus to promote the formation and mineralization of new bone matrix to replace that resorbed.

14.4   Vitamin D deficiency: rickets and osteomalacia

Rickets is a disease of young children and adolescents, resulting from a failure of the mineralization of newly formed bone. Before the deficiency is sufficiently advanced for anatomical lesions to be apparent, the impairment of mineralization can be detected by the reduced bone density on radiography (radiological rickets). More sensitive detection of early rickets is by measurement of plasma concentrations of calcidiol (which is abnormally low) or alkaline phosphatase (EC 3.1.3.1), which is abnormally elevated; see Table 14.15. In severe deficiency, the plasma concentration of calcium may fall to the level at which intracellular calcium in nerves and muscles cannot be maintained, and tetany occurs.

In infants, epiphyseal cartilage continues to grow, but is not replaced by bone matrix and mineral. The earliest sign of this is craniotabes—the occurrence of round or unossified areas in the skull, accompanied by late closure of the fontanelles. At a later stage there is enlargement of the epiphyses, initially at the costochondral junction of the ribs, giving a beading effect, the so-called rachitic rosary. This may lead to deformity of the chest, and in severe cases collapse of the rib cage, with consequent obstruction of respiration. Other epiphyseal junctions also become enlarged.

When the child begins to walk, the weight of the body deforms the defectively mineralized long bones, leading to bow legs or knock knees, as well as deformity of the pelvis. Similar problems may develop during the adolescent growth spurt.

Osteomalacia is the defective remineralization of bone during normal bone turnover in adults, so that there is a progressive demineralization, but with adequate bone matrix, leading to bone pain and skeletal deformities, with muscle weakness. Women with inadequate vitamin D status are especially at risk of osteomalacia after repeated pregnancies, as a result of the considerable drain on calcium reserves to provide for foetal bone mineralization and lactation.

Both rickets and osteomalacia are due to a lack of vitamin D, and hence low circulating concentrations of calcidiol and calcitriol, commonly associated with inadequate exposure to sunlight. Deficiency is more prevalent in northern latitudes, and commoner in urban areas than in open country. Cultural factors that reduce exposure to sunlight increase the risk of osteomalacia in women, and the house-bound elderly are especially vulnerable. Both increased exposure to sunlight (or artificial sources of UV-B irradiation) and dietary supplements of vitamin D are preventive and curative.

People of Indian and Pakistani origin living in temperate regions are especially at risk of adolescent rickets and osteomalacia. Two factors seem to be involved: relatively low exposure to sunlight (which is largely a cultural problem) and a low dietary intake of readily absorbable calcium. Vitamin D supplements are generally recommended for Asian women and children in Britain.

Similarly, the elderly are at risk of osteomalacia, both because of decreased synthesis of 7-dehydrocholesterol in the skin with increasing age (see section 14.3.1) and, more importantly, reduced exposure to sunlight. Plasma concentrations of calcidiol below 10 nmol /L are commonly seen in people aged over 75, not rising above 20 nmol /L at any time of the year. Histologically proven osteomalacia is observed in 2-5 per cent of the elderly presenting to hospital in Britain.

14.4.1 Non-nutritional rickets and osteomalacia

Induction of cytochrome P_{450} by barbiturates and other anticonvulsants can result in increased catabolism of calcidiol, and secondary, drug-induced, osteomalacia. The antituberculosis drug isoniazid inhibits cholecalciferol 25–hydroxylase, and again prolonged administration can result in osteomalacia.

Three conditions associated with defective 1-hydroxylation of calcidiol can all be treated by the administration of either calcitriol itself or 1α-hydroxycholecalciferol, which is a substrate for 25–hydroxylation in the liver (see section 14.3.2.1).

1. Strontium intoxication can cause vitamin D-resistant rickets because strontium is a potent inhibitor of calcidiol 1-hydroxylase (Omdahl and DeLuca 1971).

2. Renal failure is associated with an osteomalacia-like syndrome, renal osteodystrophy, as a result of the loss of calcidiol 1-hydroxylase activity. The condition may be complicated by defective resorption of calcium and phosphate from the urine. Furthermore, the half-life of parathyroid hormone is increased, since the principal site of its catabolism is the kidney, so that there is increased parathyroid hormone-stimulated osteoclastic action without the compensatory action of calcitriol (Mawer *et al.* 1973).

3. Hypoparathyroidism is also associated with a failure of calcidiol 1-hydroxylation, in this case because the major stimulus for induction of the 1-hydroxylase is parathyroid hormone.

There are three (rare) inherited rachitic syndromes which do not respond to normal amounts of vitamin D.

1. Familial hypophosphataemic rickets. This condition is characterized by a primary renal loss of phosphate, together with a blunting of the normal increase in calcidiol 1-hydroxylase activity in response to the resultant hypophosphataemia. Fibroblasts from affected patients show normal calcitriol receptor activity and responsiveness, and the patients respond to normal amounts of vitamin D with phosphate supplements.

2. Type I vitamin D resistant rickets. In these patients the defect is in the kidney calcidiol 1-hydroxylase, so that they form little or no calcitriol. They respond well to the administration of 1-α-hydroxycholecalciferol, which is a substrate for 25–hydroxylation in the liver, leading to normal circulating concentrations of calcitriol.

3. Type II vitamin D resistant rickets. This condition is characterized by a lack of responsiveness of target tissues to calcitriol, and is due to a defect in the calcitriol receptor (Anon 1989). Three variants are known:

> complete absence of calcitriol receptor, presumably the result of a deletion or early nonsense mutation in the receptor gene;

> poor affinity of the receptor for calcitriol, presumably the result of a mutation affecting the calcitriol binding site;

> normal receptor binding of calcitriol with impaired or absent target tissue responsiveness, presumably the result of a mutation affecting the DNA binding domain of the receptor.

14.5 Osteoporosis

Osteoporosis is a condition involving loss of bone mineral and matrix in the elderly. Unlike osteomalacia there is no defect of bone mineralization. The lower density of the bone renders it more susceptible to fracture, while in osteomalacia the incompletely mineralized bone matrix is liable to deformation rather than fracture.

The relative activities of bone resorption and formation can be estimated by measurement of the following in plasma.

1. As indices of bone formation: osteocalcin, bone isoenzyme of alkaline phosphatase, procollagen extension peptides.

2. As indices of bone resorption: pyridinium cross-link compounds of collagen, urinary hydroxyproline and hydroxylysine, tartrate-resistant acid phosphatase (largely derived from bone).

As yet there are insufficient data to permit reference ranges to be established, although there are significant differences in all of these indices between post-menopausal women receiving or not receiving hormone replacement therapy, and between those who did or did not subsequently suffer fracture of the hip (Delmas 1993; Riis 1993).

Two types of osteoporosis can be distinguished.

1. Type I osteoporosis, also known as post-menopausal osteoporosis, involves loss of trabecular bone in the vertebrae, leading to crush fracture with minimal trauma. It is essentially a condition affecting post-menopausal women, with a female:male incidence ratio of 10:1.

2. Type II osteoporosis (senile osteoporosis) is osteoporotic hip fracture. It shows only a 2:1 excess of

254 Vitamin D, calcium and phosphorus

females over males, and a geometric increase in incidence with increasing age.

These two classes are not exclusive; type I patients are more susceptible to hip fracture, while many hip fracture patients have asymptomatic vertebral crush fractures.

Although vitamin D status declines with increasing age, and there is reduced activity of calcidiol 1-hydroxylase, osteoporosis is not due to vitamin D deficiency, and does not respond to calciferol or calcitriol supplements. Indeed, there is some evidence that fractures are more common in osteoporotic patients treated with calcitriol. Equally, although there is negative calcium balance in osteoporosis, this is a result of the loss of bone, not a cause. Administration of calcium supplements has no effect on the progression of osteoporosis (Kanis and Passmore 1989; Ott and Chesnut 1989; Parfitt 1988).

The principal cause of osteoporosis seems to be the loss of oestrogen and androgen secretion with increasing age. It was noted above (see section 14.3.3.3) that osteoblasts have both oestrogen and androgen receptors. While the mechanism of action of the sex steroids is not clear, it seems likely that they act by reducing the osteoclastogenesis resulting from osteoblast activation. They may also antagonize the release of osteoblast-derived resorption factors following calcitriol and parathyroid hormone action. Hence loss of oestrogen at the menopause, and loss of testosterone with increasing age in men, results in loss of some of the normal modulation of bone resorption stimulated by calcitriol.

Osteoporosis is an inevitable consequence of ageing. The peak bone mass is achieved between the ages of 20–30, and thereafter there is a progressive loss of bone, becoming more marked post-menopausally. The condition is considerably less severe in people who enter the menopause with greater bone mass, something which is largely genetically determined, the result of genetic variation in calcitriol receptor subtypes (Morrison et al. 1994). A life-time low intake of calcium is a risk factor, and there is some evidence that a moderately high intake of calcium during early life, while the skeleton is being formed, is protective. Post-menopausal hormone replacement therapy is beneficial in reducing the rate of bone loss (Raisz and Smith 1989).

14.6   Vitamin D toxicity

Excessive intake of vitamin D, but not excessive exposure to sunlight (see section 14.3.1) causes weakness, nausea, loss of appetite, headache, abdominal pains, cramp and diarrhoea. More seriously, it also causes hypercalcaemia, with plasma concentrations of calcium between 2.75–4.5 mmol /L, compared with the normal range of 2.2–2.55 mmol /L.

The toxic threshold for adults has not been established, but most patients with clinically significant hypercalcaemia have been taking in excess of 250 µg daily, compared with a reference intake of 10 µg. Some children are known to be sensitive to hypercalcaemia and calcinosis as a result of habitual intake as low as 45 µg /day (Chesney 1990; Holick 1990). Hypercalcaemia persists for many months after the cessation of excessive intakes of vitamin D, because of the accumulation of the vitamin in adipose tissue, and its slow release into the circulation.

At plasma concentrations of calcium above 3.75 mmol /L, vascular smooth muscle may contract abnormally, leading to hypertension and hypertensive encephalopathy. Hypercalciuria may also result in the precipitation of calcium phosphates in the renal tubules and hence the development of urinary calculi. Hypercalcaemia can also result in calcinosis—the calcification of soft tissues, including kidney, heart, lungs and blood vessels. This is assumed to be the result of increased calcium uptake into tissues as a result of increased synthesis of calbindin D in response to excessive plasma concentrations of the vitamin and its metabolites.

There is a narrow margin between amounts of vitamin D adequate to ensure that rickets is prevented throughout the community and the level at which vulnerable infants will develop hypercalcaemia. This became a significant problem in Britain in the 1950s. Widespread fortification of infant foods had resulted in more or less complete eradication of what formerly had been known as 'the English disease'. By 1955 some 200 cases of hypercalcaemia had been reported. The amount of vitamin D added to infant foods was reduced, and as a result rickets reappeared. The problem is to identify those children at risk of deficiency, who therefore require additional supplements, without putting those with a low threshold for intoxication at risk of hypercalcaemia and calcinosis.

Further reading

Anderson, J.J.B. (1991). Nutritional biochemistry of calcium and phosphorus. *Journal of Nutritional Biochemistry*, **2**, 300–7.

Bender, D.A. (1992). Vitamin D. In *Nutritional Biochemistry of the Vitamins*, Chapter 3, pp. 51–86. Cambridge University Press.

Christakos, S., Gabrielides, C. and Rhoten, W.B. (1989). Vitamin D-dependent calcium binding proteins: chemistry, distribution, functional considerations and molecular biology. *Endocrine Reviews*, **10**, 3–26.

DeLuca, H.F. and Schnoes, H.K. (1983). Vitamin D: recent advances. *Annual Review of Biochemistry*, **52** 411–39.

Fraser, D.R. (1983). The physiological economy of vitamin D. *Lancet*, (I), 969–72.

Friedrich, W. (1988). Vitamin D. In *Vitamins*, Chapter 3, pp. 141–218. Walter de Gruyter, Berlin.

Lawson, D.E. (1985). Vitamin D. In *Fat-soluble Vitamins: their Biochemistry and Applications*, (ed. A.T. Diplock), Chapter 2, pp. 76–153. Heinemann, London.

Minisymposium: Osteoporosis and calcium (1992). *Journal of Internal Medicine*, **231**, 145–94.

NIH consensus conference on osteoporosis (1993). *American Journal of Medicine*, **95**, supplement 5a.

Norman, A.W. (1990). Intestinal calcium absorption: a vitamin D hormone mediated adaptive response. *American Journal of Clinical Nutrition*, **51**, 290–300.

Norman, A. W., Roth, J. and Orci, L. (1982). The vitamin D endocrine system, steroid metabolism, hormone receptors and biological response (calcium binding proteins). *Endocrine Reviews*, **3**, 331–66.

O'Malley, B.W. and Pike, J.W. (1988). Molecular biology of the vitamin D hormone. *Recent Progress in Hormone Research*, **44**, 263–97.

Pike, J.W. (1988). Vitamin D receptors and the mechanims of action of 1,25–dihydroxyvitamin D. In *Vitamin Receptors: Vitamins as Ligands in Cell Communication*, (ed. K. Dakshinamurti), Chapter 3, pp. 59–77. Cambridge University Press.

Reichel, H. and Norman, A.W. (1989). Systemic effects of vitamin D. *Annual Review of Medicine*, **40**, 71–8.

Symposium on Newly Discovered Actions of 1,25–dihydroxyvitamin D (1989). *Proceedings of the Society for Experimental Biology and Medicine*, **191**, 211–59.

Table 14.1: Average adult intakes of calcium, phosphorus and vitamin D in UK, compared with Dietary Reference Values

		men		women		threshold intake	average requirement	reference intake[1]
		mean	95% range	mean	95% range			
calcium	mg/d	937	409-1597	726	266-1299	400	550	700-800
	mmol/d	23.4	10.2-40	18.2	6.7-32	10	13.75	17.5-20
phosphorus	mg/d	1452	782-2310	1072	511-1719	300	400	550-800
	mmol/d	46.2	25-73	34.1	16-55	10	13.75	17.5-25.5
vitamin D	μg/d	3.43	0.51-9.92	2.51	0.43-6.89	-	-	5-10[2]

(1) The lower figures are the UK RNI and EU PRI; the higher figures the US RDA.
(2) US RDA for adults is 5 μg vitamin D; EU and UK have reference intake of 10 μg /day for the elderly only
Source: from data reported by Gregory *et al.* 1990; Department of Health 1991; Scientific Committee for Food 1993; National Research Council 1989.

Table: 14.2: Average intakes of vitamin D (μg/day) in UK

age	mean	median	range[1]	mean	median	range[1]	reference
1.5-2.5	1.2	0.9	0.2-4.8	1.2	0.9	0.2-4.8	Gregory *et al.* 1995
2.5-3.5	1.2	1.0	0.2-3.5	1.2	1.0	0.2-3.5	Gregory *et al.* 1995
3.5-4.5	1.4	1.1	0.3-4.6	1.3	1.1	0.3-2.9	Gregory *et al.* 1995
16-24	2.81	2.39	0.39-8.08	2.10	1.86	0.34-5.17	Gregory *et al.* 1990
25-34	3.16	2.64	0.61-9.80	2.30	2.05	0.41-6.35	Gregory *et al.* 1990
35-49	3.71	3.23	0.64-11.01	2.61	2.25	0.43-7.15	Gregory *et al.* 1990
50-64	3.80	3.24	0.37-10.67	2.82	2.34	0.55-7.13	Gregory *et al.* 1990
58-65	3.4	-	0.6-8.1	2.5	-	0.1-9.6	Davies & Holdsworth 1985
62-74	3.1	-	-	2.0	-	-	Lonergan *et al.* 1975
75-90	2.4	-	-	1.8	-	-	Lonergan *et al.* 1975

(1) The range shown is the 2.5-97.5 centile for the studies of Gregory *et al.*, and the observed extreme range for the study of Davies & Holdsworth.

Table: 14.3: Average intakes of calcium (mg /day)

(Apart from the SENECA study of the elderly, which involved 17 centres throughout Europe, all the studies quoted were in UK)

age	males			females			reference
	mean	median	range[1]	mean	median	range[1]	
1.5-2.5	637	618	-	637	618	-	Gregory *et al.* 1995
2.5-3.5	547	516	-	547	516	-	Gregory *et al.* 1995
3.5-4.5	492	472	-	504	488	-	Gregory *et al.* 1995
16-24	894	858	352-1597	675	656	240-1220	Gregory *et al.* 1990
25-34	931	908	379-1607	699	689	231-1299	Gregory *et al.* 1990
35-49	960	956	439-1683	760	737	328-1379	Gregory *et al.* 1990
50-64	949	947	420-1528	739	731	305-1131	Gregory *et al.* 1990
58-65	1013	-	551-1756	809	-	303-1536	Davies & Holdsworth 1985
62-74	958	-	-	799	-	-	Lonergan *et al.* 1975
73-78[2]	-	928 (638-1323)	220-2288	-	818 (521-1213)	216-1900	Euronut SENECA Investigators 1991
75-90	964	-	-	786	-	-	Lonergan *et al.* 1975

(1) The range shown is the 2.5-97.5 centile for the studies of Gregory *et al.*, the 10-90 centile for the SENECA study, and the observed extreme range for the study of Davies & Holdsworth.
(2) Data were reported for 17 separate centres; the mean and extreme values of the published median values are shown, with the lowest 10th centile and highest 90th centile of those reported.

Table 14.4: Sources of calcium in the average British diet

	% of total
full fat milk	23
cheese	13
other milk products	22
cereals excluding white bread	16
white bread	9
vegetables	7
meat	5
eggs	2
fish	2
confectionery	2
fruit and nuts	1

Source: Gregory *et al.* 1990.

Table 14.5: Sources of vitamin D in the average British diet

	% of total
fat spreads	30
oily fish	21
baked goods	11
eggs	9
breakfast cereals	8
milk and milk products	6
meat	4

Source: Gregory *et al.* 1990.

Table 14.6: Dietary sources of vitamin D

	µg /100g
butter[1]	0.4-0.8
margarine	0.8
cheese	0.2-0.3
milk (full cream)[1]	0.015-0.03
cod roe	2
egg	1.8
herring	22.5
liver[2]	0.2-1.1
mackerel	17.5
pilchards	8

(1) The vitamin D content of milk (and milk products) shows a two-fold variation, from a minimum at the end of winter to a maximum in summer.
(2) Liver from chickens, lamb and veal is at the lower end of this range, that from older animals (ox and pig liver) at the upper end.

Table 14.7: Reference Intakes of calcium and National Institutes of Health Optimum levels of intake (mg /day)

	US RDA (1989)	UK RNI (1991)	EU PRI (1993)	NIH optimum (1994)
birth-6m	400	525	-	400
6m-1y	600	525	400	600
1-3	800	350	400	800
4-6	800	450	450	800
7-10	800	550	550	800-1200
males				
11-14	1200	1000	1000	1200-1500
15-18	1200	1000	1000	1200-1500
19-24	1200	700	700	1200-1500
25-50	800	700	700	1000
> 50	800	700	-	-
> 65	-	-	-	1500
females				
11-14	1200	800	800	1200-1500
15-18	1200	800	800	1200-1500
19-24	1200	700	700	1200-1500
25-50	800	700	700	1000
> 50	800	700	-	
> 50 with oestrogen hrt[1]				1000
> 50 without oestrogen hrt				1500
women > 65				1500
pregnant	1200	700	700	1200-1500
lactating	1200	1250	1200	1200-1500

(1) hrt = menopausal hormone replacement therapy.
Source: National Research Council 1989; Department of Health 1991; Scientific Committee for Food 1993; NIH Consensus Development Panel 1994.

Table 14.8: Calcium metallo-enzymes and calcium binding proteins

α-amylase (EC 3.2.1.1)	salivary and pancreatic enzyme; digestion of starch (see section 7.2)
phospolipase A2 (EC 3.1.1.4)	pancreatic enzyme; intestinal digestion of phospholipids (see section 8.2)
phospholipase C (EC 3.1.4.3)	hydrolyses phosphatidylinositol bisphosphate in transmembrane signal transduction
trypsinogen (EC 3.4.21.4)	calcium enhances activation by enteropeptidase and stabilizes trypsin (see section 10.3.1)
calcium-activated muscle protease (EC 3.4.21.39)	turnover of muscle proteins; hydrolysis of troponin to tropomyosin
phosphorylase kinase (EC 2.7.1.38)	activation of glycogen phosphorylase in presence of cAMP in response to adrenaline or glucagon
protein kinase C (EC 2.7.1.123)	transmembrane signal transduction
annexins	calcium-dependent phospholipid-binding proteins involved in regulation of secretion
cadherins	calcium-dependent cell adhesion proteins; possibly important in malignancy
calbindin D	vitamin D-dependent calcium binding protein; important in intestinal calcium absorption and tissue uptake
calmodulin	calcium-dependent cell signalling; activates protein kinases when calcium is bound
osteocalcin (bone Gla protein)	vitamin K-dependent protein in bone matrix; important in bone mineral crystallization (see section 16.4.2)
prothrombin, etc.	vitamin K-dependent proteins in blood coagulation (see section 16.4.1)
troponin	control of muscle contraction; permits muscle contraction in presence of calcium ions

Table 14.9: Nomenclature of vitamin D metabolites

Trivial name	Recommended name	Abbreviation	M_r
vitamin D₃			
cholecalciferol	calciol	-	384.6
25-hydroxycholecalciferol	calcidiol	$25(OH)D_3$	400.6
1α-hydroxycholecalciferol	1(S)-hydroxycalciol	$1\alpha(OH)D_3$	400.6
24,25-dihydroxycholecalciferol	24(R)-hydroxycalcidiol	$24,25(OH)_2D_3$	416.6
1,25-dihydroxycholecalciferol	calcitriol	$1,25(OH)_2D_3$	416.6
1,24,25-trihydroxycholecalciferol	calcitetrol	$1,24,25(OH)_3D_3$	432.6
vitamin D₂			
ergocalciferol	ercalciol	-	396.6
25-hydroxyergocalciferol	ercalcidiol	$25(OH)D_2$	412.6
24,25-dihydroxyergocalciferol	24(R)-hydroxyercalcidiol	$24,25(OH)_2D_2$	428.6
1,25-dihydroxyergocalciferol	ercalcitriol	$1,25(OH)_2 D_2$	428.6
1,24,25-trihydroxyergocalciferol	ercalcitetrol	$1,24,25(OH)_3D_2$	444.6

The abbreviations shown in column 3 are not recommended, but are frequently used in the literature.

Table 14.10: Plasma concentrations of vitamin D metabolites

		nmol /L
cholecalciferol		1.3-156
24-hydroxycalcidiol		2-20
calcitriol		0.038-0.144
calcidiol	adults, summer	37-87
	adults, winter	20-45
	adults with osteomalacia	< 10
	children, summer	50-100
	children, winter	27-52
	children with rickets	< 20
	risk of hypercalcaemia	> 400

Table 14.11: Tissues in which calcitriol receptors have been identified

skeleton	osteoblasts, chondrocytes
lymphatic system	activated T and B lymphocytes, macrophages, monocytes, spleen, thymus, tonsils, lymph nodes
gastrointestinal tract	intestinal epithelial cells, parotid gland, colon, stomach
urinary tract	kidney (distal and proximal tubules), bladder
muscle	skeletal, cardiac and smooth muscle
nervous system	brain (many centres), sensory ganglia, spinal cord
reproductive system	epididymis, testis (sertoli and Leydig cells), ovary, oviduct, uterus, placenta, mammary gland
skin	epidermis, fibroblasts, hair follicles, keratinocytes, melanocytes, sebaceous glands
endocrine system	adrenal medulla and cortex, pancreas β-cells, pituitary, thyroid, parathyroid

In addition, calcitriol receptors have been identified in a wide range of tumour cells.
Source: from data reported by Hannah & Norman 1994; Walters 1992.

Table 14.12: Genes regulated by calcitriol

	increased expression	decreased expression
vitamin D metabolism	calcitriol receptor	
	calcidiol 24-hydroxylase	
mineral metabolism	calbindin D	pre-proparathyroid hormone
	osteocalcin	transferrin receptor
	osteopontin	
	plasma membrane calcium pump	
	metallothionen	
energy metabolism	glyceraldehyde 3-phosphate dehydrogenase	fatty acid binding protein
	ATP synthase	
	NADH dehydrogenase subunit I	NADH dehydrogenase subunit II
	NADH dehydrogenase subunit IV	
	cytochrome oxidase	cytochrome b
	protein kinase C	protein kinase inhibitor
		ferredoxin
regulatory peptides	nerve growth factor	histone H4
	interleukin I	interleukin II
	interleukin 6	
	interleukin III receptor	
	cachexin (tumour necrosis factor α)	γ-interferon
	monocyte-derived neutrophil-activating peptide	GM colony stimulating factor
cytoskeleton	fibronectin	α-tubulin
oncogenes	c-fms, c-fos, c-ki-ras, c-myc	c-myb
		type I collagen

Source: from data reported by Hannah & Norman 1994.

Table 14.13: Factors that affect the absorption of calcium

increased absorption	decreased absorption
increased metabolic needs in growth, pregnancy, lactation, calcium deficiency	achlorhydria associated with atrophic gastritis in the elderly
increased calcitriol	vitamin D deficiency
low intestinal luminal pH (increases solubility)	high intraluminal pH (decreases solubility)
fat (increases intestinal transit time)	free fatty acids (form soaps)
lactose (when lactase activity is normal)	lactose (in alactasic subjects)
acidic amino acids (chelate calcium for transport)	some forms of fibre (bind calcium)
	oxalate (insoluble salt)
	phytate (inositol hexaphosphate, insoluble salt)
	glucocorticoids, anticonvulsants
	excess phosphate in diet

Source: from data reported by Levenson & Bockman 1994.

Table 14.14: Turnover rates of bones in adults

	% turnover /year	
	mean	range
ribs	4.7	2.2-10
spine	8.3	3.6-20
skull	1.8	0.6-4.6
patella	3.6	2.4-5.0
ilium	6.5	5.9-7.2
proximal femur	5.7	2.6-9.4
distal femur	2.5	0.8-4.2
shaft of femur	2.0	1.5-4.2
tibia	1.1	0.4-2.6

Source: Snyder *et al.* 1975.

Table 14.15: Plasma concentrations of calcidiol, alkaline phosphatase, calcium and phosphate

	calcidiol nmol /L	alkaline phosphatase units /L	calcium mmol /L	phosphate mmol /L
infants	27-100	100-300	2.5	1.6-2.6
children with rickets	< 20	> 390	2.0-2.25	1.0
adults	20-87	57-100	2.5	1.0-1.4
adults with osteomalacia	< 10	300	2.25	0.6-1.0
adults with osteoporosis	20-87	40	2.5-3	1.3-1.6

Vitamin E and selenium

Unlike the other vitamins, vitamin E seems not to have a specific enzymic function; rather it is the major lipid-soluble, free radical-trapping antioxidant in membranes, and many of its functions can be met by synthetic antioxidants. However, some of the effects of vitamin E deficiency in experimental animals do not respond to synthetic antioxidants. The metabolic roles of vitamin E and the trace element selenium are closely related, and to a very great extent each can compensate for a deficiency of the other. The sulphur amino acids (methionine and cysteine) also have a vitamin E-sparing effect.

Deficiency of vitamin E is well established in experimental animals, resulting in reproductive failure, necrotizing myopathy, liver and kidney damage and neurological abnormalities. In man, deficiency is less well defined, and indeed it was only relatively recently that vitamin E was conclusively demonstrated to be essential in human nutrition. Deficiency is a problem only in premature infants of very low birth weight and in patients with abnormalities of lipid absorption or congenital lack of β-lipoprotein—abetalipoproteinaemia. In adults lipid malabsorption results in signs of vitamin E deficiency only after many years.

Selenium, in the form of the amino acid selenocysteine, is required in the catalytic sites of glutathione peroxidase and thyroxine deiodinase (see section 25.14.2). Glutathione peroxidase reduces hydrogen peroxide to water, and so lessens the amount of peroxide available for the generation of radicals, while vitamin E is involved in removing the products of attack by these radicals on lipids. The two nutrients therefore have complementary actions, and to a great extent the effects of deficiency of one can be prevented by adequate intake of the other.

15.1 Requirements and intakes

15.1.1 Vitamin E requirements and intakes

High intakes of polyunsaturated fatty acids increase the requirement for vitamin E. It is generally agreed that 0.4–0.5 mg vitamin E /g dietary polyunsaturated fatty acid meets requirements, although at very low levels of intake (as in very low fat diets), this may not provide enough vitamin E to protect against haemolytic anaemia.

The US RDA for vitamin E are shown in Table 15.1; neither the UK nor the EU authorities quotes reference intakes, noting that an appropriate level of intake is difficult to define, since it is the (very variable) intake of polyunsaturated fatty acids that determines requirements. This is unlikely to prove a problem in practice, since foods that are rich sources of polyunsaturated fatty acids are also naturally rich in tocopherols and tocotrienols. The main dietary sources of vitamin E are vegetable oils and cereals.

It has been suggested that plasma concentrations of vitamin E greater than are generally considered to be adequate may reduce the risk of ischaemic heart disease (Gey 1989). To maintain the suggested plasma concentration of over 4 mmol α-tocopherol /mol cholesterol would require an intake of 17–40 mg α-tocopherol equivalents /day—significantly above current average intakes (see Table 15.2), and an amount unlikely to be met from food sources.

15.1.2 Selenium requirements and intakes

Reference intakes for selenium are shown in Table 15.3, and rich sources in Table 15.4. Selenium intakes vary widely from region to region, depending on the both selenium content of the soil and its availability to plants. In New Zealand, Finland, and areas of China available soil selenium is low, and so are intakes, while in other regions of China, and parts of Venezuela, the available soil selenium is so high that plants may accumulate toxic amounts of the mineral, leading to problems of selenosis (see section 15.8). Because of the low intakes, Finland has a policy of adding selenium to fertilizers; the data in Table 15.5 were obtained before this programme was initiated.

15.2   Vitamin E vitamers and units of activity

There are eight vitamers of vitamin E; the tocopherols have a saturated side-chain, while the tocotrienols have an unsaturated side-chain. The different toco-pherols and tocotrienols (α-, β-, γ-, and δ-) differ in the methylation of the chromanol ring (see Fig. 15.1). Nutritionally, the important vitamers are α-β- and γ-tocopherol, and α-tocotrienol.

Based on biological assay in vitamin E-deficient rats, the vitamers have widely differing biological activity (see Table 15.6). The original international unit of vitamin E potency was equated with the activity of 1 mg of (synthetic) DL-α-tocopherol acetate; on this basis pure D-α-tocopherol (*RRR*-α-tocopherol,

see section 15.2.1, the most potent vitamer) is 1.49 iu /mg.

The international unit has now been abandoned as a unit of vitamin E activity. Indeed, it was based on a single synthetic preparation of DL-α-tocopherol acet-ate which is no longer available. The precise mixture of stereo-isomers in this original standard is unknown, and the different stereo-isomers have very different biological activities, so that different preparations could well differ considerably in potency. It is now usual to express the vitamin E content of foods in terms of mg equivalents of D-α-tocopherol, based on their biological activities.

For the major vitamers present in foods, the fol-lowing conversion factors are used for summing α-tocopherol equivalents:

Total α-tocopherol equivalents =

mg α-tocopherol

+ 0.5 × mg β-tocopherol

+ 0.1 × mg γ-tocopherol

+ 0.3 × mg α-tocotrienol

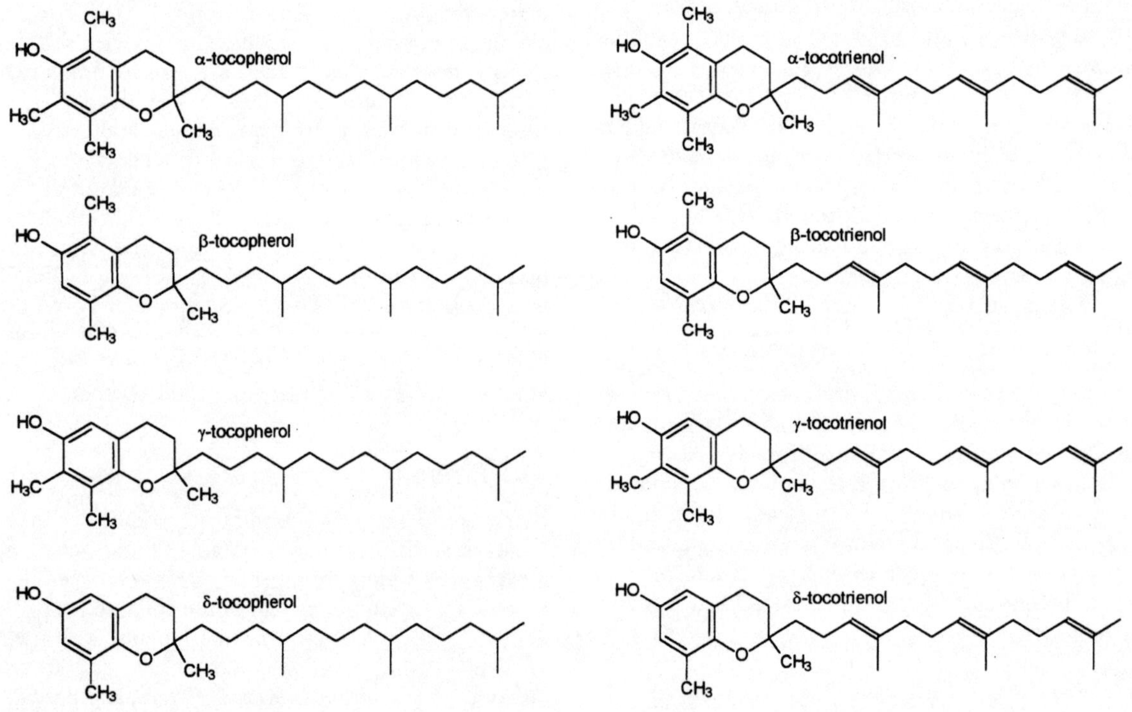

Figure 15.1 The vitamin E vitamers

The other vitamers either occur in negligible amounts in foods or have negligible vitamin activity.

In biological assays, if the test substance is administered as a bolus dissolved in vitamin E-stripped corn oil, as is usual, D-α-tocopherol acetate and succinate have higher biological activity on a molar basis than free D-α-tocopherol, because free tocopherol is susceptible to oxidation. However, this may be an artefact of the way in which the assays are performed; oral intubation in aqueous suspension together with foods shows that there is the same increase in circulating tocopherol from the free alcohol or the acetate (Burton *et al.* 1988).

15.2.1 Stereo-isomers of tocopherol

Vitamin E is unusual in that the synthetic vitamin does not have the same biological activity as the naturally occurring one, because of the complex stereochemistry of the molecule. The tocopherols have three asymmetric centres; vitamin E is one of the very few nutrients for which the systematic chemical nomenclature (*R*- and *S*-) is used to describe the spatial arrangement of groups around the asymmetric carbon atoms. The naturally occurring compound is D-α-tocopherol, in which all three asymmetric centres have the *R*-configuration (2*R*, 4'*R*, 8'*R*, or all-*R* (*RRR*)-α-tocopherol).

Chemical synthesis yields a mixture of the eight possible stereo-isomers, in which each of the asymmetric centres may have either the *R*- or *S*-configuration; this is all-*rac*-α-tocopherol. The stereo-isomers all have different potency in the rat biological assay, and the all-*rac* mixture has a relative biological activity of 0.74x that of *RRR*-α-tocopherol. The most important determinant of biological activity is the configuration of C-2; the four stereo-isomers with the 2*R* configuration are all more active than the corresponding 2*S* isomers.

15.3   Absorption and metabolism of vitamin E

Tocopherols and tocotrienols are absorbed unchanged from the small intestine, in mixed lipid micelles with other dietary lipids (see section 8.2). Esters are hydrolysed in the intestinal lumen by pancreatic esterase. Absorption is enhanced by medium chain triglycerides, and inhibited by polyunsaturated fatty acids. This latter effect may be the result of chemical interactions between tocopherols and polyunsaturated fatty acids or their peroxidation products

in the intestinal lumen, or may be because polyunsaturated fatty acids occupy relatively more space in lipoproteins, and so either displace tocopherol, or inhibit its binding.

There are few precise estimates of vitamin E absorption. In rats about 40 per cent of a single bolus of free α-tocopherol is absorbed, but 65 per cent of a slow infusion of α-tocopheryl acetate; in the few human studies that have been performed, between 20–86 per cent of a test dose may be absorbed (Bates and Heseker 1994). α-Tocopherol is better absorbed than γ-tocopherol.

The biological discrimination between the stereo-isomers of α-tocopherol begins in the gut, where esters of *SRR*-α-tocopherol are hydrolysed more slowly than esters of *RRR*-α-tocopherol. Apart from the liver, body tissues show preferential uptake of *RRR*-α-tocopherol, and in all tissues the retention of *RRR*-α-tocopherol is very much greater than that of *SRR*-α-tocopherol (Ingold *et al.* 1987)

Following oral administration of [^{2}H]-tocopherol acetate, label is observed initially in the chylomicron fraction of plasma lipoproteins, then in very low density lipoproteins (VLDL), followed by an increase in the tocopherol content of low density and high density lipoproteins (LDL and HDL), and finally in erythrocyte membranes. This is consistent with absorption in chylomicrons, followed by incorporation into VLDL secreted by the liver, and appearance in LDL and HDL as a result of the metabolism of VLDL in the circulation (Traber *et al.* 1988).

The major route of excretion is in the bile, largely as unidentified metabolites, including glucuronides and other conjugates. There may also be significant excretion of the vitamin by the skin. After the administration of chylomicron-incorporated [^{3}H]-tocopherol to rats there is not only a significant accumulation and retention of radioactivity in the skin, but also on the outer surface and in the fur (Shiratori 1974).

Tocopherol undergoes oxidation to a quinone, which may be reduced to the hydroquinone. The side-chain of the quinone and hydroquinone may be oxidized by β-oxidation, and small amounts of these oxidation products and their conjugates are excreted in the urine, accounting for only about 1 per cent of a test dose of labelled tocopherol.

15.3.1 Tissue uptake of vitamin E

There are two mechanisms for tissue uptake of vitamin E. Lipoprotein lipase releases the vitamin by hydrolysing the triacylglycerols in chylomicrons and VLDL, while separately there is uptake of LDL-bound vitamin E by means of LDL receptors (see section 8.3.2). Retention within tissues depends on binding proteins, and it is likely that the differences in biological activity and tissue retention of the vitamers and between the stereoisomers of α-tocopherol are mainly due to differential protein binding. γ-Tocopherol and α-tocotrienol bind relatively poorly, while *SRR*-α-tocopherol and *RRR*-α-tocopherol acetate do not bind to liver tocopherol-binding protein to any significant extent (Catignani 1980).

Although tocopherol binding protein is cytosolic, is seems likely that it functions to transport the vitamin into membranes, since the majority of vitamin E in tissues is associated with the membrane lipids. The stereochemistry of the side chain will also affect the incorporation of the vitamin into membranes.

15.4   Absorption and metabolism of selenium

Selenium in foods may be present as inorganic selenites (SeO_3^{2-}), selenates (SeO_4^{2-}), or selenium analogues of the sulphur amino acids, selenocysteine and selenomethionine; selenium-resistant plants growing on soils with high selenium availability also form selenomethylcysteine and selenohomocysteine, which may accumulate to as much as 5000 parts per million, posing a serious toxic hazard to animals consuming them.

Both inorganic selenium salts and organic selenium compounds seem to be well absorbed, although there is little information on the mechanism and regulation of absorption. Selenocysteine is degraded by selenocysteine β-lyase (a vitamin B_6-dependent enzyme, see section 20.4) to yield selenide (Se^{2-}) and alanine; selenate and selenite are reduced to selenide by glutathione reductase.

While some inorganic selenide may be excreted, the major fate of excess selenide is formation of dimethylselenide, $(CH_3)_2Se$ and the trimethylselonium ion $(CH_3)_3Se^+$; this latter is the major urinary selenium metabolite. Over a wide range of selenium intakes, urinary excretion represents about 55–60 per cent of intake, with less than 5 per cent in sweat and less than 1 per cent in breath. With high and toxic levels of intake, sweat and breath elimination of (foul smelling) selenium compounds becomes more important.

Total body selenium has been variously estimated as 0.17–0.25 mmol (13–20 mg) in USA and 0.05–0.13 mmol (4–10 mg) in New Zealand (Nève *et al.* 1985). Apart from the liver, muscle contains the highest concentration of selenium; skeletal muscle contains more than cardiac muscle; ranges of selenium concentration in various tissues are shown in Table 15.7.

15.4.1   The formation of selenocysteine

The metabolic function of selenium is as the selenium analogue of cysteine, selenocysteine, in the catalytic sites of glutathione peroxidase (see section 15.5.1) and thyroxine deiodinase (see section 25.14.3).

Selenocysteine is incorporated into the proteins during synthesis on the ribosome, rather than being formed by post-synthetic modification of a precursor protein. The codon for selenocysteine is UGA, which normally acts as a STOP codon (see Table 10.4), signalling the end of the gene being translated. In the synthesis of proteins that contain selenocysteine, this codon is read in a context-sensitive manner to code for selenocysteine rather than termination. This context-sensitive reading of the UGA codon is the result of a sequence of four nucleotides in the untranslated region at the 3' end of the mRNA; deletion of this sequence *in vitro* from the genes for selenoproteins abolishes the incorporation of selenocysteine, and leads to termination of translation. Conversely, introduction of the sequence into genes for other proteins results in translation of UGA as selenocysteine rather than STOP (Chambers *et al.* 1986; Shen *et al.* 1993).

Selenocysteine is formed from serine bound to tRNA, by reaction with inorganic selenide; phosphorylation of serine is not required for the reaction, which appears to be pyridoxal phosphate dependent. Serine bound to the major species of tRNA for serine is not a substrate for this reaction; only serine that is bound to the tRNA that has the anticodon to UGA undergoes reaction (Mizutani *et al.* 1991).

15.5   Metabolic functions of vitamin E and selenium

15.5.1 Antioxidant actions

Vitamin E functions as a non-enzymic lipid antioxidant both *in vitro* and *in vivo*; a number of synthetic antioxidants will prevent or cure most of the signs of vitamin E deficiency in experimental animals (see Table 15.8).

A number of highly reactive oxygen species, including hydrogen peroxide, superoxide, and other oxygen radicals (see Table 15.9) are formed during normal oxidative metabolism (see section 18.4.1), and in increased amounts in activated macrophages—the respiratory burst, part of the normal response to bacterial invasion of the body. Free radicals have an unpaired electron, and are therefore highly reactive; the unpaired electron is represented by the dot notation, as in, for example $^{\bullet}OH$, the hydroxyl radical. As shown in Table 15.9, half-lives of oxygen radicals in solution are in the range of 10^{-9}–10^{-6} sec, before they collide with another molecule, acquire an additional electron (and hence a stable chemical configuration) for themselves, and form a new radical as a result of the abstraction of an electron from the donor molecule. Radical reactions are thus self-perpetuating chain reactions.

Polyunsaturated fatty acids undergo oxidative attack by reactive oxygen species (especially superoxide and the hydroxyl radical) to yield alkylperoxyl (alkyldioxyl) radicals, which perpetuate a chain reaction in the lipid, with potentially disastrous consequences for cell membranes; apart from the direct damage to membrane lipids, the products of alkylperoxyl radical breakdown have membrane lytic activity.

Similar direct oxidative radical damage can occur to proteins and nucleic acids. More importantly, both proteins and nucleic acids are subject to attack by the reactive dialdehydes resulting from the breakdown (dismutation) of lipid alkylperoxyl radicals. Modification of proteins may result in the development of autoimmune disease, as antibodies are raised against the modified proteins, while modification of DNA leads to mutagenesis (in the germ-line cells) and initiation of carcinogenesis in other tissues.

A variety of compounds, collectively known as antioxidants, can break the lipid peroxidation chain reaction by trapping the radicals, forming non-radical products from the oxidized lipid, and themselves forming radicals which are relatively stable, because the lone electron can be delocalized in an aromatic ring or conjugated double-bond system. Stable radicals persist long enough for non-enzymic reaction between two radicals to occur, yielding a non-radical product, since the lone electrons of the two radicals form a stable pair. The major radical-trapping compounds found in plasma are shown in Table 15.10.

Phenolic compounds are especially effective as radical-trapping antioxidants, forming the stable phenoxyl radical, which may either react with a further alkylperoxyl radical to yield non-radical products, or may be reduced back to the starting phenol by reaction with a water-soluble reducing agent. Vitamin E is one of the most active such radical-trapping chain-breaking antioxidant phenols that has been investigated, and is the major lipid-soluble antioxidant in tissues (Burton and Ingold 1981, 1984).

Tocopherol acts in a catalytic manner as an antioxidant in membranes, interacting non-enzymically with ascorbate in the aqueous phase at the membrane surface. As shown in Fig. 15.2, the tocopheroxyl radical formed by reaction of α-tocopherol with a lipid peroxide radical can be reduced back to α-tocopherol by reaction with ascorbate to yield the monodehydroascorbate radical, which in turn can either be reduced back to ascorbate, or can undergo dismuta-

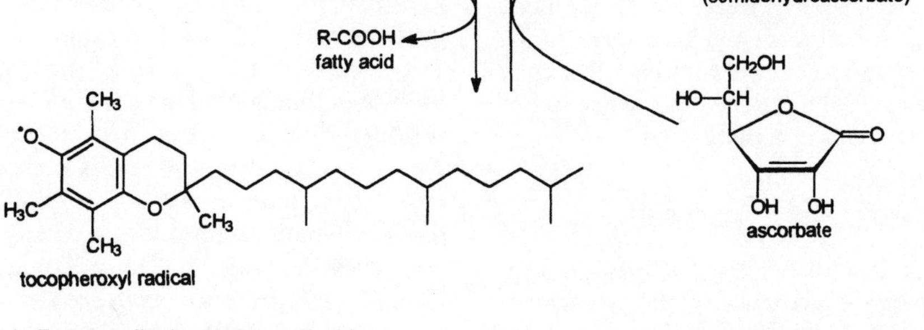

Figure 15.2 Vitamin E as a radical-trapping antioxidant·

tion to yield dehydroascorbate and ascorbate (see section 22.3.2).

The seleno-enzyme glutathione peroxidase reduces hydrogen peroxide to water, and so lowers the amount of peroxide available for the generation of radicals, while vitamin E is involved in removing the products of attack by these radicals on lipids. Thus, in vitamin E deficiency, selenium has a beneficial effect in lowering the concentrations of precursors of lipid alkylperoxyl radicals, and conversely, in selenium deficiency, vitamin E has a protective effect by removing the radicals.

When selenium is adequate but vitamin E is deficient, tissues with a low innate activity of glutathione peroxidase (e.g. the central nervous system and (rat) placenta) are especially susceptible to lipid peroxidation, while tissues with high activity of glutathione peroxidase are not. Conversely, with adequate vitamin E and inadequate selenium, membrane lipid peroxidation will be inhibited, but tissues with high peroxide production and low innate catalase activity will still be at risk from peroxidative damage, especially to sulphydryl proteins.

In the absence of ascorbate, physiological concentrations of α-tocopherol have less radical-scavenging activity than when ascorbate is present. However, the tocopheroxyl radical can be reduced to tocopherol by reaction with glutathione, catalysed by a membrane-specific isoenzyme of hydroperoxide glutathione peroxidase, which is a seleno-enzyme. Thus, in addition to its role in removing products of lipid peroxidation, selenium has a direct role in the recycling of tocopherol (Maiorino *et al.* 1989).

There may also be an effect of selenium deficiency on vitamin E nutrition. Selenium deficiency causes a specific pancreatic atrophy, which is unresponsive to vitamin E supplements; in turn this leads to impaired secretion of lipase, and hence impaired absorption of dietary lipids in general, which will affect the absorption of vitamin E (Thompson and Scott 1970).

The sulphur amino acids, methionine and cysteine, have a sparing effect on both selenium and vitamin E, presumably by permitting increased *de novo* synthesis of glutathione (GSH), and hence reducing the need for reduction and recycling of oxidized glutathione (GSSG). When tissue cysteine is limiting, this may reduce the synthesis of glutathione, and hence prejudice glutathione peroxidase activity.

15.5.2 Specific membrane functions of α-tocopherol

The differing biological activities of the isomers of α-tocopherol, and the considerably lower vitamin activity of the tocotrienols than the corresponding tocopherols (see Table 15.6) result largely from the steric requirements for incorporation of the vitamin into lipid membranes, although the affinity of intracellular binding proteins is also important for tissue uptake and retention. Diplock and Lucy (1973) proposed that in addition to its antioxidant role, α-tocopherol may have a specific physicochemical role in ordering membrane lipids, and especially phospholipids rich in arachidonic acid (see section 8.1.2 and Table 8.4).

The side-chain of *RRR*-α-tocopherol interacts closely with the methylene-interrupted *cis*-double bonds of arachidonate and other long-chain polyunsaturated fatty acids, thus stabilizing membrane structure. This will both protect membrane polyunsaturated fatty acids from oxidation and also minimize susceptibility to phospholipase attack. α-Tocopherol thus functions to preserve the impermeability of membranes, and perhaps provide some protection against phospholipase action, by preventing the liberation of fatty acids, and hence their lytic action. Obviously, the stereochemistry of the side chain will be critically important in such a function, and while the other vitamers may share the relatively non-specific antioxidant role of the vitamin, it must be assumed that only *RRR*-α-tocopherol will have the appropriate configuration to interact with membrane phospholipids.

The molar ratio of tocopherol:arachidonate in membranes is 1:500; only very small amounts of *RRR*-α-tocopherol will be required for the membrane specific actions, and it is likely that synthetic antioxidants and the other tocopherols and tocotrienols will spare *RRR*-α-tocopherol for this role.

15.5.3 Other functions of selenium

As discussed in section 25.14.2, thyroxine deiodinase is also a seleno-protein, and when iodine intake is marginal, inadequacy of selenium can lead be a factor in the development of goitre and cretinism.

Selenoprotein P is a plasma glycoprotein of unknown function which contains 7–8 selenocysteine residues /molecule. Under normal conditions some 65 per cent of plasma selenium is present in selenoprotein P; the concentration falls from 25–30 mg protein /L in selenium adequacy to < 3 mg /L in selenium deficiency. It has a rapid turnover (a half-life of 3–4 hours), and the gene is expressed in most tissues (Burk and Hill 1994).

15.6 Deficiency

15.6.1 Vitamin E deficiency in experimental animals

Vitamin E deficient female animals have an impaired ability to carry through a pregnancy. This is the basis of the commonest biological assay of the vitamin; female rats are maintained for 2–3 months on a vitamin E free diet, and are then mated. Impregnation and implantation proceed normally, but if they are not provided with vitamin E the foetuses die and are resorbed; five days after mating the animals are killed and the number of surviving foetuses gives an index of the biological activity of the test compound, relative to standard doses of α-tocopherol. Synthetic antioxidants can replace vitamin E for this function, but selenium cannot.

In male animals deficiency results in testicular atrophy, with degeneration of the germinal epithelium of the seminiferous tubules. This lesion responds to vitamin E or selenium, but not to synthetic antioxidants. There is no evidence that vitamin E deficiency has any similar effects on human fertility, and it is a considerable leap of logic from the effects of gross depletion in experimental animals to the popular, and unfounded, claims for vitamin E in enhancing human fertility and virility.

Deficiency results in the development of necrotizing myopathy, sometimes including cardiac muscle. This has been called nutritional muscular dystrophy, an unfortunate term, since deficiency of the vitamin is not a factor in the aetiology of human muscular dystrophies, and supplements of the vitamin have no beneficial effect. The necrotizing myopathy responds to selenium, but not to synthetic antioxidants (Horwitt 1965).

Vitamin E deficient animals show exudative diathesis, in which there is leakage of blood plasma from capillaries into subcutaneous tissues, apparently the result of abnormal permeability of capillary blood vessels. There is an accumulation of (usually green-coloured) fluid under the skin, and increased erythrocyte haemolysis, both of which respond to synthetic antioxidants or selenium.

Lipid peroxidation is increased in vitamin E deficiency, and subsequent catabolism of the peroxides results in the formation of malondialdehyde and other aldehydes. These can form Schiff bases with amino groups of proteins, free amino acids and nucleic acids. The resultant fluorescent pigments are called ceroid pigments, lipopigments or lipofuscin, and accumulate in increased amounts in liver and other tissues of deficient animals (Manwaring and Csallany 1988).

The nervous system is also affected in deficiency, with the development of central nervous system necrosis (nutritional encephalomacia), a condition which can be exacerbated by feeding a diet especially rich in polyunsaturated fatty acids, and, later, axonal dystrophy. This may be the result of neuronal deposition of ceroid pigments (neuronal ceroid lipofuschinosis). Synthetic antioxidants, but not selenium, can prevent these changes. The neuropathy begins from axonal membrane injury, and then develops as a distal and dying-back type of axonopathy.

15.6.2 Human vitamin E deficiency

Vitamin E is essential for man, although deficiency is not a problem even in people living on relatively poor diets. In depletion studies, very low intakes of vitamin E must be maintained for many months before there is any significant fall in circulating tocopherol, because there are relatively large tissue reserves of the vitamin. Deficiency develops in patients with severe fat malabsorption, cystic fibrosis, some forms of chronic liver disease and in rare patients with congenital abetalipoproteinaemia. These patients show neuropathy and necrotizing myopathy similar to those seen in vitamin E deficient experimental animals, and affected infants may develop retinal degeneration similar to the retrolental fibroplasia seen in premature infants suffering oxygen toxicity, as well as the accumulation of ceroid pigments (Muller *et al.* 1983; Muller 1986; Sokol 1988).

In premature infants, whose reserves of the vitamin are inadequate, vitamin E deficiency is manifest in a shortened half-life of erythrocytes, which can progress to increased intravascular haemolysis, and haemolytic anaemia. Especially where such infants are treated with hyperbaric oxygen, there is a risk of damage to the retina (retrolental fibroplasia), and vitamin E supplements may be protective, although this is not firmly established (Phelps 1987).

15.6.3 Selenium deficiency

Keshan disease is an endemic cardiac myopathy occurring in selenium-deficient areas of China, where intakes may be as low as 0.03–0.25 µmol, (2–20 µg) /day. It is characterized by cardiac insufficiency, heart enlargement, arrhythmia and electrocardiograph changes, and affects especially children and young women. Provision of supplements of 2–4 µmol /week eradicates the problem in endemic areas. Some studies have shown poor selenium status in patients in Europe with congestive cardiomyopathy either due to alcohol abuse or of unknown origin.

Kashin–Beck syndrome is an endemic osteoarthropy characterized by weakness, joint stiffness and pain, with degeneration and necrosis of joints and epiphyseal-plate cartilage of the arms and legs. Like Keshan disease, it occurs in low-selenium areas of China, and also responds favourably to selenium supplements (Ge and Yang 1993).

The role of selenium deficiency in the aetiology of endemic cretinism in areas of iodine deficiency is discussed in section 25.14.4.2.

15.7   Assessment of vitamin E and selenium nutritional status

The most commonly used index of vitamin E nutritional status is the plasma concentration of α-tocopherol; because tocopherol is transported in plasma lipoproteins this is best expressed /mol cholesterol or / mg total plasma lipids—see Table 15.11.

Gey (1989) has shown that there is an inverse relationship between plasma α-tocopherol and risk of ischaemic heart disease over a range of 2.5–4.0 mmol/mol cholesterol, and has suggested an optimum or desirable plasma concentration > 4 mmol α-tocopherol /mol cholesterol (> 3.4 μmol /g total plasma lipid).

Erythrocytes are incapable of *de novo* lipid synthesis, so peroxidative damage resulting from oxygen stress has a serious effect, shortening red cell life and possibly precipitating haemolytic anaemia in vitamin E deficiency. This has been exploited as an *in vitro* method of assessing status by measuring the haemolysis of red cells, induced by either dilute hydrogen peroxide or dialuric acid, expressed as a ratio of per centage of the haemolysis observed on incubation in water. This gives a means of assessing the functional adequacy of vitamin E intake, albeit one that will be affected by other, unrelated, factors. Plasma concentrations of α-tocopherol below 2.2 mmol /mol cholesterol or 1.1 μmol /g total plasma lipid are associated with increased susceptibility of erythrocytes to induced haemolysis *in vitro*.

An alternative method of assessing functional antioxidant status, again one that is affected by both vitamin E and other antioxidants, is by measuring the exhalation of pentane arising from the catabolism of the products of peroxidation of ω-6 polyunsaturated fatty acids or ethane arising from ω-3 polyunsaturated fatty acids. Intravenous infusion of a lipid mixture rich in linoleic acid stresses antioxidant capacity and results in increased breath pentane; this is more marked in subjects with low vitamin E status, and the administration of vitamin E reduces the exhalation of pentane (van Gossum *et al.* 1988; Tappel and Dillard 1981).

The only really useful index of selenium nutritional status is measurement of whole blood or plasma selenium; reference ranges are shown in Table 15.12. Concentrations in hair and toenails also reflect total body content, but are probably of more use for detection of selenosis than of deficiency. A number of shampoos contain selenium, which will cause falsely high results.

The activity of the erythrocyte glutathione peroxidase enzyme is only correlated with whole blood selenium below about 1 μmol /L—below the acceptable range. Thereafter there is no increase in enzyme activity with increasing selenium status. Furthermore, in addition to selenium-dependent glutathione peroxidase, there is a selenium-independent isoenzyme (Diplock 1993, Van Deel and Deelstra 1993).

15.8   Pharmacological uses and toxicity of vitamin E and selenium

Animal studies show some protective effects of tocopherol supplements against a variety of radical generating chemical toxicants, and there is evidence that relatively high levels of intake (considerably higher than those considered adequate to meet requirements, and higher than could be obtained from foods) are protective against ischaemic heart disease and some forms of cancer in human beings (Gey 1989; alpha-Tocopherol, beta-Carotene Cancer Prevention Study Group 1994).

There are no established pharmacological uses of vitamin E except for the protection of pre-term infants exposed to high partial pressure oxygen, who may develop the retinopathy of prematurity (retrolental fibroplasia); however, even here the protective effect of vitamin E is controversial and it is not routinely recommended (Phelps 1987).

Vitamin E has very low toxicity. WHO has established an Acceptable Daily Intake between 0.15–2.0 mg α-tocopherol /kg body weight, and habitual intake of supplements of up to 720 mg /day (compared with an average dietary intake of 8–12 mg /day) have no detectable adverse effects. Kappus and Diplock (1992) concluded a review of the safety of vitamin E by stating that intakes between 100–300 mg /day can be considered to be completely harmless, with a risk of adverse effects only at intakes above 3 g /day.

By contrast, selenium toxicity is a problem in areas of the world where the available soil selenium is relatively high; the first description of selenium poisoning in animals, as a result of grazing on plants that accumulate selenium is attributed to Marco Polo in the thirteenth century (Spallholz 1994).

Human toxicity (selenosis) is associated with intakes above 12 μmol (1 mg) /day, leading to thickening and loss of fingernails, erythematous bullous dermatitis, loss of hair, neurological abnormalities involving paraesthesia, paralysis and hemiplegia, as well as a garlic-like body odour. At intakes above 9.5 μmol (0.75 mg) /day there is disturbance of selenium homeostasis (Yang *et al.* 1983, 1989*a, b*).

It is suggested that the maximum safe intake of selenium from all sources should not exceed 5.7 μmol (450 μg), or 6 μg /kg body weight /day (Department of Health 1991)—only 6–8-fold higher than the reference intakes shown in Table 15.3.

Further reading

Bender, D.A. (1992). Vitamin E: tocopherols and tocotrienols. In *Nutritional Biochemistry of the Vitamins*. Chapter 4 pp. 87–105. Cambridge University Press.

Bieri, J.G. and Farrell, P.M. (1976). Vitamin E. *Vitamins and Hormones*, **34**, 31–75.

Bieri, J.G., Corash, L. and Hubbard, V.S. (1983). Medical uses of vitamin E. *New England Journal of Medicine*, **308**, 1063–1071.

Diplock, A.T. (1985). Vitamin E. In *Fat-soluble Vitamins: their Biochemistry and Applications*, (ed. A.T. Diplock), Chapter 3, pp. 154–224. Heinemann, London.

Flohé, L. (1988). The selenoprotein glutathione peroxidase, *Glutathione: Chemical Biological and Medical Aspects*, (ed. D. Dolphin, O. Avramovic, and R. Poulson), Part A, Chapter 16, pp 553–96. Wiley-Interscience, New York.

Friedrich, W. (1988). Vitamin E. In *Vitamins*, Chapter 4, pp. 219–84 Walter de Gruyter, Berlin.

Halliwell, B. and Gutteridge, J.M.C. (1984). Oxygen toxicity oxygen radicals transition metals and disease. *Biochemical Journal*, **219**, 1–14.

Muller, D.P.R. (1987). Free radical problems of the newborn. *Proceedings of the Nutrition Society*, **46**, 69–75.

Slater, T. F., Cheeseman, K. H., Davies, M. J., Proudfoot, K. and Xin, W. (1987). Free radical mechanisms in relation to tissue injury. *Proceedings of the Nutrition Society*, **46**, 1–12.

Spallholz, J.E. (1994). On the nature of selenium toxicity and carcinostatic action. *Free Radicals in Biology and Medicine*, **17**, 45–64.

Tappel, A.L. (1965). Free radical lipid peroxidation damage and its inhibition by vitamin E and selenium. *Federation Proceedings*, **24**, 73–8.

Table 15.1: Reference intakes of vitamin E

	US RDA (1989)
	mg α-tocopherol equivalent
birth-6m	3
6m-1y	4
1-3	6
4-6	7
7-10	7
males, 11-adult	10
females, 11-adult	8
pregnant	10
lactating	12

Source: National Research Council 1989.

Table 15.2: Average intakes of vitamin E (mg α-tocopherol equivalents /day) in UK

age	males mean	median	95% range	females mean	median	95% range
1.5-2.5	3.8	3.5	1.4-8.5	3.8	3.5	1.4-8.5
2.5-3.5	4.4	4.1	1.8-8.5	4.4	4.1	1.8-8.5
3.5-4.5	5.0	4.5	2.1-10.0	4.5	4.1	2.0-9.2
16-24	9.7	9.2	3.5-18.6	6.8	6.1	2.4-13.8
25-34	10.2	9.6	3.8-18.2	7.3	7.0	2.1-15.1
35-49	10.4	9.4	3.8-24.0	7.6	7.0	3.0-16.1
50-64	9.2	8.8	2.6-18.1	7.0	6.6	2.4-14.1

Source: from data reported by Gregory *et al.* 1990, 1995.

Table 15.3 Reference intakes of selenium (μg/day)

	US RDA (1989)	UK RNI (1991)	EU PRI (1993)
birth-3 m	10	10	-
3-6 m	10	13	-
7-12 m	15	10	8
1-3 y	20	15	10
4-6 y	20	20	15
7-10 y	30	30	25
males			
11-14 y	40	45	35
15-18 y	50	70	45
19-24 y	70	75	55
adults	70	75	55
females			
11-14 y	45	45	35
15-18 y	50	60	45
19-24 y	55	60	55
adults	55	60	55
pregnant	65	-	55
lactating	75	+ 15	70

Source: National Research Council 1989; Department of Health 1991; Scientific Committee for Food 1993.

Table 15.4: Rich sources of selenium

	portion (g)	μg /portion
Brazil nuts	25	383
kidney	150	165
tuna canned in oil	150	135
sardines canned in oil	150	75
shrimps	150	74
mussels	150	68
lemon sole	150	66
kipper, herring	150	65
lentils	150	60
sardines canned in tomato	150	56
plaice	150	54
cod	175	49
mackerel	150	45
trout	150	36
whiting	150	33
rabbit	150	32
crab	175	30
pilchards in tomato sauce	100	30
salmon	150	30
prawns	150	27
bread, wholemeal	70	25
mung beans (dahl)	150	24
smoked salmon	100	24
cockles	50	23
scampi	150	23
liver	150	21
pork	150	21
pork chops	150	21
bread, white	60	17
beans, red kidney	100	16
beef, canned corned	150	12
veal	150	12
chicken	150	11
egg	70	8
ham	85	7
rice	165	7

Table 15.5: Intakes of selenium and blood selenium concentrations.

	selenium intake		plasma selenium
	μmol /d	μg /day	μmol /L
China (low selenium areas)	0.14	11	0.13-0.38
New Zealand	0.35-0.40	28-32	0.57-1.14
Finland	0.38	30	0.63-1.01
Sweden	0.29-0.57	23-45	1.14-1.77
Belgium	0.63-0.76	73-60	1.20-2.10
Japan	1.12-1.27	88-100	-
USA	0.76-2.79	60-220	1.90-3.17
Canada	1.39-2.79	110-220	1.90-3.07
China and Venezuala (seleniferous areas)	> 2.79	> 220	> 4.40

Source: from data reported by Nève *et al.* 1985.

Table 15.6: Relative biological activity of the vitamin E vitamers

	M_r	iu /mg	iu /mmol	relative activity
D-α-tocopherol (*RRR*)	430.7	1.49	642	1.0
D-β-tocopherol (*RRR*)	416.7	0.75	313	0.49
D-γ-tocopherol (*RRR*)	416.7	0.15	63	0.10
D-δ-tocopherol (*RRR*)	402.7	0.05	20	0.03
D-α-tocotrienol	424.7	0.45	190	0.29
D-β-tocotrienol	410.7	0.08	33	0.05
D-γ-tocotrienol	410.7	-	-	-
D-δ-tocotrienol	396.7	-	-	-
L-α-tocopherol (SRR)	430.7	0.46	198	0.31
RRS-α-tocopherol	430.7	1.34	577	0.90
SRS-α-tocopherol	430.7	0.55	237	0.37
RSS-α-tocopherol	430.7	1.09	469	0.73
SSR-α-tocopherol	430.7	0.31	134	0.21
RSR-α-tocopherol	430.7	0.85	366	0.57
SSS-α-tocopherol	430.7	1.10	474	0.74
D-α-tocopherol acetate	488.8	1.36	664	1.03
D-α-tocopherol succinate	546.8	1.21	661	1.03
DL-α-tocopherol acetate	488.8	1.0	489	0.76

Table 15.7: Selenium content of tissues

	pmol /kg	ng /kg
muscle	3.3-7.5	260-590
liver	2.3-8.4	180-660
skin	1.5-7.9	120-620
kidney	1-1.5	80-120
lung	1-1.5	80-120
brain	0.9-1.4	70-110
testis	2-3	160-240
ovary	0.8-1.5	60-120

Source: from data reported by Dickson & Tomlinson 1967; Hamilton *et al.* 1972.

Table 15.8: Responses of experimental signs of vitamin E or selenium deficiency to vitamin E, selenium and synthetic antioxidants

	vitamin E	selenium	synthetic antioxidants
foetal resorption	+	-	+
testicular atrophy	+	+	-
necrotizing myopathy / white muscle disease	variable	+	-
cns necrosis	+	-	+
exudative diathesis	+	+	+
erythrocyte haemolysis	+	+	+
liver necrosis	variable	+	+
kidney necrosis	+	-	+

Table 15.9: Reactive oxygen species important in oxidative stress

		half-life (sec)
hydrogen peroxide	H_2O_2	stable
nitric oxide	NO^*	1-10
superoxide anion	$^\bullet O_2^-$	-
perhydroxy radical	$^\bullet HO_2$	-
hydroxyl radical	$^\bullet OH$	10^{-9}
alkoxy radical	$RO^\bullet$	10^{-6}
peroxy radical	$ROO^\bullet$	7
organic hydroperoxide	$ROOH$	-
singlet oxygen	$^iO_2$	10^{-6}

Table 15.10: Non-enzymic antioxidants in plasma

water-soluble	μmol/L
ascorbate (vitamin C)[1]	30-150
glutathione	1-2
uric acid	160-450
bilirubin	5-20
plant flavonoids[2]	variable

lipid soluble	
α-tocopherol	15-40
γ-tocopherol	3-5
total carotenoids[3]	1.1 ± 0.9
β-carotene	0.12-0.89
α-carotene	0.05-0.18
lycopene	0.01-1.05
lutein	0.1-0.3
cryptoxanthin	0.04-0.57
zeaxanthin	0.1-0.2
ubiquinol[4]	0.4-1.0
antioxidant food additives	variable

(1) See section 22.4.4.3 and 22.4.4.4
(2) See section 23.3
(3) See section 13.6.2
(4) See section 23.10

Source: from data reported by Sies *et al.*, 1992; Stahl *et al.* 1992.

Table 15.11: Indices of vitamin E nutritional status

	deficient	low	acceptable	? desirable
plasma tocopherol, μmol/L	< 12	12-16	> 16	-
plasma tocopherol, μmol /g plasma total lipid	<1.1	1.1-1.86	> 1.86	> 3.4
plasma tocopherol, mmol/mol cholesterol	< 2.2	2.2-2.25	> 2.25	> 4.0
erythrocyte fragility, ratio of haemolysis by $H_2O_2 : H_2O$	-	-	< 0.05	-

Source: from data reported by Gey 1989; Horwitt *et al.* 1972; Sauberlich *et al.* 1974.

Table 15.12: Indices of selenium nutritional status

	adequate	deficiency[1]	selenosis
whole blood selenium	1.1 μmol (90 μg) /L	0.27 μmol (21 μg) /L	> 40 μmol (3200 g) /L
plasma selenium	0.76-1.52 μmol (60-120 μg) /L	0.25-0.38 μmol (20-30 μg)/L	-
erthrocyte selenium	1.13-2.41 μmol (90-190 μg) /L	0.45 μmol (35 μg) /L	-
	1.52-8.23 nmol (120-650 ng) /g haemoglobin	1.01-1.14 nmol (80-90 ng) /g haemoglobin	-
hair selenium	4.5 nmol (360 ng) /g	< 1 nmol (80 ng) /g	> 300 nmol (24 g) /g

(1) As seen in areas with a high prevalence of Keshan disease
Source: from data reported by van Deel & Deelstra 1993; Yang *et al.* 1983.

Vitamin K was originally discovered as a result of a haemorrhagic disease in cattle fed on silage made from sweet clover, and chickens fed on solvent-extracted fat-free diets. The problem in the chickens was a lack of the vitamin in the diet, while in the cattle it was due to the presence of dicoumarol, which is an anti-metabolite of vitamin K. It soon became apparent that vitamin K was required for the synthesis of several of the proteins required for blood clotting.

It was only in 1974 (Stenflo *et al* 1974) that the metabolic role of vitamin K was elucidated, when γ-carboxyglutamate (often abbreviated to Gla) was found to be present in the vitamin K-dependent proteins, but absent from the abnormal precursors which circulate in deficiency. γ-Carboxyglutamate is chemically unstable, and undergoes spontaneous decarboxylation to glutamate under the conditions traditionally used for protein hydrolysis and amino acid analysis.

Since then a number of other proteins that undergo the same vitamin K-dependent post-translational modification (carboxylation of glutamate residues to γ-carboxyglutamate) have been discovered. All of these γ-carboxyglutamate-containing proteins bind calcium ions.

The impairment of blood clotting in response to anti-metabolites of vitamin K has been exploited in two ways: the development of clinically useful anti-coagulant drugs for patients at risk of thrombosis and, at higher doses, as rodenticides.

16.1   Vitamin K vitamers

Compounds with vitamin K activity have a 2–methyl-1,4–naphthoquinone ring. There are two naturally occurring vitamers: phylloquinone (from plants) has a 3–phytyl side chain, while the menaquinones (from bacteria) have a 3–poly-isoprenyl side chain, with up to 15 isoprenyl units (most commonly 6–10), shown by menaquinone-n (see Fig. 16.1)

Bacteria also form a variety of menaquinones with differing degrees of saturation of the side chain, variations in the positions of the double bonds and sometimes additional methylation of the naphthoquinone ring. The formation of menaquinones and ubiquinone, and the pattern of menaquinones synthesized is useful in the taxonomy and identification of bacteria. The main menaquinone synthesizing species of the intestinal flora are *Escherichia coli*, *Klebsiella pneumoniae* and *Propionobacterium* spp. (Ramotar *et al*. 1984).

The synthetic compound menadione (methylnaphthoquinone) also has vitamin activity. In the (now discarded) IUNS nomenclature, menadione was termed menaquinone, or menaquinone-0 to show that it had no side chain. In this system, phylloquinone was phytylmenaquinone and bacterial menaquinones were prenylmenaquinones. Because of the order in which they were discovered, phylloquinone is known as vitamin K_1, menaquinones are vitamin K_2 and menadione is vitamin K_3. At one time menadiol, the reduced form of menaquinone, was known as vitamin K_4; the names vitamin K_5 have been used for 4–amino-2–methyl-1–naphthol (a food preservative), vitamin K_6 for the toxic analogue 2–methyl-1,4–naphthalene diamine, and vitamin K_7 for 4–amino-3–methyl-1–naphthol.

In addition to menadione itself, menadiol diacetate (acetomenaphthone) is used in pharmaceutical preparations. Two water soluble derivatives, menadione sodium bisulphite and menadiol sodium phosphate, have been used for administration of the vitamin by injection and in patients with malabsorption syndromes which would impair the absorption of menadione, phylloquinone, and menaquinones, which are lipid soluble.

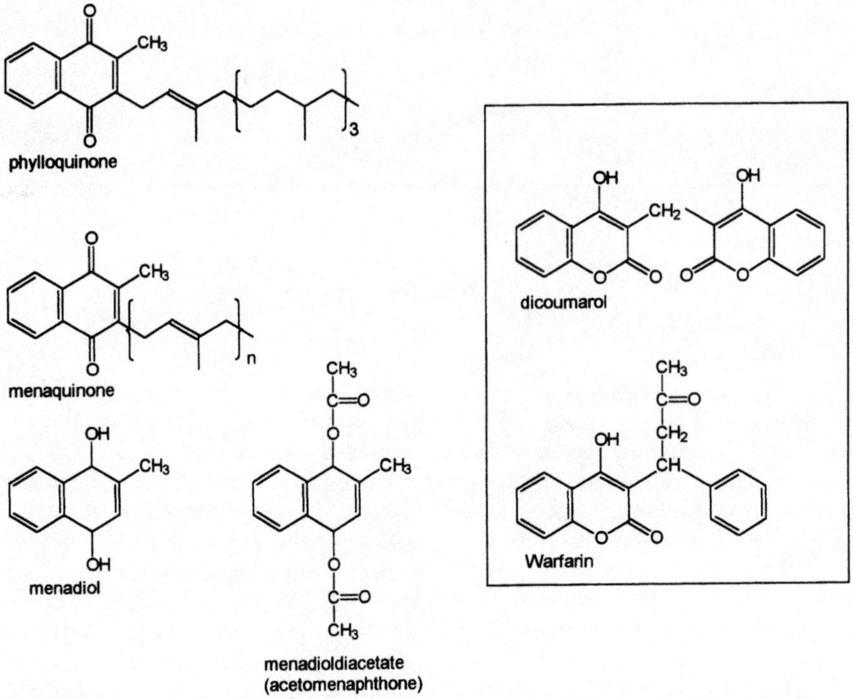

Figure 16.1 Vitamin K vitamers and antagonists
Relative molecular masses (M_r): phylloquinone 450.7, menaquinone-4 447.4, menaquinone-5 512.8, menaquinone-6 580.0, mena-quinone-7 649.0, menaquinone-8 717.1, menadione 172.2, menadiol diacetate 258.3, dicoumarol 336.3, Warfarin 308.3.

16.2   Vitamin K requirements

The determination of vitamin K requirements is complicated by the intestinal bacterial synthesis of mena-quinones, and ignorance of the extent to which these are absorbed and utilized. It is frequently suggested that about half the vitamin K requirement can be met from bacterial synthesis. There is little evidence on which to base this suggestion, other than the observation that about half the vitamin K in liver is phyllo-quinone (i.e. from dietary sources) and half a variety of menaquinones. However, the more lipophilic long-chain menaquinones may have a longer biological half-life in liver. The absorption of menaquinone from the colon is very limited, and the extent to which menaquinones are biologically active is uncertain (Shearer *et al.* 1974; Shearer 1990). Simple dietary restriction of vitamin K results in prolonged prothrombin time and increased circulating prepro-thrombin, so it is apparent that bacterial synthesis is inadequate to meet requirements in full (Suttie *et al.* 1988).

The total body pool of vitamin K is 150–200 nmol (70–100 μg); the half-life of phylloquinone is 17h,

suggesting a requirement for replacement of 50–70 μg /day. In subjects treated with neomycin to sterilize the gastro-intestinal tract, a daily intake of 0.4 μg phylloquinone is adequate to maintain normal blood clotting. On the basis of preventive studies (as opposed to earlier curative studies in deficient patients), Olson (1987a) suggested a mean daily requirement of 0.4 μg /kg body weight, and an RDA based on 0.56 g /kg body weight. Depletion / repletion studies suggest a requirement of 0.5–1 mg phylloquinone (Suttie *et al.* 1988). The US RDA, shown in Table 16.1, is based on 1 μg phylloquinone /kg body weight. The UK has published no figures for vitamin K, stating that too few studies have been performed on the variance of adult vitamin K requirements, but 1 μg /kg body weight is both safe and adequate (Department of Health 1991). The EU Working Party did not consider vitamin K (Scientific Committee for Food 1993).

16.2.1 Requirements of newborn infants

Newborn infants present a special problem with respect to vitamin K. They have low plasma levels of prothrombin and the other vitamin K-dependent clotting factors (about 30–60 per cent of the adult concentrations, depending on gestational age), and low liver reserves of vitamin K, as a result of the placental barrier which limits foetal uptake of the vitamin. Over the first 6 weeks of post-natal life the plasma concentrations of these clotting factors gradually rise to the adult level; in the meantime the infants are at risk of haemorrhagic disease of the new born. The concentration of vitamin K in human milk is relatively low, and in early infancy the intestinal flora, which at this stage are mainly *Lactobacillus* and *Bifidobacterium* spp., make no significant contribution. It is a general recommendation that newborn infants be given a prophylactic dose of 0.5–1 mg of vitamin K either orally or by injection. Because of the potential toxicity and relatively poor utilization of menadione (see section 16.7), it is usually recommended that this should be given as phylloquinone (Lane and Hathaway 1985).

16.3 Absorption and metabolism of vitamin K

Phylloquinone is absorbed in the proximal small intestine, by an apparently energy-dependent mechanism, into the lymphatic circulation; about 80 per cent of dietary intake is absorbed. Male animals are more susceptible to dietary vitamin K deprivation than females, apparently as a result of a stimulation of phylloquinone absorption by oestrogens; the administration of oestrogens increases absorption in both male and female animals (Jolly *et al.* 1977).

Menaquinones do not compete with phylloquinone for absorption, but are absorbed by passive diffusion throughout the intestinal tract, again into the lymphatic system.

Menadione is mainly absorbed by way of the portal system, although some is also absorbed in to the lymphatic system. In the liver, menadione is alkylated to menaquinone-4. The vitamin K antagonist Warfarin (see Fig. 16.1) inhibits the alkylation of menadione, although this is not its major mode of action.

Menadione that is not alkylated is rapidly metabolized, largely by reduction to menadiol, followed by the formation of the glucuronide, which is excreted in the bile, and sulphate and phosphate conjugates, which circulate in the bloodstream and are excreted in both bile and urine. Extra-hepatic tissues also form menadione conjugates. The metabolism of menadione is rapid, so that only a small proportion is converted to (biologically active) menaquinone-4.

Phylloquinone and menaquinones from the lymph are taken up by the liver, and are then released, together with menaquinone-4 formed from menadione, bound to very low density lipoprotein (see section 8.3.2); there is no specific vitamin K binding protein in plasma. After a tracer dose of radioactive phylloquinone the label is rapidly accumulated in the liver, then lost from the body with an apparent half-life of 17 hours, suggesting that there is rapid turnover and little storage of vitamin K. However, there may be considerable enterohepatic recirculation of the conjugates excreted in the bile.

The total body pool of vitamin K is 100–200 nmol (50–100 µg), of which half is in the liver. About 10 per cent of the total liver vitamin K is normally present as the epoxide, which is an intermediate in the function of the vitamin in protein carboxylation (see section 16.4).

The principal metabolites of phylloquinone and menaquinones are glucuronide conjugates of the acids which result from oxidation of the side chain. The quinone ring is reduced to the quinol to provide·a site for conjugation with glucuronic acid, phosphate or sulphate. These conjugates may then be excreted in either urine or bile. Bile normally accounts for about three times more of a test dose of $[^3H]$phylloquinone than renal excretion. After the administration of the vitamin K antagonist Warfarin there is an increase in the urinary excretion of metabolites of phylloquinone epoxide and a compensatory decrease in faecal excretion.

16.4 The metabolic function of vitamin K

The metabolic function of vitamin K is as the coenzyme in the carboxylation of protein-incorporated glutamate residues to yield γ-carboxyglutamate—a unique type of carboxylation reaction, clearly distinct from the biotin-dependent reactions discussed in section 23.1.2. Most of the vitamin K-dependent proteins are extra-cellular proteins, and therefore the major activity of vitamin K-dependent carboxylase is on the luminal side of the rough endoplasmic reticulum. However, there is also significant carboxylase activity in mitochondria. Vitamin K-dependent carboxylases are integral membrane proteins.

As shown in Fig. 16.2, the initial reaction is oxidation of vitamin K hydroquinone to the epoxide, catalysed by vitamin K epoxidase. The epoxide removes a proton from the glutamate residue to form a glutamate carbanion which then reacts non-enzymatically with carbon dioxide to form a γ-carboxyglutamate residue. The mechanism of the epoxidase is not clear; neither iron nor a flavin seems to be involved, and there is no evidence of radical intermediates (McTigue and Suttie 1983; Vidal-Cros *et al.* 1990).

Vitamin K epoxide is reduced to the quinone in a reaction involving oxidation of a dithiol to the disulphide, catalysed by epoxide reductase. The physiological dithiol substrate has not been unequivocally identified, but is assumed to be thioredoxin. Vitamin K quinone is reduced to the active hydroquinone substrate for the epoxidase reaction by either a dithiol-linked reductase similar to the epoxide reductase or NADPH-dependent quinone reductase.

It is not clear whether the epoxide reductase and the dithiol-linked quinone reductase activities are due to the same enzyme or two separate enzymes. Anticoagulants such as dicoumarol and Warfarin inhibit both vitamin K epoxide reductase and the dithiol-dependent vitamin K quinone reductase. Although resistance to Warfarin in rats is inherited as a single gene, both activities are affected, suggesting that a single enzyme might be responsible for both reactions. However, riboflavin deficiency (see section 18.5) results in decreased activity of vitamin K quinone reductase, but not of epoxide reductase. Vitamin K quinone inhibits epoxide reductase activity, although it is not clear whether this is the result of simple product inhibition, competition between two substrates for the same catalytic site, or competition for the dithiol substrate (Gurdill and Suttie 1990; Preusch and Suttie 1981, 1984).

The NADPH-dependent reduction of vitamin K quinone to the hydroquinone is not inhibited by Warfarin. In the presence of adequate amounts of vitamin K the carboxylation of glutamate residues can proceed normally, despite the presence of Warfarin, with the stoichiometric formation of vitamin K epoxide. This cannot be re-utilized, although some is reduced to 2– or 3–hydroxyvitamin K. Small amounts of vitamin K epoxide and the hydroxides are normally found in plasma; in Warfarin treated animals and patients there is a significant increase in the plasma concentration of both. There is also an increase in the urinary excretion of the products of side-chain oxidation of the epoxide and hydroxides.

16.4.1 Vitamin K-dependent blood clotting proteins

Prothrombin normally contains 10 γ-carboxyglutamate residues in the 40 amino acid sequence at the amino terminal. In the presence of high concentra-

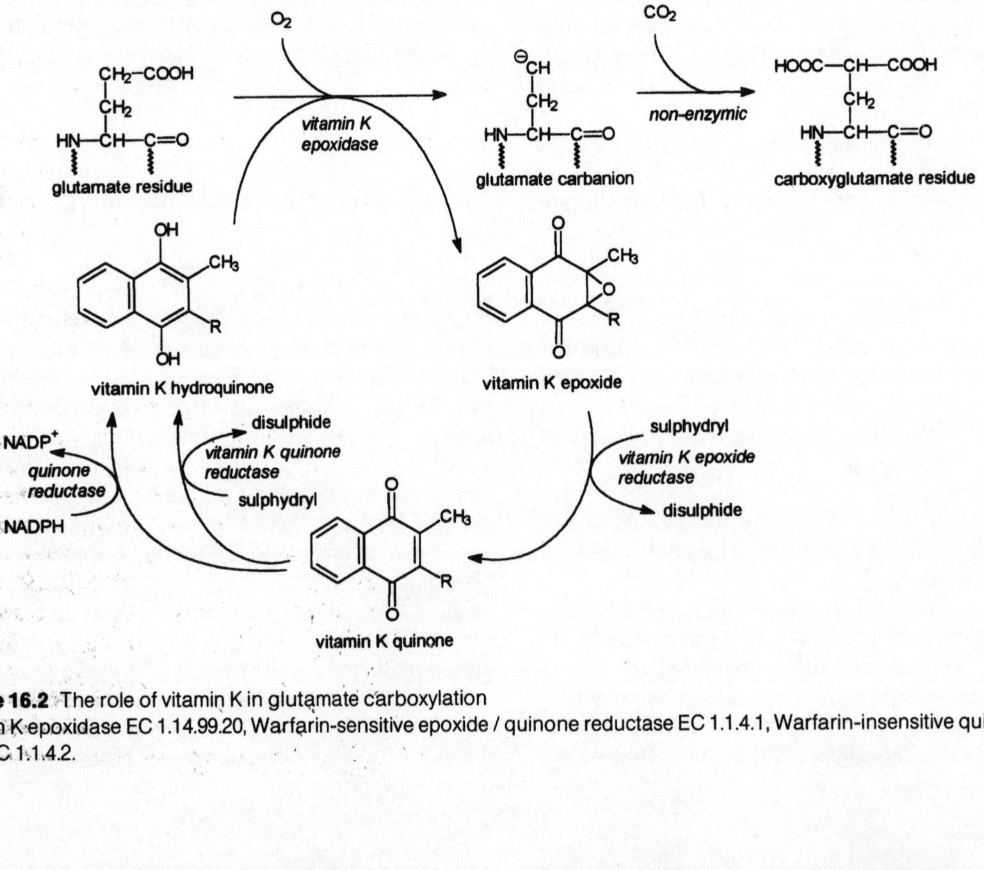

Figure 16.2 The role of vitamin K in glutamate carboxylation vitamin K epoxidase EC 1.14.99.20, Warfarin-sensitive epoxide / quinone reductase EC 1.1.4.1, Warfarin-insensitive quinone reductase EC 1.1.4.2.

tions of Warfarin, a completely uncarboxylated precursor, preprothrombin, is released into the circulation. Before the nature of this precursor protein was known, it was called 'protein induced by vitamin K absence', PIVKA, a term which is still sometimes used in the literature. At lower doses of anticoagulant partially carboxylated preprothrombins are formed.

Four vitamin K-dependent proteins involved in blood coagulation, prothrombin and Factors VII, IX, and X were discovered early in the investigations of the vitamin, as a result of the haemorrhagic disease caused by deficiency. Proteins C and S were identified later because they contain γ-carboxyglutamate. The function of γ-carboxyglutamate in these proteins is to chelate calcium, and so permit calcium-dependent binding of the proteins to negatively charged phospholipid surfaces.

The formation of blood clots is due to the conversion of the soluble protein fibrinogen into fibrin, an insoluble network of fibres. This is achieved by specific proteolysis of fibrinogen at two arginine–glycine junctions, removing two pairs of small peptides (fibrinopeptides) from fibrinogen, catalysed by thrombin. The resultant fibrin monomer aggregates into the insoluble fibrin polymer, which undergoes further covalent cross linkage, catalysed by a transa-midase, the so-called fibrin stabilizing factor or Factor XIII. Fibrin stabilizing factor is normally present as an inactive dimeric precursor, which is activated by thrombin action. The formation of an insoluble clot stops bleeding.

The initiation of the clotting process occurs on phospholipid surfaces, and the γ-carboxyglutamate residues in the various vitamin K-dependent clotting factors are essential for the calcium-dependent binding of the proteins to phospholipid.

Thrombin, which catalyses the proteolysis of fibrinogen, circulates as an inactive precursor, prothrombin, which in turn is activated by partial proteolysis to remove a peptide sequence which masks the catalytic site. There are two distinct pathways leading to the activation of prothrombin to thrombin (see Fig. 16.3 and Table 16.2).

1. The extrinsic pathway, which is initiated by thromboplastin released from injured tissues and the protease proconvertin (Factor VII).

2. The intrinsic pathway, which is initiated by the activation of Factor XII as a result of adsorption onto collagen, platelet membranes or (under laboratory conditions), glass. Factor X can also be activated by kallikrein—in turn prekallikrein

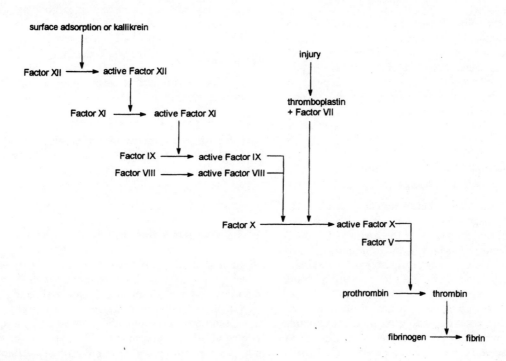

Figure 16.3 The intrinsic and extrinsic blood clotting cascades
(There is no Factor VI; what was at one time called Factor IV is calcium ions)

is activated to kallikrein by activated Factor XII, thus prolonging the initial contact activation of Factor XII. The intrinsic pathway is involved in the clotting of blood in glass tubes, and in the undesirable intravascular clotting which results in thrombosis. Control of the clotting mechanism is thus central to haemostasis, to avoid both haemorrhage and thrombosis.

Both the extrinsic and intrinsic pathways for the activation of prothrombin, and hence initiation of blood clotting, involve a number of intermediate factors. The nomenclature of the factors is based on the history of their discovery, which was largely as a result of studies in patients with various congenital defects of blood clotting.

Most of the blood clotting factors are serine proteases, which circulate as inactive zymogens. Each factor is activated by partial proteolysis, and then in turn activates the next factor—a cascade which results in considerable amplification of the original stimulus for clotting. The cascade is not a simple linear one. The concerted action of activated Factors VIII and IX is required in the intrinsic pathway for the activation of Factor X. The rate of prothrombin activation by activated Factor X alone is inadequate to meet physiological needs; an additional protein, proaccelerin or Factor V, is also required.

Like prothrombin, Factors VII, IX, and X contain γ-carboxyglutamate and hence are vitamin K-dependent, as are two further proteins: Proteins C and S, which are anticoagulants, acting to inactivate activated Factors V and VIII. Protein C is a protease which hydrolyses activated Factor V, and activates clot lysis. It circulates as a zymogen, and is activated by thrombin.

16.4.2 Osteocalcin and bone matrix γ-carboxyglutamate protein

It has long been known that treatment with Warfarin or other anticoagulants during pregnancy can lead to abnormalities of the bones of the foetus—the foetal Warfarin syndrome, which is due to impaired synthesis of osteocalcin, a γ-carboxyglutamate-containing (and hence vitamin K-dependent) protein of bone matrix.

Osteocalcin is a small calcium binding protein (46–50 amino acids depending on species), containing three γ-carboxyglutamate residues, found in bone matrix and dentine. It also contains a hydroxyproline residue, and thus undergoes both vitamin K and vitamin C-dependent post-translational mod-

ifications (see section 22.4.3). It is the most abundant of the non-collagen proteins of bone matrix, accounting for some 1–2 per cent of total bone protein. Osteocalcin synthesis is induced by physiological concentrations of calcitriol (see section 14.3.3), and release of osteocalcin into the circulation provides a sensitive marker of vitamin D action and metabolic bone disease.

Osteocalcin is synthesized in the osteoblasts as a precursor protein which then undergoes γ-carboxylation and cleavage of a peptide extension before secretion into the extracellular space, where it binds to hydroxyapatite. Its role in bone mineralization is not established, but it is associated with new bone formation rather than with resorption of existing bone matrix. It modifies the crystallization of calcium phosphates, retarding the conversion of brushite [$CaHPO_4.2H_2O$] to hydroxyapatite [$Ca_{10}(PO_4)_6(OH)_2$], and so affects the crystal structure of bone mineral.

16.4.3 Other vitamin K-dependent proteins

In addition to the blood clotting proteins and osteocalcin, γ-carboxyglutamate-containing proteins are found in.

(1) the inter-membrane space of mitochondria, where they may have a role in the mitochondrial accumulation of calcium (Gardeman and Domagk 1983);

(2) the kidney cortex;

(3) hydroxyapatite and calcium oxalate-containing urinary stones;

(4) atherosclerotic plaque (atherocalcin);

(5) soft tissues in a variety of pathological conditions involving abnormal mineralization, such as scleroderma and dermatomyositis.

16.5   Vitamin K deficiency

Vitamin K is widely distributed in green leafy vegetables and other foods, and dietary deficiency is unknown, other than under experimental conditions.

Vitamin K deficiency results in prolonged prothrombin time, and eventually haemorrhagic disease, as a result of the impairment of synthesis of the vitamin K-dependent blood clotting proteins. Although osteocalcin synthesis is similarly impaired, the effects on blood clotting predominate, and effects of vitamin

K deficiency on bone mineralization can only be demonstrated in experimental animals if they are transfused with preformed blood clotting factors. Otherwise they suffer fatal haemorrhage before there is any detectable effect on osteocalcin and bone metabolism.

The coumarin anticoagulants act as vitamin K antimetabolites, inhibiting vitamin K quinone reductase and epoxide reductase and hence causing functional vitamin K deficiency. The inhibition of vitamin K quinone reductase does not prevent the formation of the hydroquinone for epoxidase activity, since Warfarin-insensitive enzymes also catalyse the reaction. Provision of high intakes of vitamin K will overcome the inhibition of glutamate carboxylation caused by anticoagulants by permitting more or less stoichiometric utilization of the vitamin, with excretion of metabolites of the epoxide. This may cause problems with patients receiving anticoagulant therapy who take supplements of vitamin K. High dietary intakes of vitamin K, rather than supplements, are unlikely to have any significant effect on anticoagulant action; daily consumption of some 250 g of vitamin K-rich vegetables such as spinach or broccoli is required to affect prothrombin time (Karlson *et al.* 1986).

A number of antibiotics, if administered for prolonged periods, can cause or exacerbate vitamin K deficiency, and can result in bleeding defects. To some extent this may be the result of antibiotic-induced reduction in the numbers of intestinal flora, so reducing the amount of menaquinone synthesized and available for absorption. However, not all antibiotics have the same effect. Cyclosporins are especially associated with coagulopathy, and there is evidence they have a direct inhibitory effect on vitamin K epoxide reductase, acting in the same way as the coumarin anticoagulants (Matsubara *et al.* 1989).

Abnormally high intakes of vitamins A and E (such as might be obtained from dietary supplements, but considerably higher than would be expected from foods) may also result in vitamin K deficiency. Feeding chicks on diets providing 300 μg retinol /kg diet leads to an increase in prothrombin time which can be reversed by injection of menadione (Woodward and March 1974). Similarly, chicks fed on diets providing more than 1.5 g of α-tocopherol / kg diet show increased prothrombin time which responds to the administration of vitamin K, apparently as a result of competition between tocopherol quinone and vitamin K (March *et al* 1973; Rao and Mason 1975).

16.6 Assessment of vitamin K nutritional status

16.6.1 Prothrombin time and preprothrombin measurement

The usual method of assessing vitamin K nutritional status, or monitoring the efficacy of anticoagulant therapy, is a functional test of blood clotting, and hence of the ability to synthesize the vitamin K-dependent clotting factors. The standard assay measures the time taken for the formation of a fibrin clot in citrated plasma after the addition of Ca^{2+} ions and thromboplastin to activate the extrinsic clotting system—termed the prothrombin time.

Measurement of plasma concentrations of preprothrombin permits a more sensitive means of detecting marginally inadequate vitamin K status than simple determination of prothrombin time. Preprothrombin is not activated by thromboplastin, although it is a substrate for the protease from snake venom, which does not require phospholipid binding of the substrate for activity. When so activated, descarboxythrombin will catalyse clot formation from fibrinogen. This provides a means of determining the relative amounts of prothrombin and preprothrombin in blood samples. If snake venom protease is used instead of thromboplastin, the prothrombin time will be shorter, depending on how much preprothrombin is present. In normal subjects the ratio of prothrombin time using thromboplastin to that using snake venom protease is >0.6, while in vitamin K deficient or anticoagulant treated subjects it is lower (Allison *et al.* 1987).

Preprothrombin can be determined immunologically, using antibodies to prothrombin, after adsorption of the γ-carboxylated protein onto barium carbonate, or using antibodies against preprothrombin that do not cross-react with prothrombin. Circulating concentrations of preprothrombin in vitamin K deficiency are of the order of 150–1500 nmol / L, whereas it is virtually undetectable under normal conditions. If the elevated preprothromin is due to vitamin K deficiency then it will fall on administration of the vitamin, whereas if it is the result of liver disease then vitamin K supplements will have no effect (Blanchard *et al* 1981; Shearer 1990).

16.6.2 Plasma concentrations of vitamin K

The normal plasma concentration of phylloquinone in human beings has been reported as being between 0.7–5.8 nmol /L, with considerable variations between different studies. Shearer (1990) has suggested that the higher values may be erroneous, and true circulating concentrations of phylloquinone may be of the order of 1.2 nmol /L. In subjects on a restricted intake of the vitamin a fall in the plasma concentration to below 1.2 nmol /L is associated with an increase in circulating preprothrombin, and increased prothrombin time in some cases (Suttie *et al.* 1988). Because phylloquinone is transported in very low density lipoproteins, the plasma concentration is correlated with triglycerides and vitamin E (Sadowski *et al* 1989). Small amounts of menaquinones also circulate in plasma, although these are frequently below the limits of reliable determination by HPLC methods.

16.6.3 Urinary excretion of γ-carboxyglutamate

The urinary excretion of γ-carboxyglutamate, as both the free amino acid and in small peptides, also reflects functional vitamin K status, since γ-carboxyglutamate released by the catabolism of proteins is neither reutilized nor metabolized. The normal range of γ-carboxyglutamate excretion is 0.2–0.6 mol /mol creatinine in adults. Children excrete more, presumably reflecting greater turnover of osteocalcin. In patients receiving anticoagulants the urinary excretion of γ-carboxyglutamate falls to half as the prothrombin time increases 2–3–fold (Suttie *et al.* 1988).

16.7   Toxicity of vitamin K

Even large intakes of phylloquinone have no apparent toxic effects, although as discussed in section 16.5, they may be dangerous in patients receiving anticoagulant therapy.

Menadione and its water-soluble derivatives are potentially toxic in excess, causing haemolytic anaemia, hyperbilirubinaemia and kernicterus in the newborn; for this reason it is recommended that newborn infants should be given phylloquinone rather than menadione as prophylaxis against haemorrhagic disease of the newborn.

In perfused liver, menadione causes oxidation of NADPH and glutathione, and may result in considerable excretion of oxidized glutathione in the bile. In isolated hepatocytes, menadione is cytotoxic, depleting NADPH and glutathione and oxidizing thiol groups in actin, leading to anatomical abnormalities of the cytoskeleton and cell membrane. It also impairs oxidative phosphorylation by reacting directly with components of the electron transport chain, and may enter into oxygen radical-generating reactions as a result of single electron reduction to the auto-oxidizable semiquinone radical (Lind *et al.* 1982; Mirabelli *et al.* 1988; Redegeld *et al.* 1989).

Further reading

Bender, D.A. (1992). Vitamin K. In *Nutritional Biochemistry of the Vitamins*, Chapter 5, pp. 106–27. Cambridge University Press.

Friedrich, W. (1988). Vitamin K. In *Vitamins*, Chapter 5, pp. 285–338. Walter de Gruyter, Berlin.

Furie, B. and Furie, B.C. (1988). The molecular basis of blood coagulation. *Cell*, 53, 505–18.

Hauschka, P. V., Lian, J. B., Cole, D.E.C. and Gundberg, C.M. (1989). Osteocalcin and matrix Gla protein: vitamin K-dependent proteins in bone. *Physiological Reviews*, 69, 990–1047.

Olson, R.E. (1984). The function and metabolism of vitamin K. *Annual Review of Nutrition*, 4, 281–337.

Price, P.A. (1988). Role of vitamin K-dependent proteins in bone matrix. *Annual Review of Nutrition*, 8, 565–83.

Ratnoff, O.D. and Bennett, B. (1973). The genetics of hereditary disorders of blood coagulation. *Science*, 179, 1291–8.

Suttie, J.W. and Jackson, C.M. (1977). Prothrombin structure, activation and biosynthesis. *Physiological Reviews*, 57, 1–70.

Suttie, J.W. (1985). Vitamin K-dependent carboxylase. *Annual Review of Biochemistry*, 54, 459–77.

Suttie, J.W. (1985). Vitamin K. In *Fat-soluble Vitamins: their Biochemistry and Applications*, (ed. A.T. Diplock), Chapter 4, pp. 225–312. Heinemann, London.

Suttie, J.W. (1988). Vitamin K-dependent carboxylation of glutamyl residues in proteins. *Biofactors*, 1, 55–60.

Vermeer, C. (1990). γ-Carboxyglutamate-containing proteins and the vitamin K-dependent carboxylase. *Biochemical Journal*, 266, 625–36.

Table 16.1: Reference intakes of vitamin K

	US RDA (1989)
	μg
birth-6 m	5
7-12 m	10
1-3 y	15
4-6	20
7-10	30
males	
11-14	45
15-18	65
19-24	70
adult	80
females	
11-14	45
15-18	55
19-24	60
adult	65
pregnant	65
lactating	65

Source: National Research Council 1989.

Table 16.2: Proteins of the intrinsic and extrinsic blood clotting cascades.

Factor I	fibrinogen
Factor II	prothrombin (vitamin K dependent)
Factor III	thromboplastin
Factor V	proaccelerin
Factor VII	proconvertin (vitamin K dependent)
Factor VIII	anti-haemophilic factor
Factor IX	Christmas factor (vitamin K dependent)
Factor X	Stuart factor (vitamin K dependent)
Factor XI	plasma thromboplastin
Factor XII	Hageman factor
Factor XIII	fibrin stabilizing factor
Factor XIV	protein C (vitamin K dependent)

(What was at one time called Factor IV is calcium; no factor has been assigned number VI).

17

Thiamin (vitamin B$_1$)

The peripheral nervous system disease beriberi, due to thiamin deficiency, has been known sporadically for some 1300 years; it became a major problem of public health in the Far East in the nineteenth century with the introduction of the steam-powered rice mill, which resulted in more widespread consumption of highly milled (polished) rice. Thiamin was discovered as the factor in the discarded polishings which protected against the disease, and was initially called aneurine, the anti-neuritic vitamin.

While now largely eradicated, beriberi remains a problem in some parts of the world among people whose diet is especially rich in carbohydrate. A different condition, affecting the central rather than peripheral nervous system, the Wernicke–Korsakoff syndrome, also due to thiamin deficiency, occurs in developed countries, especially among alcoholics and narcotic addicts.

Thiamin was the first of the vitamins to be shown to have a clearly defined metabolic function as a coenzyme; indeed the studies of Peters' group in the 1920s and 1930s laid the foundations not only of nutritional biochemistry but also of modern metabolic biochemistry and neurochemistry. Despite this, the mechanism by which thiamin deficiency results in central or peripheral nervous system lesions remains unclear; in addition to its established coenzyme role, thiamin seems to have a role in nervous transmission.

17.1 Thiamin requirements and intake

Thiamin has a central role in energy-yielding, and especially carbohydrate, metabolism; requirements depend mainly on carbohydrate intake, and have been related to 'non-fat calories'. In practice, requirements and reference intakes are calculated on the basis of total energy intake, assuming that the average diet provides 40 per cent of energy from fat. For diets that are lower in fat content, and hence higher in

carbohydrate and protein, thiamin requirements are somewhat higher.

From depletion / repletion studies, an intake of at least 0.2 mg of thiamin /1000 kcal is required to prevent the development of deficiency signs and maintain normal urinary excretion, but an intake of 0.23 mg /1000 kcal is required for a normal transketolase activation coefficient (see section 17.6.4). At low levels of energy intake there will be a requirement for metabolism of endogenous substrates, and to maintain nervous system thiamin triphosphate.

Reference intakes (see Table 17.1) are based on 0.5 mg /1000 kcal for adults consuming more than 2000 kcal /day; the US RDA assumes a minimum requirement of 1 mg /day at low energy intake, and the UK PRI a minimum requirement of 0.8 mg /day. The EU PRI is based on an allowance of 100 µg /MJ energy expenditure, again with a minimum intake of 0.8 mg/day for people with a low energy intake.

Table 17.2 shows average intakes of thiamin in UK, and Table 17.3 the main sources in the average diet. Table 17.4 shows rich sources of thiamin.

17.2 The chemistry of thiamin

As shown in Fig. 17.1, thiamin consists of pyrimidine and thiazole rings, linked by a methylene bridge; the alcohol group of the side chain can be esterified with one, two or three phosphates, yielding thiamin monophosphate (TMP), thiamin diphosphate (TDP, also known as thiamin pyrophosphate, TPP, the metabolically active coenzyme) and thiamin triphosphate (TTP).

The free base is unstable, and two derivatives of thiamin are commonly used in food enrichment and pharmaceutical preparations: thiamin chloride hydrochloride (generally known simply as thiamin hydrochloride) and thiamin mononitrate. The mononitrate is less hygroscopic than the chloride hydro-

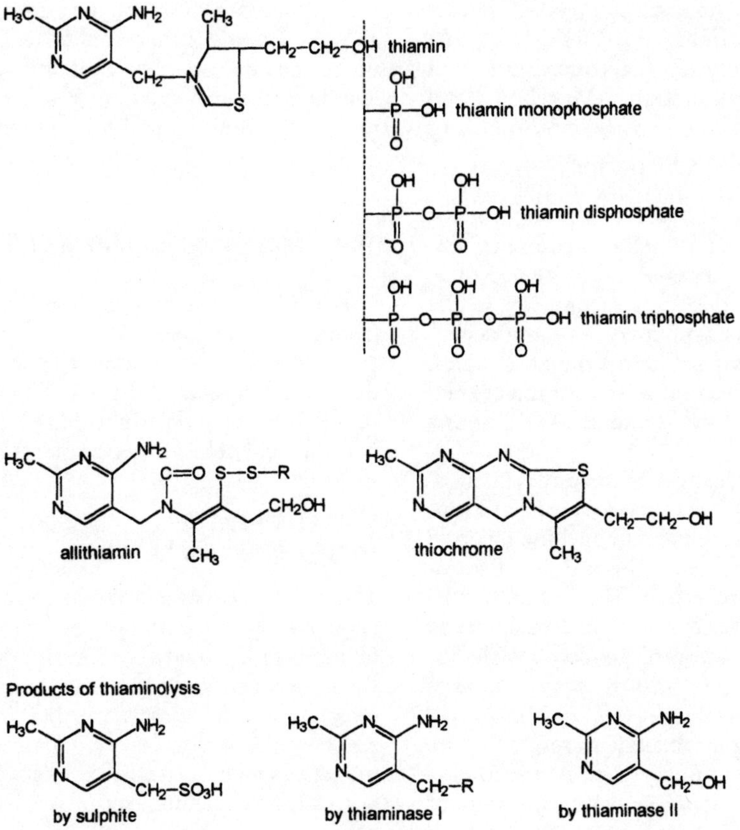

Figure 17.1 Thiamin and thiamin metabolites
Relative molecular masses (M_r): thiamin 266.4, thiamin chloride-hydrochloride 337.3, thiamin monophosphate 345.3, thiamin diphosphate 425.3, thiamin triphosphate 505.3, thiochrome 262.3.

chloride, and is the preferred form for food enrichment.

Oxidative cleavage of the thiazole ring occurs in alkaline solution, forming a reactive sulphydryl group (thiamin thiol, see Fig. 17.1), which can be reacted with other thiols, forming thiamin alkyl disulphides—allithiamins. A number of allithiamins occur in plants (especially members of the genus *Allium*). They are lipid soluble and biologically active; on reductive cleavage of the disulphide bridge they spontaneously dehydrate to yield thiamin. However, they do not undergo alkali-catalysed ring closure to thiochrome (see Fig. 17.1), which is the basis of the most commonly used method for determining thiamin chemically, so may be overlooked in chemical analysis.

Thiamin is labile to sulphite, which cleaves the methylene bridge (see Fig. 17.1). The reaction is slow at acid pH, but rapid above pH 6. Sulphite treatment of dried fruit and other foods (e.g. sausage meat and chipped potatoes) results in more or less complete loss of the thiamin.

17.3 Absorption and metabolism of thiamin

Thiamin phosphates are hydrolysed by intestinal phosphatases. The resultant free thiamin is absorbed by a sodium-independent active process in the duodenum and proximal jejunum, with little absorption in the rest of the small intestine. The transport system is saturated at relatively low concentrations of thiamin (about 2 μmol /L), so limiting the amount of thiamin that can be absorbed. At high concentrations there is some passive absorption of the vitamin, which makes only a minor contribution to thiamin nutrition. In adequately nourished subjects, increasing test doses of thiamin from 2.5 to 20 mg have only a negligible effect on the plasma concentration of thiamin or urinary excretion (Morrison and Campbell 1960). By contrast, passive absorption of the lipid soluble allithiamins is not limited.

Some thiamin is phosphorylated to thiamin monophosphate in the intestinal mucosa, although this is not essential for uptake, and isolated membrane vesicles will accumulate free thiamin against a concentration gradient. Thiamin does not accumulate in the mucosal cells; there is an (apparently sodium dependent) active efflux mechanism across the baso-lateral membrane, so that the mucosal concentration of thiamin is lower than that in the serosal fluid (Rindi and Ventura 1972).

The absorption of thiamin is impaired in alcoholics (see section 9.3.3.1). *In vitro* preparations show normal uptake of the vitamin into the mucosal cells in the presence of ethanol, but impaired transport to the serosal compartment. The sodium-potassium dependent ATPase of the baso-lateral membrane which is believed to be responsible for the active efflux of thiamin into the serosal fluid is inhibited by ethanol (Hoyumpa *et al.* 1977).

Both free thiamin and thiamin monophosphate circulate in plasma; about 60 per cent of the total is the monophosphate. Although a significant amount of newly absorbed thiamin is phosphorylated in the liver, all tissues can take up both thiamin and thiamin monophosphate, and are able to phosphorylate them to thiamin di- and triphosphates. In most tissues it is free thiamin that is the immediate precursor of thiamin diphosphate, which is formed by a pyrophosphokinase; the monophosphate arises mainly as a result of sequential hydrolysis of thiamin tri- and diphosphate.

Thiamin that is not bound to plasma proteins (mainly albumin) is rapidly filtered at the glomerulus, and there is apparently no tubular resorption of thiamin or the small amounts of phosphates which are excreted. Diuresis increases the excretion of the vitamin. Sweat may contain up to 30–56 nmol of thiamin /L, and in very hot conditions this may represent a significant loss of the vitamin.

A small amount of thiamin is excreted in the urine unchanged, accounting for about 3 per cent of a test dose, together with small amounts of thiamin monophosphate and diphosphate; one of the major excretory products is thiochrome; cyclization to thiochrome is the basis of the normal method of determining thiamin, so most reports of thiamin excretion are actually of thiamin plus thiochrome. In addition, urine contains small amounts of thiamin

disulphide, formed by the oxidation of thiamin thiol, as well as about 20 metabolites which are the result of side-chain oxidation, and cleavage of the methylene bridge with oxidation of the side chains of the resultant pyrimidine and thiazole products.

17.4   Metabolic functions of thiamin

The studies of Peters in the 1920s and 1930s (summarized in Peters 1963) established the coenzyme role of thiamin diphosphate in the oxidative decarboxylation of 2–oxo-acids and transketolase. In addition, thiamin triphosphate has a role (as yet inadequately defined) in nervous transmission.

17.4.1 Oxidative decarboxylation of pyruvate, 2–oxoglutarate and branched-chain amino acids

Thiamin diphosphate is the coenzyme for three mitochondrial multi-enzyme complexes which are involved in the oxidative decarboxylation of 2–oxoacids: pyruvate dehydrogenase (EC 1.2.4.1) and 2–oxoglutarate dehydrogenase (EC 1.2.4.2) in central energy-yielding metabolic pathways and the branched-chain oxo-acid dehydrogenase (EC 1.2.4.4) in the catabolism of leucine, isoleucine and valine.

The reaction of the pyruvate dehydrogenase complex is shown in Fig. 17.2; the reactions of the 2–oxoglutarate and branched chain oxo-acid dehydrogenase complexes follow the same sequence, and the multi-enzyme complexes have similar composition. Thiamin binds the oxo-acid substrate, decarboxylating it to an 'active aldehyde' intermediate. This is then transferred to enzyme-bound lipoamide, reducing the disulphide bridge of the lipoamide and forming a thio-ester. The resultant acyl group is transferred to CoA, and the dithiol lipoamide is re-oxidized by NAD^+.

Branched-chain oxo-acid decarboxylase is the enzyme that is affected in maple syrup urine disease (branched-chain oxo-aciduria, see Table 10.39). While a variety of different mutations are involved in different forms of the disease, at least some are due to impaired affinity of the enzyme for thiamin diphosphate. Patients with this variant of the disease respond to supplements of relatively large amounts of thiamin, of the order of several hundred mg /day, despite the limited absorption of high intakes of the vitamin. A thiamin-responsive inborn error of 2–oxoglutarate dehydrogenase has been reported, which results in anaemia because of the failure to form suf-

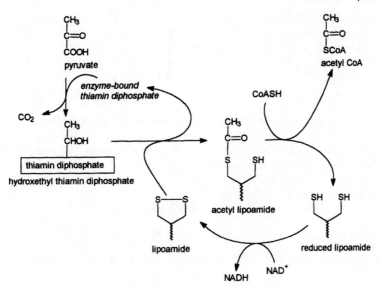

Figure 17.2 The role of thiamin in pyruvate dehydrogenase (EC 1.2.4.1)

ficient succinyl CoA for haem synthesis (Abboud *et al.* 1985).

17.4.2 Transketolase

Transketolase (EC 2.2.1.1) is a key enzyme in the pentose phosphate pathway of carbohydrate metabolism. It catalyses the transfer of a two-carbon unit from a donor ketose onto an acceptor aldose sugar. The donor ketose forms a transient intermediate with thiamin diphosphate, which then undergoes cleavage to release an aldose two carbons smaller than the ketose substrate, leaving enzyme-bound dihydroxy-ethyl thiamin diphosphate. This reacts with an acceptor aldose to form a ketose two carbons larger.

The pentose phosphate pathway is the major pathway of carbohydrate metabolism in some tissues, and a significant alternative to glycolysis (see Fig. 5.1) in all tissues. The main importance of the pathway is in the production of NADPH for use in biosynthetic reactions (and especially lipogenesis, see Fig. 5.6), and the *de novo* synthesis of ribose for nucleotide synthesis.

17.4.3 The neuronal function of thiamin triphosphate

As shown in Table 17.5, 2–3 per cent of the thiamin in nervous tissue is present as the triphosphate, which is not an intermediate in the formation or catabolism

of thiamin diphosphate. Thiamin triphosphate also occurs in significant amounts in skeletal muscle, and especially in fast-twitch muscle fibres. Unlike the nervous system, where the triphosphate is found exclusively in the 'membrane' fraction, a significant proportion of muscle thiamin triphosphate is apparently cytosolic.

The total thiamin content of different regions of the central nervous system varies; the cerebellum has the highest thiamin content, yet the lowest rate of glucose and oxygen utilization. The development of neurological abnormalities in experimental thiamin deficiency does not follow the same time-course as the impairment of pyruvate and 2–oxoglutarate dehydrogenase or transketolase activities, and the regions in which metabolic disturbances are most marked are not those that are vulnerable to anatomical lesions in deficiency.

Thiamin triphosphate in nervous tissue is protected in thiamin deficiency. While total brain thiamin falls to some 20 per cent of the control level within 4 weeks in deficient animals, with similar falls in free thiamin, and the mono- and diphosphates, there is little loss of thiamin triphosphate (Thornber *et al.* 1980). A variety of compounds which affect ion movements in nerve tissue, and electrical stimulation of isolated nerve preparations, all result in a fall in membrane thiamin triphosphate, and the release of free thiamin (Itokawa and Cooper 1970*a, b*). In isolated nerve preparations, UV illumination, which destroys thiamin, leads to loss of the action potential; addition of thiamin to the superfusion medium restores the action potential, with a time lag that is apparently due to the time taken for uptake of thiamin and phosphorylation to thiamin triphosphate (Eichenbaum and Cooper 1971).

All of this suggests that thiamin triphosphate has a role in the nervous system which is separate from the coenzyme function of thiamin diphosphate; although the mechanism is unclear, it is likely that it has a role in the nerve membrane ion pump mechanism, possibly acting as phosphate donor for the phosphorylation of one of the proteins of the sodium channel (Schoffeniels *et al.* 1984).

17.5   Thiamin deficiency

Thiamin deficiency can result in three distinct syndromes: a chronic peripheral neuritis, beriberi, which may or may not be associated with heart failure and oedema; acute pernicious (fulminating) beriberi (shoshin beriberi), in which heart failure and metabolic abnormalities predominate, with little evidence of peripheral neuritis; and Wernicke's encephalopathy with Korsakoff's psychosis, a thiamin-responsive condition associated especially with alcoholism and narcotic abuse.

In general a relatively acute deficiency is involved in the central nervous system lesions of the Wernicke–Korsakoff syndrome, and a high energy intake, as in alcoholics, is also a predisposing factor. Dry beriberi is associated with a more prolonged, and presumably less severe, deficiency, with a generally low food intake, while higher carbohydrate intake and physical activity predispose to wet beriberi.

17.5.1 Anorexia in thiamin deficiency

In experimental animals, thiamin deficiency is associated with severe anorexia; indeed, one of the problems in interpreting the literature on thiamin deficiency is distinguishing between effects of thiamin deficiency *per se* and effects due to general lack of food and inanition. Even more than with other vitamins, studies of thiamin deficiency require strict pair-feeding of control animals with those receiving the deficient diet. The mechanism of the anorexia is unclear. Its development shows a clear correlation with the loss of transketolase activity in the intestinal mucosa, but not the loss of pyruvate or 2–oxoglutarate dehydrogenase activity. Animals treated with the antagonist oxythiamin, which does not cross the blood brain barrier, and therefore has little effect on central nervous system metabolism, show anorexia. This suggests that the effect is on the intestinal mucosa rather than the central nervous system. In addition, it is possible that changes in GABA and 5–hydroxytryptamine turnover in thiamin deficiency may be involved in the aetiology of anorexia, since potentiation of GABA and 5–hydroxytryptamine activity is part of the action of a number of clinically used appetite suppressants (see section 6.4 and Table 11.32).

17.5.2 Dry beriberi

Chronic deficiency of thiamin, especially associated with a high carbohydrate diet, results in beriberi, which is a symmetrical ascending peripheral neuritis. Initially the patient complains of weakness, stiffness and cramps in the legs, and is unable to walk more than a short distance. There may be numbness of the dorsum of the feet and ankles, and vibration sense may be diminished. As the disease progresses, the ankle jerk reflex is lost, and the muscular weakness spreads upwards, involving first the extensor muscles of the foot, then the muscles of the calf, and finally the extensors and flexors of the thigh. At this stage there is pronounced toe and foot drop—the patient is unable to keep either the toe or the whole foot extended off the ground. When the arms are affected there is a similar inability to keep the hand extended—wrist drop.

The affected muscles become tender, numb and hyperaesthetic. The hyperaesthesia extends in the form of a band around the limb, the so-called stocking and glove distribution, and is followed by anaesthesia. There is deep muscle pain, and in the terminal stages, when the patient is bed-ridden, even slight pressure, as from bed clothes, causes considerable pain.

In thiamin-deficient rats, electron microscopy of the sciatic and plantar nerves shows distally pronounced axonal degeneration, with an increase in the number of mitochondria and proliferation of vesicular elements of the endoplasmic reticulum. This is followed by disintegration of neurotubules and neurofilaments, and finally axonal shrinkage and myelin disruption (Pawlik *et al.* 1977).

17.5.3 Wet beriberi

The heart may also be affected in beriberi, with dilatation of arterioles, rapid blood flow and increased pulse rate and pressure, and increased jugular venous pressure leading to right-sided heart failure and oedema—so-called wet beriberi.

The signs of chronic heart failure may be seen without peripheral neuritis. The arteriolar dilatation, and possibly also the oedema, probably result from high circulating concentrations of lactate and pyruvate, a result of impaired activity of pyruvate dehydrogenase. Together with the fall in pyruvate dehydrogenase, there is a fall in the concentration of ATP in the heart (McCandless *et al.* 1970), although in most tissues the ratio of ATP:ADP is not affected by thiamin deficiency.

17.5.4 Acute pernicious (fulminating) beriberi—shoshin beriberi

Heart failure without increased cardiac output, and no peripheral oedema, may also occur acutely, associated with severe lactic acidosis. This was a common presentation of deficiency in Japan, where it was called shoshin (acute) beriberi; in the 1920s some 26 000 deaths a year were recorded.

With improved knowledge of the cause, and improved nutritional status, the disease has become more or less unknown, although it has reappeared among Japanese adolescents consuming a diet based largely on such high carbohydrate, low nutrient, foods as sweet carbonated drinks, 'instant' noodles and polished rice (Kawai *et al.* 1980). It also occurs among alcoholics, when the lactic acidosis may be life threatening, without clear signs of heart failure (Campbell 1984). Acute beriberi has also been reported when previously starved subjects are given intravenous glucose.

Acute infantile beriberi in infants breast fed by deficient mothers may involve high output cardiac failure, as in shoshin beriberi, as well as signs of central nervous system involvement similar to those seen in Wernicke's encephalopathy.

17.5.5 The Wernicke-Korsakoff syndrome

Although the classical signs of beriberi are of peripheral neuritis, most of the biochemical studies (Peters 1963) were performed on the central nervous system of pigeons, since these birds show obvious central nervous system abnormalities in thiamin deficiency, as well as signs of peripheral neuritis. While peripheral neuritis and, as noted above, acute cardiac beriberi and lactic acidosis, occur in thiamin deficiency associated with alcohol abuse, the more usual presentation is as the Wernicke–Korsakoff syndrome, due to central nervous system lesions. Similar lesions are seen in opiate addicts, apparently associated with a high intake of sweet carbohydrate foods and low thiamin intake.

Initially there is a confused state, Korsakoff's psychosis, which is characterized by confabulation and loss of recent memory, although memory for past events may be unimpaired. Later, clear neurological signs develop—Wernicke's encephalopathy. This is characterized by nystagmus and extra-ocular palsy. *Post mortem* examination shows haemorrhagic and oedematous lesions in the thalamus, pontine tegmentum and mammillary body, with severe damage to astrocytes, neuronal dendrites and myelin sheaths (Watanabe *et al.* 1981).

Wernicke's encephalopathy may be more common than is believed on clinical grounds. Harper (1979) reported that 1.7 per cent of all *post mortem* examinations in Western Australia over a four year period showed clear anatomical evidence of the disease, yet only 13 per cent of these patients had been diagnosed as suffering from the condition before they died.

Like shoshin beriberi, Wernicke's encephalopathy can develop acutely, without the more gradual development of Korsakoff's psychosis, among previously starved patients given intravenous glucose and seriously ill patients given parenteral hyperalimentation (Handler and Perkin 1982).

17.5.6 Metabolic effects of thiamin deficiency

17.5.6.1 Carbohydrate metabolism

The role of thiamin diphosphate in pyruvate dehydrogenase means that in deficiency there is impaired conversion of pyruvate to acetyl CoA, and hence impaired entry of pyruvate into the citric acid cycle (see Fig. 5.2). Especially in subjects on a relatively high carbohydrate diet, this results in increased plasma concentrations of lactate and pyruvate, which, as discussed above, may lead to life-threatening lactic acidosis. The increase in plasma lactate and pyruvate after a test dose of glucose has been used as a means of assessing thiamin nutritional status (see section 17.6.1).

A genetic defect of pyruvate dehydrogenase has been described in children who showed intermittent attacks of cerebellar ataxia and elevation of plasma and urine lactate, pyruvate and alanine. Both the clinical signs and the neurological damage are different from those seen in thiamin deficiency, which is further evidence that while pyruvate decarboxylation is deranged in deficiency, this is not the underlying metabolic lesion (Blass *et al.* 1976).

Transketolase is more severely affected by deficiency than is pyruvate dehydrogenase, and the reduction of transketolase activity is anatomically correlated with vulnerability to lesions. However, apo-transketolase is susceptible to proteolysis, and the tissue content of the apo-enzyme falls in deficiency. The administration of thiamin to deficient animals corrects the clinical signs without restoring transketolase activity (Giguère and Butterworth 1987). Under normal conditions there seems to be a considerable excess of transketolase activity, so that even relatively severe impairment of activity has little or no effect on metabolic flux through the pentose phosphate pathway (McCandless *et al.* 1976).

17.5.6.2 Oxoglutarate dehydrogenase and the tricarboxylic acid cycle: the GABA shunt

The activity of 2–oxoglutarate dehydrogenase, a key enzyme of the citric acid cycle (see Fig. 5.2) is also impaired in thiamin deficiency. It falls more in those regions of the brain that are vulnerable to lesions, and both the development of clinical signs and their resolution on repletion with thiamin are correlated with 2–oxoglutarate activity (Butterworth *et al.* 1986). Despite this, there is not the expected lack of ATP in affected tissues, suggesting that alternative metabolic pathways, bypassing thiamin-dependent steps, may be important in energy-yielding metabolism in deficiency.

The formation and catabolism of the neurotransmitter γ-aminobutyric acid (GABA) provides an alternative to 2–oxoglutarate dehydrogenase—the so-called GABA shunt. 2–Oxoglutarate is aminated to glutamate, which is decarboxylated to GABA. GABA is inactivated by transamination to succinic semialdehyde, which is oxidized to succinate, an intermediate in the tricarboxylic acid cycle. Glutamate decarboxylase (EC 4.1.1.15) and GABA aminotransferase (EC 2.6.1.19) are found in regions of the central nervous system other than those in which GABA has a neurotransmitter role, and also in non-neuronal tissues, including liver and kidney. There is evidence of an increase in the rate of GABA turnover in thiamin deficiency, suggesting that the GABA shunt may be a significant alternative to 2–oxoglutarate dehydrogenase in energy-yielding metabolism, permitting continued tricarboxylic acid cycle activity despite the impairment of 2–oxoglutarate dehydrogenase (Page *et al.* 1989).

17.5.7 Thiaminases and thiamin antagonists

Thiaminolytic enzymes are found in a variety of micro-organisms and foods, and a number of thermostable compounds present in foods (especially polyphenols) cause oxidative cleavage of thiamin, as does sulphite, which is widely used in food processing. The products of thiamin cleavage by sulphite and thiaminases are shown in Fig. 17.1.

In people whose thiamin intake is marginal, colonization of the gastro-intestinal tract with thiaminolytic micro-organisms may be a factor in the development of beriberi. The thiaminases present in raw fish can result in so-called Chastek paralysis of foxes and mink, as a result of destruction of thiamin, and may be important in parts of the world where much of the apparent thiamin intake is from fish eaten raw or fermented. The polyphenols and thiaminase in bracken fern can cause thiamin deficiency (blind staggers) in horses, and tannic acid in tea and betel nut have been associated with human thiamin deficiency.

There are two classes of thiaminase.

1. Thiaminase I catalyses a base exchange reaction between the thiazole moiety of thiamin and a variety of bases, commonly primary, secondary or tertiary amines, but also nicotinamide and other pyridine derivatives, and sometimes proline and sulphydryl compounds. Thiaminase I is relatively widespread in a variety of micro-organisms, plants and fish. In addition to depleting thiamin, the products of base exchange catalysed by thiaminase I are structural analogues of the vitamin, and may have antagonistic effects (Edwin and Jackman 1970).

2. Thiaminase II is restricted to a small number of micro-organisms; it catalyses a simple hydrolysis, releasing thiazole and methoxypyrimidine (toxopyrimidine, which has some anti-vitamin B₆ antimetabolic activity).

The destruction of thiamin by polyphenols is not a stoichiometric reaction, and reducing compounds such as ascorbate and cysteine inhibit the reaction. In alkaline conditions the thiazole ring of thiamin undergoes a reversible cleavage to the thiol (see Fig. 6.1). Thiamin thiol can react with a variety of thiol or disulphide compounds to form alkyl thiamin derivatives (allithiamins), some of which have biological activity. However, the thiol can also undergo oxidation catalysed by polyphenols, resulting in the formation of thiamin disulphide, which has no biological activity.

17.6 Assessment of thiamin nutritional status

17.6.1 Blood lactate and pyruvate

The impairment of pyruvate dehydrogenase activity in thiamin deficiency results in a considerable increase in the plasma concentrations of lactate and pyruvate. This has been exploited as a means of assessing thiamin nutritional status, by measuring changes in the plasma concentrations of lactate, pyruvate and glucose after an oral dose of glucose and mild exercise (Horwitt and Kreisler 1949). The test is not specific for thiamin deficiency; a variety of other conditions can also result in metabolic acidosis. While it may be useful in depletion / repletion studies, it is little used nowadays in screening or assessment of nutritional status.

17.6.2 Urinary excretion of thiamin and thiochrome

Although there are a number of urinary metabolites of thiamin, a significant amount of the vitamin is excreted unchanged, especially if intake is adequate, and therefore the urinary excretion of the vitamin can provide useful information on nutritional status. Excretion decreases proportionally with intake in adequately nourished subjects, but at low intakes there is a threshold below which further reduction in intake has little effect on excretion. Reference ranges for urinary excretion are shown in Table 17.6.

The excretion of a test dose of thiamin has also been used as an index of status; following a parenteral dose of 5 mg (19 μmol) of thiamin, adequately nourished subjects excrete more than 300 nmol of the vitamin over 4 hours, while deficient subjects excrete less than 75 nmol (Sauberlich *et al.* 1974*a*).

17.6.3 Blood concentration of thiamin

In experimental animals and in depletion studies, measurement of the concentration of thiamin in plasma or whole blood provides an indication of the progression of deficiency. Whole blood total thiamin below 150 nmol /L is considered to indicate deficiency (Sauberlich *et al.* 1974a). However, the changes observed in depletion studies are small. Even in patients with frank beriberi the total thiamin concentration in erythrocytes is only 20 per cent lower than normal; whole blood thiamin is not a sensitive index of status.

17.6.4 Erythrocyte transketolase activation

The activation of apo-transketolase in erythrocyte lysate by thiamin diphosphate added *in vitro* has become the most widely used and accepted index of thiamin nutritional status. Apo-transketolase is unstable both *in vivo* and *in vitro*, so problems may arise in the interpretation of results, especially if samples have been stored for any appreciable time. An activation coefficient >1.25 is indicative of deficiency, and <1.15 is considered to reflect adequate thiamin nutrition (Brin 1964).

17.7 Toxicity of thiamin

There is no evidence of any toxic effect of high intakes of thiamin, although high parenteral doses have been reported to cause respiratory depression in animals and anaphylactic shock in human beings. Hypersensitivity and contact dermatitis have been reported in pharmaceutical workers handling thiamin. Absorption of thiamin is limited, and no more than about 10 μmol (2.5 mg) can be absorbed from a single dose; free thiamin is rapidly filtered by the kidneys and excreted.

Further reading

Bender, D.A. (1984). B vitamins in the nervous system. *Neurochemistry International*, 6, 297–321.

Bender, D.A. (1992). Vitamin B$_1$: thiamin, In *Nutritional Biochemistry of the Vitamins*, Chapter 6, pp. 128–55. Cambridge University Press.

Butterworth, R.F. (1982). Neurotransmitter function in thiamine deficiency. *Neurochemistry International* 4, 449–65.

Cooper, J. and Pincus, J.H. (1979). The role of thiamine in nervous tissue. *Neurochemical Research*, 4, 223–39.

Evans, W.C. (1975). Thiaminases and their effects on animals. *Vitamins and Hormones*, 33, 467–504.

Friedrich, W. (1988). Thiamin, vitamin B$_1$, aneurine. In *Vitamins*, Chapter 6, pp. 339–403. Walter de Gruyter, Berlin.

Haas, R.H. (1988). Thiamin and the brain. *Annual Review of Nutrition*, 8, 483–515.

Reuker, J.B., Girard, D.E. and Cooney, T.G. (1985). Wernicke's encephalopathy. *New England Journal of Medicine*, 312, 1035–8.

Table 17.1: Reference intakes for thiamin

	US RDA (1989)	UK RNI (1991)	EU PRI (1993)
	mg	mg	mg
birth—6 m	0.3	0.2	-
7—9 m	0.4	0.2	0.3
9m—1y	0.4	0.3	0.3
1—3 y	0.7	0.5	0.5
4—6	0.9	0.7	0.7
7—10	1.0	0.7	0.8
males			
11—14	1.3	0.9	1.0
15—18	1.5	1.1	1.2
19—24	1.5	1.0	1.1
25—50	1.5	1.0	1.1
> 50	1.2	0.9	-
females			
11—14	1.1	0.7	0.9
15—18	1.1	0.8	0.9
19—24	1.1	0.8	0.9
25—50	1.1	0.8	0.9
> 50	1.0	0.8	-
pregnant	1.5	+0.1	1.0
lactating	1.6	+0.2	1.1

Source: National Research Council 1989; Department of
Health 1991; Scientific Committee for Food 1993.

Table: 17.2: Average intakes of thiamin (mg /day)

(Apart from the SENECA study of the elderly, which involved 17 centres throughout Europe, all the studies quoted were in UK)

age	mean	males median	range[1]	mean	females median	range[1]	reference
1.5-2.5	0.7	0.7	0.4-1.3	0.7	0.7	0.4-1.3	Gregory *et al.* 1995
2.5-3.5	0.8	0.7	0.4-1.5	0.8	0.7	0.4-1.5	Gregory *et al.* 1995
3.5-4.5	0.9	0.9	0.4-1.4	0.8	0.8	0.4-1.3	Gregory *et al.* 1995
16-24	1.72	1.68	0.72-2.85	1.26	1.23	0.52-2.30	Gregory *et al.* 1990
25-34	1.66	1.57	0.85-2.96	1.21	1.18	0.55-2.02	Gregory *et al.* 1990
35-49	1.71	1.65	0.79-2.85	1.25	1.24	0.57-1.98	Gregory *et al.* 1990
50-64	1.70	1.69	0.78-2.83	1.25	1.23	0.70-2.05	Gregory *et al.* 1990
58-65	1.3	-	0.7-2.3	1.1	-	0.4-1.7	Davies & Holdsworth 1985
62-74	0.9	-	-	0.8	-	-	Lonergan *et al.* 1975
73-78[2]	-	1.12 (0.64-1.58)	0.46-2.13	-	0.89 (0.71-1.21)	0.44-2.11	Euronut SENECA Investigators 1991
75-90	0.9	-	-	0.7	-	-	Lonergan *et al.* 1975

(1) The range shown is the 2.5-97.5 centile for the studies of Gregory *et al.*, the 10-90 centile for the SENECA study, and the
observed extreme range for the study of Davies & Holdsworth.
(2) Data were reported for 17 separate centres; the mean and extreme values of the published median values are shown, with
the lowest 10th centile and highest 90th centile of those reported.

Table 17.3: Sources of thiamin in the average British diet

	% of average intake
potatoes	17
other vegetables	8
white bread	10
wholemeal and other bread	10
breakfast cereals	12
other cereal products	5
milk and milk products	9
bacon and ham	5
other meat	13
fruit and nuts	3
fish	2
eggs	1

Source: Gregory *et al.* 1990.

Table 17.4: Rich sources of thiamin

	portion (g)	mg /portion
cod roe, hard	100	1.3
pork, roast	150	1.0
gammon joint	150	0.9
pork chops	150	0.9
bacon joint	150	0.6
beans, red kidney	100	0.5
duck	150	0.5
kidney	150	0.5
oatmeal	100	0.5
plaice	150	0.5
ham	85	0.4
bacon rashers	85	0.3
Brazil nuts	25	0.3
liver	150	0.3
milk	560	0.3
oranges	250	0.3
peanuts	25	0.3
potato chips	265	0.3
salmon	150	0.3
venison	150	0.3
beans, haricot	100	0.2
bread, wholemeal	70	0.2
chestnuts	75	0.2
chicken	150	0.2
chickpeas	150	0.2
cod	175	0.2
crab	175	0.2
eel	150	0.2
herring roe, soft	100	0.2
lamb	150	0.2
lemon sole	150	0.2
lentils	150	0.2
lobster	150	0.2
mackerel	150	0.2
milk, skimmed	560	0.2
mung beans (dahl)	150	0.2
orange juice	200	0.2
peas	75	0.2
scampi	150	0.2
sweet potato	150	0.2
sweetcorn kernels	75	0.2
turkey	150	0.2
whiting	150	0.2

Table 17.5: Thiamin and thiamin phosphates in nervous tissues of the rat.

	total (µmol/g)	free thiamin	% of total thiamin present as monophosphate	diphosphate	triphosphate
whole brain	11-12	3.7	9.4	84	2.8
membrane fraction	-	0	11.5	71.9	16.6
mitochondria	-	0	10.9	81.6	7.5
cytosol	-	8.9	31.4	59.1	0.7
sciatic nerve	5.24	3.1	8.2	86.2	2.4

Source: Bender 1984.

Table 17.6: Indices of thiamin nutritional status

	adequate	marginal	deficient
intake			
mmol /1000kcal	> 1.1	0.75 -1.1	< 0.75
mmol /MJ	> 0.27	0.18 -0.27	< 0.18
mg /1000 kcal	> 0.3	0.2-0.29	< 0.2
µg /MJ	> 72	48-72	< 48
urinary excretion			
mmol /mol creatinine	> 28	11-27	< 11
mg /g creatinine	> 66	27-65	< 27
nmol /24h	> 375	150-375	< 150
µg /24h	> 100	40-99	< 40
urinary excretion over 4 h after a 19 nmol (5 mg) parenteral dose			
nmol	> 300	75-300	< 75
µg	> 80	20-79	< 20
transketolase activation coefficient	< 1.15	1.15-1.24	> 1.25
erythrocyte thiamin diphosphate			
nmol /L	> 150	120-150	< 120
µg /L	> 64	50-64	< 50

Source: from data reported by Brin 1964; Sauberlich *et al.* 1974; Finglas 1993.

Riboflavin (vitamin B₂)

Riboflavin has a central role as a redox cofactor in energy-yielding metabolism. Dietary deficiency is relatively widespread, yet is apparently never fatal; there is not even a clearly characteristic riboflavin deficiency disease. This does not seem to be the result of intestinal bacterial synthesis of the vitamin, rather there is very efficient conservation and reutilization of riboflavin in tissues in deficiency. Riboflavin coenzymes are tightly enzyme bound, in some cases covalently, and control of tissue flavins is largely at the level of synthesis and catabolism of flavin-dependent enzymes.

18.1   Riboflavin requirements and intakes

On the basis of depletion/repletion studies the minimum adult requirement for riboflavin is 0.5–0.8 mg/day. In population studies, normal values of the erythrocyte glutathione reductase activation coefficient (see section 18.6) are seen in subjects whose habitual intake of riboflavin is between 1.2–1.5 mg/day. At intakes between 1.1–1.6 mg/day urinary excretion rises sharply, suggesting that tissue reserves are saturated.

Because of the central role of flavin coenzymes in energy-yielding metabolism, reference intakes (see Table 18.1) are sometimes calculated on the basis of energy intake—0.14–0.19 mg/MJ (0.6–0.8 mg/1000 kcal). However, in view of the wide range of riboflavin-dependent reactions, in addition to those of energy-yielding metabolism, it is difficult to justify this basis for the calculation of requirements.

Average intakes of riboflavin are shown in Table 18.2, major sources in the average diet in Table 18.3 and rich sources in Table 18.4. Because of its intense yellow colour and low toxicity, riboflavin is widely used as a food colour (E-101).

18.2   Riboflavin and the flavin coenzymes

As shown in Fig. 18.1, riboflavin consists of a tricyclic dimethyl-isoalloxazine ring conjugated to the sugar alcohol ribitol. The metabolically active coenzymes are riboflavin 5′-phosphate and flavin adenine dinucleotide (FAD); in some enzymes the prosthetic group is riboflavin, bound covalently at the catalytic site.

The ribityl moiety is not linked to the isoalloxazine ring by a glycosidic linkage, so it is not strictly correct to call FAD a dinucleotide. Nevertheless, this trivial name is accepted, as indeed is the even less correct term flavin mononucleotide (FMN) for riboflavin phosphate.

Riboflavin phosphate and FAD may be either covalently or non-covalently bound at the catalytic sites of enzymes. Even in those enzymes where the binding is not covalent, the flavin is tightly bound, and in many cases it has a role in maintaining or determining the conformation of the enzyme protein.

As shown in Fig. 18.1, a variety of amino acid residues may be involved in covalent binding of flavin coenzymes to enzymes:

(1) flavin 8–α-carbon linkage to imidazole N-3 of a histidine residue;

(2) flavin 8–α-carbon linkage to imidazole N-1 of a histidine residue;

(3) flavin 8–α-carbon thio-ether linkage to a cysteine residue;

(4) flavin 8–α-carbon thio-hemiacetal linkage to a cysteine residue;

(5) flavin 8–α-carbon O-tyrosyl ether linkage;

(6) linkage from carbon-6 of the flavin to a cysteine residue.

It is not known whether the formation of 8–α-methyl linkage is enzymic or autocatalytic.

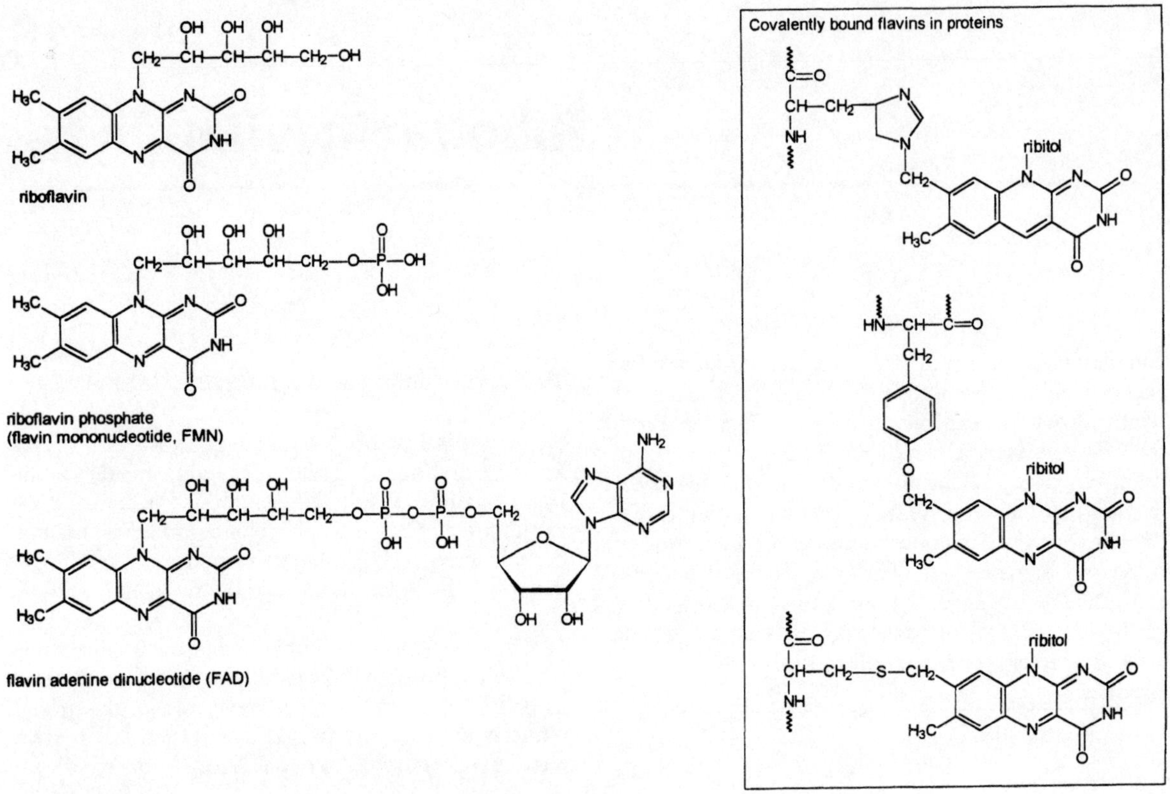

Figure 18.1 Riboflavin and the flavin coenzymes
Relative molecular masses (M_r): riboflavin 376.4, riboflavin phosphate 456.6, FAD 785.6

Although 8–hydroxymethyl-riboflavin is formed by microsomal mixed function oxidases (see section 18.4), it is not known whether or not this is a precursor of covalently bound flavin coenzymes. In some cases the flavin is incorporated into the nascent polypeptide chain while it is still attached to the ribosome, while in others a flavin-free apo-enzyme is synthesized and accumulates in riboflavin deficiency.

Although the ribitol moiety is not involved in the redox function of the flavin coenzymes, both the stereochemistry and nature of the sugar alcohol are important. While some riboflavin analogues have some vitamin action, most are inactive or have anti-vitamin activity, although they may be active in microbiological assays. The galactitol (dulcitol) analogue, galactoflavin, has been widely used as a means of inducing riboflavin deficiency in animal and human studies.

18.2.1 Photolytic destruction of riboflavin

Photolysis of riboflavin leads to the formation of lumiflavin (in alkaline solution) and lumichrome (in acidic or neutral solution) (see Fig 18.2). Because lumiflavin is chloroform extractable, photolysis in alkaline solution followed by chloroform extraction and fluorimetric determination is the basis of commonly used chemical methods of assaying riboflavin. This may explain why it was only relatively recently that it was demonstrated that only some 25 per cent of apparent urinary riboflavin is actually riboflavin; the remainder is largely a variety of lumichrome derivatives (Ohkawa *et al*. 1983*a*, 1986).

Exposure of milk in clear glass bottles to sunlight or fluorescent light (with a peak wavelength of 400–550 nm) can result in the loss of significant amounts of riboflavin as a result of photolysis. This is potentially nutritionally important, since, as shown in Table 18.3, more than a quarter of average of riboflavin intake is from milk and milk products. The resultant lumiflavin and lumichrome catalyse the oxidation of vitamin C, so that even relatively brief exposure to light, causing little loss of riboflavin, can lead to a considerable loss of vitamin C. This is nutritionally unimportant, since milk is normally an insignificant source of vitamin C. Lumiflavin and

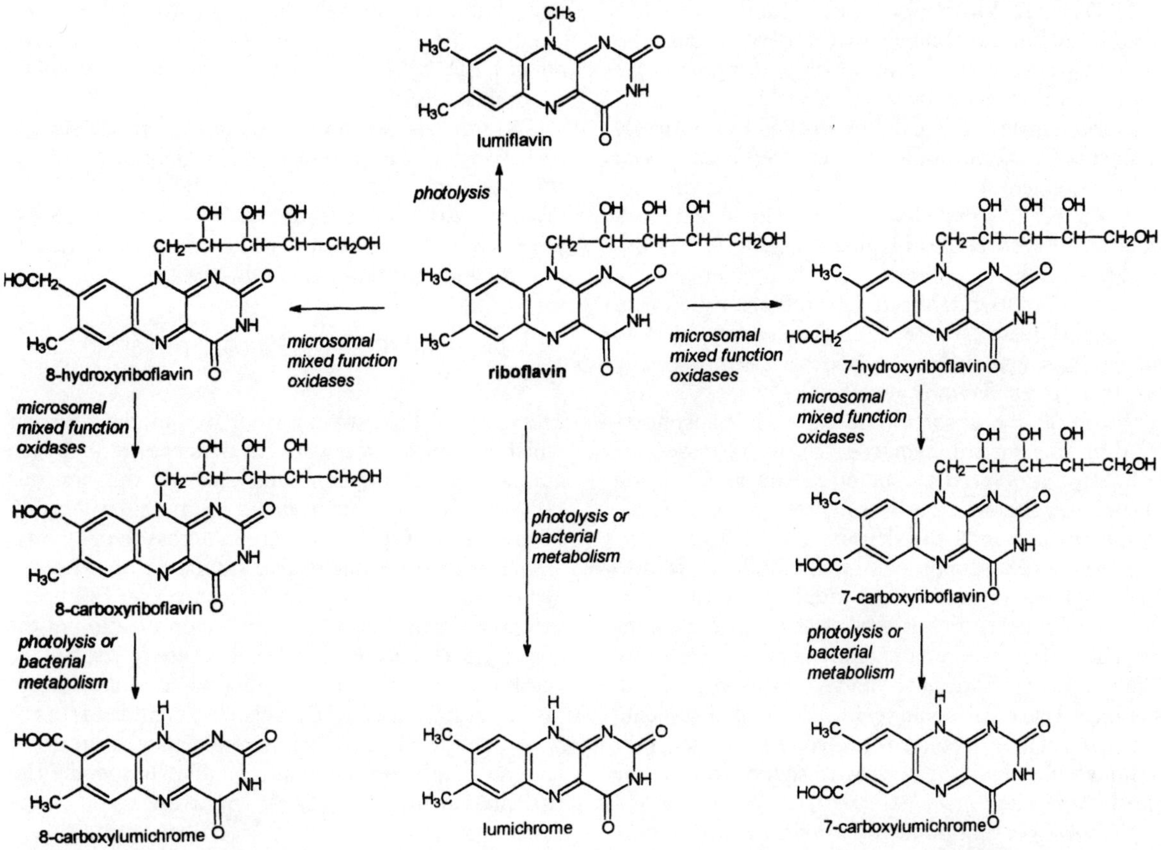

Figure 18.2 Riboflavin metabolism

lumichrome also catalyse oxidation of lipids (to lipid peroxides) and methionine (to methional), resulting in the development of an unpleasant flavour—the so-called 'sun-light' flavour. Light of 400–550 nm can penetrate both clear glass bottles and cardboard cartons; cartons for milk include a protective lining that is opaque at this wavelength.

Similar photolysis of riboflavin occurs *in vivo* during phototherapy for neonatal hyperbilirubinaemia. The peak wavelength for photolysis of bilirubin is 450 nm, the same as that for photolysis of riboflavin. Infants undergoing phototherapy show biochemical evidence of riboflavin depletion. Provision of additional riboflavin to maintain plasma concentrations enhances the photolysis of bilirubin, apparently as a result of reactive oxygen radicals generated by the products of photolysis of riboflavin. However, even relatively low concentrations of riboflavin can cause damage to DNA under conditions of photolysis, with damage to deoxyguanosine in isolated DNA, and

activation of DNA repair mechanisms in cells in culture. It is therefore not desirable to give riboflavin supplements as an adjunct to phototherapy of neonatal hyperbilirubinaemia (Gromisch *et al.* 1977; Speck *et al.* 1975).

There is no evidence that normal exposure to sunlight results in significant photolysis of riboflavin, although it is possible that some of the lumichromes found in urine may arise in this way.

18.3 Riboflavin metabolism

18.3.1 Absorption and availability

Apart from milk and eggs, which contain relatively large amounts of free riboflavin bound to specific binding proteins, most of the vitamin in foods is as flavin coenzymes bound to enzymes, some 60–90 per cent as FAD.

FAD and riboflavin phosphate in foods are hydrolysed in the intestinal lumen by a variety of phosphatases, to yield free riboflavin, which is absorbed in the upper small intestine by a sodium-dependent saturable mechanism. There is no uptake of riboflavin against a concentration gradient, and the peak plasma concentration is related to the dose only up to about 40–50 μmol (15–20 mg); thereafter there is little or no absorption of higher single doses of riboflavin.

Although intestinal bacteria synthesize riboflavin, and faecal losses of the vitamin may be 5–6-fold higher than intake, little or none of the intestinally synthesized riboflavin is absorbed.

Much of the absorbed riboflavin is phosphorylated in the intestinal mucosa by flavokinase (EC 2.7.1.26), and enters the blood-stream as riboflavin phosphate, although this does not seem to be essential to the absorption of the vitamin.

Parenterally administered free riboflavin is also largely phosphorylated in the intestinal mucosa. It is not clear whether this is the result of enterohepatic recycling of the vitamin or simply uptake of free riboflavin into the intestinal mucosa from the blood-stream. There is some evidence that significant amounts of free riboflavin are secreted in the bile, although this may be of greater significance in the rat than in man.

About 7 per cent of dietary riboflavin is covalently bound to proteins (mainly as riboflavin-8-α-histidine or riboflavin-8-α-cysteine). Neither the riboflavin nor the amino acid in the complexes released by proteolysis is biologically available; although they are absorbed from the gastrointestinal tract, they are excreted in the urine in competition with free riboflavin (Chia *et al.* 1978).

18.3.2 Tissue uptake of riboflavin

The total riboflavin concentration in plasma is very low compared with most tissues (see Table 18.5). About 50 per cent of plasma riboflavin is free riboflavin, which is the main transport form, with 44 per cent as FAD and the remainder as riboflavin phosphate. The vitamin is largely protein bound in plasma; free riboflavin binds to both albumin and α- and β-globulins; both riboflavin and the coenzymes also bind to immunoglobulins.

Most tissues contain very little free riboflavin, and except in the kidney, where 30 per cent is as riboflavin phosphate, more than 80 per cent is present as FAD, almost all bound to enzymes. Uptake into tissues is by passive carrier-mediated transport of free riboflavin, followed by metabolic trapping by phosphorylation to riboflavin phosphate, catalysed by flavokinase (EC 2.7.1.26). This is followed by onward metabolism to FAD, catalysed by FAD pyrophosphorylase (EC 3.6.1.18).

FAD that is not protein bound is rapidly hydrolysed to riboflavin phosphate by nucleotide pyrophosphatase; unbound riboflavin phosphate is similarly rapidly hydrolysed to riboflavin by non-specific phosphatases, and free riboflavin will diffuse out of tissues into the bloodstream (Aw *et al.* 1983).

18.3.3 Plasma riboflavin binding protein in pregnancy

There is a distinct plasma riboflavin binding protein which is induced by oestrogens; it is present in female animals in varying amounts through the oestrous cycle, but is not found in males or immature females. It serves to transport the vitamin across the placenta, which is impermeable to free riboflavin or the coenzymes, and is essential for foetal uptake. In experimental animals passive immuno-neutralization of the protein causes a considerable decrease in the uptake of riboflavin by the foetus, and a 90 per cent decrease in the formation of FAD. This results in death of the foetus and termination of the pregnancy, although it has no effect on maternal riboflavin metabolism (Krishnamurthy *et al.* 1984; Muniyappa and Adiga 1980).

In pregnant women there is a progressive increase in the erythrocyte glutathione reductase activation coefficient (an index of functional riboflavin nutritional status, see section 18.6), with a return to normal on parturition despite the daily secretion of 0.5–1 μmol (200–400 μg) of riboflavin into milk. This suggests that the oestrogen-induced riboflavin binding protein can sequester the vitamin for foetal uptake, even at the expense of causing functional deficiency in the mother.

In laying hens induction of this riboflavin protein results in a 100–fold increase in plasma riboflavin compared with males or non-laying females. A similar protein occurs in eggs, and has been exploited for radio-ligand binding assay of riboflavin. Because binding to the protein quenches the native fluorescence of riboflavin, it can be exploited for a direct titrimetric fluorescence assay of the vitamin in urine and other biological samples.

18.3.4 Catabolism and excretion of riboflavin

Riboflavin and riboflavin phosphate that are not bound to plasma proteins are filtered at the glomerulus; the phosphate is generally dephosphorylated in the bladder. Renal tubular resorption of riboflavin is saturated at normal plasma concentrations. There is also active tubular secretion of the vitamin, which does not appear to be saturable (i.e. the K_m is considerably higher than normal plasma concentrations). Urinary excretion of riboflavin after high doses can be 2–3–fold greater than the glomerular filtration rate.

Under normal conditions about 25 per cent of the urinary excretion of riboflavin is as the unchanged vitamin, with a small amount as a variety of glycosides of riboflavin and its metabolites. Riboflavin-8–α-histidine and riboflavin-8–α-cysteine arising from the catabolism of enzymes in which the coenzyme is covalently bound are excreted unchanged.

Liver cytochrome P_{450}-linked mixed function oxidases result in the production of 7– and 8–hydroxymethylriboflavin, both of which are substrates for flavokinase. There is some evidence that 8–hydroxymethylriboflavin may have biological activity; it is not known whether or not it is involved in the formation of 8–amino acid covalent links in proteins. Significant amounts of both of these hydroxylated derivatives, and their onward oxidation products (7– and 8–carboxyriboflavin) are excreted in the urine (see Fig. 18.2). Intestinal bacterial cleavage of the ribityl side chain results in the formation of 10–hydroxyethylflavin (an oxidation product of lumiflavin), lumichrome and 7– and 8–carboxy-lumichromes, which are also excreted in the urine. Some of the lumichromes detected in urine may also result from photolytic cleavage of riboflavin and its metabolites (Chastain and McCormick 1987; Ohkawa *et al.* 1983*a, b*, 1986).

18.3.5 Riboflavin balance

There is no evidence of any significant storage of riboflavin; apart from the limitation on absorption, any surplus intake is excreted rapidly, so that once metabolic requirements have been met urinary excretion of riboflavin and its metabolites reflects intake until intestinal absorption is saturated. In depleted animals, the maximum growth response is achieved with intakes which give about 75 per cent saturation of tissues, and the intake to achieve tissue saturation is that at which there is quantitative urinary excretion of the vitamin.

Equally, there is very efficient conservation of tissue riboflavin in deficiency. There is only a four-fold difference between the minimum concentration of flavins in the liver in deficiency and the level at which saturation occurs. In the central nervous system there is only a 35 per cent difference between deficiency and saturation.

Control over tissue concentrations of riboflavin coenzymes seems to be largely by control of the activity of flavokinase and the synthesis and catabolism of flavin-dependent enzymes. Almost all the vitamin in tissues is enzyme-bound, and free riboflavin phosphate and FAD are rapidly hydrolysed to riboflavin. If this is not rephosphorylated, it rapidly diffuses out of tissues and is excreted.

In deficiency, almost the only loss of riboflavin from tissues will be the small amount that is covalently bound to enzymes; the 8–α-linkage is not cleaved by mammalian enzymes and 8–α-derivatives of riboflavin are not substrates for flavokinase and cannot be reutilized.

18.3.6 Thyroid hormones and riboflavin metabolism

The activities of a variety of flavin-dependent enzymes are depressed in hypothyroidism, and are increased by the administration of thyroxine or triiodothyronine (see section 25.14.3). The effect of thyroid hormones is not blocked by protein synthesis inhibitors, and seems to be the result of increased synthesis of riboflavin phosphate and FAD, leading to increased saturation of enzyme proteins with coenzymes; this increases the stability of the enzymes against proteolysis, and so increases activity (Rivlin and Langdon 1966).

Tissue concentrations of flavin coenzymes in hypothyroid animals may be as low as in those fed a riboflavin deficient diet. In hypothyroid patients erythrocyte glutathione reductase activity may be as low, and its activation by FAD added *in vitro* (see section 18.6) as high as in vitamin deficient patients. Tissue concentrations of flavin coenzymes and erythrocyte glutathione reductase are normalized by the administration of thyroid hormones with no increase in riboflavin intake (Cimino *et al.* 1987).

Hypothyroid animals and patients have low tissue levels of flavin coenzymes, and reduced activity of flavokinase. Tissue concentrations of free riboflavin are also low, presumably reflecting the rapid clearance of free riboflavin from tissues, and the fact that there is normally only a transient pool of free riboflavin as a result of the turnover of flavin coenzymes. The loss of free riboflavin will lower the activity of flavokinase, since this enzyme is unstable in the absence of its substrate, and activity falls markedly in deficiency. The administration of thyroid hormones to hypothyroid animals results in a rapid increase in flavokinase activity. This is not the result of enzyme induction, but rather the activation of an inactive precursor protein; as flavokinase activity increases, so there is a parallel decrease in the tissue content of an apparently inactive riboflavin binding protein (Lee and McCormick 1985; Rivlin 1970).

Hyperthyroidism is not associated with elevated tissue concentrations of flavin coenzymes, despite increased activity of flavokinase. Again this demonstrates the importance of the enzyme binding of flavin coenzymes and the rapid hydrolysis of unbound FAD and riboflavin phosphate in the regulation of tissue concentrations of the vitamin.

18.4   Metabolic functions of the flavin coenzymes

The metabolic function of the flavin coenzymes is as electron carriers in a wide variety of oxidation and reduction reactions central to all metabolic processes, including the mitochondrial electron transport chain, and key enzymes in fatty acid and amino acid oxidation, and the citric acid cycle. Unlike the nicotinamide nucleotide coenzymes (see section 19.2), which act as cosubstrates, leaving the catalytic site of the enzyme after reaction, the flavin coenzymes remain bound to the enzyme throughout the catalytic cycle. The majority of flavoproteins have FAD as the prosthetic group rather than riboflavin phosphate; some have both flavin coenzymes, and some have other prosthetic groups as well.

As shown in Fig. 18.3, flavins can undergo a one-electron reduction to the semiquinone radical or a two-electron reduction to dihydroflavin. In some enzymes formation of dihydroflavin occurs by two single-electron steps, with intermediate formation of the semiquinone radical. Dihydroflavin can be oxidized by reaction with a substrate, NAD(P)⁺, or cytochromes in a variety of dehydrogenases, or can react with molecular oxygen in oxygenases and mixed function oxidases (hydroxylases).

18.4.1 Flavins and oxidative stress

As shown in Table 18.6, re-oxidation of the reduced flavin in oxygenases and mixed-function oxidases proceeds by way of formation of the flavin radical and flavin hydroperoxide, with the intermediate gen-

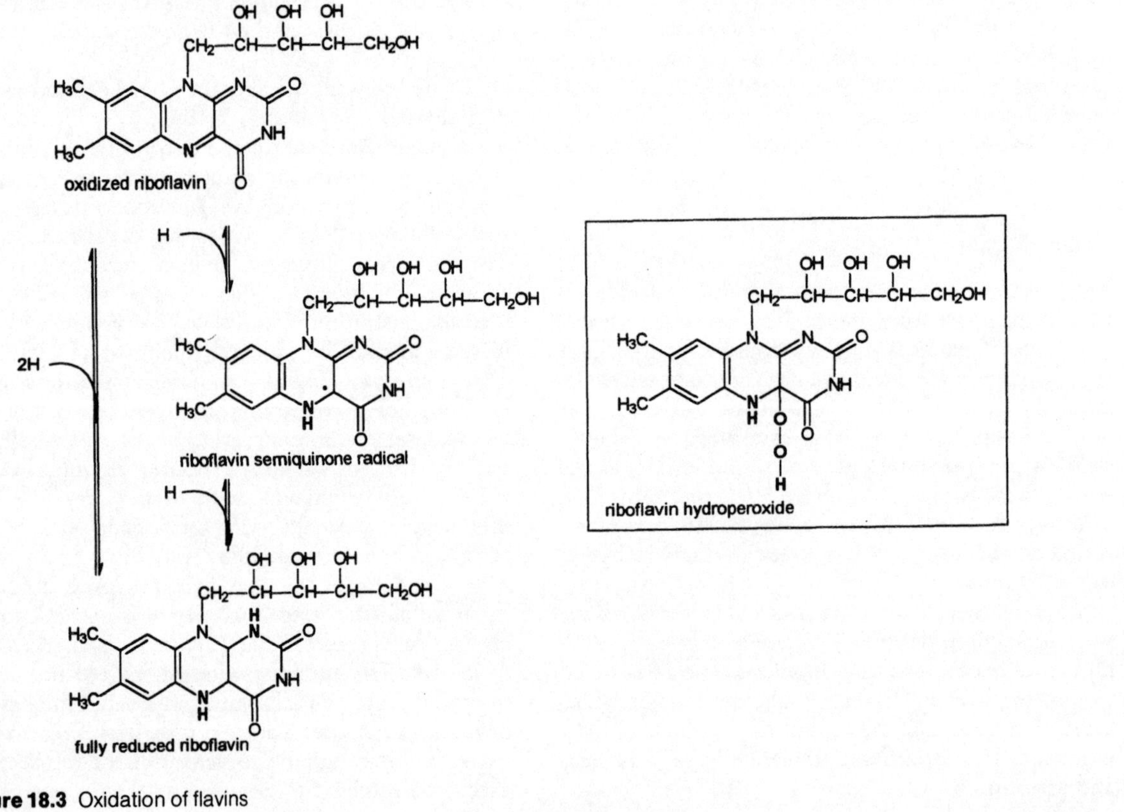

Figure 18.3 Oxidation of flavins

eration of superoxide and perhydroxyl radicals and hydrogen peroxide. Because of this, flavin oxidases make a significant contribution to the total oxidant stress of the body (see section 15.5.1). Overall, some 3–5 per cent of the daily consumption of about 30 mol of oxygen by an adult human being is converted to singlet oxygen, hydrogen peroxide and the super-oxide, perhydroxyl and hydroxyl radicals, rather than undergoing complete reduction to water in the electron transport chain. There is thus a total production of some 1.5 mol of reactive oxygen species daily, potentially capable of causing damage to membrane lipids, proteins and nucleic acids.

18.5 Riboflavin deficiency

Riboflavin deficiency is relatively common, yet there is no clear deficiency disease and the condition seems never to be fatal. This presumably reflects the high degree of conservation of riboflavin in tissues (see section 18.3.5).

Riboflavin deficiency is characterized by lesions of the margin of the lips (cheilosis) and corners of the mouth (angular stomatitis), a painful desquamation of the tongue, so that it is red, dry and atrophic (magenta tongue) and a sebhorroeic dermatitis, with filiform excrescences, affecting especially the naso-labial folds, eyelids and ears, with abnormalities of the skin around the vulva and anus and at the free border of the prepuce. The lesions of the mouth may respond to either riboflavin or vitamin B_6 in apparently riboflavin deficient subjects (Lakshmi and Bamji 1974; see section 20.3 for a discussion of the role of riboflavin in vitamin B_6 metabolism).

There may also be conjunctivitis with vascularization of the cornea, and opacity of the lens. This last is the only lesion of ariboflavinosis for which the biochemical basis is known—glutathione is important in maintaining the normal clarity of crystallin in the lens, and glutathione reductase is a flavoprotein which is particularly sensitive to riboflavin depletion.

18.5.1 Impairment of lipid metabolism in riboflavin deficiency

The main effect of riboflavin deficiency is on lipid metabolism. Riboflavin deficient animals have a lower metabolic rate than controls, and require a 15–20 per cent higher food intake to maintain body weight. Feeding a high fat diet leads to more marked impairment of growth, and a higher requirement for riboflavin to restore growth.

Within a day of initiating a riboflavin-free diet in weanling rats there is a 35 per cent decrease in the oxidation of palmitoyl CoA. All three mitochondrial acyl CoA dehydrogenases are affected, although it is the short chain acyl CoA dehydrogenase which is most severely impaired, and which becomes the rate-limiting step of fatty acid oxidation (see Fig. 5.3). The accumulated short chain fatty acyl CoA derivatives may undergo microsomal ω-oxidation to dicarboxylic acids. As a result, a number of dicarboxylic acids, including adipic, suberic, sebacic, octenedioic, hexenedioic and decendioic acids are excreted in the urine. It is not known to what extent riboflavin deficient human beings show similar organic aciduria, but there are a number of riboflavin-responsive organic acidurias that are due to impairment of one or other of the acyl CoA dehydrogenases (Goodman 1981; Veitch *et al.* 1988).

In animals, the production of $^{14}CO_2$ from [^{14}C]adipic acid is significantly reduced in riboflavin deficiency, and responds rapidly to repletion with vitamin. It has been suggested that the ability to metabolize a test dose of [^{13}C]adipic acid may provide a sensitive means of investigating riboflavin nutritional status in human beings (Bates 1989, 1990).

18.5.2 Resistance to malaria in riboflavin deficiency

A number of studies have noted that in areas where malaria is endemic, riboflavin deficient subjects are relatively resistant and have a lower parasite burden than adequately nourished subjects. Dietary deficiency of riboflavin, hypothyroidism, which induces functional riboflavin deficiency by lowering the synthesis of flavokinase (see section 18.3.6), or the administration of chlorpromazine, which inhibits flavokinase and can cause functional riboflavin deficiency all inhibit the growth of malarial parasites in experimental animals (Dutta *et al.* 1985).

The biochemical basis of this resistance to malaria in riboflavin deficiency is not known, but a number of possible mechanisms have been proposed:

1. The malarial parasites may have a particularly high requirement for riboflavin. A number of flavin analogues have anti-malarial action.

2. The impairment of glutathione reductase activity may result in lower availability of glutathione in erythrocytes, so that the parasites are unable to meet their requirements. However, there is no evidence of either a decrease in erythrocyte glutathione in riboflavin deficiency nor any change

in the ratio of reduced:oxidized glutathione; there is normally a considerable excess of glutathione.

3. As a result of impaired antioxidant activity in erythrocytes, there may be increased fragility of erythrocyte membranes or reduced membrane fluidity. As in sickle cell trait, which also protects against malaria, this may result in exposure of the parasites to the host's immune system at a vulnerable stage in their development, resulting in the production of protective antibodies.

18.5.3 Secondary micronutrient deficiencies in riboflavin deficiency

Riboflavin deficiency is sometimes associated with hypochromic anaemia as a the result of impaired iron absorption (see section 24.2.3). A greater proportion of a test dose of iron is retained in the intestinal mucosal cells bound to ferritin, and hence lost in the faeces, rather than being absorbed. The mobilization of iron bound to ferritin, in either intestinal mucosal cells or the liver, for transfer to transferrin, requires oxidation of Fe^{2+} to Fe^{3+}, a reaction catalysed by a flavin-dependent enzyme (Adelakan and Thurnham 1986).

Riboflavin depletion decreases the oxidation of dietary vitamin B_6 to pyridoxal (see section 20.3); pyridoxine oxidase (EC 1.1.1.65) is a flavoprotein, which is very sensitive to riboflavin depletion (Rasmussen *et al.* 1979). It is not clear to what extent there is functional vitamin B_6 deficiency in riboflavin deficiency. This is partly because vitamin B_6 nutritional status is generally assessed by the metabolism of a test dose of tryptophan (see section 20.6.4), and kynurenine hydroxylase (EC 1.14.13.9) in the tryptophan oxidative pathway (see Fig. 19.4) is a flavoprotein; riboflavin deficiency can therefore disturb tryptophan metabolism quite separately from its effects on vitamin B_6 nutritional status. In riboflavin-deficient animals, despite a decrease in pyridoxine oxidase to 15 per cent of the control activity, and an increase in the concentration of pyridoxine in tissues, there is no significant decrease in the tissue concentration of pyridoxal phosphate (Lakshmi and Bamji 1974). However, Greb *et al.* (1993) have shown that riboflavin deficiency does impair hepatic vitamin B_6 metabolism

The disturbance of tryptophan metabolism in riboflavin deficiency, due to impairment of kynurenine hydroxylase, can also result in reduced synthesis of NAD from tryptophan, and may therefore be a factor in the aetiology of pellagra (see section 19.5).

18.5.4 Drug-induced riboflavin deficiency

The phenothiazines such as chlorpromazine, used in the treatment of schizophrenia, and the tricyclic antidepressant drugs such as imipramine, are structural analogues of riboflavin, and inhibit flavokinase. In experimental animals administration of these drugs at doses equivalent to those used clinically results in an increase in the erythrocyte glutathione reductase activation coefficient (see section 18.6), and increased urinary excretion of riboflavin, with reduced tissue concentrations of riboflavin phosphate and FAD, despite feeding diets providing more riboflavin than is needed to meet requirements (Pinto *et al.* 1981). While there is no evidence that patients treated with these drugs for a prolonged period develop clinical signs of riboflavin deficiency, long-term use of chlorpromazine is associated with a reduction in metabolic rate.

18.6   Assessment of riboflavin nutritional status

As shown in Table 18.7, the urinary excretion of riboflavin and its metabolites can be used as an index of riboflavin nutritional status. Either the basal excretion or excretion after a test dose of riboflavin reflects status. The main experimental basis for estimates of riboflavin requirements (see section 18.1) is the rapid increase in excretion once tissues are saturated.

However, riboflavin excretion is only correlated with intake in subjects who are maintaining nitrogen balance. In subjects in negative nitrogen balance there may be more urinary excretion than would be expected, largely as a result of the catabolism of tissue flavoproteins, and loss of their prosthetic groups. Higher intakes of protein than are required to maintain nitrogen balance do not affect the requirement for riboflavin or indices of riboflavin nutritional status, although, as might be expected, more riboflavin is retained in subjects in positive nitrogen balance, as a result of increased net synthesis of flavoproteins.

The plasma concentration of riboflavin does not vary reliably with status. Bates (1993) has suggested that erythrocyte riboflavin reflects tissue saturation, but there have been few studies to establish values in depletion and deficiency.

Glutathione reductase (EC 1.6.4.2) is especially sensitive to riboflavin depletion. In deficient animals the activity of glutathione reductase responds earlier and more markedly than any other index of riboflavin status apart from liver concentrations of flavin coenzymes and the activity of hepatic flavokinase (Prentice and Bates 1981). The activity of the enzyme in erythrocytes can therefore be used as an index of riboflavin status. Interpretation of the results can be complicated by anaemia, and it is more usual to use the activation of erythrocyte glutathione reductase (EGR) by FAD added *in vitro*. An activation coefficient of 1.0–1.4 reflects adequate nutritional status, >1.7 indicates deficiency.

Pyridoxine oxidase (EC 1.1.1.65) is also sensitive to riboflavin depletion. In normal subjects and in experimental animals the erythrocyte glutathione reductase and pyridoxine oxidase activation coefficients are correlated, and both reflect riboflavin nutritional status. In subjects with glucose 6–phosphate dehydrogenase deficiency (favism, see section 7.7.1) there is an apparent protection of erythrocyte glutathione reductase, so that even in riboflavin deficiency it does not lose its cofactor, and the EGR activation coefficient remains within the normal range. The mechanism of this protection is unknown. In such subjects the erythrocyte pyridoxine oxidase activation coefficient gives a response which mirrors riboflavin nutritional status (Clements and Anderson 1980).

18.7   Riboflavin toxicity

Because of its low solubility and limited absorption from the gastrointestinal tract, riboflavin has no significant or measurable toxicity by mouth. At extremely high parenteral doses (300–400 mg/kg body weight) there may be crystallization of riboflavin in the kidney because of its low solubility.

Further reading

Adiga, P.R. (1994). Riboflavin carrier protein in reproduction. In *Vitamin Receptors: Vitamins and Ligands in Cell Communication*, (ed. K. Dakshinamurti), Chapter 6, pp. 137–77. Cambridge University Press.

Bates, C.J. (1987). Human riboflavin requirements and metabolic consequences of deficiency in man and animals. *World Review of Nutrition and Dietetics*, 50, 215–65.

Bender, D.A. (1992). Vitamin B$_2$: riboflavin. In *Nutritional Biochemistry of the Vitamins*, Chapter 7, pp. 156–83. Cambridge University Press.

Friedrich, W. (1988). Vitamin B$_2$: riboflavin and its bioactive variants. In *Vitamins*, Chapter 7, pp. 403–74. Walter de Gruyter, Berlin.

Ghisla, S. and Massey, V. (1989). Mechanisms of flavoprotein-catalysed reactions. *European Journal of Biochemistry*, 181, 1–17.

Massey, V. and Hemmerich, P. (1980). Active site probes of flavoproteins. *Biochemical Society Transactions*, 8, 246–57.

McCormick, D.B. (1989). Two interconnected B vitamins: riboflavin and pyridoxine. *Physiological Reviews*, 69, 1170–98.

White, H.B. and Merrill, A.H. (1988). Riboflavin binding proteins. *Annual Review of Nutrition*, 8, 279–99.

Table 18.1: Reference intakes of riboflavin

	US RDA (1989)	UK RNI (1991)	EU PRI (1993)
	mg	mg	mg
birth-6 m	0.4	0.4	-
7-12 m	0.5	0.4	0.4
1-3	0.8	0.6	0.8
4-6	1.1	0.8	1.0
7-10	1.2	1.0	1.2
males			
11-14	1.5	1.2	1.4
15-18	1.8	1.3	1.6
19-24	1.7	1.3	1.6
25-50	1.7	1.3	1.6
> 50	1.4	1.3	-
females			
11-14	1.3	1.1	1.2
15-18	1.3	1.1	1.3
19-24	1.3	1.1	1.3
25-50	1.3	1.1	1.3
> 50	1.2	1.1	-
pregnant	1.6	+0.3	1.6
lactating	1.8	+0.5	1.7

Source: National Research Council 1989; Department of
Health 1991; Scientific Committee for Food 1993.

Table: 18.2: Average intakes of riboflavin (mg /day)

(Apart from the SENECA study of the elderly, which involved 17 centres throughout Europe, all the studies quoted were in UK)

age	mean	males median	range[1]	mean	females median	range[1]	reference
1.5-2.5	1.2	1.2	0.5-2.2	1.2	1.2	0.5-2.2	Gregory *et al.* 1995
2.5-3.5	1.2	1.1	0.4-2.3	1.2	1.1	0.4-2.3	Gregory *et al.* 1995
3.5-4.5	1.2	1.2	0.5-2.0	1.1	1.1	0.5-2.0	Gregory *et al.* 1995
16-24	1.96	1.91	0.83-3.66	1.45	1.33	0.57-2.79	Gregory *et al.* 1990
25-34	2.08	1.95	0.92-3.54	1.50	1.41	0.52-2.96	Gregory *et al.* 1990
35-49	2.14	2.03	1.00-3.69	1.64	1.54	0.66-3.05	Gregory *et al.* 1990
50-64	2.11	2.08	0.92-3.59	1.63	1.59	0.68-2.77	Gregory *et al.* 1990
58-65	2.04	-	0.96-3.62	1.76	-	0.57-4.07	Davies & Holdsworth 1985
62-74	1.7	-	-	1.2	-	-	Lonergan *et al.* 1975
73-78[2]	-	1.56 (0.94-2.00)	0.43-3.20	-	1.35 (0.88-1.70)	0.50-3.20	Euronut SENECA Investigators 1991
75-90	1.5	-	-	1.1	-	-	Lonergan *et al.* 1975

(1) The range shown is the 2.5-97.5 centile for the studies of Gregory *et al.*, the 10-90 centile for the SENECA study, and the observed extreme range for the study of Davies & Holdsworth.
(2) Data were reported for 17 separate centres; the mean and extreme values of the published median values are shown, with the lowest 10th centile and highest 90th centile of those reported.

Table 18.3: Sources of riboflavin in the average British diet

	% of average intake
milk and milk products	27
breakfast cereals	11
other cereal products	11
eggs	5
beef and veal	5
liver and liver products	6
other meat	10
vegetables	7
beer and cider	5
other beverages	6
fish	2
fruit and nuts	1

Source: Gregory *et al.* 1990.

Table 18.5: Tissue concentrations of riboflavin and coenzymes in the rat

	total, μmol/kg	% present as		
		riboflavin	riboflavin phosphate	FAD
plasma	0.064	65	7	28
liver	58.0	3	23	74
kidney	63.2	4	41	55
skeletal muscle	4.1	3	12	85

Table 18.4: Rich sources of riboflavin

	portion (g)	mg /portion
liver	150	4.6
kidney	150	3.0
milk	560	1.1
cod roe, hard	100	1.0
duck	150	0.8
eel	150	0.6
sardines canned in oil	150	0.6
beef	150	0.5
herring roe, soft	100	0.5
mackerel	150	0.5
pork	150	0.5
sardines canned in tomato	150	0.5
veal	150	0.5
yoghourt	150	0.5
almonds	25	0.3
bacon joint	150	0.3
chicken	150	0.3
chocolate, milk	125	0.3
crab	175	0.3
egg	70	0.3
ham	85	0.3
herring	150	0.3
lamb	150	0.3
pilchards in tomato sauce	100	0.3
salmon, canned	150	0.3
turkey	150	0.3
whiting	150	0.3
beans, red kidney	100	0.2
broccoli tops	75	0.2
cheese	40	0.2
chestnuts	75	0.2
cod	175	0.2
dogfish	150	0.2
halibut	150	0.2
hamburger	100	0.2
lemon sole	150	0.2
lobster	150	0.2
mushrooms	50	0.2
plaice	150	0.2
rabbit	150	0.2
salmon	150	0.2
scampi	150	0.2
skate	150	0.2
spinach	130	0.2
spring greens	75	0.2
tuna	150	0.2

Table 18.6: Flavoproteins as a source of oxygen radicals

Flavoprotein oxidases - normal oxidative metabolism

$$X\text{-}H_2 + O_2 \rightarrow X + H_2O_2$$
$$X\text{-}H_2 + flavin \rightarrow X + flavin\text{-}H_2$$
$$flavin\text{-}H_2 + O_2 \rightarrow flavin + H_2O_2$$

1. Fully reduced flavin-H$_2$ reacts with oxygen to form the flavin semiquinone radical and superoxide

$flavin\text{-}H_2 + O_2 \rightarrow flavin\text{-}H^{\bullet} + {}^{\bullet}O_2^-$

2. Flavin semiquinone and superoxide react to form flavin hydroperoxide

$flavin\text{-}H^{\bullet} + {}^{\bullet}O_2^- \rightarrow flavin\text{-}HOOH$

3. Flavin hydroperoxide slowly breaks down to yield flavin semiquinone and perhydroxyl

$flavin\text{-}HOOH \rightarrow flavin\text{-}H^{\bullet} + {}^{\bullet}O_2H$

4. Perhydroxyl decays to superoxide plus a proton

${}^{\bullet}O_2H \rightarrow H^+ + {}^{\bullet}O_2^-$

5. In the presence of H$^+$, flavin semiquinone and superoxide yield peroxide and oxidized flavin

$flavin\text{-}H^{\bullet} + H + {}^{\bullet}O_2^- \rightarrow flavin + H_2O_2$

Mixed function oxidases - metabolism of foreign compounds

$$X\text{-}H_2 + O_2 \rightarrow X\text{-}OH + H_2O$$
or
$$X + NADPH + O_2 \rightarrow X\text{-}OH + NADP^+ + H_2O$$

1. Flavin is reduced by reaction with either substrate-H$_2$ or NADPH

2. Fully reduced flavin-H$_2$ reacts with oxygen to form the flavin semiquinone radical and superoxide

$flavin\text{-}H_2 + O_2 \rightarrow flavin\text{-}H^{\bullet} + {}^{\bullet}O_2^-$

3. Flavin semiquinone and superoxide react to form flavin hydroperoxide

$flavin\text{-}H^{\bullet} + {}^{\bullet}O_2^- \rightarrow flavin\text{-}HOOH$

4. Flavin hydroperoxide reacts with substrate

$flavin\text{-}HOOH + X \rightarrow flavin\text{-}HOOH\text{-}X$

5. Intermediate complex breaks down to hydroxylated product + flavin hydroxide

$flavin\text{-}HOOH\text{-}X \rightarrow flavin\text{-}OH + X\text{-}OH$

6. Flavin hydroxide breaks down to regenerate fully oxidized flavin + H$_2$O

$flavin\text{-}OH \rightarrow flavin + H_2O$

Table 18.7: Indices of riboflavin nutritional status

		adequate	marginal	deficient
urine riboflavin	µg /g creatinine	> 80	27-80	< 27
	mol /mol creatinine	> 24	8-24	< 8
	µg /24h	> 120	40-120	< 40
	nmol /24h	>300	100-300	< 100
	mg over 4 h after 5 mg dose	>1.4	1.0-1.4	< 1.0
	µmol over 4 h after 5 mg dose	> 3.7	2.7-3.7	< 2.7
erythrocyte riboflavin	µg /g haemoglobin	> 0.45	-	-
	nmol /g haemoglobin	> 1.2	-	-
glutathione reductase	activation coefficient	< 1.4	1.4-1.7	> 1.7

Source: from data reported by Bates 1993; Sauberlich *et al.* 1974.

Niacin and tryptophan

Niacin is unusual among the vitamins in that it was discovered as a chemical compound, nicotinic acid produced by the oxidation of nicotine, in 1867—long before there was any suspicion that it might have a role in nutrition. Its metabolic function as part of what was then called Coenzyme II (NADP) was discovered in 1935—again before its nutritional significance was known. Therefore, it has never been assigned a number among the B vitamins; although it is conventionally placed between vitamins B_2 and B_6, it is not correct to refer to niacin as vitamin B_3, a name that was originally applied to what was probably pantothenic acid (see section 23.2 and Table 23.1).

It is probably not correct to regard niacin as a vitamin. Its metabolic role is as the precursor of the nicotinamide moiety of the nicotinamide nucleotide coenzymes, NAD and NADP, and this can also be synthesized *in vivo* from the essential amino acid tryptophan. At least in developed countries, average intakes of protein provide more than enough tryptophan to meet requirements for NAD synthesis without any need for preformed niacin; it is only when tryptophan metabolism is disturbed, or intake of the amino acid is inadequate, that niacin becomes a dietary essential.

It is usual to regard pellagra as a niacin deficiency disease, and tryptophan as a substitute for niacin when the dietary intake of the vitamin is inadequate. However, is not strictly correct, and pellagra should be regarded as being due to a deficiency of both tryptophan and niacin.

19.1 Requirements and intake

All estimates of niacin requirements, and hence reference intakes, are based very largely on a single large-scale depletion/repletion study performed in the 1950s (Horwitt *et al.* 1956) and there is therefore excellent agreement on reference intakes of niacin,

with an average requirement of 5.5 mg/1000 kcal (1.3 mg/MJ) energy intake, a reference intake of 6.6 mg/1000 kcal (1.6 mg/MJ), and an assumption that for people with a low energy intake an amount of niacin appropriate for expenditure of 2000 kcal should be provided, to allow for metabolism of endogenous substrates.

The depletion/repletion study that established these average requirements also established the equivalence of dietary tryptophan and preformed niacin. On the basis of urinary excretion of niacin metabolites when subjects were fed varying amounts of tryptophan, Horwitt *et al.* (1956) proposed that 60 mg tryptophan were required to replace 1 mg preformed niacin. This 60:1 ratio was a deliberate underestimate of the observed mean equivalence, so as to allow for individual variation, and provide a margin of safety. Requirements and reference intakes are expressed in niacin equivalents, where 1 mg niacin equivalent = preformed niacin + 1/60 of the tryptophan.

There is little justification for expressing niacin requirements in terms of energy intake or expenditure. Horwitt *et al.* (1956) noted that the practice began before there were any estimates of niacin requirements, and it was customary to set niacin at 10 times the intake of thiamin; as discussed in section 17.1, thiamin requirements are indeed related to energy expenditure. Although the best known function of niacin is in energy-yielding metabolism (see section 19.2.1), the nicotinamide nucleotide coenzymes are not tightly enzyme bound, but are readily interchangeable throughout the cell; as discussed in section 19.2.2, the net use of NAD is in response to oxidative damage to DNA, not in energy-yielding metabolism.

Reference intakes are shown in Table 19.1, average intakes of total niacin equivalents in Table 19.2, sources of niacin in the average diet in Table 19.4, and rich sources of niacin in Table 19.5.

There is probably little or no requirement for any preformed niacin in the diet, since it is likely that average intakes of protein (at least in developed countries) will provide enough tryptophan to meet requirements. Table 19.3 shows estimated intake of tryptophan from the major sources of dietary protein in the average (British) diet (see Table 10.13). For an adult in nitrogen balance (see section 10.1), an amount of tryptophan equivalent to virtually all of the daily intake is available for NAD synthesis; the average intake of 1 g of tryptophan is equivalent to 16.6 mg niacin, or 6.8 mg/1000 kcal, an amount equivalent to the reference intake.

19.1.1 Unavailable niacin in cereals

Chemical analysis reveals niacin in cereals (largely in the bran), but this is biologically unavailable, since it is bound as niacytin—nicotinoyl esters to a variety of macromolecules ranging between M_r 1500–17 000. In wheat bran some 60 per cent is esterified to polysaccharides, and the remainder to polypeptides and glycopeptides (Mason *et al.* 1973).

Treatment of cereals with alkali (for example soaking overnight in calcium hydroxide solution, as is the traditional method for the preparation of tortillas in Mexico) and baking with alkaline baking powder, releases much of the nicotinic acid. This may explain why pellagra has always been rare in Mexico, despite the fact that maize is the dietary staple. Roasting of whole grain maize has a similar effect, since there is enough ammonia released from glutamine to form free nicotinamide by ammonolysis.

A small fraction of the niacin in niacytin may be biologically available as a result of hydrolysis by gastric acid. About 10 per cent of the total is released as free nicotinic acid after extraction of maize or sorghum meal with 0.1 M hydrochloric acid, and Carter and Carpenter (1982) have shown that about 10 per cent of the total niacin content of maize is biologically available to man.

19.2   Niacin vitamers and coenzymes; the metabolic functions of niacin

The term niacin is the generic descriptor for the two compounds that have the biological action of the vitamin: nicotinic acid and nicotinamide (see Fig. 19.1).

Nicotinic acid was discovered and named as a product of the chemical oxidation of nicotine in 1867. There is confusion in the literature because of the North American usage of the name niacin to mean specifically nicotinic acid while the amide is known as niacinamide. The name niacin was coined

in the late 1940s when the role of deficiency in the aetiology of pellagra was realized, and it was decided that dietary staples should be fortified with the vitamin. It was felt that nicotinic acid was not a suitable name for a substance that was to be added to foods, both because of its phonetic (and chemical) relationship to nicotine, and because it is an acid.

Although, as discussed below, the amino acid tryptophan is a precursor for niacin synthesis, it is not generally regarded as a niacin vitamer.

In addition to its role as a precursor of the nicotinamide nucleotide coenzymes, nicotinic acid is believed to be the ligand for the chromium ion in the glucose tolerance factor (see section 25.9.1).

19.2.1 The nicotinamide nucleotide coenzymes, NAD and NADP

Nicotinamide is the reactive moiety of the nicotinamide nucleotide coenzymes NAD (nicotinamide adenine dinucleotide) and NADP (nicotinamide adenine

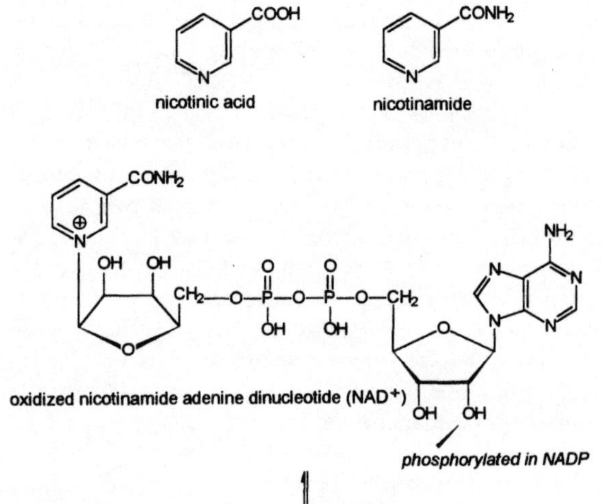

Figure 19.1 Niacin vitamers and the nicotinamide nucleotide coenzymes

Relative molecular masses (M_r): nicotinic acid 123.1, nicotinamide 122.1, NAD 663.4, NADP 743.4

dinucleotide phosphate), shown in Fig. 19.1. The notation NAD(P) is used to mean either NAD or NADP.

NAD was originally known as Coenzyme I, and later as diphosphopyridine nucleotide (DPN), and NADP as Coenzyme II, later triphosphopyridine nucleotide (TPN). Although this nomenclature was replaced in the 1960s, the coenzymes are still sometimes called the pyridine nucleotide coenzymes, although it is more correct to refer to them as the nicotinamide nucleotide coenzymes.

The major function of NAD and NADP is as coenzymes in oxidation and reduction reactions. As shown in Fig. 19.1, the oxidized coenzymes have a positive charge on the nicotinamide ring nitrogen, and undergo a two-electron reduction. The oxidized forms are conventionally shown as NAD(P)$^+$, and the reduced forms either as NAD(P)H$_2$, or, more correctly, as NAD(P)H + H$^+$, since although it is a two-electron reduction, only one proton is incorporated into the ring, the other remaining associated with the coenzyme.

In general, NAD$^+$ is involved as an electron acceptor in energy-yielding metabolism, being oxidized by the mitochondrial electron transport chain, while the major coenzyme for reductive synthetic reactions is NADPH. An exception to this general rule is the pentose phosphate pathway of glucose metabolism, which results in the reduction of NADP$^+$ to NADPH, and is the principal metabolic source of reductant for fatty acid synthesis.

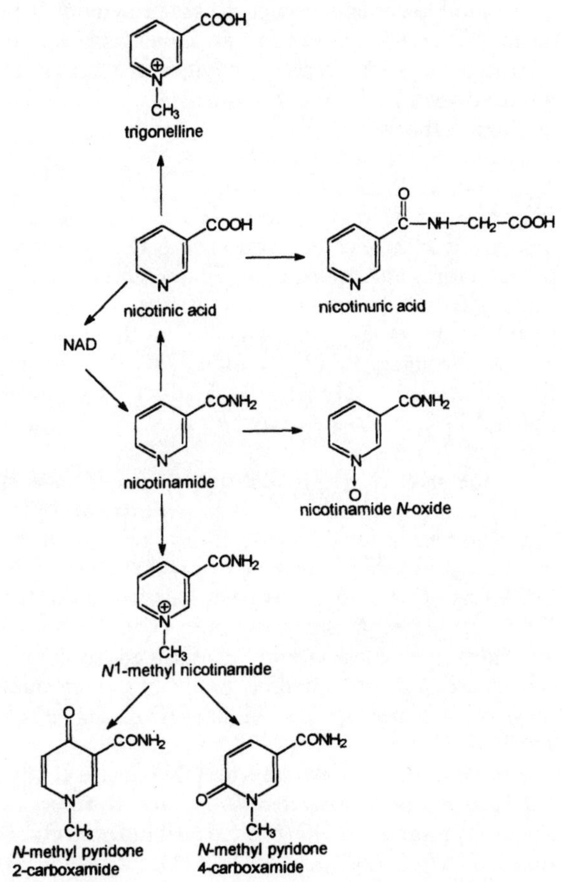

19.2.2 The role of NAD in ADP-ribosylation

In addition to its coenzyme role, NAD has a further function, as the source of ADP-ribose for the ADP-ribosylation of proteins and poly(ADP-ribosylation) of nucleoproteins involved in the DNA repair mechanism. Only NAD$^+$ is a substrate for these enzymes, not NADP, and not the reduced coenzyme.

19.2.2.1 ADP-ribosyltransferases

ADP-ribosyltransferases are enzymes of the cytosol, plasma membrane and nuclear envelope which catalyse the transfer of ADP-ribose onto arginine, lysine or asparagine residues in acceptor proteins to form N-glycosides, modifying the activity of the enzyme in the process. ADP-ribosylation is a reversible modification of proteins, and there are specific hydrolases which cleave the N-glycoside linkage.

In addition to endogenous ADP-ribosyltransferases, a number of bacterial toxins, including diphtheria and cholera toxins, *Escherichia coli* enterotoxin LT and *Pseudomonas aeruginosa* exotoxin A

Figure 19.2 Metabolites of nicotinic acid and nicotinamide

also have ADP-ribosyltransferase activity. Indeed, it was by investigation of the metabolic effects of these toxins that the endogenous ADP-ribosyltransferases were discovered.

The ribosomal elongation factor II is the acceptor protein for the ADP-ribosyltransferase activity of diphtheria toxin and *Pseudomonas aeruginosa* exotoxin A, as well as a mammalian cytosolic ADP-ribosyltransferase. ADP-ribosylation results in loss of activity. The uncontrolled action of the bacterial toxins causes the cessation of protein synthesis, and hence cell death. The more regulated action of the endogenous ADP-ribosyltransferase is presumed to be part of the normal regulation of protein synthesis.

A variety of guanine nucleotide binding proteins (G-proteins) involved with the regulation of adenylate cyclase activity are substrates for ADP-ribosyltransferases. ADP-ribosylation of the stimulatory G-protein increases its activity, while ADP-ribosylation of the inhibitory G-protein decreases its activity. The result of ADP-ribosylation of either protein is increased adenylate cyclase activity, an increase in intracellular cAMP, and the opening of membrane calcium channels.

19.2.2.2 Poly(ADP-ribose) polymerase

Poly(ADP-ribose) polymerase (EC 2.4.2.30) is primarily a nuclear enzyme, although it also occurs in mitochondria and ribosomes. The acceptor for the initial ADP-ribose moiety is a glutamate or the carboxyl group of a terminal lysine in the acceptor enzyme, forming an O-glycoside. This is followed by successive ADP-ribosyl transfer to form poly(ADP-ribose), which may be a linear or branched polymer.

In the nucleus, poly(ADP-ribose) polymerase is closely associated with chromatin, and has an absolute requirement for double-stranded DNA for activity. It is activated by binding to breakage points in DNA fragments, and is involved in activation of the DNA repair mechanism in response to strand breakage. In the immediate vicinity of a flush-ended double strand break several hundred ADP-ribose molecules may be polymerized per minute (Durkacz *et al.* 1980).

The acceptor protein may be DNA ligase II (EC 6.5.1.2), which is activated by poly(ADP-ribosylation) or a histone, resulting in reduced histone inhibition of DNA ligase II. DNA-dependent RNA polymerase is also a substrate for poly(ADP-ribosyl) polymerase, suggesting a role in the regulation of transcription, and the post-synthetic processing of transcripts to form mature mRNA, and poly-(ADP-ribose) polymerase is also involved in the condensation and decondensation of chromatin during the cell cycle and in DNA replication in cell proliferation.

Poly-ADP-ribosylation of proteins is reversed by the action of poly(ADP-ribose)glycohydrolase, which removes ADP-ribose units from the polymer sequentially, and ADP-ribose-protein lyase, which removes the initial, protein-bound, ADP-ribose moiety.

19.3   Metabolism of niacin

19.3.1 Digestion and absorption

Niacin is present in tissues, and therefore in foods, largely as the nicotinamide nucleotides. The *post mortem* hydrolysis of NAD(P) is extremely rapid in animal tissues, so it is likely that much of the niacin of meat (a major dietary source of the vitamin) is free nicotinamide. Cereals contain what is presumably a

storage form of the vitamin in the form of niacytin, which is largely biologically unavailable. In calculation of niacin intakes, it is conventional to ignore the niacin content of cereals completely, although, as discussed in section 19.1.1, 10 per cent of niacytin may be biologically available.

Nicotinamide nucleotides present in the intestinal lumen are not absorbed as such, but undergo hydrolysis to free nicotinamide. Both nicotinic acid and nicotinamide are absorbed from the small intestine by a sodium-dependent saturable process, although at unphysiologically high concentrations there is also a significant amount of passive diffusion across the intestinal mucosa. A number of intestinal bacteria have high nicotinamide deamidase activity, and a significant proportion of dietary nicotinamide may be deamidated in the intestinal lumen.

19.3.2 Synthesis of the nicotinamide nucleotide coenzymes.

As shown in Fig. 19.2, NAD(P) can be synthesized from either of the niacin vitamers, and from quinolinic acid, an intermediate in the metabolism of tryptophan (see section 19.4).

In liver there is little utilization of preformed niacin for nucleotide synthesis. Although isolated hepatocytes will take up both vitamers from the incubation medium, they seem not to be used for NAD synthesis, and cannot prevent the fall in intracellular NAD(P) which occurs during incubation (Bender and Olufunwa 1988). The enzymes for nicotinic acid and nicotinamide utilization, nicotinamide deamidase (EC 3.5.1.19), nicotinamide (EC 2.4.2.12) and nicotinic acid (EC 2.4.2.11) phosphoribosyltransferases, are more or less saturated with their substrates at normal concentrations in the liver, and hence are unlikely to be able to use additional niacin for nucleotide synthesis (Bender *et al.* 1982).

By contrast, incubation of isolated hepatocytes with tryptophan results in a considerable increase in the synthesis of NAD(P), and accumulation of nicotinamide and nicotinic acid in the incubation medium. Similarly, feeding experimental animals on diets providing high intakes of nicotinic acid or nicotinamide has relatively little effect on the concentration of NAD(P) in the liver, while high intakes of tryptophan lead to a considerable increase. It thus seems likely that the major role of the liver is to synthesize NAD(P) from tryptophan, followed by hydrolysis to release niacin into the circulation for use by extra-hepatic tissues (Bender *et al.* 1982; Bender and Olufunwa 1988; McCreanor and Bender 1986).

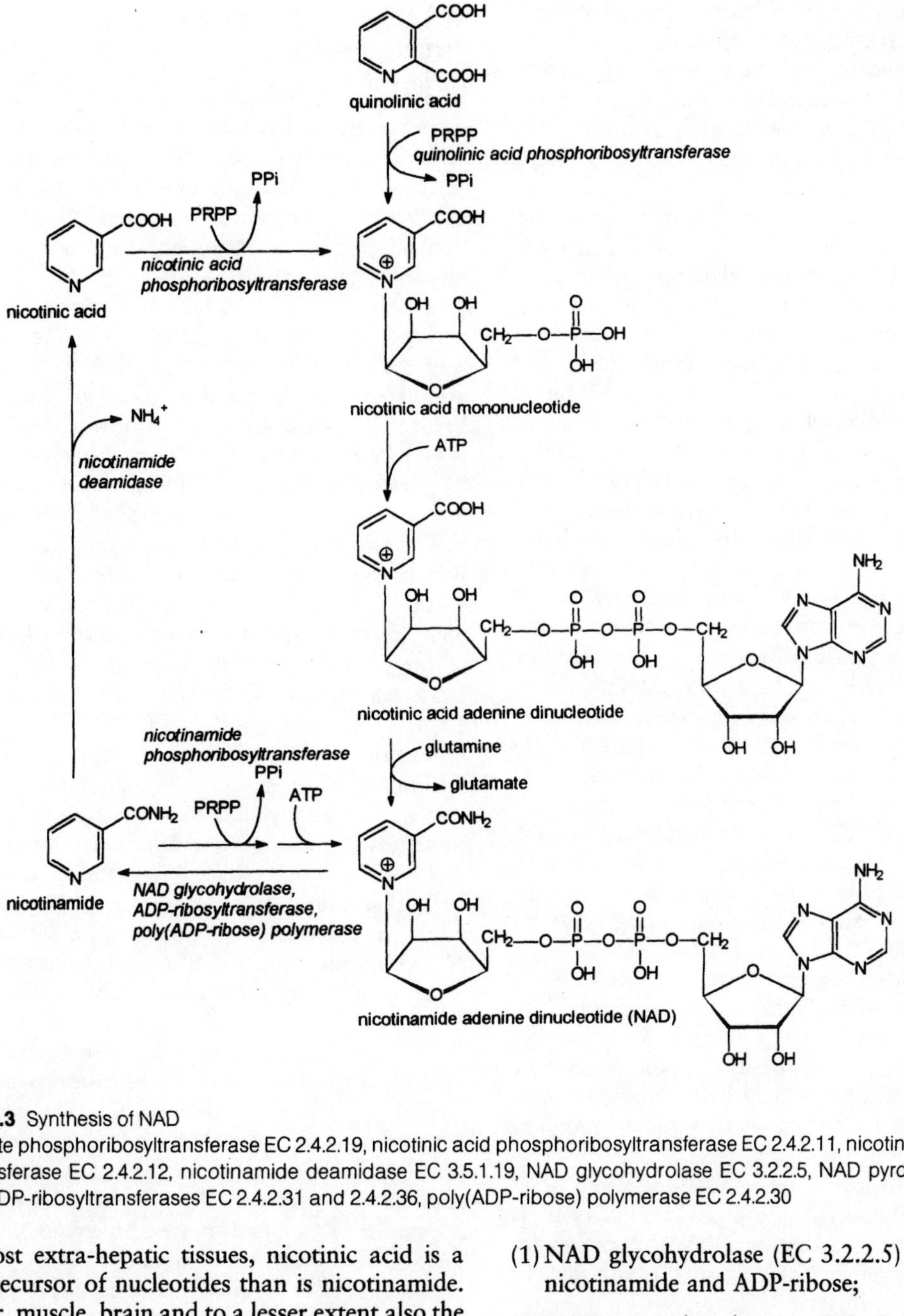

Figure 19.3 Synthesis of NAD

Quinolinate phosphoribosyltransferase EC 2.4.2.19, nicotinic acid phosphoribosyltransferase EC 2.4.2.11, nicotinamide phosphoribosyltransferase EC 2.4.2.12, nicotinamide deamidase EC 3.5.1.19, NAD glycohydrolase EC 3.2.2.5, NAD pyrophosphatase EC 3.6.1.22, ADP-ribosyltransferases EC 2.4.2.31 and 2.4.2.36, poly(ADP-ribose) polymerase EC 2.4.2.30

In most extra-hepatic tissues, nicotinic acid is a better precursor of nucleotides than is nicotinamide. However, muscle, brain and to a lesser extent also the testis, are able to take up nicotinamide from the blood-stream effectively, and apparently utilize it without prior deamidation (Gerber and Deroo 1970).

19.3.3 Catabolism of NAD(P)

The catabolism of NAD$^+$ is catalysed by four enzymes:

(1) NAD glycohydrolase (EC 3.2.2.5) which releases nicotinamide and ADP-ribose;

(2) NAD pyrophosphatase (EC 3.6.1.22), which releases nicotinamide mononucleotide. This can either be hydrolysed by NAD glycohydrolase to release nicotinamide, or can be a re-utilized to form NAD;

(3) ADP-ribosyltransferase(s) (EC 2.4.2.31 and 2.4.1.36);

(4) poly(ADP-ribose) polymerase (EC 2.4.2.30).

All of these enzymes act only on the oxidized coenzymes, and not on the reduced forms. Maintenance of experimental animals under conditions of modest hypoxia not only results in the expected shift in the NAD(P)H:NAD(P)$^+$ ratio, but also in a considerable increase in the total nicotinamide nucleotide concentration in liver and other tissues, as a result of reduced catabolism. Hyperoxia leads to increased turnover of the coenzymes, and increased urinary excretion of end-products of nicotinamide metabolism (McCreanor and Bender 1983). In cultured cells, oxidative stress leads to both NAD depletion and DNA strand breakage (Janero *et al.* 1993), and in human volunteers vitamin C depletion is associated with depletion of red cell NAD(P) and a doubling of the amount of 8–hydroxyguanine in sperm DNA, suggesting failure of DNA repair (Jacob *et al.* 1991).

The activation of ADP-ribosyltransferase and poly(ADP-ribose) polymerase by toxins, oxidative stress or DNA damage may result in considerable depletion of intracellular NAD(P), and may indeed provide a protective suicide mechanism to ensure that cells that have suffered very severe damage die, as a result of NAD(P) depletion. The administration of DNA-breaking carcinogens to experimental animals results in the excretion of large amounts of nicotinamide metabolites, and depletion of tissue NAD(P); addition of the compounds to cells in culture has a similar effect. Chronic exposure to such carcinogens and mycotoxins may be a contributory factor in the aetiology of pellagra when dietary intakes of tryptophan and niacin are marginal (Chu and Lawley 1975; Paine *et al.* 1982).

The total NADase activity of tissues, due to NAD glycohydrolase, ADP-ribosyltransferase and poly (ADP-ribose) polymerase, is very high. Were no regulatory factors involved, the total tissue content of nicotinamide nucleotides could be hydrolysed within a few minutes. Two factors prevent this *in vivo*:

1. NAD glycohydrolase is mainly a microsomal enzyme and poly(ADP-ribose) polymerase is mainly nuclear, so that membrane permeability barriers may prevent access of the enzymes to much of their substrate.

2. The values of K_m of the enzymes are of the same order of magnitude as those of many of the NAD(P)-dependent enzymes in the cell, so that there is considerable competition for the nucleotides. Only that relatively small proportion of the nicotinamide nucleotide pool in the cell that is free at any one time will be immediately available for hydrolysis.

19.3.4 Urinary excretion of niacin and metabolites

Under normal conditions there is little or no urinary excretion of either nicotinamide or nicotinic acid. This is because both vitamers are actively resorbed from the glomerular filtrate. It is only when the concentration is so high that the resorption mechanism is saturated that there is any significant excretion.

A considerable amount of nicotinamide may be released into the glomerular filtrate (and normally resorbed) by the very active NAD glycohydrolase associated with the renal tubule brush border membrane. The metabolic function of this is unclear, but it may be associated with the phosphaturic response to parathyroid hormone. Increasing the tissue content of NAD(P), either hormonally or by feeding high-niacin diets, leads to increased urinary excretion of phosphate. This is apparently not a direct effect of NAD on the renal mechanism for phosphate resorption, but rather the result of saturation of the phosphate carrier with the additional phosphate released by hydrolysis of NAD(P) (Berndt *et al* 1981; Tenenhouse and Chu 1982).

The metabolites of niacin are shown in Fig. 19.3. Nicotinamide in excess of requirements for NAD synthesis is methylated by nicotinamide N-methyltransferase (EC 2.1.1.1), an S-adenosylmethionine dependent enzyme which is present in most tissues. Very high intakes of nicotinamide may deplete tissue pools of one-carbon fragments (see section 21.4). N^1-methyl nicotinamide is actively secreted into the urine by the proximal renal tubules (Ross *et al.* 1975).

N^1-Methyl nicotinamide can also be metabolized further, to yield methyl pyridone-2–carboxamide and methyl pyridone-4–carboxamide. The extent to which this oxidation occurs, and the relative proportions of the two pyridones formed, varies not only from one species to another, but also between different strains of the same species. Aldehyde oxidase (EC 1.2.3.1) catalyses the formation of both pyridones, and some additional 2–pyridone arises from the activity of xanthine oxidase (EC 1.1.3.22); both of these enzymes are molybdenum-dependent flavoproteins (see section 25.19).

Nicotinamide can also undergo oxidation to nicotinamide N-oxide. This is normally a minor metabolite, unless large amounts (about 200 mg) of nicotinamide are ingested. At high levels of nicotinamide intake, some 6–hydroxynicotinamide may also be excreted.

Nicotinic acid can be conjugated with glycine to form nicotinuric acid (nicotinoyl-glycine), or may be methylated to trigonelline (N^1-methyl nicotinic acid). Small amounts of 6–hydroxynicotinic acid may also be formed.

It is not clear to what extent urinary excretion of trigonelline reflects endogenous methylation of nicotinic acid, since there are significant amounts of trigonelline in foods, which may be absorbed, but cannot be utilized as a source of niacin, and are excreted unchanged. In addition, trigonelline is formed by intestinal bacterial methylation of niacytin (Mason and Kodicek 1970). Trigonelline in coffee beans is demethylated to nicotinic acid during roasting, and moderate coffee consumption may meet a significant proportion of niacin requirements.

19.4 The synthesis of nicotinamide nucleotides from tryptophan

The oxidative pathway of tryptophan metabolism is shown in Fig. 19.4. Under normal conditions almost all of the dietary intake of tryptophan, apart from the small amount that is used for net new protein synthesis, is metabolized by this pathway, and hence is potentially available for NAD synthesis. About 1 per cent of tryptophan metabolism is by way of 5–hydroxylation and decarboxylation to 5–hydroxytryptamine (serotonin), which is excreted mainly as 5–hydroxyindoleacetic acid.

A number of studies have investigated the equivalence of dietary tryptophan and preformed niacin as precursors of the nicotinamide nucleotides, generally by determining the excretion of N^1-methyl nicotinamide and methyl pyridone carboxamide in response to test doses of the precursors, in subjects maintained on deficient diets. The most extensive such study was that of Horwitt *et al.* (1956). They found that there was a considerable variation between subjects in the response to tryptophan and niacin, and it was in order to allow for this individual variation that they proposed the ratio of 60 mg of tryptophan equivalent to 1 mg of preformed niacin.

Changes in hormonal status may result in considerable changes in this ratio, with between 7–30 mg of dietary tryptophan equivalent to 1 mg of preformed niacin in late pregnancy (Wertz *et al.* 1958). The intake of tryptophan also affects the ratio, and at low intakes 1 mg of tryptophan may be equivalent to only 1/125 mg preformed niacin (Nakagawa *et al.* 1969).

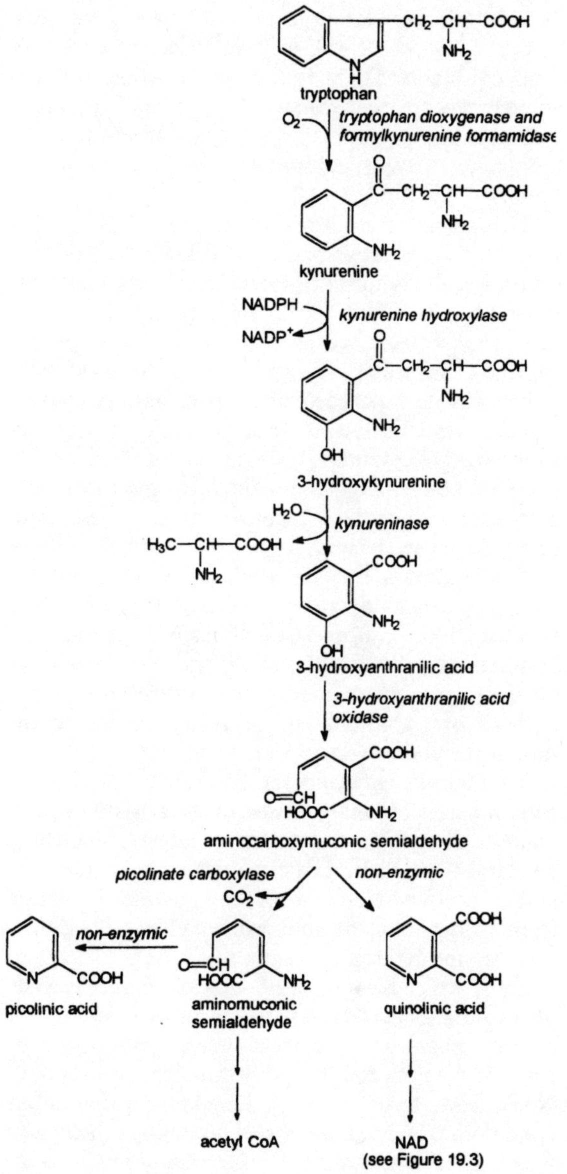

Figure 19.4 The oxidative metabolism of tryptophan Tryptophan dioxygenase EC 1.13.11.11, formylkynurenine formamidase EC 3.5.1.9, kynurenine hydroxylase EC 1.14.13.9, kynureninase EC 3.7.1.3, 3-hydroxyanthranilate oxidase EC 1.10.3.5, picolinate carboxylase EC 4.1.1.45

19.4.1 Picolinate carboxylase and non-enzymic cyclization to quinolinic acid

The synthesis of NAD from tryptophan involves the non-enzymic cyclization of aminocarboxymuconic semialdehyde to quinolinic acid. The alternative metabolic fate of aminocarboxymuconic semialdehyde is decarboxylation, catalysed by picolinate carboxylase (EC 4.1.1.45), leading to acetyl CoA and total oxidation. There is thus competition between an enzyme-catalysed reaction, which has hyperbolic, saturable kinetics, and a non-enzymic reaction which has linear, first order, kinetics (Ikeda *et al.* 1965; Mehler *et al.* 1964).

The result of this is that at low rates of flux through the oxidative pathway, which result in concentrations of aminocarboxymuconic semialdehyde below that at which picolinate carboxylase is saturated, most metabolism will be by way of the enzyme-catalysed pathway, leading to oxidation. There will be little accumulation of aminocarboxymuconic semialdehyde to undergo non-enzymic cyclization for NAD synthesis. As the rate of formation of aminocarboxymuconic semialdehyde increases, and picolinate carboxylase becomes more or less saturated, so an increasing proportion will be available to undergo non-enzymic cyclization to quinolinic acid, and hence onward metabolism to NAD. There is thus not a simple stoichiometric relationship between tryptophan and niacin, and the equivalence of the two coenzyme precursors will vary as the amount of tryptophan to be metabolized and the rate of metabolism vary.

As might be expected, the synthesis of NAD from tryptophan is inversely related to the activity of picolinate carboxylase. Inhibition results in increased availability of aminocarboxymuconic semialdehyde, and increased NAD formation, while induction leads to depletion of aminocarboxymuconic semialdehyde, and reduced formation of NAD.

Cats, which have some 30–50–fold higher activity of picolinate carboxylase than other species, are entirely reliant on a dietary source of preformed niacin, and are not capable of any significant synthesis of NAD from tryptophan. A hereditary pellagra-like condition has been described in human beings in which there is no significant excretion of niacin metabolites in response to a test dose of tryptophan, but no accumulation of any of the intermediates of the tryptophan oxidative pathway, suggesting that the defect was the result of increased activity of picolinic carboxylase (Salih *et al.* 1985).

It is thus apparent that the utilization of tryptophan as a precursor for NAD synthesis depends on both the amount of tryptophan to be metabolized and also the rate of metabolic flux through the pathway. The activities of three enzymes, tryptophan dioxygenase, kynurenine hydroxylase and kynureninase, may all affect the rate of formation of aminocarboxymuconic semialdehyde, as may the rate of uptake of tryptophan into the liver. Impairment of

kynurenine hydroxylase and kynureninase activities by oestrogen metabolites may account for the observed two-fold excess of females over males in most reports of outbreaks of pellagra (see section 19.5.1).

19.4.2 Tryptophan dioxygenase

Tryptophan dioxygenase (EC 1.13.11.11, also known as tryptophan oxygenase or tryptophan pyrrolase), is the enzyme that controls the entry of tryptophan into the irreversible oxidative pathway; control of its activity forms part of the regulation of the catabolic drive proposed by Millward and Rivers (1988) to explain the basis of protein requirements (see section 10.8.3.1).

Tryptophan dioxygenase has a short half-life (of the order of 2 hours) and is subject to regulation by three mechanisms: saturation with its haem cofactor, hormonal induction and feed-back inhibition and repression by NAD(P).

19.4.2.1 Stabilization of tryptophan dioxygenase by the haem cofactor

Unlike most other haem enzymes, the haematin of tryptophan dioxygenase behaves more like a dissociating cofactor than a tightly bound prosthetic group. The holo-enzyme is considerably more resistant to proteolysis than is the apo-enzyme, and in the presence of relatively large amounts of haem both the activity of the enzyme and the total amount of immuno-reactive tryptophan dioxygenase protein in the liver are increased. Induction of the rate-limiting enzyme of haem synthesis, δ-amino-laevulinate synthetase, for example by progesterone and synthetic progestagens, is associated with increased hepatic tryptophan dioxygenase and increased oxidative metabolism of tryptophan. This is not induction of tryptophan dioxygenase apo-enzyme, but the result of reduced catabolism of the enzyme protein (Schimke *et al.* 1965a, b).

Oduho *et al.* (1994) have shown that in iron-deficient chicks there is an impaired ability to utilize tryptophan, but not preformed niacin, as a precursor of the nicotinamide nucleotides, reflecting the sensitivity of tryptophan dioxygenase to the availability of haem.

Tryptophan and a number of tryptophan analogues increase the activity of tryptophan dioxygenase by promoting conjugation of the apo-enzyme with haematin, and stabilizing the holo-enzyme. The analogues which promote haem conjugation are not substrates, neither do they compete with tryptophan at the catalytic site of the enzyme. They appear to bind to a domain on the enzyme protein which is distinct from the catalytic site. The conjugation promoting site of the mammalian liver apo-enzyme has a relatively broad specificity, and a K_m for tryptophan of 26 μM, while the catalytic site on the holo-enzyme binds only L-tryptophan, and has a ten-fold higher K_m.

19.4.2.2 Hormonal control of tryptophan dioxygenase
Tryptophan dioxygenase is sensitive to induction by both glucocorticoid hormones and glucagon; the mechanisms involved are different, and the effects are at least partially additive.

The synthesis of tryptophan dioxygenase is induced by glucocorticoid hormones (cortisol in man and corticosterone in the rat). This is true induction of new mRNA and protein synthesis, with up to a 10–fold increase in tryptophan dioxygenase mRNA in response to glucocorticoid administration. Because of this, the activity of tryptophan dioxygenase in the liver mirrors the diurnal variation in endogenous cortisol secretion.

Glucagon (mediated by cAMP) increases the synthesis of tryptophan dioxygenase following the administration of glucocorticoids, although it has little effect in unstimulated animals. The effect of glucagon appears to be the result of an increase in the rate of translation of mRNA rather than an increase in transcription, and is antagonized by insulin. Insulin also partially antagonizes the induction of tryptophan dioxygenase by glucocorticoids, possibly by antagonising a permissive effect of glucagon. Feeding experimental animals with glucose both lowers the basal activity of tryptophan dioxygenase in the liver and reduces the maximum induction achievable by the administration of glucocorticoids (Altar *et al* 1983; Nakamura *et al.* 1980).

19.4.2.3 Feed-back control of tryptophan dioxygenase by nicotinamide nucleotides.
High concentrations of the nicotinamide nucleotide coenzymes, and especially NADPH, both inhibit preformed tryptophan oxygenase and also repress its synthesis. It is not clear how important this is in terms of physiological regulation, since the concentrations of the nucleotides required to achieve significant inhibition are relatively high, but some of the effects of alcohol on tryptophan metabolism may be due to the increase in NADH and NADPH that follows the ingestion of relatively large amounts of alcohol (Cho-Chung and Pitot 1967; Wagner 1964).

19.4.3 Kynurenine metabolism

The activities of both kynurenine hydroxylase (EC 1.14.13.9) and kynureninase (EC 3.7.1.3) are only slightly higher than that of tryptophan dioxygenase under basal conditions, and increased tryptophan dioxygenase activity is accompanied by increased accumulation and excretion of kynurenine, hydroxykynurenine and their transamination products, kynurenic and xanthurenic acids (see Fig. 20.4).

Impairment of the activity of either enzyme may impair the onward metabolism of kynurenine, and so reduce the accumulation of aminocarboxymuconic semialdehyde, and hence the synthesis of NAD.

19.4.3.1 Kynurenine hydroxylase
Kynurenine hydroxylase is an FAD-dependent mixed function oxidase of the outer mitochondrial membrane, which uses NADPH as the reductant. The activity of kynurenine hydroxylase in the liver of riboflavin deficient rats is only 30–50 per cent of that in control animals, and deficient rats excrete abnormally large amounts of kynurenic and anthranilic acids after the administration of a loading dose of tryptophan, and correspondingly lower amounts of quinolinate and niacin metabolites. Riboflavin deficiency (see section 18.5.3) may thus be a contributory factor in the aetiology of pellagra when intakes of tryptophan and niacin are marginal.

In a number of studies, sexually mature women show a higher ratio of urinary kynurenine:hydroxykynurenine than do children, post-menopausal women or men, suggesting inhibition of kynurenine hydroxylase by endogenous oestrogens or their metabolites. In experimental animals the administration of oestrogens results in a very considerable reduction in kynurenine hydroxylase activity, to about 30 per cent of the control activity. The mechanism of this effect is unclear, since the addition of oestrogens or their metabolites has no effect on the enzyme *in vitro* (Bender and McCreanor 1985).

19.4.3.2 Kynureninase
Kynureninase is a pyridoxal phosphate-dependent enzyme, and its activity is extremely sensitive to vitamin B_6 depletion. Indeed, the ability to metabolize a test dose of tryptophan has been used to assess vitamin B_6 nutritional status (see section 20.6.4). Deficiency of vitamin B_6 will lead to severe impairment of NAD synthesis from tryptophan.

Kynureninase is also inhibited by oestrogen metabolites; the importance of this is shown not only by the many reports of abnormal tryptophan metabolism in women receiving oral contraceptive steroids, but, more importantly, by the two-fold excess of women over men suffering from pellagra in areas where the disease is an important problem (Miller 1978)—see section 19.5.1.

19.5   Pellagra—a disease of tryptophan and niacin deficiency

The disease of pellagra was first described as *la mal de la rosa* in Asturias in central Spain by Casal in 1735. He observed that the condition was apparently related to diet and was distinct from scurvy, syphilis, and other then known causes of apparently similar dermatitis. The name pellagra was coined by the Italian physician Frapolli in 1771, to describe the most striking feature of the disease, the roughened sunburn-like appearance of the skin.

Pellagra became common in Europe when maize was introduced from the New World as a convenient high-yielding dietary staple, and by the nineteenth century it was widespread throughout southern Europe and north Africa. The disease was unknown in southern Africa until the outbreak of rinderpest in 1897, which led to wide-spread death of cattle, and a major change in the dietary habits of the Bantu. From being a meat and milk-eating community, they became, and have remained, largely maize eaters, and pellagra continues to be a major problem of public health nutrition in South Africa.

The other region where pellagra was a major problem at the beginning of this century was the southern part of the United States of America. The social and economic upheaval of the American Civil War led to a poor maize-based diet for large sections of the population, and it was not until the entry of the United States into the Second World War that increasing employment and a rise in the general standard of living solved the dietary problem. Although Casal had considered pellagra to be due to a dietary deficiency, the investigations at the beginning of this century started from the assumption that, like other diseases, it was due to an infection. It was the pioneering studies of Goldberger and coworkers in the United States that showed that the condition was neither contagious nor infectious, and could indeed be prevented or cured by dietary means.

After it had been established that pellagra was a deficiency disease, the next problem was to discover the missing nutrient. Additional dietary protein was shown to be beneficial, so it was concluded that pellagra was due to protein deficiency. This view, and later that it was more specifically due to a deficiency

of tryptophan, was held for some time. In 1938 Spies and coworkers showed that nicotinic acid would cure pellagra, and thereafter it was gradually accepted that it was a niacin deficiency disease.

Pellagra is characterized by a photosensitive dermatitis, like severe sunburn, typically with a butterfly-like pattern of distribution over the face, affecting all parts of the skin that are exposed to sunlight. Similar skin lesions may also occur in areas not exposed to sunlight, but subject to pressure, such as the knees, elbows, wrists and ankles. Advanced pellagra is also accompanied by dementia (more correctly a depressive psychosis), and there may be diarrhoea. Untreated pellagra is fatal.

Despite our understanding of the biochemistry of niacin, we still cannot account for the characteristic photosensitive dermatitis in terms of the known metabolic lesions. There is no apparent relationship between reduced availability of tryptophan and niacin and sensitivity of the skin to UV light. The only biochemical abnormalities that have been reported in the skin of pellagrins involve increased catabolism of the amino acid histidine, leading to a reduction in the concentration of urocanic acid, a histidine metabolite which is the major UV absorbing compound in normal dermis.

The other characteristic feature of pellagra is the development of a depressive psychosis, superficially similar to schizophrenia and the organic psychoses, but clinically distinguishable by the sudden lucid phases which alternate with the most florid psychiatric signs. It is probable that these mental symptoms can be explained by a relative deficit of the essential amino acid tryptophan, and hence reduced synthesis of the neurotransmitter serotonin, and not to a deficiency of niacin *per se* (Lehman 1972). However, there are anatomical lesions in the central nervous system and EEG abnormalities which can be attributed to depletion of NAD(P) and can be mimicked by the administration of nicotinamide analogues which are incorporated into NAD(P) analogues by the transglycosidase activity of NAD glycohydrolase.

19.5.1 Additional factors in the aetiology of pellagra

Although the nutritional aetiology of pellagra is well established, and additional tryptophan or niacin will prevent or cure the disease, there are a number of reports that suggest that additional factors may be involved.

Carpenter and Levin (1985) re-examined the diets associated with the development of pellagra in the US during the early part of this century, and showed that the total intake of tryptophan and niacin was apparently adequate, as judged by current knowledge of requirements. They suggest that deficiency of riboflavin (and hence impaired activity of kynurenine hydroxylase), or vitamin B_6 (and hence impaired activity of kynureninase), may be important when intakes of tryptophan and niacin are only marginally adequate.

During the first half of the present century, of the 87 000 people who died from pellagra in the United States, there were twice as many women as men (Miller 1978). Reports of individual outbreaks of pellagra, both in USA and more recently elsewhere, show a similar sex ratio. As discussed above, this may well be the result of inhibition of kynureninase, and impairment of the activity of kynurenine hydroxylase, by oestrogen metabolites, and hence reduced synthesis of NAD from tryptophan (Bender and Totoe 1984a, b).

Zinc deficiency (see section 25.26.2), in association with alcoholism (see section 9.3.1) may also be a factor in the aetiology of pellagra. Vannuchi and Moreno (1989) showed that when alcoholics were treated with a defined enteral feeding mixture devoid of tryptophan and niacin, the addition of zinc salts led to an increase in urinary excretion of N^1-methylnicotinamide and methyl pyridone carboxamide, with a corresponding fall in plasma tryptophan. It is likely that this reflects the role of zinc in glucocorticoid (and other steroid hormone) receptors—the increase in tryptophan metabolism in response to zinc supplementation is presumably due to increased receptor synthesis and hence increased sensitivity to the induction of tryptophan dioxygenase by cortisol (see section 25.26).

19.5.1.1 Possible pellagragenic toxins

Woolley (1946) reported the isolation of an unidentified lipid-soluble toxin from some samples of maize that was pellagragenic in experimental animals. More recently, Schoental (1983) has suggested that mycotoxins resulting from fungal spoilage of maize and other grain stored under damp conditions may have been responsible for some major outbreaks of pellagra. Certainly, the only known outbreak of the disease in Mexico can be traced to a consignment of maize that was shipped under damp conditions and had a significant fungal over-growth.

As discussed above (see section 19.2.3.2) a number of bacterial, fungal and environmental toxins activate ADP-ribosyltransferase or poly(ADP-ribose) polymerase, and it is possible that chronic exposure to such toxins will deplete tissue NAD(P) and hence be

a contributory factor in the development of pellagra when intakes of tryptophan and niacin are marginal.

Chronic exposure to high levels of lead may also precipitate pellagra. Zerez *et al.* (1990) showed that NAD synthetase is inhibited by relatively low concentrations of lead acetate *in vitro*, and the activity of this enzyme was abnormally low in erythrocytes from people who had been occupationally exposed to lead. They suggested that measurement of erythrocyte NAD synthetase might provide a sensitive marker of lead exposure; it is equally likely that normal environmental and occupational exposure to lead may compromise niacin status.

19.5.1.2 The pellagragenic effect of excess dietary leucine

Pellagra continues to be a major problem in parts of India where jowar (*Sorghum vulgare*) is the dietary staple. Gopalan and Srikantia (1960) suggested that the relative excess of leucine in the proteins of jowar might be a contributory factor in the aetiology of pellagra. They noted that the intake of tryptophan and niacin is as great as that of rice eaters, yet pellagra is a common problem among jowar eaters, and not in rice eating communities. Certainly, the tryptophan content of sorghum proteins is higher than that of maize, the cereal traditionally associated with endemic pellagra.

Belavady and Rao (1979) showed that there was a good correlation between the leucine content of different varieties of sorghum and the induction of black tongue disease (the canine equivalent of pellagra) in dogs, and a number of other studies from the Indian National Institute for Nutrition Research in Hyderabad have demonstrated depletion of nicotinamide nucleotides in human beings and experimental animals by feeding a modest excess of leucine. The effect is apparently on the synthesis of NAD from tryptophan, and not on the utilization of preformed dietary niacin (Gopalan and Rao 1975).

A number of workers from other centres have challenged the Hyderabad findings. Nakagawa and coworkers (1975) were unable to show any effect of the administration of leucine on the urinary excretion of niacin metabolites in volunteers who were fed on a diet in which the sole source of nitrogen was a mixture of amino acids. Manson and Carpenter (1978a, b) showed no effect of excess leucine on the growth of dogs, chicks or rats, or on the urinary excretion of N^1-methyl nicotinamide. Yamada *et al.* (1979) showed a significant decrease in the liver content of nicotinamide nucleotides when rats were fed on diets providing 5 or 10 per cent casein and 5 per cent leucine, but only when the diet was free from niacin. Magboul and Bender (1983) showed that when rats were fed on diets that were only marginally adequate with respect to tryptophan and niacin, the addition of 1.5 per cent leucine led to a significant depletion of liver and blood nicotinamide nucleotides. This effect was only apparent when the niacin content of the diet was such that it provided less than half the minimum requirement and was most marked when the diets provided virtually no preformed niacin. This again suggests that the effect of leucine is on the metabolism of tryptophan, and not on the utilization of niacin.

Studies with [^{14}C]tryptophan in both intact animals and isolated hepatocytes show that leucine does indeed inhibit the synthesis of NAD from tryptophan, inhibiting metabolism at the level of kynurenine hydroxylase and kynureninase, causing the accumulation of intermediates. In isolated hepatocytes, the more important effect seems to be at the level of uptake of tryptophan into the cells; leucine and tryptophan share a common transport mechanism with the other large neutral amino acids (Bender 1983, 1989; Salter *et al.* 1985).

The effects of leucine in these studies were only apparent in rats maintained for 5–7 weeks on diets that provided a minimally adequate amount of tryptophan to permit limited synthesis of NAD(P); the restriction was so severe that the control animals (receiving the same diet but without the added burden of 1.5 per cent excess leucine) had greatly impaired growth compared with controls. These constraints would seem to explain why other workers have reported no effect of a dietary excess of leucine. In addition, leucine seems to activate NAD glycohydrolase, and therefore urinary excretion of niacin metabolites might be normal despite decreased synthesis and reduced tissue concentrations of the nucleotides.

It is likely that leucine is a factor in the aetiology of pellagra only when the dietary intakes of both tryptophan and niacin are extremely low—a condition that may occur when sorghum is the dietary staple, especially at times of food shortage.

19.5.1.3 Non-nutritional pellagra

Table 19.6 shows those inborn errors of metabolism that are associated with the development of pellagra despite an apparently adequate intake of both tryptophan and niacin; all are defects of tryptophan metabolism, suggesting that endogenous synthesis from tryptophan is the more important source of NAD. In most cases the pellagra-like signs resolve with (relatively high) niacin supplements, although there are notes in some of the case reports that the affected infants could not tolerate niacin.

Hartnup disease is a rare genetic condition in which there is a defect of the membrane transport mechanism for tryptophan and other large neutral amino acids. As a result the intestinal absorption of free tryptophan is impaired, although dipeptide absorption is normal (see section 10.3.2). There is a considerable urinary loss of tryptophan (and other amino acids) as a result of failure of the normal resorption mechanism in the renal tubules—renal aminoaciduria. In addition to neurological signs that can be attributed to a deficit of tryptophan for the synthesis of 5–hydroxytryptamine in the central nervous system, the patients show clinical signs of pellagra, which respond to the administration of niacin.

Carcinoid is a tumour of the enterochromaffin cells which normally synthesize 5–hydroxytrytophan and 5–hydroxytryptamine. The carcinoid syndrome is seen when there are significant metastases of the primary tumour, normally in the liver. It is characterized by much increased gastrointestinal motility and diarrhoea, as well as regular periodic flushing. These symptoms can be attributed to systemic release of large amounts of 5–hydroxtryptamine, and can be controlled with inhibitors of tryptophan hydroxylase. The synthesis of 5–hydroxytryptamine in advanced carcinoid syndrome may be so great that as much as 60 per cent of the body's tryptophan metabolism proceeds by this pathway, compared with about 1 per cent under normal conditions. A significant number of patients with advanced carcinoid syndrome develop clinical signs of pellagra, because of this diversion of tryptophan away from the oxidative pathway of metabolism (Castiello and Lynch 1972; Lehmann 1972).

19.5.1.4 Drug-induced pellagra

The anti-tuberculosis drug isoniazid (iso-nicotinic acid hydrazide) can lead to the development of pellagra, by forming a biologically inactive complex with pyridoxal phosphate, the metabolically active form of vitamin B$_6$, and hence reducing the activity of kynureninase. This isoniazid-induced pellagra responds to the administration of niacin supplements. However, isoniazid may also cause peripheral neuropathy, which responds to vitamin B$_6$ and not niacin, and therefore it has become common practice to give vitamin B$_6$ supplements together with isoniazid.

During the 1960s the doses of isoniazid used in the treatment of tuberculosis were considerably reduced, as a result of the introduction of other effective antimycobacterial agents in therapeutic cocktails and it was no longer thought necessary to give patients supplements of vitamin B$_6$. There have been some reports of the development of pellagra in patients treated with relatively low doses of isoniazid; the patients were of Indian origin, and it is likely that they were genetically slow acetylators of isoniazid, so that an apparently low dose of the drug was, for them, high. Up to 60 per cent of Indians are slow acetylators of isoniazid.

In addition to its role as a pyridoxal phosphate-trapping reagent, isoniazid may also inhibit the metabolism of niacin directly; there have been reports of cases of pellagra developing in isoniazid-treated patients despite vitamin B_6 supplementation. Isoniazid is a substrate for the transglycosidase activity of NAD glycohydrolase, yielding a product that not only has no coenzyme activity, but may also inhibit nicotinamide nucleotide-dependent enzymes.

Although no case of clinical pellagra has been unequivocally reported, there have been a number of cases of pellagra-like conditions among patients receiving two anti-Parkinsonian drugs, Benserazide and Carbidopa. Both drugs inhibit the oxidative metabolism of tryptophan, and Parkinsonian patients treated with these drugs excrete less N^1-methyl nicotinamide than control patients with similarly severe disease but receiving different medication (Bender *et al.* 1979)

19.6   Assessment of niacin nutritional status

Although the nicotinamide nucleotide coenzymes function in a large number of oxidation and reduction reactions, this cannot be exploited as a means of assessing the state of the body's niacin reserves, because the coenzymes are not firmly attached to their apo-enzymes, as are thiamin pyrophosphate, riboflavin and pyridoxal phosphate, but act as cosubstrates of the reactions, binding to and leaving the enzyme as the reaction proceeds. No specific metabolic lesions associated with NAD(P) depletion have been identified.

The two methods of assessing niacin nutritional status are measurement of blood nicotinamide nucleotides and the urinary excretion of niacin metabolites, neither of which is wholly satisfactory. Criteria for interpreting the results are shown in Table 19.7.

19.6.1 Tissue and whole blood concentrations of nicotinamide nucleotides

Measurement of liver and other tissue concentrations of NAD(P) gives a precise estimate of niacin nutritional status and seems to be the most sensitive indicator in experimental animals. Measurement of the whole blood concentration of NAD(P) may serve the same purpose; there is a good correlation between blood and liver concentrations of nicotinamide nucleotides in experimental animals. The sensitivity of the method is such that reproducible determinations can be carried out on finger-prick samples of 200 µL of blood (Bender *et al.* 1982).

Fu *et al.* (1990) have shown that erythrocyte NAD falls during niacin depletion and rises during repletion in human subjects. Erythrocyte NADP was unaffected, and they suggested that the ratio of NAD:NADP might prove to be a useful index of niacin nutritional status, with a ratio <1.0 indicating deficiency.

Srikantia *et al.* (1968) showed that there is less NAD(P) and more nicotinamide mononucleotide in erythrocytes from pellagrins than control subjects, but this does not seem to have been confirmed or investigated further as a possible means of determining niacin nutritional status.

19.6.2 Urinary excretion of N^1-methyl nicotinamide and methyl pyridone carboxamide

The most widely used method for assessing niacin nutritional status is measurement of the urinary excretion of N^1-methyl nicotinamide, which is relatively simple to determine.

The excretion of methyl pyridone carboxamide is more severely reduced in marginal niacin inadequacy than is that of N^1-methyl nicotinamide. The excretion of methyl pyridone carboxamide decreases rapidly in subjects fed on a niacin deficient diet, and virtually ceases several weeks before the appearance of clinical signs of deficiency; by contrast, a number of studies have shown continuing excretion of N^1-methyl nicotinamide even in pellagrins.

De Lange and Joubert (1964) suggested that a better indication of niacin nutritional status can be obtained by determining the ratio of methyl pyridone carboxamide:N^1-methyl nicotinamide in urine. The ratio of these two metabolites is relatively constant, between 1.3–4.0 in adequately nourished subjects, despite the administration of loading doses of tryptophan or niacin. They suggested that a ratio of less than 1.0 would indicate depletion of niacin reserves.

19.7   Pharmacological uses and toxicity of niacin

Nicotinic acid is used clinically in large doses (of the order of 1–3 g /day) as a hypolipidaemic agent. It reduces both triglycerides and total cholesterol by about 20 per cent, acting as an inhibitor of cholesterol synthesis. It has a more marked effect on cholesterol in low density and very low density lipoproteins, and increases high density lipoprotein cholesterol (Parsons 1961a).

Nicotinic acid in modest doses causes a marked vasodilatation, with flushing, burning and itching of the skin. Very large single doses of nicotinic acid may cause sufficient vasodilatation to lead to hypotension; after the administration of 1–3 g of nicotinic acid daily for several days the effect wears off to a considerable extent. A number of nicotinoyl esters have been developed in order to permit sensitive patients to benefit from the hypolipidaemic effect of nicotinic acid without the vasodilatation (see Table 8.16). Nicotinamide does not have this effect.

At intakes in excess of 1 g of niacin /day there is evidence of toxicity. Parsons (1961) reported changes in liver function tests, carbohydrate tolerance and uric acid metabolism which were reversible on withdrawal of niacin. Baggenstoss *et al.* (1967) reported changes in liver ultra-structure in patients receiving high doses of niacin, namely dilatation of the endoplasmic reticulum with the formation of vesicles and sacs, and a diminution in the parallel arrays of rough endoplasmic reticulum, with fewer ribosomes on the outer surface. There was also elongation of the mitochondria, with bud-like projections and crystalloid inclusions. The mechanism of niacin hepatotoxicity is not known. Sustained release preparations, as compared with simple crystalline preparations, are associated with more severe liver damage and clinical liver failure, presumably because they permit more prolonged maintenance of blood and tissues concentrations of the vitamin, whereas after an acute high dose there is normally considerable excretion of unchanged nicotinic acid and nicotinamide, as the renal threshold is exceeded.

Supplements of tryptophan have been used with some success in the treatment of depressive diseases, apparently without ill effect. However, some 1300 cases of a potentially fatal eosinophilia-myalgia syndrome associated with the use of tryptophan supplements were been reported to the US Center for Disease Control in 1989 and early 1990 (Medsger 1990), and there have been reports from other countries. The problem was due to a contaminant, tentatively identified as ethylidene-*bis*-tryptophan, in a single batch of tryptophan, rather than to toxicity of tryptophan *per se.*

Further reading

Bender, A.E. and Bender, D.A. (1986). Niacin and tryptophan metabolism: the biochemical basis of niacin requirements and recommendations. *Nutrition Abstracts and Reviews* 56, 695–719.

Bender, D.A. (1983). Biochemistry of tryptophan in health and disease. *Molecular Aspects of Medicine*, 6, 101–97.

Bender, D.A. (1992). Niacin. In *Nutritional Biochemistry of the Vitamins*, Chapter 8, pp. 184–222. Cambridge University Press.

Frei, B. and Richter, C. (1988). Mono-(ADP-ribosylation) in rat liver mitochondria. *Biochemistry*, 27, 529–35.

Friedrich, W. (1988). Niacin: nicotinic acid, nicotinamide, NAD(P). In *Vitamins*, Chapter 8, pp. 475–542. Walter de Gruyter, Berlin.

Moss, J. and Vaughan, M. (1988). ADP-ribosylation of guanyl nucleotide binding regulatory proteins by bacterial toxins. *Advances in Enzymology*, 61, 303–79.

Roe, D.A. (1973). *A Plague of Corn: the Social History of Pellagra*. Cornell University Press, Ithaca, NY.

Rose, D.P. (1972). Aspects of tryptophan metabolism in health and disease. *Journal of Clinical Pathololology*, 25, 17–25.

Sydenstricker, V.P. (1958). The history of pellagra, its recognition as a disease of nutrition, and its conquest. *American Journal of Clinical Nutrition*, 6, 409–14.

Ueda, K. and Hayaishi, O. (1985). ADP-ribosylation. *Annual Review of Biochemistry*, 54, 73–100.

Table 19.1: Reference intakes of niacin (total niacin equivalents)

	US RDA (1989)	UK RNI (1991)	EU PRI (1993)
	mg	mg	mg
birth-6m	5	3	-
7-9 m	6	4	5
9m-1y	6	5	5
1-3 y	9	8	9
4-6	12	11	11
7-10	13	12	13
males			
11-14	17	15	15
15-18	20	18	18
19-24	19	17	18
25-50	19	17	14
> 50	15	16	-
females			
11-14	15	12	14
15-18	15	14	14
19-24	15	13	14
25-50	15	13	14
> 50	13	12	-
pregnant	17	-	14
lactating	20	+2	16

Source: National Research Council 1989; Department of Health 1991; Scientific Committee for Food 1993.

Table 19.2: Intakes of total niacin equivalents, mg/day, in UK

	males			females		
age	mean	median	95% range	mean	median	95% range
1.5-2.5	14.9	14.3	8.2-24.7	14.9	14.3	8.2-24.7
2.5-3.5	16.4	16.0	8.2-29.4	16.4	16.0	8.2-29.4
3.5-4.5	18.2	18.1	9.6-30.1	17.5	16.5	8.6-32.4
16-24	39.0	38.3	19.7-60.5	27.3	27.1	12.3-42.3
25-34	40.2	39.8	22.8-62.2	27.7	27.3	13.2-45.2
35-49	40.5	39.7	21.9-65.8	29.5	28.9	14.7-47.4
50-64	39.5	38.9	20.3-61.9	28.7	28.3	14.7-47.4

(1) The range shown is the 2.5-97.5 centile.
Source: from data reported by Gregory *et al.* 1990, 1995.

Table 19.3: Estimated intake of tryptophan in western diets

	% of protein intake	g protein /day	tryptophan mg/g protein	tryptophan intake mg/d
meat	36	30.6	12.0	367
cereals	23	19.6	12.3	241
milk and milk products	17	14.5	14.1	204
vegetables	9	7.7	9.6	74
fish	6	5.1	11.2	57
eggs	4	3.4	17.6	60
total		85		1003

Table 19.4: Sources of niacin in the average British diet

	% of average intake
beef and veal	8
poultry	7
other meat	18
vegetables	10
milk and milk products	9
white bread	7
wholemeal and other bread	7
breakfast cereals	8
other cereal products	6
fish	5
eggs	3
fruit and nuts	1
beverages	8

Source: Gregory *et al.* 1990.

Table 19.5: Rich sources of niacin

	portion (g)	mg niacin equivalents / portion
tuna	150	20
liver	150	18
chicken	150	12
mackerel	150	12
sardines canned in oil	150	12
salmon	150	11
turkey	150	11
veal	150	11
beef	150	9
dogfish	150	8
duck	150	8
kidney	150	8
lamb	150	8
pilchards in tomato sauce	100	8
pork	150	8
sardines canned in tomato	150	8
bloater	150	6
gammon joint	150	6
herring	150	6
rabbit	150	6
eel	150	5
lemon sole	150	5
plaice	150	5
shrimps	150	5
whiting	150	5
crab	175	4
peanuts	25	4
skate	150	4
bacon rashers	85	3
bread, wholemeal	70	3
cod	175	3
ham	85	3
pearl barley	100	3
potato chips	265	3
artichokes, globe	220	2
beans, broad	75	2
beans, red kidney	100	2
beer	560	2
bread, brown	60	2
lobster	150	2
mushrooms	50	2
peas	75	2
potatoes	140	2
scampi	150	2

Table 19.6: Conditions associated with the development of non-nutritional pellagra

	mechanism	reference
carcinoid syndrome	diversion of tryptophan to serotonin synthesis	Castiello and Lynch 1972
Hartnup disease	failure of tryptophan absorption	Baron *et al.* 1956
tryptophanuria	tryptophan dioxygenase (EC 1.13.11.11) deficiency	Tada *et al.* 1963; Snedden *et al.* 1983; Wong *et al.* 1976
xanthurenic aciduria	kynureninase (EC 3.7.1.3) deficiency	Komrower *et al.* 1964.
kynureninuria	kynurenine hydroxylase (EC 1.14.13.9) deficiency	Price *et al.* 1967
hereditary lethal pellagra	? elevated picolinic carboxylase (EC 4.1.1.45)	Salih *et al.* 1985
isoniazid treatment	inihibition of kynureninase (EC 3.7.1.3)	Knapp *et al.* 1958; Standal *et al.* 1974
dopa decarboxylase inhibitors	inihibition of kynureninase (EC 3.7.1.3)	Bender *et al.* 1979

Table 19.7: Indices of niacin nutritional status

	elevated	adequate	marginal	deficient
N^1-methyl nicotinamide				
μmol /24 h	> 48	17-47	5.8-17	< 5.8
mg /g creatinine	> 4.4	1.6-4.3	0.5-1.6	< 0.5
mmol /mol creatinine	> 4.0	1.3-3.9	0.4-1.3	< 0.4
methyl pyridone carboxamide				
μmol /24 h	-	> 18.9	6.4-18.9	< 6.4
mg /g creatinine	-	> 4.0	2.0-3.9	< 2.0
mmol /mol creatinine	-	> 4.4	0.44-4.3	< 0.44
ratio, methyl pyridone carboxamide : N^1-methyl nicotinamide				
	-	1.3-4.0	1.0-1.3	< 1.0
ratio, erythrocyte NAD : NADP	-	> 1.0	-	< 1.0

Source: from data reported by de Lange and Joubert 1964; Fu *et al.* 1990; Gontzea *et al.* 1976; Kelsay 1969.

20

Vitamin B₆

Vitamin B$_6$ has a central role in the metabolism of amino acids: in transaminase reactions (and hence the interconversion and catabolism of amino acids and the synthesis of non-essential amino acids); in decarboxylation to yield biologically active amines; and in a variety of elimination and replacement reactions. It is also the cofactor for glycogen phosphorylase and a variety of other enzymes.

In addition, pyridoxal phosphate, the metabolically active vitamer, has a role, as yet inadequately defined, in the release of steroid hormone receptors from tight nuclear binding. Vitamin B$_6$ thus affects the responsiveness of target tissues to hormone action.

The vitamin is widely distributed in foods, and clinical deficiency is virtually unknown, apart from an outbreak during the 1950s, which resulted from over-heating of infant milk formula (see section 20.5). Marginal inadequacy, affecting amino acid metabolism and possibly also steroid hormone responsiveness, may be relatively common. A number of vitamin B$_6$-dependency syndromes have been reported—inborn errors of metabolism in which the defect is in the coenzyme binding site of the affected enzyme (see section 20.5.1).

Oestrogens cause abnormalities of tryptophan metabolism which resemble those seen in vitamin B$_6$ deficiency, and the vitamin is widely used to treat the side-effects of oestrogen administration and oestrogen-associated symptoms of the premenstrual syndrome, although there is little evidence of its efficacy. High doses of the vitamin, of the order of 50–100 times requirements, cause peripheral sensory neuropathy.

20.1 Vitamin B₆ requirements and intake

Most studies of vitamin B$_6$ requirements have followed the development of abnormalities of tryptophan (see section 20.6.4) and methionine (see section 20.6.6) metabolism during depletion and normalization during repletion with graded intakes of the vitamin. While the tryptophan load test is unreliable as an index of vitamin B$_6$ nutritional status in field studies, under the controlled conditions of depletion / repletion studies it does give a useful indication of the state of vitamin B$_6$ nutrition.

Since the major role of vitamin B$_6$ is in amino acid metabolism it is likely that protein intake will affect vitamin B$_6$ requirements. Adults maintained on vitamin B$_6$-deficient diets develop abnormalities of tryptophan and methionine metabolism faster, and their blood vitamin B$_6$ falls more rapidly, when their protein intake is relatively high (80–160 g/day in various studies) than on low protein intakes (30–50 g/day). Similarly, during repletion of deficient subjects, tryptophan and methionine metabolism and blood vitamin B$_6$ are normalized faster at low than at high levels of protein intake (Canham *et al.* 1969; Kelsay *et al.* 1968a; Miller and Linkswiler 1967).

From such studies the mean requirement for vitamin B$_6$ is estimated to be 13 μg /gram dietary protein, and reference intakes (see Table 20.1) are based on 15–16 μg /g dietary protein. This allowance may not hold at very low intakes of protein, or under conditions of severely restricted food intake, because of the need for pyridoxal phosphate for the metabolism of amino acids released by catabolism of muscle proteins. However, in prolonged fasting pyridoxal phosphate is released from muscle by the breakdown of glycogen phosphorylase, and is available for redistribution to other tissues (see section 20.3.1).

Table 20.2 shows average intakes of vitamin B$_6$, and Table 20.3 foods that are rich sources (but see section 20.2.1 for a discussion of the biological availability of pyridoxine glucoside in foods).

There have been some attempts to estimate vitamin B$_6$ requirements from the size of the total body pool and its metabolic turnover. Short-term studies with isotopic tracers suggest a total body content of between 160–600 μmol (40–150 mg), with a half life of 33 days, suggesting a minimum requirement for replacement between 0.6–2.27 mg/day. However, some 80 per cent of the total body vitamin B$_6$ is in skeletal muscle glycogen phosphorylase, with a relatively slow turnover. Based on longer-term tracer studies, Coburn (1990) has suggested a total body pool of 250 mg, or 15 nmol (3.7 µg)/g body weight, with a loss of about 0.13 per cent /day, and hence a minimum requirement for replacement of 0.02 µmol (5 µg)/kg body weight—some 350 µg/day for a 70 kg adult. This is considerably lower than the requirement to normalize tryptophan or methionine metabolism in depletion / repletion studies, and may reflect dilution of the small pool associated with amino acid metabolism, which has a rapid turnover, by the larger and more stable pool associated with glycogen phosphorylase.

20.1.1 Requirements of infants

Estimation of the vitamin B$_6$ requirements of infants presents a problem, and there is a clear need for further research. Human milk, which must be assumed to be adequate for infant nutrition, provides only some 2.5–3 µg of vitamin B$_6$/g protein—very much lower than the requirement for adults, although there is no reason why infants should have a lower requirement.

Based on the body content of 15 nmol (3.7 µg) of vitamin B$_6$/g body weight, and the rate of weight gain, Coburn (1990) suggested that a minimum requirement for infants over the first 6 months of life is 100 µg (417 nmol)/day to establish tissue reserves, and an additional 20 per cent to allow for metabolic turnover. Even if the mother receives daily supplements of 2.5 mg of vitamin B$_6$ throughout lactation, thus more than doubling the normal intake, the infant's intake ranges from 100–300 µg/day over the first 6 months of life. At 1 month this is only 8.5 µg/g protein, rising to 15 g/g by 2 months (Borschel *et al.* 1986).

A first approximation to the vitamin B$_6$ needs of infants came from studies of those who convulsed as a result of gross deficiency caused by over-heated infant milk formula (see section 20.5). At intakes of 60 µg/day the incidence of convulsions was 0.3 per cent. Provision of 260 µg/day prevented or cured convulsions, but 300 µg/day was required to normalize tryptophan metabolism (Bessey *et al.* 1957). This is almost certainly a considerable overestimate of requirements, since pyridoxyl-lysine, formed by heating the vitamin with proteins, has antivitamin activity, and would therefore result in a higher apparent requirement.

20.2 Vitamin B$_6$ vitamers and nomenclature

The generic descriptor vitamin B$_6$ includes six vitamers: the alcohol pyridoxine, the aldehyde pyridoxal, the amine pyridoxamine and their 5'-phosphates. There is some confusion in the literature, because at one time 'pyridoxine' was used as a generic descriptor, with 'pyridoxol' as the specific name for the alcohol. Since 1973 the official IUPAC-IUB and IUNS nomenclature has been as shown in Fig. 20.1. The vitamers are metabolically interconvertible and, as far as is known, they have equal biological activity; 4–pyridoxic acid is a biologically inactive end-product of vitamin B$_6$ metabolism.

20.2.1 Biologically unavailable vitamin B$_6$ in foods

Two groups of vitamin B$_6$ derivatives that may be present in foods have low biological availability, and have some antivitamin antimetabolic activity as well: pyridoxine glucosides that are naturally present in plant foods, and the products of reaction of pyridoxal with lysine in proteins that have been heated severely. Overall, it is estimated that some 70–80 per cent of dietary vitamin B$_6$ is biologically available (Kabir *et al.* 1983; Reynolds 1988).

20.2.1.1 Pyridoxine glucosides

A considerable proportion of the vitamin B$_6$ in plant foods may be present as pyridoxine glucosides; up to 50 per cent in some foods, see Table 20.4, mainly as pyridoxine-5–β-D-glucoside, although other glucosides are present in some foods. The biological availability of these glucosides is uncertain. They are absorbed, but, at least in laboratory animals, are then excreted in the urine unchanged. Isotope studies in human beings suggest that about 50–60 per cent of the glucosides is available, possibly as a result of intestinal bacterial glucosidases, since intravenously administered pyridoxine glucoside is significantly less available. There is some evidence, from animal studies, that the glucoside modifies the metabolism and tissue retention of vitamin B$_6$ (Gregory *et al.* 1991; Gilbert and Gregory 1992).

20.2.1.2 Pyridoxyl-lysine

When foods are heated, pyridoxal and pyridoxal phosphate can react with the ε-amino groups of lysine to form a Schiff base (aldimine), which may either be stabilized by metal ion chelation or be reduced to the aldamine. This renders both the vita-

pyridoxine

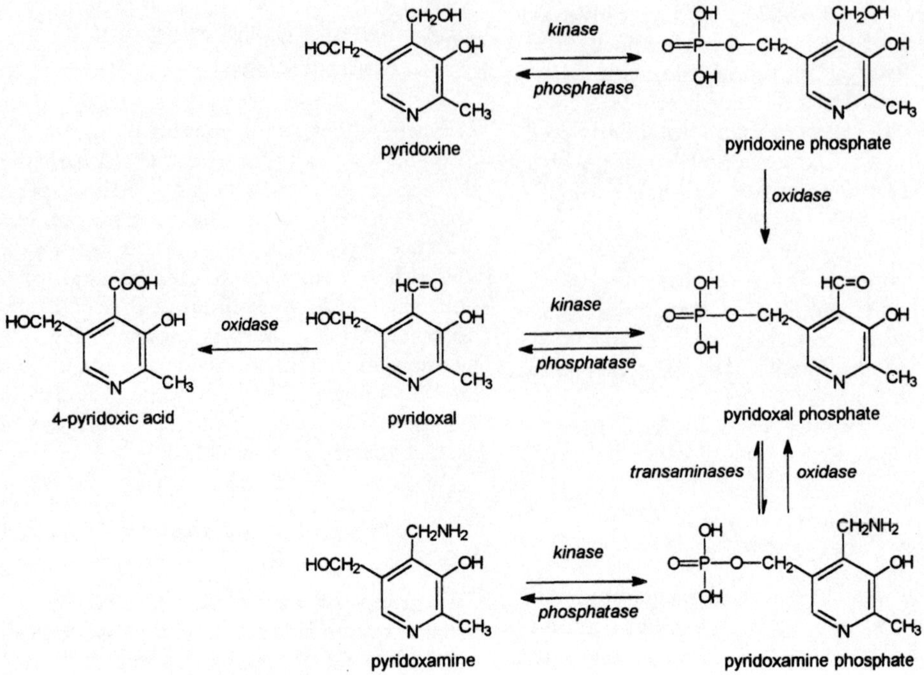

pyridoxine phosphate

kinase

phosphatase

oxidase

4-pyridoxic acid

pyridoxal

pyridoxal phosphate

oxidase

kinase

phosphatase

transaminases   *oxidase*

pyridoxamine

pyridoxamine phosphate

kinase

phosphatase

Figure 20.1 Metabolic interconversion of the vitamin B$_6$ vitamers
Relative molecular masses (M$_r$): pyridoxine 169.3, pyridoxal 168.2, pyridoxamine 169.3, pyridoxal phosphate 247.1, pyridoxamine phosphate 248.2, 4-pyridoxic acid 184.2. Pyridoxal kinase EC 2.7.1.38, pyridoxine oxidase EC 1.1.1.65, pyridoxamine phosphate oxidase 1.4.3.5, pyridoxal oxidase EC 1.1.3.12.

min B$_6$ and the lysine biologically unavailable (see Fig. 10.5); more importantly, the pyridoxyl-ε-amino-lysine released during digestion is absorbed, and has antivitamin B$_6$ antimetabolite activity (Gregory and Kirk 1977; Gregory 1980*b*).

Both pyridoxal and pyridoxamine can also react with the sulphydryl group of cysteine, pyridoxamine can react with reducing sugars, and in the presence of ascorbic acid (vitamin C) inactive 6–hydroxypyridoxine may be formed (Bates and Heseker 1994).

20.3 Absorption and metabolism of vitamin B$_6$

The phosphorylated vitamers are dephosphorylated by membrane-bound alkaline phosphatase in the intestinal mucosa; pyridoxal, pyridoxamine and pyridoxine are all absorbed rapidly by passive diffusion. Intestinal mucosal cells have pyridoxine kinase, pyridoxine phosphate oxidase and phosphatases (see Fig. 20.1), so that there is net accumulation of pyridoxal phosphate by metabolic trapping. Much of the

ingested pyridoxine is released into the portal circulation as pyridoxal, after dephosphorylation at the serosal surface. Unlike other B vitamins, there seems to be no limitation on the amount of vitamin B$_6$ that is absorbed.

Most of the absorbed vitamin is taken up by the liver, although other tissues can also take up the unphosphorylated vitamers from the circulation. Uptake is by passive diffusion, followed by metabolic trapping as phosphate esters. Pyridoxine and pyridoxamine phosphates are oxidized to pyridoxal phosphate, as shown in Fig. 20.1. All tissues have pyridoxine kinase activity, but pyridoxine phosphate oxidase is found only in liver, kidney and brain, with low activity in erythrocytes. Plasma concentrations of the vitamin B$_6$ vitamers are shown in Table 20.5.

Pyridoxine phosphate oxidase is a flavoprotein, it is sensitive to riboflavin depletion, and activation of the erythrocyte apoenzyme by riboflavin phosphate *in vitro* can be used as an index of riboflavin nutritional status. The effects of riboflavin deficiency on vitamin B$_6$ nutritional status are discussed in section 18.5.3.

Pyridoxine is rapidly converted to pyridoxal phosphate in liver and other tissues. Pyridoxal phosphate does not cross cell membranes, and efflux of the vitamin from most tissues is as pyridoxal. Pyridoxal phosphate is exported from the liver bound to albumin. Much of the free pyridoxal phosphate in the liver (i.e. that which is not protein bound) is hydrolysed to pyridoxal, which is also exported, and circulates bound to both albumin and haemoglobin in erythrocytes. Free pyridoxal remaining in the liver is rapidly oxidized to 4–pyridoxic acid, which is the main excretory product of the vitamin (Lumeng *et al.* 1974).

Extra-hepatic tissues take up both pyridoxal and pyridoxal phosphate from the plasma. Pyridoxal phosphate is hydrolysed to pyridoxal, which can cross cell membranes, by extracellular alkaline phosphatase, then trapped intracellularly by phosphorylation.

Tissue concentrations of pyridoxal phosphate are controlled by the balance between phosphorylation and dephosphorylation. The activity of phosphatases acting on pyridoxal phosphate is greater than that of the kinase in most tissues. This means that pyridoxal phosphate which is not bound to enzymes is readily dephosphorylated. The total pyridoxal phosphate content of liver and brain falls on adrenalectomy, apparently as a result of the loss of glucocorticoid induction of pyridoxal phosphate-dependent enzymes, so that less of the vitamin is protein bound, and more is available for dephosphorylation. Conversely, the administration of glucocorticoid hormones increases tissue pyridoxal phosphate by inducing pyridoxal phosphate-dependent enzymes which then bind the coenzyme and protect it from dephosphorylation.

Free pyridoxal either leaves the cells or is oxidized to 4–pyridoxic acid by aldehyde dehydrogenase (which is present in all tissues) and also by hepatic and renal aldehyde oxidase. 4–Pyridoxic acid is the main excretory product of vitamin B$_6$ and its excretion reflects recent intake more than the state of underlying tissue reserves of the vitamin. Small amounts of pyridoxal and pyridoxamine are also excreted in the urine, although much of the active vitamin B$_6$ which is filtered in the glomerulus is resorbed in the kidney tubules.

20.3.1 Muscle pyridoxal phosphate

Some 80 per cent of the body's total vitamin B$_6$ is as pyridoxal phosphate in muscle, and some 80 per cent of this is associated with glycogen phosphorylase (see section 20.4.2). This does not seem to function as a reserve of the vitamin and is not released from muscle in times of deficiency. The normal muscle concentration of pyridoxal phosphate is of the order of 10 nmol /g; in patients with McArdle's disease (glycogen storage disease due to congenital lack of glycogen phosphorylase) the muscle content of pyridoxal phosphate is reduced to one fifth of this. Patients with McArdle's disease do not show any signs of vitamin B$_6$ deficiency, nor are they more susceptible to vitamin B$_6$ depletion than normal subjects (Haller *et al.* 1983).

Muscle pyridoxal phosphate is released into the circulation (as pyridoxal) in starvation, as muscle glycogen reserves are exhausted and there is less requirement for glycogen phosphorylase activity. Under these conditions it is available for redistribution to other tissues, and especially liver and kidney, to meet the increased requirement for gluconeogenesis from amino acids (Black *et al.* 1975, 1978). Muscle pyridoxal phosphate does fall during vitamin B$_6$ depletion in experimental animals, but this is largely a response to lower food intake, and hence lower muscle glycogen reserves. During acute repletion of deficient animals, the pyridoxal phosphate content of most tissues returns to normal within a few hours, while muscle pyridoxal phosphate only increases slowly, over several days, as glycogen phosphorylase is restored.

20.4 Metabolic functions of vitamin B$_6$

The metabolically active vitamer is pyridoxal phosphate, which is involved in many reactions of amino acid metabolism where the carbonyl group is the reactive moiety; in glycogen phosphorylase, where it is the phosphate group that is important in catalysis; and in the recycling of steroid hormone receptors from tight nuclear binding, where again it is the carbonyl group that is important.

Pyridoxal phosphate has a clear role in lipid metabolism as the coenzyme for phosphatidylserine decarboxylation, leading to the formation of phosphatidylethanolamine, and thence to phosphatidylcholine (see section 23.6.1). In addition there is some evidence that it is involved in the metabolism of polyunsaturated fatty acids, based on the observation that when linoleate-depleted animals are repleted there is greater formation of arachidonate if they are also supplied with vitamin B$_6$ supplements. There is also evidence that carnitine synthesis (see section 23.5.1) is pyridoxal phosphate dependent; again it is largely indirect evidence based on changes in carnitine metabolism in vitamin B$_6$ deficiency, and no pyridoxal phosphate-dependent reaction has been identified.

20.4.1 Pyridoxal phosphate in amino acid metabolism

The various reactions of pyridoxal phosphate in amino acid metabolism all depend on the same chemical principle—the ability to stabilize amino acid carbanions, and hence to weaken bonds about the α-carbon of the substrate. This is achieved by reaction of the α-amino group with the carbonyl group of the coenzyme.

In the absence of the amino acid substrate, pyridoxal phosphate is bound to enzymes by the formation of a Schiff base (aldimine) with the ε-amino group of a lysine residue at the active site. The first reaction with the substrate is transfer of the aldimine linkage from the ε-amino group of the lysine residue to the α-amino group of the substrate. Depending on the reactive groups in the active site of the enzyme, and from which bond(s) around the α-carbon of the amino acid electrons are withdrawn, the amino acid

may undergo decarboxylation, racemization, transamination or one of a variety of side-chain modifications, see Fig. 20.2.

20.4.1.1 Decarboxylation
If the electron withdrawing effect of the heterocyclic nitrogen is primarily centred on the α-carbon-carboxyl bond, the result is decarboxylation of the amino acid aldimine and release of CO$_2$. The resultant carbanion is then protonated, and the primary amine corresponding to the amino acid is displaced by the lysine residue at the active site, with reformation of the internal Schiff base. The biologically important amines formed by decarboxylation of amino acids are shown in Table 20.6.

20.4.1.2 Racemization
Amino acid racemases are important in bacterial metabolism, since several D-amino acids are required for the synthesis of cell wall mucopolysaccharides. There is no evidence that there are any significant mammalian amino acid racemases; such utilization of D-amino acids as occurs (see section 10.2.1) is

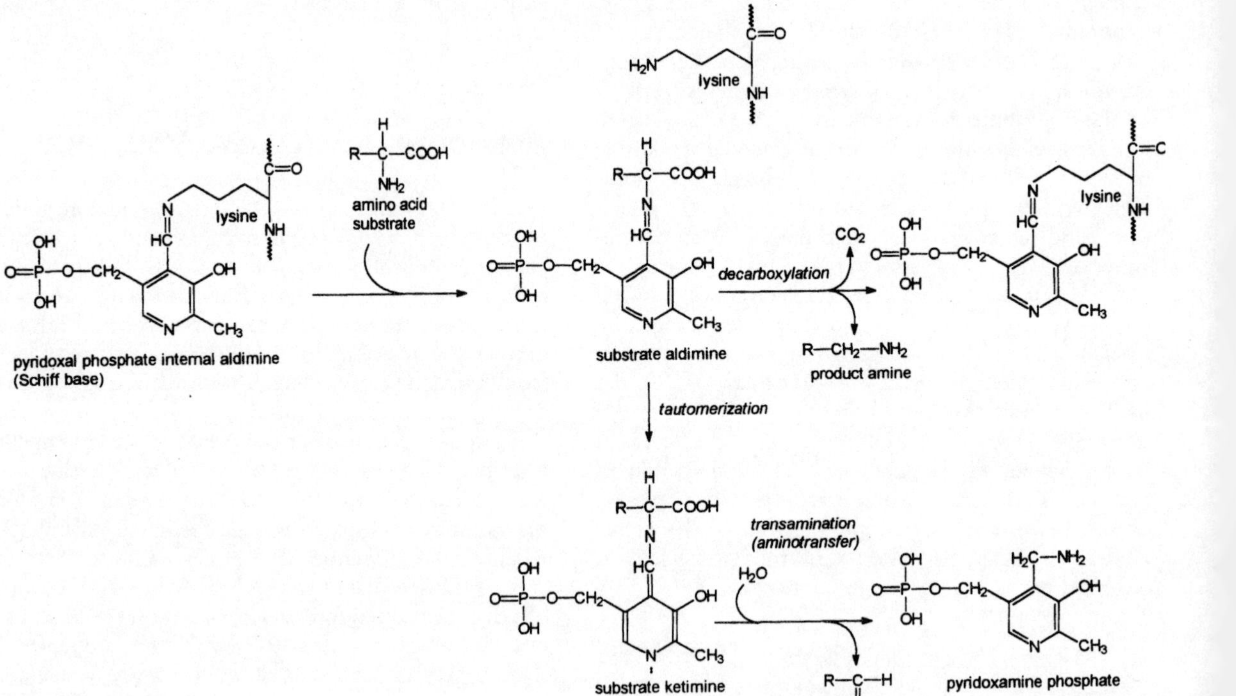

Figure 20.2 Reactions of amino acids in pyridoxal phosphate-dependent enzymes

probably due to the action of D-amino acid oxidase to form the symmetrical 2–oxo-acid which is then a substrate for stereospecific aminotransfer.

Deprotonation of the α-carbon of the amino acid leads to tautomerization of the Schiff base to the quinonoid ketimine, as shown in Fig. 20.2. The simplest reaction that the ketimine can undergo is reprotonation at the now symmetrical α-carbon.

20.4.1.3 Transamination

Transamination, the reversible formation of 2–oxo-acids (α-keto-acids) from amino acids, is of central importance in amino acid metabolism, providing pathways for the catabolism of all amino acids other than lysine (which does not undergo transamination in mammalian tissues), although pathways other than transamination may be more important for the catabolism of some amino acids.

Many of the transaminase reactions are linked to the amination of 2–oxo-glutarate to glutamate or glyoxylate to glycine, which are substrates for oxidative deamination, reforming the oxo-acids. This thus provides a pathway for the net deamination of most amino acids. Equally, transamination provides a pathway for the synthesis of those amino acids for which there is an alternative source of the oxo-acid (the non-essential amino acids, see sections 10.2.1 and 10.6.2). The reaction of transamination is shown in Fig. 20.3, and the oxo-acids corresponding to the protein amino acids in Table 20.7.

Hydrolysis of the α-carbon-amino bond of the ketimine results in the release of the 2–oxo-acid corresponding to the amino acid substrate, and leaves pyridoxamine phosphate at the catalytic site of the enzyme. This is the half reaction of transamination. The process is completed by reaction of pyridoxa-mine phosphate with a second oxo-acid substrate, forming an intermediate ketimine, then by the reverse of the reaction sequence shown in Fig. 20.2, releasing the amino acid corresponding to this second substrate after displacement from the aldimine by the reactive lysine residue to reform the internal Schiff base.

20.4.1.4 Transamination reactions catalysed by other pyridoxal phosphate enzymes

In addition to their main reactions, a number of pyridoxal phosphate dependent enzymes also catalyse the half reaction of transamination as an undesirable side-reaction, occurring perhaps once in 10 000 reaction cycles. Such enzymes include most of the amino acid decarboxylases, serine hydroxymethyltransferase (see section 21.1.4.1), and kynureninase (see section 20.6.4).

The result of this transamination is the formation of pyridoxamine phosphate at the active site of the enzyme, and hence loss of activity. Pyridoxamine phosphate dissociates from the active site, so that it is only if adequate pyridoxal phosphate is available that the resultant apo-enzyme can be reactivated. This probably explains why some enzymes, such as kynureninase, are especially sensitive to vitamin B₆ depletion.

20.4.1.5 Side-chain elimination and replacement reactions

The third bond in the Schiff base aldimine that can be labilized by the electron-withdrawing effect of the ring nitrogen is that between the α-carbon and the side chain of the amino acid, resulting in a variety of elimination and replacement reactions, such as the reactions of serine dehydratase (EC 4.2.1.13); serine hydroxymethyltransferase (see section 21.1.4.1); cysteine lyase (EC 4.4.1.10), which replaces the sul-

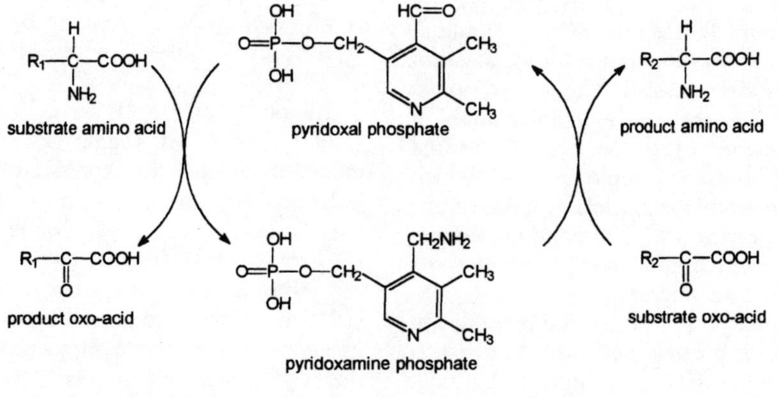

Figure 20.3 The reaction of transamination

phydryl group of cysteine with SO$_3$, releasing H$_2$S; selenocysteine lyase (EC 4.4.1.16), which cleaves selenocysteine to release H$_2$Se and alanine (see section 15.4.1); and cystathionine β-synthetase (EC 4.2.1.22, see Fig. 20.5). The reaction may also involve β-elimination, as in γ-cystathionase (EC 4.4.1.1, see Fig. 20.5).

20.4.2 The role of pyridoxal phosphate in glycogen phosphorylase

Glycogen phosphorylase (EC 2.4.1.1) catalyses the sequential phosphorolysis of glycogen to release glucose-1–phosphate; it is thus the key enzyme in the utilization of liver and muscle glycogen reserves.

Unlike other pyridoxal phosphate-dependent enzymes, in which it is the carbonyl group which is essential for catalysis, the internal Schiff base between pyridoxal phosphate and lysine in glycogen phosphorylase can be reduced with sodium borohydride without affecting catalytic activity. Thus, while pyridoxal phosphate is indeed essential for phosphorylase activity, it does not act by the same kind of mechanism as in amino acid metabolism. It is the phosphate group of the coenzyme that is essential for the reaction of glycogen phosphorylase.

The initial stage in the phosphorolysis of glycogen is protonation of the glycosidic oxygen of the polysaccharide by inorganic phosphate. The resultant oxycarbonium ion is stabilized by the inorganic phosphate. The role of pyridoxal phosphate is as a proton shuttle or buffer to stabilize the oxycarbonium-phosphate ion pair, permitting covalent binding of the phosphate to the oxycarbonium ion, to form glucose 1–phosphate (Palm *et al.* 1990).

20.4.3 The role of pyridoxal phosphate in nuclear hormone action

Steroid hormones, thyroid hormone (see section 25.14.3), and vitamins D (see section 14.3.3) and A (see section 13.3.3) act by modulating the synthesis of specific proteins in target tissues. The steroid enters the nucleus and alters the rate of transcription of DNA to mRNA. Target tissue specificity is ensured by the presence of hormone receptor proteins which are responsible for both the nuclear uptake of the steroid and the interaction with DNA and nucleoproteins; as discussed in section 25.26.1, these receptor proteins all contain 'zinc fingers'.

Pyridoxal phosphate reacts with a lysine residue in the hormone receptor protein, and extracts the hormone-receptor complex from tight nuclear binding. *In vitro*, reaction with pyridoxal phosphate also inhibits the binding of receptor protein to isolated DNA and chromatin. The effect is specific for the phosphorylated vitamer, suggesting that there may be a specific pyridoxal phosphate binding site on the receptor proteins, and it is apparent at low concentrations of pyridoxal phosphate, of the same order of magnitude as occur in tissues under normal conditions.

The specificity of the effects of pyridoxal phosphate, but not pyridoxal, and the low concentrations at which the effect can be observed, led Cidlowski and Thanassi (1981) to propose that pyridoxal phosphate may have a physiological role in the action of steroid hormones. They suggested that it might act as a cofactor in the release of hormone-receptor complexes from tight nuclear binding, resulting in release of the steroid from the nucleus, and freeing or recycling receptors for further uptake of steroid.

In experimental animals, vitamin B$_6$ deficiency results in increased and prolonged nuclear uptake and retention of oestradiol in the uterus and testosterone in the prostate. Coupled with the increased and prolonged nuclear accumulation of steroid hormones in target tissues in vitamin B$_6$ deficiency, there is evidence of enhanced sensitivity to oestrogen and testosterone activity *in vivo*. Deficient animals show greater induction of uterine peroxidase, and considerably greater suppression of the hypothalamic secretion of luteinizing hormone, by oestrogens than do vitamin B$_6$-supplemented controls. In vitamin B$_6$ deficient male animals there is an increased mitotic response in the prostate to low doses of testosterone. Deficient male animals have a higher activity of ornithine decarboxylase (an androgen-induced enzyme) in the liver, and deficient females have higher renal ornithine transaminase (an oestrogen-induced enzyme). The induction of hepatic tyrosine transaminase and tryptophan dioxygenase by glucocorticoids is also enhanced in vitamin B$_6$ deficient animals. (Bender 1987, 1994; Bowden *et al.* 1986; Symes *et al.* 1984).

Allgood *et al.* (1990) and Allgood and Cidlowski (1992) have shown that pyridoxal phosphate does indeed modulate gene expression in response to steroid hormones. Using a series of gene constructs of various hormone-response elements with a reporter gene transfected into a variety of cell types in culture, they showed that acute vitamin B$_6$ depletion of the cells led to increased gene expression in response to hormone action, while supplementation with pyridoxal phosphate led to greatly reduced gene expression after hormone stimulation.

20.5 Vitamin B$_6$ deficiency

Clinical deficiency of vitamin B$_6$ is rare. The vitamin is widely distributed in foods, and intestinal flora synthesize relatively large amounts, at least some of which is believed to be absorbed and hence available. Nevertheless, as shown in Table 20.8, a significant proportion of people in developed countries show biochemical evidence of being inadequately supplied with vitamin B$_6$. It is noteworthy that in only one of the studies listed in Table 20.8 were the same subjects assessed by two criteria of adequacy: plasma pyridoxal phosphate and erythrocyte aspartate aminotransferase activation coefficient (see section 20.6.3). As shown in Table 20.9, few subjects appeared to be inadequately supplied with the vitamin by both criteria (Bender 1993).

It is apparent from discussion of the role of pyridoxal phosphate in steroid hormone action (see section 20.4.3) that moderate vitamin B$_6$ deficiency will enhance the responses of target tissues to steroid hormones. This may be important in the induction and subsequent development of hormone-dependent cancer of the breast and prostate, and may therefore affect the prognosis. Vitamin B$_6$ supplementation may be a useful adjunct to other therapy in these common cancers; certainly there is evidence that poor vitamin B$_6$ nutritional status is associated with a poor prognosis in women with breast cancer (Bell 1980).

In vitamin B$_6$-deficient experimental animals there are more or less specific skin lesions (e.g. acrodynia in the rat) and fissures or ulceration at the corners of the mouth and over the tongue, as well as a number of endocrine abnormalities, defects in the metabolism of tryptophan (see section 20.6.4), methionine (see section 20.6.6) and other amino acids, hypochromic microcytic anaemia (the first step of haem biosynthesis is pyridoxal phosphate dependent), changes in leukocyte count and activity, a tendency to epileptiform convulsions and peripheral nervous system damage resulting in ataxia and sensory neuropathy.

Much of our knowledge of human vitamin B$_6$ deficiency is derived from an outbreak in the early 1950s, which resulted from an infant milk preparation which had undergone severe heating in manufacture. This was the first clear evidence that vitamin B$_6$ was a dietary essential for human beings. Heating led to the formation of pyridoxyl-lysine by reaction between pyridoxal phosphate and the ε-amino groups of lysine in proteins. As discussed in section 10.2.1.2, pyridoxyl-lysine has little biological activity, and may also be an antimetabolite of vitamin B$_6$,

so exacerbating the deficiency. In addition to a number of metabolic abnormalities, many of the affected infants convulsed. They responded to the administration of vitamin B$_6$ supplements.

Investigation of the neurochemical basis of the convulsions seen in vitamin B$_6$ deficiency revealed the role of GABA (γ-aminobutyrate, which is synthesized by the decarboxylation of glutamate) as an inhibitory neurotransmitter. More recent studies have suggested that the accumulation of hydroxykynurenine in the brain in deficiency may be the critical factor precipitating convulsions. GABA is depleted in the brains of deficient adult and neonate animals, while hydroxykynurenine accumulation is considerably more marked in neonates than adults—only neonates convulse in vitamin B$_6$ deficiency. GABA depletion may be a necessary, but not sufficient, condition for convulsions in vitamin B$_6$ deficiency (Guilarte and Wagner 1987).

20.5.1 Vitamin B$_6$ dependency syndromes

A small number of cases have been reported of patients with genetic defects that result in an abnormally high requirement for vitamin B$_6$ in order to maintain the activity of the affected enzyme. The conditions, and the enzymes affected, are shown in Table 20.10. The molecular basis of the defects appears to be a grossly impaired affinity of the defective enzyme for its cofactor, and the patients respond well to doses of 50–1000 mg of vitamin B$_6$/day. Apart from the affected enzyme, other biochemical indices of vitamin B$_6$ nutritional status are normal in these patients (Frimpter et al. 1969; Mudd 1971).

20.5.2 Enzyme responses to vitamin B$_6$ deficiency

Some pyridoxal phosphate-dependent enzymes appear to be relatively protected against deficiency, and are always saturated with cofactor, showing the same activity on assay in vitro whether additional pyridoxal phosphate is present in the incubation medium or not. Examples of this class of enzymes include liver cysteine sulphinate decarboxylase (EC 4.1.1.29, which is involved in the synthesis of taurine from cysteine, see section 23.9.1) and the brain and liver glutamate and aspartate aminotransferases.

Other enzymes appear not to be fully saturated with cofactor, and show increased activity in vitro when additional pyridoxal phosphate is present in the incubation medium; examples of these enzymes include brain glutamate decarboxylase (EC 4.1.1.15), liver kynureninase and cystathionase, and aspartate aminotransferase from red blood cells. The activities of these enzymes thus varies with vitamin B$_6$ nutritional status, although, as discussed above (see section 20.4.1.4), those enzymes which, like glutamate decarboxylase and kynureninase, undergo transamination and mechanism-dependent inactivation, may show increased inactivation under conditions of vitamin B$_6$ deficiency, and an exaggerated response to the addition of pyridoxal phosphate. When the intake of vitamin B$_6$ is increased to a relatively high level, these apo-enzymes are activated *in vivo*, resulting in increased activity of enzymes that may well be primary or secondary rate-limiting enzymes of metabolic pathways.

In deficiency, the synthesis and catabolism of some pyridoxal phosphate dependent enzymes is altered. For example, within a few days of feeding a vitamin B$_6$-free diet to animals there is a fall in the activity of cysteine sulphinate decarboxylase in liver; after two weeks the amount of the enzyme protein has fallen to extremely low levels. It is likely that these enzymes are 'sacrificed' to release pyridoxal phosphate for other, more essential, enzymes. Other enzymes show the opposite response—apparent induction of the apo-enzyme in vitamin B$_6$ deficiency, presumably in an attempt to trap as much of the available pyridoxal phosphate as possible. An example of such a response is the considerable increase in apo-glutamate decarboxylase in the brains of vitamin B$_6$ deficient rats (Bayoumi *et al.* 1972). Since the product of glutamate decarboxylase, γ-amino butyrate (GABA), is a central neurotransmitter, it is obviously important to maintain its synthesis for as long as possible. By contrast, the aromatic amino acid decarboxylase (EC 4.1.1.28) that is involved in the synthesis of the catecholamine neurotransmitters and 5–hydroxytryptamine, is unaffected in vitamin B$_6$ deficiency. This enzyme has a very high affinity for pyridoxal phosphate, and is normally fully saturated with cofactor (Eberle and Eiduson 1968).

20.6   Assessment of vitamin B$_6$ nutritional status

20.6.1 Plasma concentrations of the vitamin

Fasting plasma total vitamin B$_6$ (measured microbiologically), or more specifically pyridoxal phosphate, is widely used as an index of vitamin B$_6$ nutritional status. The generally accepted criteria of adequacy are shown in Table 20.11.

Conditions that involve increased plasma activity of alkaline phosphatase may result in reduced plasma concentrations of pyridoxal phosphate, without affecting vitamin B$_6$ nutritional status or tissue concentrations of pyridoxal phosphate. In such conditions there is a compensatory increase in the circulating concentration of pyridoxal, which is the main form for extra-hepatic uptake of vitamin B$_6$. Barnard *et al.* (1986) have shown that despite the fall in plasma pyridoxal phosphate in pregnancy, which has been widely interpreted as indicating vitamin B$_6$ depletion or a greatly increased requirement for the vitamin, the plasma concentration of pyridoxal phosphate plus pyridoxal is unchanged. This suggests that determination of plasma pyridoxal phosphate alone may not be a reliable index of vitamin B$_6$ nutritional status.

There is an increase in circulating pyridoxal phosphate in response to moderately severe exercise. Leklem and Schultz (1983) reported a 16–37 per cent increase in plasma pyridoxal phosphate in young men after a 4.5 km run. The changes in blood volume and circulating transaminase activities were too small to account for this, and they suggested that there was release of the vitamin from muscle as a result of breakdown of glycogen phosphorylase, as is seen in starvation. This suggests that any recent relatively severe physical exertion will affect the determination of vitamin B$_6$ nutritional status by measurement of the plasma concentration of pyridoxal phosphate, masking a possible deficiency. There is no evidence of increased vitamin B$_6$ requirements in severe exercise, and supplements of the vitamin have no effect on athletic performance or work output.

20.6.2 Urinary excretion of vitamin B$_6$

Some biologically active vitamin B$_6$ is excreted in the urine, and a number of studies have assessed nutritional status by microbiological measurement of this excretion; it is difficult to interpret the results in terms of underlying nutritional status rather than as a reflection of recent intake, although the excretion does fall in deficiency (Sauberlich *et al.* 1972). A possibly important source of error here is that minor renal damage, resulting in even slight albuminuria, will result in a considerable increase in urinary albumin-bound pyridoxal phosphate.

About half of the normal dietary intake of vitamin B$_6$ is excreted as 4–pyridoxic acid (see Fig. 20.1). Urinary excretion of 4–pyridoxic acid will largely reflect recent intake of the vitamin rather than underlying nutritional status; the generally accepted criteria for assessment of 4–pyridoxic acid excretion are shown in Table 20.11.

20.6.3 Coenzyme saturation of transaminases

A number of studies have measured the activation of plasma transaminases by pyridoxal phosphate added *in vitro*; however, it is difficult to interpret the results, since plasma transaminases arise largely accidentally, as a result of cell turnover, and the amount released will depend on tissue damage. Furthermore, there is a considerable amount of pyridoxal phosphate in plasma, largely associated with serum albumin, and the extent to which plasma transaminases are saturated will depend largely on the relative affinity of albumin and the enzyme concerned for the coenzyme, rather than reflecting the availability of pyridoxal phosphate for intracellular metabolism.

Studies on erythrocyte transaminase activation coefficient are easier to interpret, since the extent to which the enzymes are saturated depends mainly on the availability of pyridoxal phosphate. The reference ranges for erythrocyte aspartate and alanine transaminase activation coefficients are shown in Table 20.11.

Erythrocyte transaminase activation does not respond to acute vitamin B$_6$ depletion as rapidly as do other indices (Donald and Bosse 1979). This presumably reflects the avidity with which pyridoxal phosphate-dependent enzymes retain their coenzyme. Erythrocytes that are released into the circulation containing holo-enzyme will not lose coenzyme, so that the activation coefficient will only change as newly formed erythrocytes containing inadequate amounts of pyridoxal phosphate enter the circulation, replacing older cells. Under normal circumstances, circulating erythrocytes have a life of some 100 days, so it is unlikely that relatively acute depletion studies (typically periods of about 28 days have been used) would result in any significant change in transaminase activation coefficient, although other indices of vitamin B$_6$ nutritional status show the expected changes. The converse of this is that an abnormally elevated erythrocyte transaminase activation coefficient can be taken as evidence of a continuing relatively long-term deficiency.

In deficient subjects who are given vitamin B$_6$ there is the expected fall in the transaminase activation coefficient, reflecting increased enzyme saturation with coenzyme, since circulating erythrocytes are able to take up the vitamin from plasma, and can thus respond to an improvement in availability of the vitamin.

20.6.4 The tryptophan load test

The tryptophan load test for vitamin B$_6$ nutritional status (the ability to metabolize a test dose of tryptophan) is one of the oldest metabolic tests for functional vitamin nutritional status. It was developed as a result of observation of the excretion of an abnormal coloured compound, later identified as the tryptophan metabolite xanthurenic acid, in the urine of deficient animals.

Under normal conditions, the rate-limiting enzyme of the oxidative pathway of tryptophan metabolism (see Fig. 19.4) is tryptophan dioxygenase, and the activities of succeeding enzymes are such that there is little accumulation of intermediates. In vitamin B$_6$ deficiency the activity of kynureninase, which is a pyridoxal phosphate dependent enzyme, is lower than that of tryptophan oxygenase, the normal rate-limiting enzyme of the pathway. This means that there is a considerable accumulation of both hydroxykynurenine and kynurenine, sufficient to permit greater metabolic flux than usual through kynurenine transaminase (EC 2.6.1.7), resulting in increased formation of kynurenic and xanthurenic acids (see Fig. 20.4). Although kynurenine transaminase is also pyridoxal phosphate dependent, it seems to be little affected in vitamin B$_6$ deficiency; this may be because it binds its coenzyme more tightly than does kynureninase, or because it has a slower rate of turnover, or possibly simply that as a mainly intra-mitochondrial enzyme it is relatively protected compared with cytosolic enzymes.

Xanthurenic and kynurenic acids, and kynurenine and hydroxykynurenine, are easy to measure in urine, so the tryptophan load test (the ability to metabolize a test dose of 2–5 g (150–380 µmol /kg body weight) of tryptophan) has been widely adopted as a convenient and very sensitive index of vitamin B$_6$ nutritional status. However, because of the multiple factors that affect tryptophan dioxygenase activity (see section 19.4.2), abnormal results of the tryptophan load test must be regarded with caution, and cannot automatically be interpreted as indicating vitamin B$_6$ deficiency. Increased entry of tryptophan into the pathway will overwhelm the capacity of kynureninase (and perhaps also kynurenine hydroxylase), leading to increased formation of xanthurenic and kynurenic acids.

In patients suffering from a wide variety of different conditions, including Hodgkins' lymphoma, rheumatoid arthritis, schizophrenia, porphyria, renal tuberculosis, and aplastic anaemia, there is abnormal excretion of kynurenine metabolites after a test dose of tryptophan (Altman and Greengard 1966; Coon and Nagler 1969). It is unlikely that such disparate conditions would all be associated with vitamin B$_6$ deficiency. Furthermore, there are no clinical signs of deficiency, such as dermatitis or hypochromic

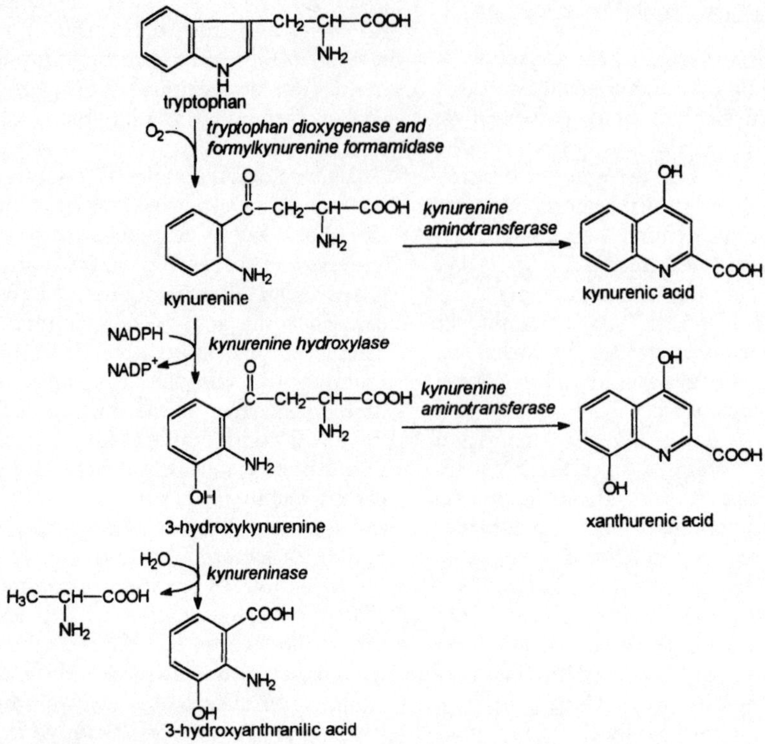

Figure 20.4 The tryptophan load test for vitamin B$_6$ nutritional status
Tryptophan dioxygenase EC 1.13.11.11, formylkynurenine formamidase EC 3.5.1.9, kynurenine hydroxylase EC 1.14.13.9, kynureninase EC 3.7.1.3, kynurenine aminotransferase EC 2.6.1.7 and 2.6.1.63

anaemia, associated with these conditions. Liver biopsy shows elevated tryptophan dioxygenase activity, presumably due to increased glucocorticoid secretion as a result of the general stress of illness.

Induction of extrahepatic indoleamine dioxygenase (EC 1.13.11.42, which catalyses the same reaction as tryptophan dioxygenase, albeit by a different mechanism) by bacterial lipopolysaccharides and interferon-γ , may result in the production of relatively large amounts of kynurenine and hydroxykynurenine in tissues which lack the enzymes for onward metabolism. Kidney has kynurenine transaminase activity, and therefore extrahepatic metabolism of tryptophan may result in significant excretion of kynurenic and xanthurenic acids even when vitamin B$_6$ nutrition is adequate.

Coon and Nagler (1969) noted that the administration of vitamin B$_6$ supplements to nutritionally normal subjects resulted in reduced urinary excretion of kynurenine and its metabolites after a test dose of tryptophan, reflecting the activation of apo-kynureninase in tissues. They concluded that normalization of

tryptophan metabolism by vitamin B$_6$ supplements cannot be regarded as evidence of vitamin B$_6$ deficiency.

20.6.5 Oestrogens and vitamin B$_6$ nutritional status

Rose (1966*a, b*) was the first to report apparent vitamin B$_6$ deficiency in women taking combined progestagen-oestrogen oral contraceptives. He showed increased urinary excretion of xanthurenic acid after a tryptophan load, and normalization after the administration of relatively high doses of vitamin B$_6$.

Since 1966 there have been many reports of abnormal tryptophan metabolism in women taking oral contraceptives and as menopausal hormone replacement therapy. These have been widely interpreted as evidence of oestrogen-induced vitamin B$_6$ deficiency or depletion. In most cases the metabolism of tryptophan has only been normalized by the administration of vitamin B$_6$ supplements of the order of 20–50 mg/day—some 10–20–fold higher than requirements. Where other indices of vitamin B_6 nutritional status have been reported, they have generally been unaffected by contraceptive use. It is likely that oestrogens do not cause vitamin B_6 deficiency, but rather that the abnormalities of tryptophan metabolism result from a direct effect of oestrogens or their metabolites on one or more of the enzymes of tryptophan metabolism. Three possible sites of action have been identified: tryptophan oxygenase, kynureninase and kynurenine hydroxylase.

20.6.5.1 Oestrogen effects on tryptophan dioxygenase

Hormonal induction of tryptophan dioxygenase can lead to abnormalities of tryptophan metabolism superficially similar to those seen in vitamin B_6 deficiency, since the rate of kynurenine formation exceeds its rate of onward metabolism. It has been widely assumed that oestrogens induce tryptophan oxygenase, in the same way as do glucocorticoids. There is, however, little experimental evidence to support this assumption; while oestrogens may induce tryptophan dioxygenase indirectly, by displacing glucocorticoid hormones from plasma protein binding, they have little or no effect on tryptophan dioxygenase activity in experimental animals (Bender 1983).

Conversely, the normalization of excretion of tryptophan metabolites following high doses of vitamin B_6 may be due to reduced activity of tryptophan dioxygenase, possibly as a result of decreased sensitivity to glucocorticoid induction (Allgood *et al.* 1990; Allgood and Cidlowski 1992; Bender and Totoe 1984*a*, *b*, and see section 20.4.3).

20.6.5.2 Oestrogen effects on kynureninase

The abnormalities of tryptophan metabolism in response to oestrogens suggest a direct effect on kynureninase. It has been suggested that there might be specific displacement of the coenzyme, pyridoxal phosphate, from kynureninase, by oestrogens or their metabolites. Competition between pyridoxal phosphate and oestrogen metabolites would explain the correction of tryptophan metabolism in oral contraceptive users by the administration of relatively large amounts of the vitamin by reactivating the apo-enzyme. While some unphysiological oestrogen derivatives do compete with pyridoxal phosphate, there is no such competition from physiological oestrogen metabolites.

Oestrone sulphate and glucuronide are uncompetitive inhibitors of the reaction between apo-kynureninase and pyridoxal phosphate, a mechanism of action that would not be expected to result in removal of the coenzyme from holo-enzyme, or indeed significant inhibition of the activation of apo-enzyme. However, steroid conjugates inhibit the reaction of the holo-enzyme competitively with respect to the substrate, suggesting that in response to administered oestrogens there might be significant inhibition (Bender and Wynick 1981).

It is thus apparent that the abnormalities of tryptophan metabolism in women receiving oestrogens are not the result of vitamin B_6 depletion or deficiency, but rather due to an artefact—direct inhibition of kynureninase, the enzyme that is central to the tryptophan load test, by oestrogen metabolites. Nevertheless, the administration of relatively large amounts of vitamin B_6 (20–25 mg/day) does correct tryptophan metabolism in women receiving oestrogens (Luhby *et al.* 1971). This is presumably because there is a relatively large amount of apo-kynureninase in the liver, which is inactive under normal conditions; in response to a high intake of the vitamin this apo-enzyme will be activated, and so despite the inhibition by oestrogen conjugates, there will be an increase in the total kynureninase activity.

20.6.5.3 Oestrogen effects on kynurenine hydroxylase

Bender and McCreanor (1985) reviewed a number of published studies of tryptophan load tests from which it was possible to calculate ratios of kynurenine:hydroxykynurenine as an index of the relative activity of kynurenine hydroxylase (EC 1.14.13.9). In general, sexually mature women show a higher ratio of kynurenine:hydroxykynurenine than do children, post-menopausal women or men, suggesting inhibition of kynurenine hydroxylase by endogenous oestrogens. In experimental animals the administration of oestrogens (oestrone sulphate or ethynyl-oestradiol) results in a very considerable reduction in kynurenine hydroxylase activity. The mechanism of this effect is unclear, since addition of oestrone sulphate, oestradiol or ethynyl-oestradiol to the incubation mixture has no effect on the activity of the partially purified enzyme. Nevertheless, oestrogens do reduce tryptophan metabolism at the level of kynurenine hydroxylase in addition to the inhibition of kynureninase. The result is an increase in the urinary excretion of kynurenine and its metabolites in response to the administration of oestrogens.

20.6.6 The methionine load test

The metabolism of methionine, shown in Fig. 20.5, includes two pyridoxal phosphate dependent steps: cystathionine synthetase (EC 4.2.1.22) and cystathionase (EC 4.4.1.1). Cystathionine synthetase is little affected by vitamin B_6 deficiency, presumably since it has a high affinity for its cofactor, and possibly also a slow rate of turnover. However, cystathionase activity falls in vitamin B₆ deficiency, and there is an increase in the tissue content of inactive apo-enzyme.

The result of this is that in vitamin B₆ deficiency there is an increase in the urinary excretion of cystathionine, both after a loading dose of methionine and under basal conditions (Linkswiler 1981). The ability to metabolize a test dose of methionine is therefore a useful test of vitamin B₆ nutritional status, and there is good agreement between impairment of methionine metabolism and other indices of vitamin B₆ nutritional status. The metabolism of methionine does not seem to be subject to the same artefacts as does the tryptophan load test.

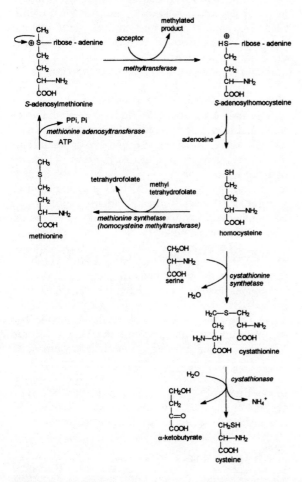

Figure 20.5 Methionine metabolism as a test for vitamin B₆ nutritional status
Methionine adenosyltransferase EC 2.5.1.6, methionine synthetase EC 2.1.1.13 (vitamin B₁₂ dependent), 2.1.1.5 (betaine as methyl donor), cystathionine synthetase EC 4.2.1.22, cystathionase EC 4.4.1.1

20.7 Pharmacological uses and toxicity of vitamin B₆

Supplements of vitamin B₆ ranging from 25–100 mg / day, and sometimes up to 2000 mg /day or higher, have been recommended for a variety of conditions, including post-natal depression, depression and other side-effects associated with oral contraceptives, hyperemesis of pregnancy, the premenstrual syndrome and the carpal tunnel syndrome.

Doses of 50–200 mg of vitamin B₆ /day have an anti-emetic effect, and the vitamin is widely used, alone or in conjunction with other anti-emetics, to minimize the nausea associated with radiotherapy and to treat pregnancy sickness. There is no evidence that vitamin B₆ has any beneficial effect in pregnancy sickness, nor that women who suffer from morning sickness have lower vitamin B₆ nutritional status than other pregnant women (Schuster *et al.* 1985).

Doses of vitamin B₆ of 100 mg /day have been reported to be beneficial in the treatment of the carpal tunnel syndrome, or what has been called tenosynovitis (Ellis *et al.* 1979). However, most of the reports originate from one centre, and there appears to be little independent confirmation of the usefulness of the vitamin in this condition.

Although, as discussed above (see section 20.6.5), oestrogens do not cause vitamin B₆ deficiency, the administration of supplements of the vitamin has beneficial effects on some of the side-effects of both administered and endogenous oestrogens. These effects are in two main areas: in normalizing glucose tolerance, both in women taking (high oestrogen) oral contraceptives and in gestational diabetes, and as an anti-depressant.

20.7.1 Vitamin B₆ and gestational diabetes

Mild impairment of glucose tolerance is common in pregnancy, and may indeed be severe enough to be classified as diabetes mellitus. This gestational diabetes generally resolves at parturition, although in some subjects it may persist, pregnancy having been the trigger for the development of maturity-onset type II diabetes (see section 7.7.2). Wynn and Doar (1966) showed that 18 per cent of women taking oral contraceptive steroids for more than three months had impaired glucose tolerance, which returned to normal on withdrawal of the steroids. Both in women taking oral contraceptives and in gestational diabetes, supplements of 100 mg vitamin B₆ /day result in improved glucose tolerance (Adams *et al.* 1976; Benninck and Schreurs 1975; Spellacy *et al.* 1977).

The relatively high accumulation of xanthurenic acid in tissues in response to both oestrogen administration and vitamin B_6 deficiency may account for the impairment of glucose tolerance. Kotake and coworkers (1975) have demonstrated that xanthurenic acid forms a complex with insulin which has little or no hormonal activity, although it cross-reacts with anti-sera. The beneficial effect of vitamin B_6 on glucose tolerance would then be the result of normalization of tryptophan metabolism by activating apo-kynureninase, as discussed above. The relevance of elevated xanthurenic acid to impaired glucose tolerance has been challenged by Cornish and Tesoriero (1975), who demonstrated that the administration of relatively large amounts of xanthurenic acid to rats had no effect on glucose tolerance.

Other tryptophan metabolites that accumulate following inhibition of kynureninase, including xanthurenic and kynurenic acids, inhibit the synthesis of pro-insulin (but not other proteins) in isolated pancreatic islets (Noto and Okamoto 1978). Similarly, hydroxykynurenine inhibits (leucine-stimulated) release of insulin from isolated pancreatic islets. Circulating concentrations of all of these tryptophan metabolites would be reduced following supplementation with vitamin B_6, and thus it is possible that impairment of insulin synthesis and secretion may be involved in the impairment of glucose tolerance in response to oestrogens, and its alleviation by vitamin B_6.

20.7.2 The antidepressant action of vitamin B_6

One of the relatively common side-effects of oestrogenic oral contraceptives is depression, affecting about 6 per cent of women in some studies. This frequently responds well to the administration of relatively large amounts of vitamin B_6 (generally in excess of 40 mg /day, although abnormalities of tryptophan metabolism are corrected by intakes of 20–25 mg /day). Post-natal depression also responds to similar supplements of vitamin B_6 in some studies.

The generally accepted view of the biochemical basis of depressive illness is that it is due to impaired synthesis of one or more neurotransmitter amines. Two groups of neurotransmitters are implicated, serotonin (5–hydroxytryptamine) and the catecholamines (dopamine, noradrenaline and adrenaline); many of the clinically effective anti-depressants act by increasing the synthesis or decreasing the catabolism of these compounds in the central nervous system.

The synthesis of both serotonin and the catecholamines involves a pyridoxal phosphate dependent

step—decarboxylation of the hydroxylated amino acid precursor to the active amine. However, although the brain concentration of serotonin falls in severe deficiency in experimental animals, the decarboxylase is not the rate-limiting step for serotonin synthesis, and is little affected by vitamin B_6 depletion. Furthermore, in patients in renal failure undergoing dialysis, while brain pyridoxal phosphate falls to about half normal, and brain concentrations of GABA are reduced, there is no reduction in the concentrations of serotonin or catecholamine metabolites (Perry *et al.* 1985).

This suggests that some mechanism other than correction of a marginal deficiency of vitamin B_6 must be involved in the anti-depressant action of the vitamin. Bender and Totoe (1984a) showed that the administration to rats of relatively large amounts of vitamin B_6 (10 mg /kg body weight) led to a significant reduction of tryptophan dioxygenase activity *in vivo*, presumably as a result of impairment of the permissive action of glucocorticoid hormones in synthesis of the enzyme, by high concentrations of pyridoxal phosphate (see section 20.4.3). This was accompanied by a relatively large increase in the circulating concentration of tryptophan, an increase in the brain tryptophan concentration and in the rates of brain tryptophan uptake and serotonin synthesis.

If the depression associated with oestrogens is indeed the result of impairment of serotonin synthesis then such a mechanism, possibly together with reduced competition for tryptophan transport by kynurenine, would account for the anti-depressant action of vitamin B_6.

20.7.3 Vitamin B_6 in the premenstrual syndrome

The studies showing a beneficial action of vitamin B_6 in overcoming depression associated with oral contraceptives have led to the use of the vitamin in depression and other psychopathology associated with endogenous oestrogens, in the premenstrual syndrome. There is no evidence of poorer vitamin B_6 nutritional status in women who suffer from the premenstrual syndrome (van den Berg *et al.* 1986).

There are few well-controlled studies of the effects of vitamin B_6 in premenstrual syndrome. In general, those that have been properly controlled report little benefit from doses between 50–200 mg/day compared with placebo, although some studies do claim a beneficial effect (Gunn 1985). Despite the lack of evidence, vitamin B_6 is widely prescribed (and self-prescribed) for the treatment of the premenstrual syndrome.

20.7.4 Toxicity of vitamin B$_6$

As a water-soluble vitamin which is rapidly metabolized and excreted, B$_6$ might be expected to have low toxicity. However, animal studies have demonstrated the development of signs of peripheral neuropathy, with ataxia, muscle weakness and loss of balance in dogs given 200 mg pyridoxine/kg body weight for 40–75 days (Phillips *et al.* 1978), and the development of a swaying gait and ataxia within 9 days at a dose of 300 mg/kg body weight (Krinke *et al.* 1980). At a dose of 50 mg/kg body weight, there are no clinical signs of toxicity, but histologically there is a loss of myelin in dorsal nerve roots. At higher doses there is more wide spread neuronal damage, with loss of myelin and degeneration of sensory fibres in peripheral nerves, the dorsal columns of the spinal cord and the descending spinal tract of the trigeminal nerve. The clinical signs of vitamin B$_6$ toxicity in animals regress within 3 months after withdrawal of these massive doses, but sensory nerve conduction velocity, which decreases during the development of the neuropathy, does not recover fully (Schaeppi and Krinke 1982).

Schaumburg *et al.* (1983) reported the development of sensory neuropathy in 7 patients taking 2–7 g of pyridoxine HCl /day. Although there was some residual damage in some patients, withdrawal of these extremely high doses resulted in a considerable recovery of sensory nerve function. Other reports have suggested that intakes as low as 50 mg/day are associated with neurological damage, although these have been based on patients' reporting of symptoms rather than detailed neurological examination.

The mechanism of pyridoxine neurotoxicity is not known. It has been suggested that high concentrations of pyridoxine compete with pyridoxal for phosphorylation; pyridoxine phosphate is oxidized to pyridoxal phosphate in only a few tissues. The result of this would be depletion of peripheral nerve pyridoxal phosphate and accumulation of pyridoxine phosphate. It is noteworthy that none of the reviews of patients with vitamin B$_6$ dependency syndromes (see Table 20.10), who are treated with between 50–1000 mg /day, mentions the development of peripheral sensory neuropathy.

Further reading

Bender, D.A. (1987). Oestrogens and vitamin B$_6$ — actions and interactions. *World Review of Nutrition and Dietetics*, 51, 140–88.

Bender, D.A. (1989). Vitamin B$_6$ requirements and recommendations. *European Journal of Clinical Nutrition*, 43, 289–309.

Bender, D.A. (1992). Vitamin B$_6$ In *Nutritional Biochemistry of the Vitamins*, Chapter 9, pp. 223–68. Cambridge University Press.

Dakshinamurti, K. (1982). Neurobiology of pyridoxine. *Advances in Nutritional Research*, 4, 143–79.

Fasella, P.M. (1967). Pyridoxal phosphate. *Annual Review of Biochemistry*, 36, 185–210.

Friedrich, W. (1988). Vitamin B$_6$. In *Vitamins*, Chapter 9, pp. 543–618. Walter de Gruyter, Berlin.

Hayashi, H., Wada, H., Yoshimura, T., Esaki, N. and Soda, K. (1990). Recent topics in pyridoxal 5'-phosphate enzyme studies. *Annual Review of Biochemistry*, 59, 87–110.

Ink, S.L. and Henderson, L.M. (1984). Vitamin B$_6$ metabolism. *Annual Review of Nutrition*, 4, 455–70.

Wiss, O. and Weber, F. (1964). Biochemical pathology of vitamin B$_6$ deficiency. *Vitamins and Hormones*, 22, 495–501.

Table 20.1: Reference intakes of vitamin B_6

	US RDA (1989)	UK RNI (1991)	EU PRI (1993)
	mg	mg	mg
birth—6 m	0.3	0.2	-
7—9 m	0.6	0.3	0.4
9m—1 y	0.6	0.4	0.4
1—3 y	1.0	0.7	0.7
4—6	1.1	0.9	0.9
7—10	1.4	1.0	1.1
males			
11—14	1.7	1.2	1.3
15—18	2.0	1.5	1.5
> 19	2.0	1.4	1.5
females			
11—14	1.4	1.0	1.1
15—18	1.5	1.2	1.1
> 19	1.6	1.2	1.1
pregnant	2.2	-	1.3
lactating	2.1	-	1.4

Source: National Research Council 1989; Department of Health 1991; Scientific Committee for Food 1993.

Table 20.2: Average intakes of vitamin B_6 (mg /day)

(Apart from the SENECA study of the elderly, which involved 17 centres throughout Europe, all the studies quoted were in UK)

	males			females			reference
age	mean	median	range1	mean	median	range1	
1.5-2.5	1.1	1.1	0.5-1.9	1.1	1.1	0.5-1.9	Gregory *et al.* 1995
2.5-3.5	1.2	1.2	0.5-2.4	1.2	1.2	0.5-2.4	Gregory *et al.* 1995
3.5-4.5	1.4	1.3	0.6-2.4	1.3	1.2	0.6-2.7	Gregory *et al* 1995
16-24	2.57	2.47	1.15-5.15	1.63	1.63	0.73-2.83	Gregory *et al.* 1990
25-34	2.53	2.48	1.24-4.18	1.54	1.53	0.64-2.56	Gregory *et al.* 1990
35-49	2.49	2.39	1.17-4.60	1.60	1.57	0.76-2.74	Gregory *et al.* 1990
50-64	2.34	2.17	1.21-4.47	1.53	1.47	0.70-2.53	Gregory *et al.* 1990
58-65	1.38	-	0.54-2.43	1.14	0.55-2.23	-	Davies & Holdsworth 1985
62-74	1.3	-	-	1.2	-	-	Lonergan *et al.* 1975
73-782	-	1.44 (1.07-1.71)	0.78-2.45	-	1.20 (0.75-1.48)	0.48-2.32	Euronut SENECA Investigators 1991
75-90	0.9	-		0.9	-	-	Lonergan *et al.* 1975

(1) The range shown is the 2.5-97.5 centile for the studies of Gregory *et al.*, the 10-90 centile for the SENECA study, and the observed extreme range for the study of Davies & Holdsworth.
(2) Data were reported for 17 separate centres; the mean and extreme values of the published median values are shown, with the lowest 10th centile and highest 90th centile of those reported.

Table 20.3: Rich sources of vitamin B$_6$

	portion (g)	mg /portion
salmon	150	1.1
mackerel	150	1.0
venison	150	1.0
bloater	150	0.9
herring	150	0.9
rabbit	150	0.8
tuna	150	0.8
liver	150	0.7
sardines canned in oil	150	0.7
cod	175	0.6
crab	175	0.6
goose	150	0.6
mung beans (dahl)	150	0.6
plaice	150	0.6
potatoes	140	0.6
avocado	130	0.5
beef, roast	150	0.5
kidney	150	0.5
pork	150	0.5
sardines canned in tomato	150	0.5
trout	150	0.5
turkey	150	0.5
veal	150	0.5
bacon joint	150	0.4
bananas	135	0.4
beans, red kidney	100	0.4
beef	150	0.4
chicken	150	0.4
duck	150	0.4
eel	150	0.4
lentils	150	0.4
Brussels sprouts	75	0.3
chestnuts	75	0.3
halibut	150	0.3
milk	560	0.3
oatmeal	100	0.3
oranges	250	0.3
pears	150	0.3
pilchards in tomato sauce	100	0.3
plantain, green	85	0.3

Table 20.4: Vitamin B_6 vitamers in plant foods

	total vitamin B_6	pyridoxal phosphate	pyridoxamine phosphate	pyridoxal	pyridoxine	pyridoxamine	glucosides
	mg /100g			% of total			
cauliflower	230	35	7	8	7	1	41
broccoli	269	21	4	20	20	6	28
carrots	226	21	3	8	8	1	59
kohlrabi	79	8	9	39	0	0	45
paprika	262	3	19	8	6	38	26
potato	270	10	4	31	13	10	31
white cabbage	86	19	3	38	5	4	31
apple	104	32	0	24	23	5	15
orange	84	29	9	16	15	3	28
hazelnuts	315	0	1	68	15	2	14
almonds	137	0	5	25	69	1	0
sunflower seeds	605	9	5	24	5	5	52
millet	492	22	16	17	22	8	15
rye flour	390	8	2	16	46	12	16
wholemeal bread	79	29	9	5	22	6	30
wheat flour	296	10	4	23	18	17	28

Source: from data reported by Schramm & Bitsch 1993; Reynolds 1988.

Table 20.5: Plasma concentrations of vitamin B_6 vitamers

	nmol/L	µg/L	% of total
total vitamin B_6	244	50	-
pyridoxal phosphate	90	22	54
pyridoxine phosphate	6	1.5	3.4
pyridoxamine phosphate	12	3.0	5
pyridoxal	38	6.4	15.2
pyridoxine	41	6.9	15.1
pyridoxamine	18	3.0	7.9
4-pyridoxic acid	39	7.2	-

Source: from data reported by Leklem 1990; McChrisley & Thye 1988.

Table 20.6: Amines formed by pyridoxal phosphate-dependent decarboxylases

amine	parent amino acid	enzyme	EC number
agmatine	arginine	arginine decarboxylase	4.1.1.19
dopamine[1] (dihydroxyphenylethylamine)	dopa (3,4-dihydroxyphenylalanine)	aromatic amino acid decarboxylase	4.1.1.28
phosphatidylethanolamine[2]	phosphatidylserine	phosphatidylserine decarboxylase	4.1.1.65
GABA (γ-amino-butyric acid)	glutamate	glutamate decarboxylase	4.1.1.15
histamine	histidine	histidine decarboxylase	4.1.1.22
phenylethylamine	phenylalanine	bacterial phenylalanine decarboxylase	4.1.1.53
putrescine[3]	ornithine	ornithine decarboxylase	4.1.1.17
serotonin (5-hydroxytryptamine)	5-hydroxytryptophan	aromatic amino acid decarboxylase	4.1.1.28
tryptamine	tryptophan	bacterial tryptophan decarboxylase	4.1.1.28
tyramine	tyrosine	bacterial tyrosine decarboxylase	4.1.1.25

(1) Dopamine is also the precursor for noradrenaline and adrenaline biosynthesis
(2) Phosphatidylethanolamine is the precursor for choline synthesis, see section 23.6.1
(3) Putrescine is the precursor for synthesis of spermine and spermidine by reaction with decarboxylated S-adenosylmethionine.

Table 20.7: Transamination products of the amino acids

amino acid	oxo-acid
alanine	pyruvate
arginine	α–oxo-γ-guanidoacetate
aspartic acid	oxaloacetate
cysteine	β-mercaptopyruvate
glutamic acid	α-oxo-glutarate
glutamine	α-oxo-glutaramic acid
glycine	glyoxylate
histidine	imidazolepyruvate
isoleucine	α-oxo-β-methylvalerate
leucine	α-oxo-isocaproate
[lysine[1]	α-oxo-ε-aminocaproate $\rightarrow$ pipecolic acid]
methionine	S-methyl-β-thiol 1α-oxopropionate
ornithine	glutamic-γ-semialdehyde
phenylalanine	phenylpyruvate
proline	γ-hydroxypyruvate
serine	hydroxypyruvate
threonine	α-oxo-β-hydroxybutyrate
tryptophan	indolepyruvate
tyrosine	*p*-hydroxyphenylpyruvate
valine	α-oxo-isovalerate

(1) Lysine does not usually undergo transamination; if it does, the product, α-oxo-ε-aminocaproate, undergoes spontaneous dehydration and cyclization to pipecolic acid.

Table 20.8: Biochemical evidence of vitamin B_6 deficiency in developed countries

	n	% deficient	criterion	reference
breast-fed infants	84	10	pyridoxal phosphate	Wilson & Davies 1984
preschool children	35	9	pyridoxal phosphate	Fries *et al.* 1981
young women embarking on contraceptive study	129	0.8	pyridoxal phosphate	Bender 1993
young women embarking on contraceptive study	129	13.2	aspartate transaminase activation	Bender 1993
adolescent girls	127	13	alanine transaminase activation	Kirksey *et al.* 1978
pregnant adolescents	122	17	alanine transaminase activation	Martner-Hawes *et al.* 1986
low income pregnant women	127	68	alanine transaminase activation	Schuster *et al.* 1981
pregnant women	458	42	aspartate transaminase activation	Heller *et al.* 1973
hospital patients	650	25	aspartate transaminase activation	Lemoine *et al.* 1980
free-living elderly	198	27	pyridoxal phosphate	Schrijver *et al.* 1987
free-living elderly	198	26	aspartate transaminase activation	Schrijver *et al.* 1987
elderly men undergoing prostate surgery	94	4.3	pyridoxal phosphate	Bender 1993
elderly men undergoing prostate surgery	94	8.5	aspartate transaminase activation	Bender 1993
hospitalized elderly	153	19	aspartate transaminase activation	Hoorn *et al.* 1975
hospitalized elderly	102	28	alanine transaminase activation	Vir & Love 1978
men, various ages	617	25	pyridoxal phosphate	Rose *et al.* 1976

Table 20.9: Lack of concordance between two criteria of vitamin B_6 nutritional status

	elderly men		young women	
	% marginal	% deficient	% marginal	% deficient
plasma pyridoxal phosphate	15.9	4.3	21.7	0.8
erythrocyte aspartate aminotransferase activation coefficient	32.9	8.5	31.8	13.2
both criteria	9.6	1.1	6.9	0

Source: from data reported by Bender 1993.

Table 20.10: Vitamin B_6 responsive inborn errors of metabolism

	enzyme affected	EC number
convulsions of the newborn	glutamate decarboxylase ($\downarrow$ GABA synthesis)	4.1.1.15
cystathioninuria	cystathionase (see Figure 20.5)	4.4.1.1
gyrate atrophy with ornithinuria	ornithine-δ-aminotransferase	2.6.1.13
homocystinuria	cystathionine synthase (see Figure 20.5)	4.2.1.22
primary hyperoxaluria, type I	peroxisomal alanine-glyoxylate transaminase	2.6.1.44
sideroblastic anaemia	δ-aminolevulinate synthase ($\downarrow$ haem synthesis)	2.3.1.37
xanthurenic aciduria	kynureninase (see Figure 20.4)	3.7.1.3

Table 20.11: Indices of vitamin B_6 nutritional status

	adequate status
plasma total vitamin B_6	> 40 nmol (10 µg) /L
plasma pyridoxal phosphate	> 30 nmol (7.5 µg) /L
erythrocyte alanine aminotransferase activation coefficient	< 1.25
erythrocyte aspartate aminotransferase activation coefficient	< 1.80
erythrocyte aspartate aminotransferase	> 0.13 units (8.4 µkat) /L
urine 4-pyridoxic acid	> 3.0 µmol /24h
	> 1.3 mmol /mol creatinine
urine total vitamin B_6	> 0.5 µmol /24h
	> 0.2 mmol /mol creatinine
urine xanthurenic acid after 2 g tryptophan load	< 65 µmol /24 h increase
urine cystathionine after 3 g methionine load	< 350 µmol /24 h increase

Source: from data reported by Bitsch 1993; Leklem 1990; McChrisley & Thye 1988.

Folic acid and vitamin B$_{12}$

Folic acid functions in the transfer of one-carbon fragments in a wide variety of biosynthetic and catabolic reactions; it is therefore metabolically closely related to vitamin B$_{12}$, which also functions in one-carbon transfer. Deficiency of either vitamin has similar clinical effects, and the main effects of vitamin B$_{12}$ deficiency are exerted by effects on folate metabolism.

Although folate is widely distributed in foods, dietary deficiency is not uncommon, and a number of commonly used drugs can cause folate depletion. By contrast, dietary deficiency of vitamin B$_{12}$ is rare, despite the fact that the vitamin is found only in animal foods and some bacteria; rather, pernicious anaemia due to vitamin B$_{12}$ lack is normally the result of a defect in the mechanism for intestinal absorption of the vitamin.

Two other pterin cofactors are chemically related to folate: biopterin (see section 23.4) and molybdopterin (see section 25.19). They are coenzymes in mixed function oxidases, and are not vitamins, but can be synthesized in the body. It is the linkage of the pteridine ring to p-aminobenzoyl-poly-γ-glutamate which renders folate a dietary essential; it is the ability to condense p-aminobenzoate to a pteridine, rather than to synthesize the pteridine nucleus itself, which has been lost by higher animals.

21.1   Requirements and intakes

21.1.1 Folate requirements

Depletion/repletion studies to determine folate requirements using methyl-tetrahydrofolate suggest a requirement of the order of 80–100 µg (170–220 nmol)/day. The total body pool of folate in adults is some 17 µmol (7.5 mg), with a biological half-life of 101 days. This suggests a minimum requirement for replacement of 85 nmol (37 µg) per day. Studies of the urinary excretion of acetamido-p-aminobenzoyl

glutamate in subjects maintained on folate-free diets suggest that there is catabolism of some 170 nmol (80 µg) of folate/day (Herbert 1987a; McPartlin et al. 1992, 1993).

Because of the problems of determining the biological availability of the various folate polyglutamate conjugates found in foods (see section 21.3), reference intakes allow a wide margin of safety, and are based on an allowance of 3 µg (6.8 nmol)/kg body weight (see Table 21.1). Average intakes of folate are shown in Table 21.2, and rich sources in Table 21.3.

21.1.2 Folate in pregnancy

During the 1980s a considerable body of evidence accumulated that spina bifida and other neural tube defects were associated with low intakes of folate, and that increased intake during pregnancy might be protective. The US and UK reference intakes for folate were published before the results of intervention trials were available, and before the publication of evidence that folate catabolism is considerably increased in pregnancy (McPartlin et al. 1993). It is now established that supplements of folate in early pregnancy result in a significant reduction in the incidence of neural tube defects (Czeizel 1993; MRC Research Group 1991), and it is recommended that intakes be increased by 400 µg/day in early pregnancy. The studies were conducted using methyl-tetrahydrofolate, and it is unlikely that an equivalent increase in intake could be achieved from unfortified foods; supplements are recommended. As shown in Table 3.2, closure of the neural tube occurs by day 28 of pregnancy, which is before the woman knows she is pregnant. The advice therefore is that all women who are, or may be about to become, pregnant, should take folate supplements.

Neural tube defects occur in about 0.75–1 per cent of pregnancies. It can be argued that fortification of foods would be more appropriate than recommending supplements. However, high intakes of folate can prevent the development of megabloblastic anaemia in elderly subjects with vitamin B_{12} deficiency due to gastric atrophy, so that the first presenting sign is irreversible degeneration of the spinal cord. Very high intakes of folate also antagonize the anticonvulsants used to control epilepsy (a condition that affects some 2 per cent of the population), so increasing the frequency of attacks. Enrichment of common foods with sufficient folate to ensure adequate intakes to minimize the risk of neural tube defect might put some of these other vulnerable groups at risk of excessive intake.

21.1.3 Vitamin B_{12} requirements

Most estimates of vitamin B_{12} requirements are based on the amounts given parenterally to maintain normal health in patients with pernicious anaemia due to a failure of vitamin B_{12} absorption (see section 21.6.1). This overestimates normal requirements, since there is considerable enterohepatic circulation of vitamin B_{12}; in people with defective absorption, the vitamin that is excreted in the bile will be lost in the faeces, whereas it is normally almost completely re-absorbed.

The total body pool of vitamin B_{12} is of the order of 2.5 mg (1.8 µmol), with a minimum desirable body pool of about 1 mg (0.3 mol). The daily loss is about 0.1 per cent of the body pool in subjects with normal enterohepatic circulation of the vitamin; on this basis requirements are about 1–2.5 µg/day (Herbert 1987*b*).

The only group of people at risk of dietary deficiency are strict vegetarians (Vegans), since there are no plant sources of the vitamin. Vitamin B_{12} deficiency is rare in India, where there is a large Vegan population, and it has been suggested that the trace amounts present in faecal contamination of food and water are adequate to meet requirements and establish adequate body reserves. It takes some 10–15 years before Vegan immigrants to north America and northern Europe develop signs of dietary deficiency. It is therefore likely that the requirement is considerably lower than 1 µg/day.

Average intakes of omnivores (see Table 21.5) are considerably higher than the reference intakes shown in Table 21.4; rich sources of vitamin B_{12} are shown in Table 21.6.

21.2   Folate vitamers and nomenclature

As shown in Fig. 21.1, folic acid consists of a reduced pterin linked to *p*-aminobenzoic acid, forming pteroic

acid. The carboxyl group of the *p*-aminobenzoic acid moiety is linked by a peptide bond to the α-amino group of glutamate, forming pteroylglutamate (PteGlu). The coenzymes may have up to 7 additional glutamate residues linked by γ-peptide bonds, forming pteroyldiglutamate (PteGlu$_2$), pteroyltriglutamate (PteGlu$_3$), etc., collectively known as folate or pteroyl polyglutamate conjugates (PteGlu$_n$)

'Folate' is the preferred trivial name for pteroylglutamate, although both 'folate' and 'folic acid' may also be used as a generic term to include various polyglutamates. PteGlu$_2$ is sometimes referred to as folic acid diglutamate, PteGlu$_3$ as folic acid triglutamate, etc.

The pteridine ring of folic acid is normally fully reduced, as tetrahydrofolate (tetrahydropteroylglutamate, H$_4$PteGlu), although the oxidized form, dihydrofolate (dihydropteroylglutamate, H$_2$PteGlu) is an important metabolic intermediate, and in the reactions of thymidylate synthetase and methylene tetrahydrofolate reductase (see section 21.4.3.1), the pteridine ring has a redox role in the reaction.

Tetrahydrofolate can carry one-carbon fragments attached to N-5 (formyl, formimino or methyl groups), N-10 (formyl) or bridging N-5–N-10 (methylene or methenyl groups). 5–Formyl-folate is more stable to atmospheric oxidation than folate itself, and is therefore commonly used in pharmaceutical preparations; it is also known as folinic acid, and the synthetic (racemic) compound as leucovorin.

21.3   Absorption and metabolism of folate

About 80 per cent of dietary folate is as polyglutamates; a variable amount may be substituted with various one-carbon fragments or be present as dihydrofolate derivatives. The biological availability and hence nutritional value of the various polyglutamate conjugates and one-carbon derivatives of folate is not known; values ranging between 40–70 per cent of the availability of pteroylmonoglutamate have been reported for different foods (Bates and Heseker 1994).

21.3.1 Intestinal conjugase and enterohepatic circulation of methyl-tetrahydrofolate

Folate conjugates are hydrolysed in the small intestine by pteroylpolyglutamate hydrolase (conjugase, EC 3.4.22.12), a zinc-dependent peptidase of the pancreatic juice, bile and mucosal brush border. Because conjugase is a zinc metallo-enzyme, zinc defi-

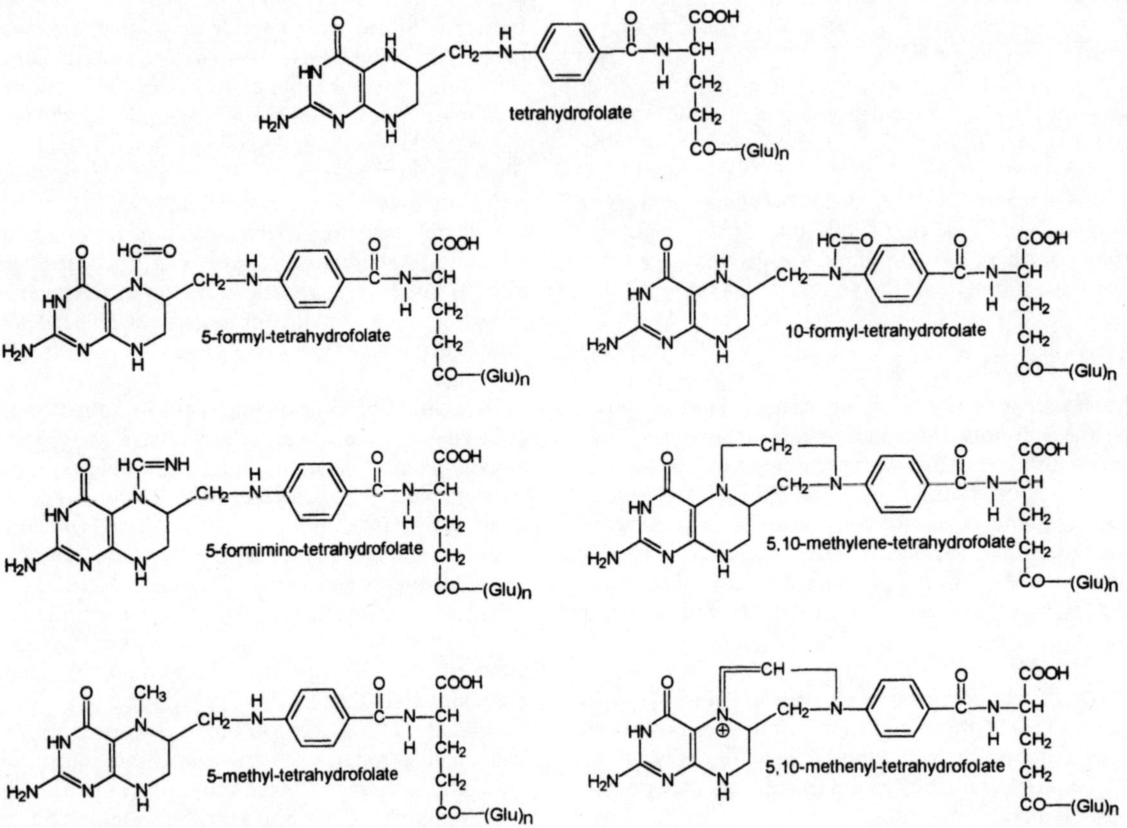

Figure 21.1 Folic acid vitamers
Relative molecular mass (M$_r$) of tetrahydrofolate = 445.4,

ciency can impair folate absorption; Canton and Cremin (1990) have suggested that the absorption of test doses of folate polyglutamates may provide a sensitive index of zinc nutritional status (see section 25.26.3). The absorption of folate monoglutamates (from pharmaceutical preparations or foods) is not affected by zinc status.

Free folate, released by conjugase action, is absorbed by active transport in the jejunum. The folate in milk is mainly bound to a specific binding protein; the protein-folate complex is absorbed intact, mainly in the ileum, by a mechanism which is distinct from the active transport system for the absorption of free folate. The biological availability of folate from milk, or of folate from diets to which milk has been added, is considerably greater than that of unbound folate (Mason and Selhub 1988; Swiatlow *et al.* 1990).

Much of the dietary folate undergoes methylation and reduction within the intestinal mucosa, so that what enters the portal bloodstream is largely 5–methyl-tetrahydrofolate. Other substituted and unsubstituted folate monoglutamates, and dihydrofolate are also absorbed; they are reduced and methylated in the liver, then secreted in the bile. The liver also takes up various folates released by tissues; again these are reduced, methylated and secreted in the bile.

The total daily enterohepatic circulation of folate is equivalent to about one-third of the dietary intake; in experimental animals bile drainage for 6 hours results in a reduction of serum folate to 30–40 per cent of normal (Steinberg *et al.* 1979). Despite this, there is very little faecal loss of folate; jejunal absorption of methyl-tetrahydrofolate is a very efficient process, and the faecal excretion of some 450 nmol (200 μg) of folates per day represents synthesis by intestinal flora and does not reflect intake to any significant extent.

21.3.2 Tissue uptake and polyglutamylation of folate

Methyl-tetrahydrofolate circulates bound to albumin, and is available for uptake by extra-hepatic tissues. Small amounts of other one-carbon substituted folate also circulate (about 10–15 per cent of plasma folate is 10–formyl-tetrahydrofolate), and will also enter cells by the same carrier-mediated process, where they are trapped by formation of polyglutamates, which do not cross cell membranes.

The metabolically active folates are polyglutamates. Folate monoglutamate crosses cell membranes readily, while polyglutamates do not, hence rapid formation of at least a diglutamate enhances tissue uptake and retention of folate. Further elongation of the polyglutamate chain to form metabolically active coenzymes can proceed in a more leisurely fashion.

A single enzyme catalyses the stepwise addition of glutamate (in γ-glutamyl peptide linkage) to tetrahydrofolate. 5–Formyl and 5–methyl H_4PteGlu are substrates to only a limited extent; other substituted tetrahydrofolates and dihydrofolate are not substrates. The immediate product is released to compete with other intracellular folate conjugates for enzyme binding, rather than undergoing further glutamyl transfer while remaining enzyme bound. Because of this, the diglutamate is the main product at high concentrations of folate; increasing amounts of tri- tetra- and penta- and hexaglutamates are formed as the concentration of tetrahydrofolate is reduced.

The main circulating folate is methyl-tetrahydrofolate, which is a poor substrate for polyglutamylation, demethylation by the action of methionine synthetase (see section 21.7.2) is required for effective metabolic trapping of folate. In vitamin B_{12} deficiency, when methionine synthetase activity is impaired, there will therefore be impairment of the retention of folate in tissues.

Under normal conditions the predominant folates in liver are pentaglutamates, with small amounts of tetra- and hexaglutamates. The extent of polyglutamylation is controlled to a great extent by the availability of folate; in deficient animals hexa- to octaglutamates predominate, while in supplemented animals liver folate is mainly as the tri- to pentaglutamates.

Red blood cells accumulate several hundred-fold higher concentrations of folate than plasma, as polyglutamates bound to haemoglobin at a specific site

which competes with the 2,3–bisphophoglycerate binding site. The function of this haemoglobin binding is not known, but it probably represents a storage form of the vitamin rather than a mechanism for regulating haemoglobin function; under normal conditions there is only about 1 mmol of folate /10 mol of haemoglobin (Benesch *et al.* 1985).

Demethylated tetrahydrofolate monoglutamate is released by extrahepatic tissues, and is transported bound to a plasma folate binding protein. This has a very low affinity for methyl-tetrahydrofolate and other one-carbon substituted derivatives, and functions mainly to return folate to the liver. While extra-hepatic tissues will take up unsubstituted tetrahydrofolate in free solution, they do not take up protein-bound tetrahydrofolate. In the liver tetrahydrofolate is either conjugated for storage or remethylated and secreted in the bile, in the same way as newly absorbed folate.

21.3.3 Folate excretion

There is very little urinary loss of folate—only some 5–10 nmol of microbiologically active material per day. Not only is most folate in plasma bound to proteins (either folate-binding protein for unsubstituted folate or albumin for methyl-tetrahydrofolate), and thus protected from glomerular filtration, but the renal brush border has a high concentration of folate-binding protein which acts to reabsorb any filtered in the urine.

The catabolism of folate is largely by cleavage of the C-9–N-10 bond, catalysed by carboxypeptidase G (EC 3.4.17.11). The *p*-aminobenzoic acid moiety is amidated and excreted in the urine as *p*-acetamidobenzoate and *p*-acetamidobenzoyl-glutamate; pterin is excreted either unchanged or as isoxanthopterin and other biologically inactive compounds (Saleh *et al.* 1982).

21.4 Metabolic functions of folate

The metabolic role of folate is as a carrier of one-carbon fragments, both in catabolism and in biosynthetic reactions. As shown in Fig. 21.1, these may be carried as formyl, formimino, methyl, methylene or methylene residues. The major sources of these one-carbon fragments and their major uses, as well as the interconversions of the substituted folates, are shown in Fig. 21.2.

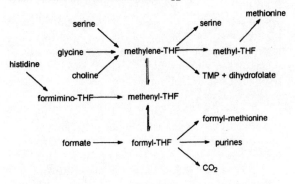

Figure 21.2 Metabolic interconversions of one-carbon substituted folates

21.4.1 Sources of one-carbon substituted folates

The major point of entry for one-carbon fragments into substituted folates is methylene-tetrahydrofolate, which is formed by the catabolism of glycine, serine and choline.

21.4.1.1 Serine hydroxymethyltransferase

Serine hydroxymethyltransferase (EC 2.1.2.1) is a pyridoxal phosphate-dependent aldolase which catalyses the cleavage of serine to glycine and methylene-tetrahydrofolate. In this reaction the one-carbon fragment which is transferred is already in the appropriate oxidation state.

While folate is required for the catabolism of variety of compounds, serine is the most important source of substituted folates for biosynthetic reactions, and the activity of serine hydroxymethyltransferase is regulated by the state of folate substitution and the availability of folate rather than by the state of serine metabolism. Methyl-tetrahydrofolate is a potent inhibitor of the enzyme, so when there is an adequate concentration of substituted folates from other sources, serine can be spared for energy-yielding metabolism or gluconeogenesis. While the hydroxymethyltransferase is the major route of serine catabolism under normal conditions, the reaction is freely reversible, and under appropriate conditions in liver it functions mainly to form serine from glycine, as a substrate for gluconeogenesis (Snell 1984).

21.4.1.2 The glycine cleavage system

The glycine cleavage system is a multi-enzyme complex consisting of the following:

1. A pyridoxal phosphate-dependent glycine dehydrogenase (EC 1.4.4.2).

2. A lipoamide-containing aminomethyltransferase (EC 2.1.2.10) which is reduced to the disulphydryl form during the reaction and is subsequently reoxidized by the dihydrolipoyl dehydrogenase component of the complex. This protein serves to oxidize the one-carbon fragment to the appropriate level to form methylene-tetrahydrofolate.

3. The methylene-tetrahydrofolate synthesizing protein, which accepts the carbon from the aminomethyltransferase, releasing the amino group as ammonium.

21.4.1.3 Dimethylglycine and sarcosine dehydrogenases

Choline (see section 23.6) is oxidized to betaine (trimethylglycine), then the first methyl group is transferred directly to homocysteine, forming methionine (see section 21.7.2). The resultant dimethylglycine is demethylated to methylglycine (sarcosine) by an iron-flavoprotein, dimethylglycine dehydrogenase (1.5.99.2), which oxidizes the methyl group to formaldehyde before transferring it to tetrahydrofolate to form methylene-tetrahydrofolate. The demethylation of sarcosine to glycine, catalysed by sarcosine dehydrogenase (EC 1.5.99.1) also yields methylene-tetrahydrofolate.

21.4.1.4 Histidine catabolism

As shown in Fig. 21.3, the catabolism of histidine leads to the formation of formiminoglutamate. The formimino group is transferred onto tetrahydrofolate to form formimino-tetrahydrofolate, which is subsequently deaminated to form methenyl-tetrahydrofolate. A single bifunctional enzyme catalyses the FIGLU formiminotransferase and formiminofolate cyclodeaminase reactions, so there is little or no free formimino-tetrahydrofolate in tissues under normal conditions. The two catalytic sites are separate, and with tetrahydrofolate monoglutamate there is release of the formimino derivative. However, when polyglutamates are used there is channelling of the intermediate between the two sites, and no release of the formimino derivative (MacKenzie and Baugh 1980; Paquin *et al.* 1985).

While the catabolism of histidine is not a major source of substituted folate, the reaction is of interest because it has been exploited as a means of assessing folate nutritional status. In folate deficiency the activity of the formiminotransferase is impaired by lack of cofactor, and, especially after a loading dose of histidine, there is impaired oxidative metabolism of histidine and accumulation of formiminoglutamate (FIGLU), which is excreted in the urine (see section 21.9.4).

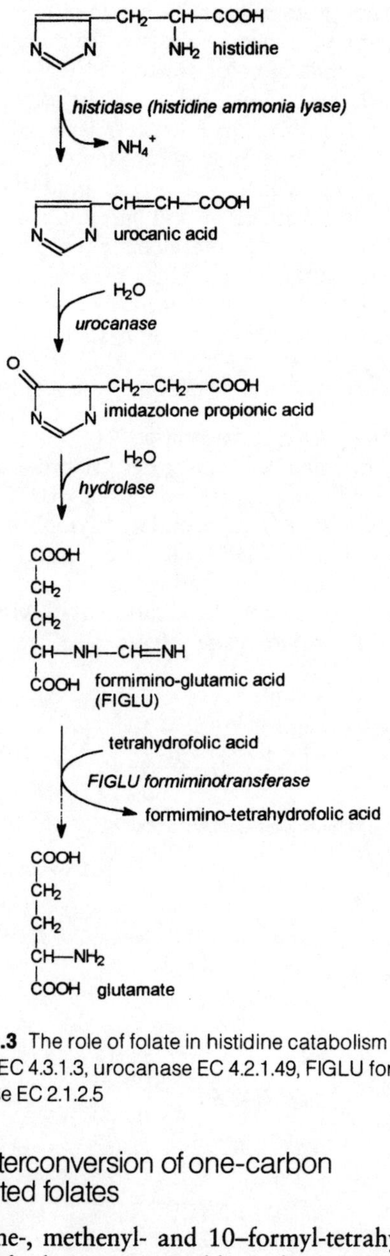

Figure 21.3 The role of folate in histidine catabolism
Histidase EC 4.3.1.3, urocanase EC 4.2.1.49, FIGLU formiminotransferase EC 2.1.2.5

21.4.2 Interconversion of one-carbon substituted folates

Methylene-, methenyl- and 10–formyl-tetrahydrofo-
lates are freely interconvertible. In liver some 33 per
cent of the folate is present as unsubstituted tetrahydrofolate, with 37 per cent as methyl-tetrahydrofolate, 23 per cent as 10–formyl-tetrahydrofolate and
7 per cent as 5–formyl-tetrahydrofolate (Wilson and
Horne 1984).

The two activities involved, methylene tetrahydrofolate dehydrogenase (EC 1.5.1.15) and methenyl-tetrahydrofolate cyclohydrolase (EC 3.5.4.9) form a
trifunctional enzyme with 10–formyl-tetrahydrofolate synthetase (EC 6.3.4.3) (Paukert *et al.* 1976).

This means that single carbon fragments entering
the folate pool in any form other than as methyl-tetrahydrofolate (see below) can readily be available for
any of the biosynthetic reactions shown in Fig. 21.2.
Equally, when there is a greater entry of single carbon
units into the folate pool from the catabolic reactions
discussed above than is required for biosynthetic
reactions, the surplus can be oxidized to CO_2 by
way of 10–formyl-tetrahydrofolate, thus ensuring a
continuing supply of tetrahydrofolate for catabolic
reactions. 10–Formyl-tetrahydrofolate dehydrogenase is inhibited by free tetrahydrofolate, and its activity is regulated by the ratio of formyl-
tetrahydrofolate:free tetrahydrofolate in the tissue.

The reduction of methylene-tetrahydrofolate to
methyl-tetrahydrofolate is catalysed by methylene-
tetrahydrofolate reductase, an FAD-dependent
enzyme; during the reaction the pteridine ring of the
substrate is oxidized to dihydrofolate, then reduced
to tetrahydrofolate by the flavin, which is reduced by
NADPH (Matthews 1982). The reaction is irreversible under physiological conditions, and to some
extent methyl-tetrahydrofolate can be regarded as
an end-product of one-carbon metabolism.

Methyl-tetrahydrofolate is also the major form in
which folate enters cells, as discussed above (see section 21.3.1); most dietary folates are reduced and
methylated either during absorption or as a result
of enterohepatic circulation. Methyl-tetrahydrofolate
can only be used for other folate requiring reactions
after demethylation in the reaction catalysed by
homocysteine methyltransferase (see section 21.7.2).

21.4.3 Utilization of one-carbon substituted folates

As shown in Fig. 21.2, 10–formyl tetrahydrofolate
and methylene tetrahydrofolate are donors of one-
carbon fragments in a number of biosynthetic reactions, including especially the synthesis of purines,
pyrimidines, porphyrins, the methylation of homocysteine to methionine and the formylation of
methionyl tRNA to yield formylmethionyl tRNA
for the initiation of protein synthesis.

In most cases the reaction is a simple transfer of
the one-carbon group from substituted tetrahydrofolate onto the acceptor substrate. Two reactions are of
especial interest: thymidylate synthetase and methionine synthetase (see section 21.7.2).

21.4.3.1 Thymidylate synthetase and dihydrofolate reductase

The methylation of deoxyuridine monophosphate
(dUMP) to thymidine monophosphate (TMP), cata-

lysed by thymidylate synthase (EC 2.1.1.45) is essential for the synthesis of DNA, although preformed TMP can be reutilized by salvage from the catabolism of DNA (see section 21.4.3.2).

As shown in Fig. 21.4, the methyl donor is methylene tetrahydrofolate; the reaction involves reduction of the one-carbon fragment to a methyl group at the expense of the folate, which is oxidized to dihydrofolate. Under normal conditions, dihydrofolate is rapidly reduced to tetrahydrofolate, a reaction catalysed by dihydrofolate reductase (EC 1.5.1.3). There is some evidence that thymidylate synthase and dihydrofolate reductase form a multi-enzyme complex.

Thymidylate synthase and dihydrofolate reductase are especially active in tissues with a high rate of cell division, and hence a high rate of DNA replication and a high requirement for thymidylate. Because of this, inhibitors of dihydrofolate reductase have been exploited as anti-cancer drugs. The most successful of these is methotrexate, the 4-amino analogue of 10-methyl-tetrahydrofolate. Chemotherapy consists of alternating periods of administration of methotrexate and folate (normally as 5-formyl-tetrahydrofolate, leucovorin) in order to replete the normal tissues and avoid induction of folate deficiency—so-called 'leucovorin rescue'. As well as depleting tissue pools of tetrahydrofolate, methotrexate leads to the accumulation of relatively large amounts of 10-formyl-dihydrofolate, which is a potent inhibitor of both thymidylate synthetase and glycinamide ribotide transformylase, an intermediate step in purine nucleotide synthesis. It is likely that this, rather than simple depletion of tetrahydrofolate, is the basis of the cytotoxic action of methotrexate (Baram *et al.* 1988).

21.4.3.2 The dUMP suppression test

Rapidly dividing cells can either use preformed TMP or can synthesize it *de novo* from dUMP. Isolated bone marrow cells or stimulated lymphocytes incubated with [³H]TMP will incorporate label into DNA. In the presence of adequate amounts of methylene-tetrahydrofolate, the addition of dUMP as a substrate for thymidylate synthetase reduces the

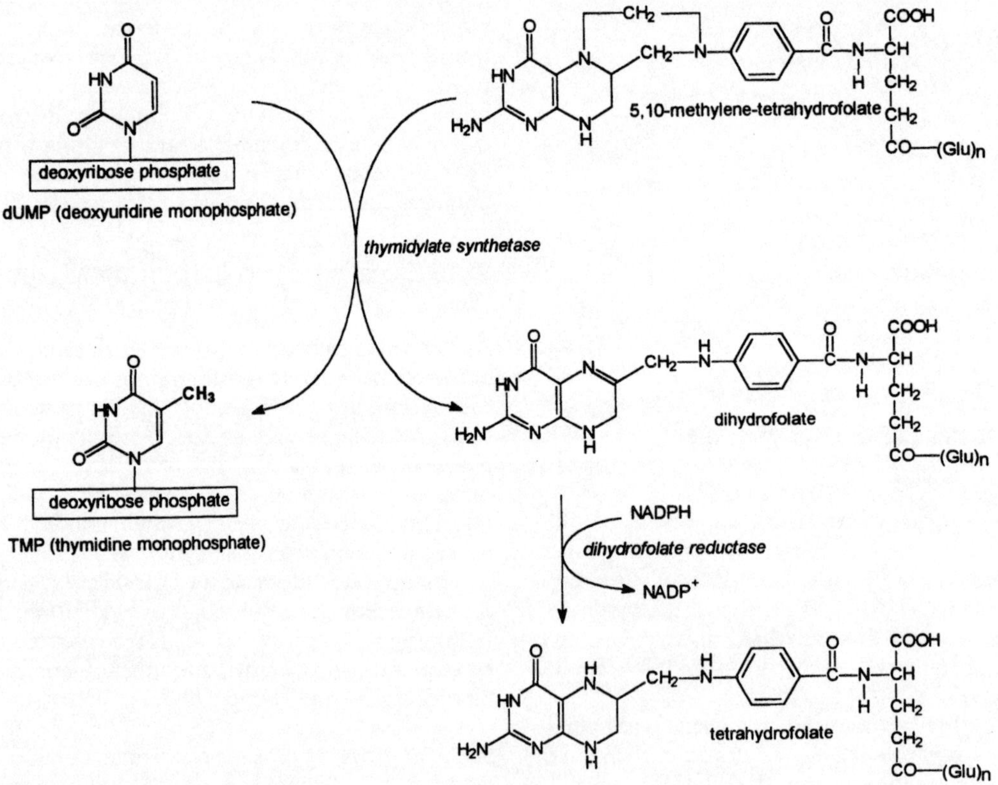

Figure 21.4 The reaction of thymidylate synthetase and dihydrofolate reductase
Thymidylate synthetase EC 2.1.1.45, dihydrofolate reductase EC 1.5.1.3

incorporation of [³H]TMP as a result of dilution of the pool of labelled material by newly synthesized TMP. The extent to which dUMP suppresses the incorporation of [³H]TMP into DNA thus reflects folate nutritional status (see section 21.9.5).

21.5 Vitamin B$_{12}$ vitamers and nomenclature

The structure of vitamin B$_{12}$ is shown in Fig. 21.5. The term corrinoid is used as a generic descriptor for cobalt-containing compounds of this general structure, which, depending on the substituents in the pyrrole rings, may or may not have vitamin activity. Some of the corrinoids that are growth factors for micro-organisms not only have no vitamin B$_{12}$ activity, but may be antimetabolites of the vitamin.

The term 'vitamin B$_{12}$' is used as a generic descriptor for the cobalamins—those corrinoids having the biological activity of the vitamin. Chemically, cobalamins are corrinoids which have a dimethylbenzimidazole nucleotide attached to the D ring, and chelating the central cobalt atom.

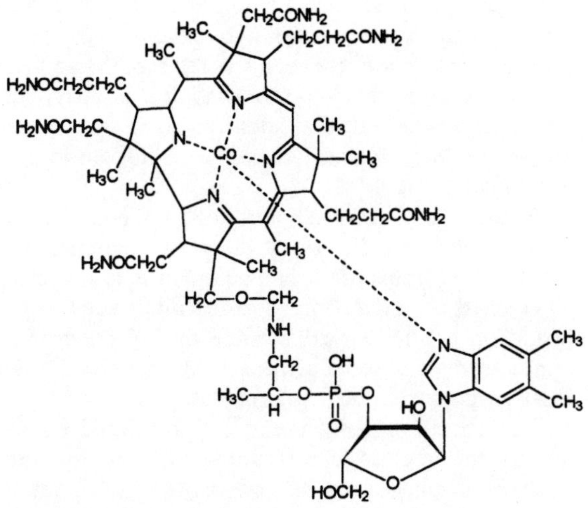

Figure 21.5 Vitamin B$_{12}$
Four coordination sites on the central cobalt atom are occupied by the nitrogen atoms of the corrin ring, and one by the nitrogen of the dimethylbenzimidazole nucleotide. The sixth coordination site may be occupied by:
CN⁻ cyanocobalamin, M$_r$ = 1355.4
OH⁻ hydroxocobalamin, M$_r$ = 1346.4
H$_2$O aquocobalamin, M$_r$ = 1347.4
-CH$_3$ methylcobalamin, M$_r$ = 1344.4
5'-deoxyadenosine adenosylcobalamin, M$_r$ = 1579.6

Four of the six chelation sites of the cobalt atom of cobalamin are occupied by the nitrogens of the corrin ring, and one by the nitrogen of the dimethylbenzimidazole nucleotide side chain. The sixth site may be occupied by the following ligands in biologically active vitamers:

(1) cyanide (CN⁻, cyanocobalamin);

(2) hydroxide (OH⁻, hydroxocobalamin);

(3) water (H$_2$O, aquocobalamin);

(4) methyl (CH$_3$, methylcobalamin);

(5) 5'-deoxy-5'adenosine (adenosylcobalamin).

Sulphitocobalamin, with a sulphite (SO$_3^{2-}$) ligand, occurs in some foods as a result of processing, but is poorly absorbed.

The cobalt atom is in the Co^{3+} oxidation state in hydroxo-, aquo-, methyl and cyano-cobalamins, and in the Co$^+$ oxidation state in adenosylcobalamin and, transiently, in the demethylated prosthetic group of methionine synthetase (see section 21.7.2).

Although cyanocobalamin was the first form in which vitamin B$_{12}$ was isolated, it is not an important naturally occurring vitamer, but rather an artefact due to the presence of cyanide in the charcoal used in the extraction procedure. It is more stable to light than the other vitamers, and hence is commonly used in pharmaceutical preparations. Photolysis of cyanocobalamin in solution leads to the formation of aquocobalamin or hydroxocobalamin, depending on pH. Hydroxocobalamin is also used in pharmaceutical preparations, and is better retained after parenteral administration than is cyanocobalamin.

Small amounts of cyanocobalamin are found in the bloodstream (about 2 per cent of total plasma vitamin B$_{12}$) apparently as part of the metabolism of cyanide derived from food (and tobacco smoke), but not in erythrocytes or tissues. If it is not converted to aquo- or hydroxocobalamin, cyanocobalamin may have antivitamin action, and has been implicated in the neurological damage associated with chronic cyanide intoxication seen in parts of West Africa where the dietary staple, cassava, is rich in cyanogenic glycosides (see section 7.6).

The major plasma vitamer is methylcobalamin, accounting for some 60–80 per cent of plasma vitamin B$_{12}$, with up to 20 per cent as adenosylcobalamin and the remainder mainly hydroxocobalamin. In tissues the major vitamer is adenosylcobalamin (about 70 per cent in liver), with about 25 per cent as hydroxocobalamin, and less than 5 per cent as methylcobalamin.

Vitamin B$_{12}$ is synthesized only by bacteria. There are no plant sources of this vitamin, which comes only from animal foods. The legal method of determining vitamin B$_{12}$ is a microbiological growth assay, using *Lactobacillus leichmannii*; a number of corrinoids found in plants are growth factors for this organism, and hence are measured as 'vitamin B$_{12}$', although they have no vitamin activity in human beings, and indeed may even be antimetabolites of the vitamin (Herbert 1988).

21.6   Absorption and metabolism of vitamin B$_{12}$

21.6.1 Absorption

Very small amounts of vitamin B$_{12}$ can be absorbed by passive diffusion across the intestinal mucosa, but under normal conditions this is insignificant, accounting for less than 1 per cent of large oral doses; the major route of vitamin B$_{12}$ absorption is by way of attachment to a specific binding protein in the intestinal lumen.

This binding protein is 'intrinsic factor', so called because in the early studies of pernicious anaemia (see section 21.8), it was found that two curative factors were involved—an extrinsic or dietary factor, which we now know to be vitamin B$_{12}$, and an intrinsic or endogenously produced factor. Intrinsic factor is a glycoprotein (M_r 44 000, containing 15 per cent carbohydrate) secreted by the gastric parietal cells, which also secrete hydrochloric acid; the secretion of both intrinsic factor and gastric acid is stimulated by vagus nerve stimulation, histamine, gastrin and insulin (see section 6.1.2).

Gastric acid and pepsin have a role in vitamin B$_{12}$ nutrition, serving to release the vitamin from protein binding, and so make it available. Atrophic gastritis is a relatively common problem of advancing age; in the early stages there is failure of acid secretion but more or less normal secretion of intrinsic factor. This can result in vitamin B$_{12}$ depletion due to failure to release the vitamin from dietary proteins, but the absorption of a test dose of free vitamin B$_{12}$ (the Schilling test, see section 21.9.2) will be normal.

In the stomach, vitamin B$_{12}$ binds to cobalophilin, a binding protein secreted in the saliva. The cobalophilins are a group of antigenically related, relatively unspecific, corrinoid-binding proteins, formerly known as R-proteins because of their rapid mobility on electrophoresis compared with other cobalamin-binding proteins.

In the duodenum cobalophilin is hydrolysed, releasing the vitamin B$_{12}$ for binding to intrinsic factor. Pancreatic insufficiency can therefore be a factor in the development of vitamin B$_{12}$ deficiency, since failure to hydrolyse cobalophilin will result in the excretion of cobalophilin-bound vitamin B$_{12}$ rather than transfer to intrinsic factor.

Intrinsic factor binds the various vitamin B$_{12}$ vitamers with equal affinity, but not other corrinoids. There is one vitamin B$_{12}$ binding site per mol of intrinsic factor, and on binding the vitamin the protein undergoes a conformational change, resulting in dimerization, and greatly enhanced resistance to proteolysis. Considerably more intrinsic factor is secreted than is needed for the binding and absorption of dietary vitamin B$_{12}$, which requires only about 1 per cent of the total intrinsic factor available.

Vitamin B$_{12}$ is absorbed from the distal third of the ileum. There are intrinsic factor-vitamin B$_{12}$ binding sites on the brush border of the mucosal cells in this region; free intrinsic factor does not interact with these receptors. It is not certain whether the intrinsic factor-vitamin B$_{12}$ complex enters the mucosal cells intact or whether the vitamin is transferred from the complex to intracellular binding, leaving apo-intrinsic factor at the mucosal surface. Although there is good evidence for receptor-mediated endocytosis of the intrinsic factor-vitamin B$_{12}$ complex into enterocytes, there seems to be no lysosomal involvement in the release of free vitamin B$_{12}$, unlike other receptor-mediated endocytosis, and histochemical studies show intrinsic factor only at the mucosal surface (Donaldson 1985; Robertson and Gallagher 1985).

At the serosal surface, vitamin B$_{12}$ emerges bound to transcobalamin II, one of the plasma vitamin B$_{12}$ binding and transport proteins; again it is not clear whether the attachment to transcobalamin occurs inside or at the serosal surface of the enterocyte, although there is some evidence that transcobalamin II is synthesized in ileal enterocytes.

The absorption of vitamin B$_{12}$ is limited by the number of intrinsic factor-vitamin B$_{12}$ binding sites in the ileal mucosa, so that not more than about 1–1.5 µg (0.7–1.1 nmol) from a single oral dose of the vitamin can be absorbed. The absorption is also slow; peak blood concentrations of the vitamin are not achieved until some 6–8 hours after an oral dose.

21.6.2 Plasma vitamin B$_{12}$ binding proteins (transcobalamins)

The initial binding of vitamin B$_{12}$, after either intestinal absorption or parenteral administration, is to transcobalamin II, which circulates mainly as the apo-protein. This seems to be the major protein for vitamin B$_{12}$ uptake into tissues; the half-life of holo-transcobalamin II in plasma is of the order of 1.5 hours, and all cells have surface receptors for holo-transcobalamin II. Tissue uptake is by receptor-mediated endocytosis, followed by lysosomal proteolysis to release hydroxocobalamin. Hydroxocobalamin may either undergo methylation to methylcobalamin in the cytosol, or it may enter the mitochondria and undergo a two-step reduction, catalysed by a flavoprotein reductase to yield Co$^+$-cobalamin, and reaction with ATP, catalysed by adenosyltransferase (EC 2.5.1.17) to form adenosyl-cobalamin.

Although transcobalamin II is the metabolically important pool of plasma vitamin B$_{12}$, it accounts for only a small proportion of the total circulating vitamin. About 90 per cent is bound to transcobalamin I; the function of this binding protein is not well understood, but it seems to act as a storage form of the vitamin. Holo-transcobalamin I has a relatively long half-life (7–10 days), and does not seem to be involved in tissue uptake or inter-tissue transport of the vitamin.

21.6.3 Enterohepatic circulation of vitamin B$_{12}$

There is a considerable enterohepatic circulation of vitamin B$_{12}$. A third plasma vitamin B$_{12}$ binding protein, transcobalamin III, is rapidly cleared by the liver, with a plasma half-life of the order of 5 minutes. This seems to provide a mechanism for returning vitamin B$_{12}$ and its metabolites from peripheral tissues to the liver, as well as for clearance of other corrinoids without vitamin activity, which may arise either from foods or the products of intestinal bacterial action, and be absorbed passively across the lower gut.

These corrinoids are then secreted into the bile, bound to cobalophilins. 3–8 μg (2.25–6 nmol) of vitamin B$_{12}$ may be secreted in the bile each day, about the same as the dietary intake. Like dietary vitamin B$_{12}$ bound to salivary cobalophilin, the biliary cobalophilins are hydrolysed in the duodenum, and the vitamin released binds to intrinsic factor, so permitting reabsorption in the ileum. While cobalophilins and transcorrin III have low specificity, and will bind a variety of corrinoids, intrinsic factor binds only cobalamins, and so only the biologically active vitamin will be reabsorbed to any significant extent.

21.7 Metabolic functions of vitamin B$_{12}$

In mammals there are three vitamin B$_{12}$-dependent reactions: methylmalonyl CoA mutase, leucine aminomutase (EC 5.4.3.7), and methionine synthetase.

21.7.1 Methylmalonyl CoA mutase

Methylmalonyl CoA arises directly as an intermediate in the catabolism of valine, and is formed by the carboxylation of propionyl CoA arising in the catabolism of isoleucine, cholesterol and (rare) fatty acids with an odd number of carbon atoms. Normally it undergoes an adenosylcobalamin-dependent rearrangement to succinyl CoA, catalysed by methylmalonyl CoA mutase (EC 5.4.99.2, see Fig. 21.6). In vitamin B$_{12}$ deficiency the activity of this enzyme is greatly reduced, although there is induction of the apo-enzyme to some 1.5–5–fold above that seen in control animals.

As a result of this impairment of the mutase, there is an accumulation of methylmalonyl CoA, some of which is hydrolysed to yield methylmalonic acid, which is excreted in the urine; urinary excretion of methylmalonic acid provides a means of assessing vitamin B$_{12}$ nutritional status (see section 21.9.3).

Methylmalonyl CoA inhibits the synthesis of fatty acids from acetyl CoA at concentrations of the order of those found in tissues of vitamin B$_{12}$ deficient animals. It is a substrate for fatty acid synthesis, leading to the formation of branched-chain and odd-carbon fatty acids (Cardinale *et al.* 1970).

Propionyl CoA inhibits glutamate N-acetyltransferase (EC 2.3.1.1) competitively with respect to acetyl CoA, forming N-propionylglutamate. Unlike N-acetylglutamate, this is not an activator of carbamyl phosphate synthetase, and as a result of impaired

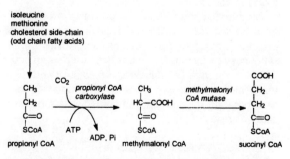

Figure 21.6 The reaction of methylmalonyl CoA mutase Propionyl CoA carboxylaes EC 6.4.1.3, methylmalonyl CoA mutase EC 5.4.99.2

urea synthesis, vitamin B$_{12}$ deficiency may be associated with protein intolerance and hyperammonaemia.

Methylmalonic aciduria can also occur without any evidence of vitamin B$_{12}$ deficiency, as a result of a genetic defect of either methylmalonyl CoA mutase or the synthesis of adenosylcobalamin. In some cases the condition is a vitamin dependency syndrome, and responds to very high intakes of vitamin B$_{12}$. Although patients show mental retardation, failure to thrive, intermittent hypo- or hyperglycaemia and protein intolerance, they do not develop either the megaloblastic anaemia or the neurological degeneration associated with vitamin B$_{12}$ deficiency (see section 21.8).

21.7.2 Homocysteine methyltransferase (methionine synthetase) and the methyl-folate trap

In addition to its role in the synthesis of proteins and the polyamines spermidine and spermine, methionine, as the *S*-adenosyl derivative, acts as a methyl donor in a wide variety of biosynthetic reactions. The resultant homocysteine may either be metabolized to yield cysteine (see Fig. 20.5) or may be remethylated to yield methionine.

Two enzymes catalyse the methylation of homocysteine to methionine:

(1) methionine synthetase (EC 2.1.1.13), a vitamin B$_{12}$-dependent methyltransferase, for which the methyl donor is methyl tetrahydrofolate;

(2) homocysteine methyltransferase (EC 2.1.1.5), which utilizes betaine (an intermediate in the catabolism of choline, see section 23.6) as the methyl donor, and is not vitamin B$_{12}$-dependent.

Both enzymes are found in most tissues, but only the vitamin B$_{12}$-dependent methionine synthetase is found in the central nervous system.

Methionine synthetase is inactivated irreversibly by nitrous oxide, which oxidizes the cobalt of the prosthetic group to Co^{2+}. Inactivation of methionine synthetase by nitrous oxide has been used as an acute model of vitamin B$_{12}$ deficiency in experimental animals, and chronic exposure to nitrous oxide may cause vitamin B$_{12}$ deficiency in man; dentists are especially at risk.

21.7.2.1 The methyl-folate trap hypothesis

The reduction of methylene-tetrahydrofolate to methyl-tetrahydrofolate is irreversible, and the major source of folate for tissues is methyl-tetrahydrofolate (see section 21.3.2). The only metabolic role of methyl-tetrahydrofolate is the methylation of homocysteine to methionine, and this is the only way in which methyl-tetrahydrofolate can be demethylated to yield free tetrahydrofolate in tissues. Methionine synthetase thus provides the link between the physiological functions of folate and vitamin B$_{12}$. Impairment of methionine synthetase activity, for example in vitamin B$_{12}$ deficiency or after prolonged exposure to nitrous oxide, will result in the accumulation of methyl-tetrahydrofolate which can neither be utilized for any other one-carbon transfer reactions nor demethylated to provide free tetrahydrofolate.

Experimental animals that have been exposed to nitrous oxide to deplete vitamin B$_{12}$ show an increased proportion of liver folate present as methyl-tetrahydrofolate (85 per cent rather than the normal 45 per cent), largely at the expense of unsubstituted tetrahydrofolate, and increased urinary loss of methyl-tetrahydrofolate. (Horne *et al.* 1989; Lumb *et al.* 1982). Tissue retention of folate is impaired because methyl-tetrahydrofolate is a poor substrate for polyglutamylfolate synthetase compared with unsubstituted tetrahydrofolate. As a result of this, vitamin B$_{12}$ deficiency is frequently accompanied by biochemical evidence of functional folate deficiency, including impaired metabolism of histidine, excretion of formiminoglutamate and impaired thymidylate synthetase activity (as shown by abnormally low dUMP suppression), although plasma concentrations of methyl-tetrahydrofolate are normal or elevated.

This functional deficiency of folate is exacerbated by the associated low concentrations of methionine and *S*-adenosyl methionine, although most tissues (apart from the central nervous system) also have betaine-homocysteine methyltransferase, which may be adequate to maintain tissue pools of methionine. Under normal conditions *S*-adenosyl methionine inhibits methylene-tetrahydrofolate reductase, and so prevents the formation of further methyl-tetrahydrofolate; relief of this inhibition results in increased reduction of one-carbon substituted tetrahydrofolates to methyl-tetrahydrofolate.

The activity of 10–formyl tetrahydrofolate dehydrogenase (EC 1.5.1.6), which catalyses the oxidation of 10–formyl tetrahydrofolate to CO$_2$ and tetrahydrofolate, is reduced at times of low methionine availability, as a means of conserving valuable one-carbon fragments. There is therefore no sink for one-carbon substituted tetrahydrofolate, and increasing amounts of folate are trapped as methyl-tetrahydrofolate which cannot be used because of the lack of vitamin B$_{12}$ (Krebs *et al.* 1976).

This has been called the methyl-folate trap, and appears to explain many of the similarities between the symptoms and metabolic effects of folate and vitamin B$_{12}$ deficiency. However, it does not provide a completely satisfactory explanation of the effects of vitamin B$_{12}$ deficiency (Chanarin *et al.* 1985).

21.8 Deficiency of folate and vitamin B$_{12}$

Deficiency of either folate or vitamin B$_{12}$ results in a clinically similar megaloblastic anaemia; because of the neurological damage which accompanies the megaloblastic anaemia of vitamin B$_{12}$ deficiency, the condition is generally known as pernicious anaemia.

Table 21.7 shows the sequence of events in the development of folate deficiency, and Table 21.8 the development of vitamin B$_{12}$ deficiency.

Both vitamin B$_{12}$ and folate deficiency are associated with psychiatric illness, although the underlying mechanisms are not clear. Herbert (1962) noted insomnia, forgetfulness and irritability during the development of self-imposed folate deficiency, which responded well to the administration of the vitamin. Up to 16 per cent of patients with pernicious anaemia show psychotic illness, and a larger number have lesser mental changes. A significant number of vitamin B$_{12}$-deficient patients have psychiatric or neurological abnormalities which respond well to parenteral vitamin B$_{12}$, but no haematological abnormalities. It has been suggested that these patients may have vitamin B$_{12}$ deficiency with an intake of folate adequate to prevent depletion as a result trapping as methyl-folate.

Folic acid deficiency is relatively common; some 8–10 per cent of the population of developed countries have low or marginal folate stores, as assessed by measurement of erythrocyte folate. By contrast, dietary deficiency of vitamin B$_{12}$ is rare and most deficiency is due to failure of secretion of intrinsic factor, leading to failure of absorption of the vitamin. Pernicious anaemia affects some 0.13 per cent of the population, with a slight excess of females over males, and an incidence increasing with age, as a result of atrophic gastritis.

Failure of intrinsic factor secretion is commonly a result of auto-immune disease; 90 per cent of patients with pernicious anaemia have complement-fixing antibodies to the cytosol of the gastric parietal cells. Similar auto-antibodies are found in 30 per cent of the relatives of pernicious anaemia patients, suggesting that there is a genetic or familial basis for the condition.

About 70 per cent of patients also have anti-intrinsic factor antibodies in plasma, saliva and gastric juice. These can be either blocking antibodies which prevent the binding of vitamin B$_{12}$ to intrinsic factor, or precipitating antibodies which precipitate both free intrinsic factor and intrinsic factor-vitamin B$_{12}$ complex. Some patients have both types of anti-intrinsic factor antibody. Although the oral administration of partially purified preparations of intrinsic factor will restore the absorption of vitamin B$_{12}$ in many patients with pernicious anaemia, this can result eventually in the production of anti-intrinsic factor antibodies, so parenteral administration of vitamin B$_{12}$ is the preferred means of treatment. For patients who secrete anti-intrinsic factor antibodies in the saliva or gastric juice, oral intrinsic factor will be of no benefit.

Dietary deficiency of vitamin B$_{12}$ does occur, rarely, in strict vegetarians, since there are no plant foods that are sources of vitamin B$_{12}$. The small amounts that have been reported in some plants and algae are almost certainly either due to contamination with vitamin B$_{12}$ producing bacteria, or the result of analytical error (see section 21.5).

The rarity of vitamin B$_{12}$ deficiency among people who have no apparent dietary source of the vitamin suggests that significant amounts can be made by gut flora and may be absorbed by passive diffusion across the lower gut. Small numbers of such organisms have been found in faecal samples, but much of the microbiologically active vitamin B$_{12}$ they produce may be inactive corrinoids, and cobalamin is not well absorbed from the colon. More probably, bacterial contamination of soil, water, and foods with vitamin B$_{12}$-producing organisms will provide small, but adequate, amounts of the vitamin. The fruit bat develops vitamin B$_{12}$ deficiency when fed on washed fruit under laboratory conditions, but in the wild microbial contamination of the outside of the fruit provides an adequate intake of the vitamin.

21.8.1 Megaloblastic anaemia

In man, deficiency of either folic acid or vitamin B$_{12}$ results in megaloblastic anaemia—the release into the circulation of immature erythrocytes due to a failure of the normal process of maturation in the bone marrow. There may also be a low white cell and platelet count, as well as increased numbers of hyper-segmented neutrophils. Iron deficiency may mask megaloblastic anaemia due to folate or vitamin B$_{12}$ deficiency.

The cause of the megaloblastosis is depressed DNA synthesis, as a result of impaired activity of thymidylate synthetase, a folate-dependent enzyme (see section 21.4.3.1), but more or less normal synthesis of RNA. While it is obvious that folic acid deficiency will result in impaired thymidylate synthesis, it is less easy to see how vitamin B$_{12}$ deficiency results in impaired thymidylate synthesis without invoking the methyl-folate trap hypothesis—functional deficiency of folate in vitamin B$_{12}$ deficiency as a result of trapping as methyl-folate (see section 21.7.2)

The megaloblastic response to vitamin B$_{12}$ deficiency seems to be unique to man; deficient animals develop neuropathy, but have unimpaired haemopoeisis. It may be that man is more reliant on the *de novo* synthesis of thymidylate, and less able to salvage it from DNA breakdown, than other species. The normal suppression of the incorporation of [^{3}H]thymidine into DNA by added dUMP is less than 3 per cent in the fruit bat, 23 per cent in the rat and 65 per cent in man (see section 21.9.5).

21.8.2 Neurological degeneration

Vitamin B$_{12}$ deficiency is accompanied by neurological degeneration in about two-thirds of cases—either peripheral neuropathy or sub-acute combined degeneration of the spinal cord. The neurological damage can occur in the absence of haematological signs of deficiency, especially if the intake of folate is adequate. The lesion is a demyelination, and is reversible in its early stages. Folic acid deficiency is only rarely associated with similar neurological degeneration, and indeed it was believed at one time that the effect on myelination was a specific result of vitamin B$_{12}$ deficiency.

Supplementation with methionine protects against the aggravating effect of folate in vitamin B$_{12}$ deficient fruit bats (van der Westhuyzen *et al.* 1982), and can prevent the development of sub-acute combined degeneration of the spinal cord in nitrous oxide treated monkeys (Scott *et al.* 1981).

The cause of the demyelination and sub-acute combined degeneration of the spinal cord is a specific failure of methylation of arginine 107 of myelin basic protein. The protective effect of methionine supplements can possibly be accounted for by increasing the availability of S-adenosyl methionine as methyl donor for this reaction. Inhibition of S-adenosyl methionine dependent methylation by chronic administration of cyclo-leucine also causes demyelinating neuropathy with a similar failure of methylation of arginine 107.

21.8.3 Drug-induced folate deficiency

A number of folate antimetabolites are used clinically, as cancer chemotherapy (e.g. methotrexate),

and as anti-bacterial (trimethoprim) and anti-malarial (pyrimethamine) agents; they act as inhibitors of dihydrofolate reductase (see section 21.4.3.1). Although drugs such as trimethoprim and pyrimethamine owe much of their clinical usefulness to considerably higher affinity for the dihydrofolate reductase of the target organism than the human enzyme, their prolonged use can result in (iatrogenic) folate deficiency.

A number of anti-epileptic drugs, including diphenylhydantoin (phenytoin), and sometimes phenobarbital and primidone, can also cause folate deficiency. While overt megaloblastic anaemia affects only some 0.75 per cent of treated epileptics, there is some degree of macrocytosis in 40 per cent. The mechanism of this drug-induced folic acid deficiency is not clear, although a number of effects have been reported.

1. Diphenylhydantoin and other anticonvulsants impair the intestinal absorption of folates. This may be by inhibition of intestinal conjugase—however, the evidence from various studies is conflicting.

2. Diphenylhydantoin causes an increased rate of catabolism of folate and increased excretion of folate metabolites (Kelly *et al.* 1979).

3. Chronic treatment of experimental animals with primidone depletes liver folate pentaglutamates, suggesting inhibition of folate polyglutamate synthetase (Carl *et al.* 1987). This would be expected to lead to increased excretion of folate metabolites.

4. Administration of diphenylhydantoin leads to decreased activity of methylene tetrahydrofolate reductase and an increased rate of oxidation of formyl tetrahydrofolate (increased oxidation of formate and histidine), with a fall in methylene and methyl tetrahydrofolates—the reverse of the effect of the methyl-folate trap (Billings 1984).

The megaloblastosis responds to folic acid supplements, but in about 50 per cent of such patients treated with relatively high supplements for 1–3 years there is an increase in the frequency of epileptic fits (Reynolds 1967). In normal subjects the concentration of folate in the cerebrospinal fluid is some 2–3 times higher than in plasma; in epileptics taking diphenylhydantoin the cerebrospinal fluid and plasma concentrations of folate are approximately equal. This suggests that the mechanism of action of the anticonvulsants may involve folic acid antagonism. There is some evidence that very large amounts of folate have a convulsant effect in animals, although this is only at extremely high intakes or by direct intra-cerebral administration of unphysiologically large amounts, and is not relevant to dietary or supplement intakes of the vitamin.

21.9 Assessment of folate and vitamin B$_{12}$ nutritional status

A number of methods have been developed to permit assessment of folate and vitamin B$_{12}$ nutritional status and differentiation between deficiency of folic acid or vitamin B$_{12}$ as a cause of megaloblastic anaemia. Obviously, detection of antibodies to intrinsic factor or gastric parietal cells will confirm autoimmune pernicious anaemia rather than nutritional deficiency of either vitamin. Indices of folate and vitamin B$_{12}$ nutritional status are shown in Table 21.9.

21.9.1 Blood concentrations of the vitamins

Measurement of plasma concentrations of the two vitamins is probably the method of choice, and a number of simple and reliable radio-ligand binding assays have been developed, some of which permit simultaneous determination of the two vitamins. Nevertheless, there are a number of problems involved in radio-ligand binding assays, especially for folate, and in some centres microbiological determination of plasma or whole blood folates is the preferred technique. Radio-ligand binding assays for vitamin B$_{12}$ may give falsely high values if the binding protein is cobalophilin, which binds a number of metabolically inactive corrinoids as well as cobalamins; more precise determination of true vitamin B$_{12}$ comes from assays in which the binding protein is purified intrinsic factor, although this may still detect some corrinoids without vitamin activity.

A serum concentration of vitamin B$_{12}$ below 110 pmol /L is associated with megaloblastic bone marrow, incipient anaemia and myelin damage. Below 150 pmol /L there are early bone marrow changes, abnormalities of the dUMP suppression test and methylmalonic aciduria after a valine load.

Serum folate below 7 nmol /L or erythrocyte folate below 320 nmol /L indicates negative folate balance and early depletion of body reserves. At this stage the first bone marrow changes are detectable (Bailey 1990).

About 30 per cent of vitamin B$_{12}$ deficient subjects have elevated serum folate. This is mainly methyl-tetrahydrofolate, the result of the methyl-folate trap (see section 21.7.2). About one third of folate-deficient subjects have low serum vitamin B$_{12}$; the reason for this is not clear, but it responds to the administration of folate supplements.

21.9.2 The Schilling test for vitamin B$_{12}$ absorption

The absorption of vitamin B$_{12}$ can be determined by the Schilling test. An oral dose of [^{57}Co] or [^{58}Co]vitamin B$_{12}$ is given with a parenteral flushing dose of 1 mg of non-radioactive vitamin to saturate body reserves, and the urinary excretion of radioactivity is followed as an index of absorption of the oral material. Normal subjects excrete 16–45 per cent of the radioactivity over 24 hours, while patients lacking intrinsic factor excrete less than 5 per cent.

The test can be repeated, giving intrinsic factor orally together with the radioactive vitamin B$_{12}$; if the impaired absorption was due to a simple lack of intrinsic factor, and not to anti-intrinsic factor antibodies in saliva or gastric juice, or some other cause, then a normal amount of the radioactive material should be absorbed and excreted.

A modified technique permits the absorption in the presence and absence of exogenous intrinsic factor to be determined at the same time, giving [^{57}Co]vitamin B$_{12}$-intrinsic factor complex and free [^{58}Co]vitamin B$_{12}$ together and measuring the amount of each isotope excreted in the urine.

21.9.3 Methylmalonic aciduria

Modest vitamin B$_{12}$ deficiency results in increased accumulation of methylmalonyl CoA, and hence methylmalonic aciduria. This can be exploited both as a means of detecting subclinical deficiency and monitoring vitamin B$_{12}$ status in patients with pernicious anaemia who have been treated with parenteral vitamin—as they become depleted, so the excretion of methylmalonic acid, especially after a loading dose of valine, will provide a sensitive index of depletion of vitamin B$_{12}$ reserves.

Methylmalonyl CoA mutase is especially sensitive to vitamin B$_{12}$ depletion, so methylmalonic aciduria is the most sensitive index of vitamin B$_{12}$ status. Folate deficiency does not cause methylmalonic aciduria. However, up to 25 per cent of patients with confirmed pernicious anaemia excrete normal amounts of methylmalonic acid even after a loading dose of valine (Chanarin *et al.* 1973).

21.9.4 Histidine metabolism—the FIGLU test

The ability to metabolize a test dose of histidine provides a sensitive functional test of folate nutritional status; as shown in Fig. 21.3, formiminoglutamate (FIGLU) is an intermediate in histidine catabolism, and is metabolized by the tetrahydrofolate dependent enzyme formiminoglutamate formiminotransferase. In folate deficiency the activity of this enzyme is impaired, and formiminoglutamate accumulates and is excreted in the urine, especially after a test dose of histidine—the so-called FIGLU test. In experimental animals the test can be rendered more sensitive by measuring the production of $^{13}CO_2$ from [^{13}C]histidine, which is considerably reduced in folate deficiency.

Although the FIGLU test depends on folate nutritional status, the metabolism of histidine will also be impaired, and hence a positive result obtained, in vitamin B$_{12}$ deficiency, because of the secondary deficiency of free folate. About 60 per cent of vitamin B$_{12}$-deficient subjects show increased FIGLU excretion after a histidine load.

21.9.5 The dUMP suppression test

The ability of deoxyuridine to suppress the incorporation of [^3H]thymidine into DNA in rapidly dividing cells can be used to give an index of functional folate nutritional status. Bone marrow biopsy samples provide the best source, so this has been generally a research tool rather than a screening test; however, transformed lymphocytes can also be used. The dUMP suppression test is probably the most sensitive index of folate depletion; abnormalities are apparent within 5 weeks of initiating folate deprivation, whereas detectably high urinary FIGLU occurs only after 13 weeks depletion, and bone marrow is overtly megaloblastic at 19 weeks (Herbert 1962, 1987a). The dUMP suppression test shows abnormal results when folate falls below 4.5 pmol / 10^6 cells.

Cells that have been pre-incubated with deoxyuridine, then exposed to [^3H]thymidine incorporate little or none of the labelled material into DNA. This is because of both dilution of the labelled material in the larger intracellular pool of newly synthesized TMP, and also inhibition of thymidylate kinase by thymidine triphosphate. In normal cells the incorporation of [^3H]thymidine into DNA after pre-incubation with dUMP is 1.4–1.8 per cent of that without pre-incubation. By contrast, cells that are deficient in folate form little or no thymidine from dUMP, and hence incorporate nearly as much of the

[^3H]thymidine after incubation with dUMP as they do without pre-incubation.

Again either a primary deficiency of folic acid or functional deficiency secondary to vitamin B$_{12}$ deficiency will have the same effect. In folate deficiency, addition of any biologically active form of folate, but not vitamin B$_{12}$, will normalize the dUMP suppression of [^3H]thymidine incorporation. In vitamin B$_{12}$ deficiency, addition of vitamin B$_{12}$ or methylene-tetrahydrofolate, but not methyl-tetrahydrofolate, will normalize dUMP suppression (Killman 1964; Pelliniemi and Beck 1980).

21.10   Toxicity of folate

There is some evidence that folate supplements in excess of 350 µg /day may impair zinc absorption, and intakes in excess of 5 mg /day have been associated with increased fit frequency in epileptics. At moderately high levels of intake, folate supplements may mask the anaemia of vitamin B$_{12}$ deficiency so that subacute combined degeneration of the spinal cord is the first sign of deficiency. High supplements of folate are thus not recommended for strict vegetarians or the elderly who are at risk of vitamin B$_{12}$ deficiency.

Further reading

Bender, D.A. (1992). Folic acid and other pterins and vitamin B$_{12}$. In *Nutritional Biochemistry of the Vitamins*, Chapter 10, pp. 269–315. Cambridge University Press.

Darcy-Vrillon, B., Selhub, J., and Rosenberg, I.H. (1988). Analysis of sequential events in intestinal absorption of folylpolyglutamate. *American Journal of Physiology*, 255, G361–6.

Davis, R.E. and Nicol, D.J. (1988). Minireview—Folic acid. *International Journal of Biochemistry*, 20, 133–9.

Friedrich, W. (1988). Folic acid and unconjugated pteridines. In *Vitamins*, Chapter 10, pp. 619–752. Walter de Gruyter, Berlin.

Friedrich, W. (1988). Vitamin B$_{12}$. In *Vitamins*, Chapter 13, pp. 837–928. Walter de Gruyter, Berlin.

Herbert, V. (1987). Making sense of laboratory tests of folate status: folate requirements to sustain normality. *American Journal of Haematology*, 26, 199–207.

Hitchings, G.H. and Smith, S.L. (1980). Dihydrofolate reductases as targets for inhibitors. *Advances in Enzyme Regulation*, 18: 349–71.

Kapadia, C.R. and Donaldson, R.M. (1985). Disorders of cobalamin (vitamin B$_{12}$) absorption and transport. *Annual Review of Medicine*, 36, 93–110.

Lambie, D.G. and Johnson, R.H. (1985). Drugs and folate metabolism. *Drugs*, 30, 145–55.

Metz, J. (1992). Cobalamin deficiency and the pathogenesis of nervous system disease. *Annual Review of Nutrition*, 12, 59–70.

Schneider, Z. and Stroinski, A. (1987). *Comprehensive B₁₂: Chemistry, Biochemistry, Nutrition, Ecology, Medicine.* Walter de Gruyter, Berlin.

Scott, J. and Weir, D. (1994). Folate / vitamin B_{12} interrelationships. *Essays in Biochemistry*, 28, 63–72.

Scott, J., Kirke, P., Molloy, M., Daly, L. and Weir, D. (1994). The role of folate in the prevention of neural tube defect. *Proceedings of the Nutrition Society*, 53, 631–6.

Seetharam, B. and Alpers, D.H. (1994). Cobalamin binding proteins and their receptors. *Vitamin Receptors: Vitamins and Ligands in Cell Communication*, (ed. K. Dakshinamurti), Chapter 4, pp. 78–105. Cambridge University Press.

Steinberg, S.E. (1984). Mechanisms of folate homeostasis. *American Journal of Physiology*, 246, G319–24.

Weitman, S., Anderson, R. G.W. and Kamen, B.A. (1994). Folate binding proteins. In *Vitamin Receptors: Vitamins and Ligands in Cell Communication*, (ed. K. Dakshinamurti), Chapter 5, pp. 106–36. Cambridge University Press.

Table 21.1: Reference intakes for folate

	US RDA (1989)	UK RNI (1991)	EU PRI (1993)
	µg	µg	µg
birth–6 m	25	50	-
7–12 m	35	50	50
1–3 y	50	70	100
4–6	75	100	130
7–10	100	150	150
males			
11–14	150	200	180
15–18	200	200	200
adult	200	200	200
females			
11–14	150	200	180
15–18	180	200	200
adult	180	200	200
pregnant[1]	400	+100	400
lactating	280	+60	350

(1) Supplements of folate of 400 µg /day are recommended in pregnancy to minimize the risk of neural tube defect.
Source: National Research Council, 1989; Department of Health, 1991; Scientific Committee for Food, 1993.

Table 21.2: Average intakes of folate (µg/day) in UK

	males			females		
age	mean	median	95% range	mean	median	95% range
1.5-2.5	120	114	59-222	120	114	59-222
2.5-3.5	133	126	61-252	133	126	61-252
3.5-4.5	143	138	59-244	138	134	63-248
16-24	302	285	140-600	198	194	85-330
25-34	317	303	164-549	206	198	84-348
35-49	321	308	138-555	220	212	105-383
50-64	300	289	156-545	218	214	101-354

Source: from data reported by Gregory *et al.* 1990, 1995.

Table 21.3: Rich sources of folate

	portion (g)	µg /portion
mung beans (dahl)	150	210
red kidney beans	100	130
spinach	130	117
kidney	150	113
Brussels sprouts	75	100
endive	30	100
parsnips	110	96
asparagus	60	93
chickpeas	150	81
beans, French	100	80
oranges	250	78
okra	80	70
broccoli	75	68
beans, runner	100	60
oatmeal	100	60
cabbage	75	56
beer, bitter	560	50
leeks	125	50
spring greens	75	50
bean sprouts	80	49
potatoes	140	49
lentils	150	45
beans, baked	200	44
beetroot	40	44
cauliflower	65	43
cheese, soft (camembert)	40	41
orange juice	200	40
salmon	150	39
grapefruit	140	36
crab	175	35
egg	70	35
milk	560	34
satsumas	100	33
cheese, hard	40	31
liver	150	30
artichokes, globe	220	29
peanuts, fresh	25	28
blackberries	80	27
bread, wholemeal	70	27
yoghourt	150	27
beef	150	26
lobster	150	26
raspberries	80	26
sweet potato	150	26
wheat bran	10	26
semolina	100	25
beans, broad	75	24
beef	150	24
bread, brown	60	24
shrimps	150	23
turkey	150	23
beer, lager or stout	560	22
mushrooms	50	22
swedes	120	22
cod	175	21
peanut butter	25	21
tangerines	100	21

Table 21.4: Reference intakes of vitamin B_{12}

	US RDA (1989)	UK RNI (1991)	EU PRI (1993)
	µg	µg	µg
birth—6 m	0.3	0.3	-
7—12 m	0.5	0.4	0.5
1—3 y	0.7	0.5	0.7
4—6	1.0	0.8	0.9
7—10	1.4	1.0	1.0
males			
11—14	2.0	1.2	1.3
15—18	2.0	1.5	1.4
adult	2.0	1.5	1.4
females			
11—14	2.0	1.2	1.3
15—18	2.0	1.5	1.4
adult	2.0	1.5	1.4
pregnant	2.2	-	+0.2
lactating	2.6	+0.5	+0.5

Source: National Research Council, 1989; Department of Health, 1991; Scientific Committee for Food, 1993.

Table: 21.5: Average intakes of vitamin B_{12} (µg /day) in UK

	males			females		
age	mean	median	95% range	mean	median	95% range
1.5-2.5	2.9	2.5	0.8-6.7	2.9	2.5	0.8-6.7
2.5-3.5	2.8	2.4	0.9-7.2	2.8	2.4	0.9-7.2
3.5-4.5	2.8	2.6	0.8-6.2	2.8	2.4	0.9-6.2
16-24	6.2	5.1	1.7-19.8	4.4	3.4	1.3-17.4
25-34	7.1	5.7	2.7-24.7	4.5	3.5	1.1-16.4
35-49	7.6	5.9	2.4-26.7	5.6	4.1	1.5-18.6
50-64	7.8	5.9	2.6-23.6	5.8	4.3	1.6-16.4

Source: from data reported by Gregory *et al.* 1990, 1995.

Table 21.6: Rich sources of vitamin B_{12}

	portion (g)	µg /portion
liver	150	50.0
kidney	150	46.5
sardines canned in oil	150	42.0
mussels	150	33.2
sardines canned in tomato	150	21.0
rabbit	150	18.0
bloater	150	16.5
herring or kipper	150	16.5
mackerel	150	15.0
pilchards in tomato sauce	100	12.0
salmon	150	7.5
trout	150	7.4
tuna	150	7.2
duck	150	4.5
cod	175	3.5
beef	150	3.0
lamb	150	3.0
plaice	150	3.0
shrimps	150	3.0
turkey	150	3.0
goose	150	2.8
milk	560	2.2
egg	70	1.8

Table 21.7: Stages in the development of folate deficiency

	normal	negative balance	depletion	deficient erythropoeisis	anaemia
serum folate, µmol/L	> 11.3	< 6.7	< 6.7	< 6.7	< 6.7
erythrocyte folate, µmol/L	> 450	> 450	< 360	< 270	< 230
dUMP suppression test	normal	normal	normal	abnormal	abnormal
polymorphonuclear leukocyte lobe average	< 3.5	< 3.5	< 3.5	> 3.5	> 3.5
liver folate, nmol/g	> 6.8	> 6.8	< 3.6	< 2.7	< 2.3
erythrocytes	normal	normal	normal	normal	macrocytic
mean cell volume, fL	< 95	< 95	< 95	< 95	> 95
haemoglobin, g/L	> 120	> 120	> 120	> 120	< 120
plasma clearance of intravenous folate	normal	normal	normal	increased	increased
urine FIGLU after histidine load, µg /mL	< 50	-	-	-	> 50

Source: Herbert 1987.

Table 21.8: Stages in the development of vitamin B₁₂ deficiency

	normal	negative balance	depletion	deficient erythropoeisis	anaemia
holotranscorrin II, ng/L	> 22	< 15	< 15	< 9	< 9
transcorrin II saturation, %	> 54	< 5	< 2	< 1	< 1
holohaptocorrin, pmol/L	> 110	> 110	< 110	< 75	< 75
dUMP suppression test	normal	normal	normal	abnormal	abnormal
hypersegmentation	no	no	no	yes	yes
total plasma B₁₂ binding saturation, %	> 15	> 15	> 15	< 15	< 10
haptocorrin saturation, %	> 20	> 20	> 20	< 20	< 10
erythrocyte folate, µmol /L	> 360	> 360	> 360	< 320	< 320
erythrocytes	normal	normal	normal	normal	macro-ovalocytic
mean cell volume, fL	< 95	< 95	< 95	< 95	> 95
haemoglobin, g/L	> 120	> 120	> 120	> 120	< 120
transcorrin II	normal	normal	normal	elevated	elevated
methylmalonic aciduria	no	no	no	?	yes
myelin damage	no	no	no	?	?

Source: Herbert 1987.

Table 21.9: Indices of folate and vitamin B₁₂ nutritional status

	reference range		deficiency	
	nmol /L	µg /L	nmol /L	µg /L
serum folate	9.8-16.2	4.4-7.2	< 6.8	< 3
erythrocyte folate	420-620	185-270	< 320	< 140
whole blood vitamin B₁₂	0.22-0.65	0.29-0.87	-	-
serum vitamin B₁₂	0.14-0.52	0.19-0.69	< 0.075	< 0.10
erythrocyte vitamin B₁₂	0.06-0.21	0.08-0.28	-	-
transcorrin II bound vitamin B₁₂	-	-	< 0.15	< 0.22
mean cell volume		-	> 100 fL	
serum methylmalonic acid		-	> 1 µmol /L	
serum homocysteine		-	> 20 µmol /L	
urine FIGLU over 8h after histidine load		-	> 50 µg /mL	
excretion of radio-labelled vitamin B₁₂ (Schilling test)	16-45%		< 5%	

Source: from data reported by Bailey, 1990; Herbert, 1987; van den Berg, 1993.

Vitamin C (ascorbic acid)

Vitamin C is a vitamin for only a limited number of vertebrate species: man and the other primates, the guinea pig, bats, the passeriform birds and most fishes. Insects and invertebrates are incapable of ascorbate synthesis. Ascorbate is synthesised as an intermediate in the gulonolactone pathway of glucose metabolism; in those vertebrate species for which ascorbate is a vitamin, one enzyme of the pathway, gulonolactone oxidase (EC 1.11.3.8), is absent.

The vitamin C deficiency disease, scurvy, has been known for many centuries, and was described in the Ebers papyrus of 1500 BC and by Hippocrates. The Crusaders are said to have lost more men through scurvy than were killed in battle, while in some of the long voyages of exploration of the fourteenth and fifteenth centuries up to 90 per cent of the crew died from scurvy. Cartier's expedition to Quebec in 1535 was struck by scurvy; the local Indians taught him to use an infusion of swamp spruce leaves to prevent or cure the condition.

Recognition that scurvy was due to a dietary deficiency came relatively early. James Lind demonstrated in 1757 that orange and lemon juice were protective, and Cook maintained his crew in good health during his circumnavigation of the globe (1772–1775) by stopping frequently to take on fresh fruit and vegetables. In 1804 the British Navy decreed a daily ration of lemon or lime juice for all ratings, a requirement that was extended to the merchant navy in 1865.

Ascorbic acid was isolated from cabbage, lemon juice and adrenal glands by Szent-György in 1928, and identified as the anti-scorbutic factor by Waugh and King in 1932. Its structure was established by Haworth and coworkers in 1933, and the same year Haworth, in Birmingham, and Reichstein, in Switzerland, succeeded in synthesizing the vitamin.

Ascorbate is a reducing sugar, and in addition to its specific role as cofactor for a variety of redox reactions it also functions as a relatively non-specific reducing agent. Some of these non-specific reactions are physiologically important, others have led to con-fusion in the literature because *in vitro* it will enhance the activity of a number of enzymes for which it is not a cofactor.

22.1 Requirements and intakes

There have been two major studies of ascorbate requirements in depletion/repletion studies, one in Sheffield during the 1940s (Medical Research Council 1948) and the other in Iowa during the 1960s (Baker *et al.* 1969, 1971; Hodges *et al.* 1969, 1971). In addition, Kallner and coworkers have determined the body pool of ascorbate and the fractional rate of turnover under various conditions (Kallner *et al.* 1979, 1981).

22.1.1 Minimum requirements for vitamin C

The minimum requirement for vitamin C was established in the Sheffield study, which showed that an intake of 5–10 mg /day was adequate to prevent the development of scurvy, or to cure the clinical signs. Results from the Iowa study suggested that as little as 6.5 mg /day was adequate, and studies in India show that intakes as low as 10 mg /day are compatible with good health.

However, at this level of intake the subjects in the Sheffield study had impaired wound healing, as assessed by the tensile strength of scar tissue. Optimum wound healing requires a mean intake of 20 mg /day. Allowing for individual variation, this gives an RDA of 30 mg /day, which is the WHO/FAO RDA, and was the British RDA until 1991.

22.1.2 Requirements estimated from the plasma concentration of ascorbate

The plasma concentration of ascorbate shows a sigmoidal relationship with intake. Below about 30 mg /day the plasma concentration is extremely low, and does not reflect increasing intake to any significant extent. As the intake rises above 30 mg /day, so the plasma concentration begins to increase sharply, reaching a plateau of 68–85 µmol (12–15 mg) /L, at intakes between 70–100 mg /day, when the renal threshold is reached and the vitamin is excreted quantitatively with increasing intake.

The mid-point of the steep region of the curve, where the plasma concentration increases more or less linearly with increasing intake, represents a state where tissue reserves are adequate and plasma ascorbate is available for transfer between tissues. This corresponds to an intake of 40 mg /day; at this level of intake the total body pool is about 900 mg (5.1 mmol). This is the basis of the UK and EU reference intakes (see Table 22.1)

22.1.3 Requirements estimated from the metabolic turnover of ascorbate

Clinical signs of deficiency are seen when the total body pool of ascorbate is below 1.7 mmol (300 mg). The pool increases with intake, reaching a maximum of about 8.5 mmol (1500 mg) in adults, equivalent to 114 µmol (20 mg) /kg body weight. The fractional turnover rate of ascorbate is 3–4 per cent daily, suggesting a need for 45–60 mg /day for replacement.

The basis of the US RDA (see Table 22.1) of 60 mg is the observed mean fractional turnover rate of 3.2 per cent of a body pool of 20 mg /kg body weight / day, with allowances for incomplete absorption of dietary ascorbate and individual variation.

Olson and Hodges (1987) suggested that a total body pool of 900 mg (5.1 mmol) is adequate; it is three-fold higher than the minimum pool required to prevent scurvy, and there is no evidence that there are any health benefits from a body pool greater than 600 mg. They noted that the figure of 1500 mg which is the basis of the US and other RDA, was found in subjects consuming a self-selected diet, with a relatively high intake of vitamin C, and therefore could not be considered to represent any index of requirement. On the basis of a mean catabolic rate of 2.7 per cent /day, and allowing for efficiency of absorption and individual variation, they proposed an RDA of 40 mg.

Because the mean fractional turnover rate of 3.2 per cent /day was observed during a depletion study, and the rate of ascorbate catabolism varies with intake, it has been suggested that this implies a rate of 3.6 per cent /day before depletion. On this basis, and allowing for incomplete absorption and indivi-

dual variation, some national authorities arrive at reference intake of 80 mg.

22.1.4 Higher recommendations

There is a school of thought that believes that human requirements for vitamin C are considerably higher than those discussed above. Pauling (1970) determined the vitamin C intake of gorillas in captivity, assumed that this was the same as their intake in the wild (where they eat considerably less fruit than under zoo conditions), and then assumed, unjustifiably, that because they had this intake, it was their requirement. Scaling this to human beings, he suggested a requirement of 1–2 g /day.

Intakes in excess of about 80–100 mg /day lead to a quantitative increase in urinary excretion of unmetabolized vitamin C with increasing intake, indicating that at this level tissue reserves are saturated. It is difficult to justify a requirement in excess of tissue storage capacity.

22.1.4.1 Smoking

The rate of ascorbate catabolism is up to 40 per cent greater in smokers than non-smokers (Kallner *et al.* 1981), and therefore that their vitamin C requirement may be almost twice that of non-smokers. In general, smokers have lower plasma and leukocyte concentrations of ascorbate than non-smokers, but in most surveys they also have a lower intake.

22.1.5 Intakes and sources of vitamin C

Table 22.2 shows average intakes of vitamin C, Table 22.3 the proportion of average intakes provided by various foods, and Table 22.4 rich sources.

22.2   Vitamin C vitamers and nomenclature

The physiologically important compound is L-ascorbic acid. It can undergo oxidation to the monodehydroascorbate free radical and onwards to dehydroascorbate, both of which have vitamin activity because they can be reduced to ascorbate (see Fig. 22.1).

Further oxidation in the presence of oxygen, and especially under alkaline conditions, or in the presence of heavy metal ions which are substrates for reduction, results in the formation of dioxogulonic acid (diketogulonic acid), which has no biological activity.

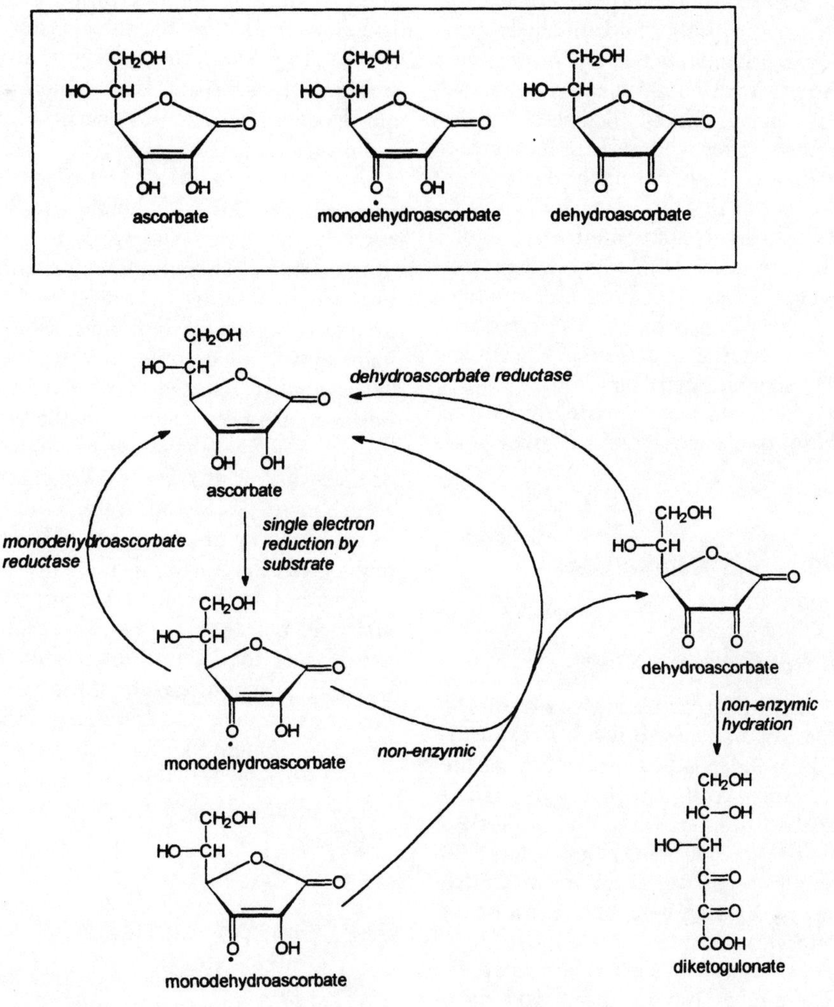

Figure 22.1 Vitamin C vitamers
Relative molecular mass (M_r) of ascorbate = 176.1. Dehydroascorbate (monodehydroascorbate) reductase EC 1.6.5.4

D-Iso-ascorbic acid (erythorbic acid) also has vitamin activity. *In vivo* it has only about 5 per cent of the biological activity of ascorbate, but this seems to be due to poor intestinal absorption and tissue uptake. It is not a naturally occurring compound, but it is widely used, interchangeably with ascorbic acid, in cured meats and as an antioxidant in a variety of foods.

Vitamin C is used in food processing as the free acid (E-300), the sodium (E-301) and calcium (E-302) salts and as ascorbyl palmitate (E-304), a lipid soluble antioxidant. While most of the ascorbate used as a flour improver and in bread making by the Chorleywood process is destroyed in baking, a considerable number of other processed foods provide significant amounts of the vitamin because of its use as an antioxidant and meat-curing aid.

22.2.1 Assay of vitamin C

Because it is a potent reducing agent, vitamin C is commonly determined by titrimetric or potentiometric redox methods. Such methods underestimate the amount of the vitamin present because dehydroascorbate, which has vitamin activity, and is formed by atmospheric oxidation of ascorbate in the sample, is not detected by redox assay methods.

Vitamin C can also be determined colorimetrically, after oxidation to dehydroascorbate, by reaction with dinitrophenylhydrazine. Under appropriate conditions neither ascorbic acid itself nor potentially interfering sugars, reacts with dinitrophenylhydrazine. However, dioxogulonate, which has no vitamin activity, does react with dinitrophenylhydrazine under the same conditions. Unless dioxogulonate is determined separately after sulphide reduction of dehydroascorbate to ascorbate, this method over estimates the vitamin.

Ascorbic acid and dehydroascorbate form a fluorescent quinolaxine derivative with o-phenylene diamine. This provides a very sensitive and specific fluorimetric assay procedure, which is the preferred method of analysis (Deutsch and Weeks 1965). An HPLC method for separate determination of ascorbate, dehydroascorbate and isoascorbate, applicable to foods, has been published by Vanderslice and Higgs (1993).

22.3 Absorption and metabolism of vitamin C

22.3.1 Absorption and tissue uptake

There is sodium-dependent active transport of the vitamin at the intestinal mucosal brush border membrane, with a sodium-independent mechanism at the basolateral membrane. Both ascorbate and dehydroascorbate are absorbed across the buccal mucosa by carrier-mediated passive processes. Intestinal absorption of dehydroascorbate is carrier mediated, followed by reduced to ascorbate before transport across the basolateral membrane.

Some 80–95 per cent of dietary ascorbate is absorbed at usual intakes (up to about 100 mg / day). The absorption of larger amounts of the vitamin is relatively lower, falling from 50 per cent of a 1.5 g dose to 25 per cent of a 6 g and 16 per cent of a 12 g dose (Rivers 1987). The unabsorbed ascorbate from high doses is a substrate for intestinal bacterial metabolism.

About 70 per cent of blood-borne ascorbate is in plasma and erythrocytes (which do not concentrate the vitamin from plasma). The remainder is in white cells, which have a marked ability to concentrate ascorbate; mononuclear leukocytes achieve 80–fold, platelets 40–fold and granulocytes 25–fold concentration compared with the plasma concentration (see Table 22.5).

In adequately nourished subjects and those receiving supplements the ascorbate concentration in erythrocytes, platelets and granulocytes, but not in mononuclear leukocytes, is correlated with the plasma concentration. Mononuclear leukocytes seem to be able to concentrate ascorbate more or less independently of the plasma concentration (Evans *et al.* 1982). In deficiency, as plasma concentrations of ascorbate fall, mononuclear leukocyte, granulocyte and platelet concentrations of ascorbate are protected to a considerable extent.

Both ascorbate and dehydroascorbate circulate in free solution, and also bound to albumin. About 5 per cent of plasma vitamin C is normally as dehydroascorbate. Tissue uptake mechanisms for the two vitamers differ. There is active concentrative uptake of ascorbate into cells, while dehydroascorbate shows apparently concentrative uptake only because it is reduced intracellularly to ascorbate. Both vitamers are carried by the glucose transport system, and concentrations of glucose, of the order of those seen in diabetic hyperglycaemia, can inhibit ascorbate uptake significantly. In addition, because it is lipophilic at physiological pH, dehydroascorbate may enter cells by diffusion.

There is no specific storage organ for ascorbate; apart from leukocytes (which account for only 10 per cent of total blood ascorbate), the only tissues showing a significant concentration of the vitamin are the adrenal and pituitary glands (see Table 22.6). Although the concentration of ascorbate in muscle is relatively low, skeletal muscle contains much of the body's pool of 5–8.5 mmol (900–1500 mg).

22.3.2 Oxidation and reduction of ascorbate

Oxidation of ascorbic acid, for example by the reduction of superoxide to hydrogen peroxide, or Fe^{3+} to Fe^{2+}, proceeds by a one-electron process, leading to the monodehydroascorbate radical. The radical rapidly disproportionates into ascorbate and dehydroascorbate (see Fig. 22.1). Most tissues also have an NADPH-dependent monodehydroascorbate reductase (EC 1.6.5.4), a flavoprotein which reduces the radical to ascorbate. Dehydroascorbate is unstable in solution, undergoing hydrolytic ring opening to yield dioxogulonic acid. However, *in vivo* it is normally reduced to ascorbate by either a glutathione-dependent (EC 1.8.5.1) or an NADPH-dependent (EC 1.10.3.3) reductase.

In many plants there are ascorbate oxidases which form monodehydroascorbate. These enzymes, and onward non-enzymic oxidation to dioxogulonic acid, are responsible for the oxidative loss of vitamin C in vegetables after harvesting – see section 26.3.1.4.

22.3.3 Metabolism and excretion

Dehydroascorbate can undergo hydration to dioxo-gulonate and decarboxylation to xylose, thus providing a route for entry into central carbohydrate metabolic pathways via the pentose phosphate pathway. This is the major metabolic fate of ascorbate in those species for which it is not vitamin, and also in the guinea pig, where 60 per cent of the radioactivity from $[^{14}C]$ascorbate is recovered in expired carbon dioxide. Label from $[^{14}C]$ascorbic acid is also incorporated into glycogen in guinea pig liver. However, oxidation to carbon dioxide is only a minor fate of ascorbate in man. At usual intakes of the vitamin (90 mg /day) less than 1 per cent of the radioactivity from $[^{14}C]$ascorbate is recovered as carbon dioxide. While more $^{14}CO_2$ is recovered from subjects receiving high intakes of the vitamin, this seems to be the result of bacterial metabolism of unabsorbed vitamin in the intestinal lumen, rather than liver metabolism as in the guinea pig (Kallner *et al.* 1985).

The fate of the greater part of ascorbic acid is excretion in the urine, either unchanged or as dehydroascorbate and dioxogulonate. Both ascorbate and dehydroascorbate are filtered at the glomerulus, then resorbed, by sodium-independent facilitated diffusion. Resorbed dehydroascorbate is reduced to ascorbate in the kidney. It is when glomerular filtration of ascorbate and dehydroascorbate exceeds the capacity of these transport systems, at a plasma concentration of ascorbate between 70–85 µmol /L, that the vitamin is excreted in the urine in amounts proportional to intake.

22.4 Metabolic functions of vitamin C

Ascorbic acid has specific and well-defined roles in two classes of enzymes, the copper-containing hydroxylases, and the 2–oxoglutarate-linked iron-containing hydroxylases. It also increases the activity of a number of other enzymes *in vitro*, although this is a non-specific reducing action rather than reflecting any metabolic function of the vitamin. In addition it has a number of non-enzymic effects due to its action as a reducing agent and oxygen radical quencher.

22.4.1 Dopamine β-hydroxylase

Dopamine β-hydroxylase (EC 1.14.17.1) is a copper-containing enzyme involved in the synthesis of the catecholamines, noradrenaline and adrenaline, from tyrosine in the adrenal medulla and central nervous system. The enzyme contains Cu^+, which is oxidized to Cu^{2+} during the hydroxylation of the substrate; reduction back to Cu^+ specifically requires ascorbate, which is oxidized to monodehydroascorbate (Diliberto *et al.* 1982; Mennita *et al.* 1986).

22.4.2 Peptidyl glycine hydroxylase (peptide α-amidase)

A number of peptide hormones have a carboxy terminal amide which is essential for biological activity. The amide group is derived from a glycine residue which is on the carboxyl side of the amino acid which will become the amidated terminal of the mature peptide. This glycine is hydroxylated on the α-carbon by a copper-containing enzyme, peptidyl-glycine hydroxylase (EC 1.14.17.3). The α-hydroxy-glycine residue then decomposes non-enzymically to yield the amidated peptide and glyoxylate (Tajima *et al.* 1990). The copper prosthetic group is oxidized in the reaction, and as in dopamine β-hydroxylase, ascorbate is specifically required for reduction back to Cu^+.

22.4.3 Oxoglutarate-linked iron-containing hydroxylases

A number of iron-containing hydroxylases share a common reaction mechanism, in which hydroxylation of the substrate is linked to decarboxylation of 2–oxoglutarate; they are listed in Table 22.7. Many of these enzymes are involved in the modification of precursor proteins to yield the final, mature, protein. This is a process of post-synthetic modification—modification of an amino acid residue after it has been incorporated into the protein during synthesis on the ribosome. Proline and lysine hydroxylases are required for the post-synthetic modification of pro-collagen in the formation of mature, insoluble, collagen, and proline hydroxylase is also required for the post-synthetic modification of the precursor proteins of osteocalcin (see section 16.4.2) and the C1q component of complement. Aspartate β-hydroxylase is required for the post-synthetic modification of the precursor of protein C, the vitamin K dependent protease which hydrolyses activated Factor V in the blood clotting cascade (see Fig. 16.3). Trimethyllysine and γ-butyrobetaine hydroxylases are required for the synthesis of carnitine (see section 23.5).

Procollagen proline 4–hydroxylase is the best studied of this class of enzymes; it is assumed that the others have essentially the same mechanism. As shown in Fig. 22.2, the first step in the reaction is

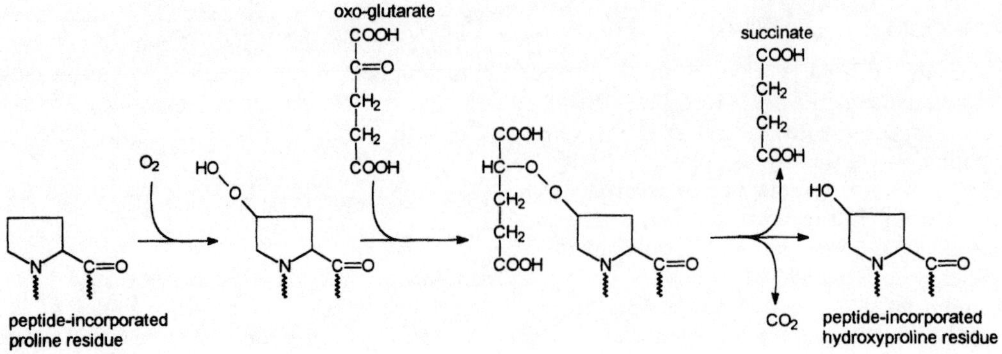

Figure 22.2 The role of vitamin C in procollagen proline hydroxylase (EC 1.14.11.2)

an attack on the substrate by oxygen, followed by condensation with 2–oxoglutarate. This is followed by release of the hydroxylated substrate and decarboxylation to release succinate. The Fe^{2+} prosthetic group of the enzyme does not undergo oxidation.

Ascorbate is oxidized during the reaction, but not stoichiometrically with the decarboxylation of 2–oxoglutarate and hydroxylation of the substrate. The purified enzyme is active in the absence of ascorbate, but after some 5–10 sec (about 15–30 cycles of enzyme action) the rate of reaction begins to fall. At this stage the iron in the catalytic site has been oxidized to Fe^{3+}, which is catalytically inactive; activity is restored by only ascorbate, which reduces it back to Fe^{2+}. Myllylä *et al.* (1978) proposed that the oxidation of Fe^{2+} is the consequence of a side-reaction rather than the main reaction of the enzyme, which would explain how 15–30 cycles of enzyme activity can occur before there is significant loss of activity in the absence of ascorbate, and why the consumption of ascorbate is not stoichiometric.

22.4.4 Non-enzymic actions of ascorbate

Over the years a number of enzymes, including tryptophan dioxygenase (EC 1.13.11.11, see section 19.4.2) and tyrosine hydroxylase (EC 1.14.16.2, see Table 10.40), have been assumed to be ascorbate-dependent, because their activity is stimulated *in vitro* by the addition of ascorbate to the incubation medium. In general these reactions are not ascorbate dependent; ascorbate is just one of a variety of reducing reagents that are able to enhance the reaction.

Scorbutic guinea pigs have elevated levels of histamine in the blood, which responds rapidly to repletion with vitamin C. Ascorbate has no effect on the synthesis or release of histamine, nor on the activity of histaminase (EC 1.4.3.6) or other amine oxidases. Rather, it seems to catalyse a non-enzymic degradation of histamine to aspartate, by imidazole N-oxygenation in the presence of oxygen and catalytic amounts of Cu^{2+} (Uchida *et al.* 1989).

22.4.4.1 The role of ascorbate in iron absorption and metabolism
As discussed in section 24.2.3, inorganic iron is absorbed as Fe^{2+}, and not as Fe^{3+}; ascorbic acid in the intestinal lumen will both maintain iron in the reduced state and also chelate it, thus increasing the amount absorbed. A dose of 25 mg of vitamin C taken together with a semi-synthetic meal increases the absorption of iron some 65 per cent, while a 1 g dose gives a 9–fold increase. This occurs only when ascorbic acid is present together with the test meal; neither intravenous administration of vitamin C nor supplements several hours before the test meal has any effect on iron absorption. The endogenous vitamin C in foods has the same effect on iron absorption (Brise and Hallberg 1962).

This is not a specific effect of ascorbate; a variety of other reducing agents also enhance the absorption of inorganic iron, including alcohol and fructose.

Ascorbate is also active in the reduction of Fe^{3+} in the plasma transport protein, transferrin, to Fe^{2+} for storage in ferritin in the liver or haem synthesis (Mazur *et al.* 1960). Again it is not known to what extent this represents specific actions of ascorbate, since other reducing reagents, including glutathione, also enhance haem synthesis, and the NADH-dependent reductase is believed to be the major factor controlling the transfer of iron between transferrin and ferritin (Zaman and Verwilghen 1977).

22.4.4.2 Inhibition of nitrosamine formation

The safety of nitrates and nitrites used in curing meat, a traditional method of preservation, has been questioned because of the formation of nitrosamines by reaction between nitrite and amines naturally present in foods under the acid conditions in the stomach. In experimental animals, nitrosamines are potent carcinogens, and some authorities have limited the amounts of these salts that are permitted, although there is no evidence of any hazard to human beings from nitrosamine formation. Ascorbate can prevent the formation of nitrosamines by reacting non-enzymically with nitrite and other nitrosating reagents, forming NO, NO_2 and N_2. Again this is an effect of ascorbate present in the stomach at the same time as the dietary nitrites and amines, rather than an effect of vitamin C nutritional status.

However, while ascorbate can deplete nitrosating compounds under anaerobic conditions, the situation may be reversed in the presence of oxygen. Nitric oxide reacts with oxygen to form N_2O_3 and N_2O_4, both of which are nitrosating reagents, and can also react with ascorbate to form NO and monodehydroascorbate. It is thus possible for ascorbate to be depleted, with no significant effect on the total concentration of nitrosating species. It remains to be determined whether or not ascorbate has any significant effect in reducing the risk of nitrosamine formation and carcinogenesis (Tannenbaum and Wishnok 1987).

22.4.4.3 Reduction of the vitamin E radical

One of the major roles of vitamin E is as a radical-trapping antioxidant at membrane surfaces (see section 15.5.1). Tocopherol reacts with lipid peroxides, forming the α-tocopheroxyl radical, which reacts with ascorbate in the aqueous phase, regenerating α-tocopherol, and forming the monodehydroascorbate radical, which reacts to yield ascorbate and dehydroascorbate (see Fig. 22.1). Vitamin C may thus have a vitamin E-sparing antioxidant action, coupling lipophilic and hydrophilic reactions. However, Burton *et al.* (1990) showed no effect of vitamin C status on the turnover of $[^2H]$-tocopherol in the guinea pig. They suggested that either vitamin C does not have a significant vitamin E-sparing action, or that other water-soluble antioxidants in plasma and extracellular fluid may also interact with the tocopheroxyl radical. During the oxidation of lipids in foods, vitamin C is oxidized before there is any significant loss of vitamin E.

22.4.4.4 Pro- and antioxidant roles of ascorbate

Ascorbate can act as a radical-trapping antioxidant, reacting with superoxide and a proton to yield hydrogen peroxide, or with the hydroxy radical to yield water. In each instance the product is the monodehydroascorbate radical. Thus, as well as reducing the tocopheroxyl radical formed by interaction of α-tocopherol in membranes with lipid peroxides, ascorbate also acts to trap the oxygen radicals which would otherwise react to form lipid peroxides.

At high concentrations, ascorbate can reduce molecular oxygen to superoxide, being oxidized to monodehydroascorbate. At physiological concentrations of ascorbate, both Fe^{3+} and Cu^{2+} ions are reduced by ascorbate, yielding monodehydroascorbate. Fe^{2+} and Cu^+ are readily reoxidized by reaction with hydrogen peroxide to yield hydroxide ions and hydroxyl radicals. Cu^+ also reacts with molecular oxygen to yield superoxide (Wayner *et al.* 1986).

Thus, as well as its antioxidant role, ascorbate has pro-oxidant action, and the net result will depend on the relative rates of formation of superoxide and hydroxyl radicals by autoxidation and metal-catalysed reactions of ascorbate, and the trapping of these radicals by ascorbate. Certainly in tissue culture ascorbate has a cytotoxic action as a result of radical-initiated DNA damage. However, Jacob *et al.* (1991) reported that in volunteers maintained on a vitamin C-free diet for a relatively short time there was a doubling of the content of 8–hydroxyguanine in sperm DNA, suggesting increased damage to DNA by radical action in the absence of adequate amounts of ascorbate.

22.5 Vitamin C deficiency, scurvy

Although there is no specific organ for storage of vitamin C in the body, signs of deficiency do not develop in previously adequately nourished subjects until they have been deprived of the vitamin for 4–6 months, by which time plasma and tissue concentrations have fallen considerably. The earliest signs of scurvy in volunteers maintained on a vitamin C-free diet are skin changes, beginning with plugging of hair follicles by horny material, followed by enlargement of the hyperkeratotic follicles and petechial haemorrhage, with significant extravasation of red cells—presumably the result of increased fragility of blood capillaries and vasodilatation caused by elevated plasma histamine (Chatterjee 1978).

At a later stage there is also haemorrhage of the gums, beginning in the interdental papillae, and progressing to generalized sponginess and bleeding. This is frequently accompanied by secondary bacterial infection and considerable withdrawal of the gum from the necks of the teeth. As the condition progresses, there is loss of dental cement, and the teeth become loose in the alveolar bone, and may be lost.

Wounds show only superficial healing in scurvy, with little or no formation of (collagen-rich) scar tissue, so that healing is delayed and wounds can readily be reopened. The scorbutic scar tissue has only about half the tensile strength of that normally formed.

Advanced scurvy is accompanied by intense pain in the bones, which can be attributed to changes in bone mineralization and demineralization as a result of abnormal collagen synthesis. Bone formation ceases and the existing bone becomes rarefied, so that the bones fracture with minimal trauma.

The name scurvy is believed to be derived from the Italian *scorbutico*, meaning an irritable, neurotic, discontented, whining and cranky person. The deficiency disease is certainly associated with listlessness and general malaise, and sometimes changes in personality and psychomotor performance and a lowering of the general level of arousal. These behavioural effects can presumably be attributed to impaired synthesis of catecholamines, as a result of low activity of dopamine β-hydroxylase (see section 22.4.1).

Most of the other clinical signs of scurvy can be accounted for by the effects of ascorbate deficiency on collagen synthesis, as a result of impaired proline and lysine hydroxylase activity (see section 22.4.3). Depletion of muscle carnitine, as a result of impaired activity of trimethyllysine and γ-butyrobetaine hydroxylases, may account for the lassitude and fatigue which precede clinical signs of scurvy.

22.5.1 Anaemia in scurvy

Anaemia is frequently associated with scurvy, and may be either macrocytic, indicative of folate deficiency (see section 21.8), or hypochromic, indicative of iron deficiency (see section 24.4) (Goldberg 1963).

Folate deficiency may be epiphenomenal, since the major dietary sources of folate are the same as those of ascorbate. However, some patients with clear megaloblastic anaemia respond to the administration of vitamin C alone, suggesting that there may be a role of ascorbate in the maintenance of normal pools of reduced folates, although there is no evidence that any of the reactions of folate (see section 21.4) is ascorbate dependent,

Iron deficiency in scurvy may well be secondary to reduced absorption of inorganic iron, and impaired mobilization of tissue iron reserves (see sections

22.4.4.1 and 24.3). At the same time, the haemorrhages of advanced scurvy will cause a considerable loss of blood.

There is also evidence that erythrocytes have a shorter half-life than normal in scurvy, possibly as a result of peroxidative damage to membrane lipids due to impairment of the reduction of tocopheroxyl radical by ascorbate (see section 22.4.4.3).

22.6   Assessment of vitamin C nutritional status

22.6.1 Urinary excretion and saturation testing

Urinary excretion of ascorbate falls to undetectably low levels in deficiency, and therefore very low excretion will indicate deficiency. However, no guidelines for the interpretation of urinary ascorbate have been established, and because of non-enzymic oxidation and breakdown to oxalate in urine samples (Chalmers *et al.* 1986), basal urinary excretion of ascorbate is rarely used in the assessment of status. During depletion / repletion studies, urinary excretion increases before tissue saturation has been achieved (Sauberlich 1975).

At a daily intake of 30 mg /day, some 1–3 mg of unmetabolized ascorbate are excreted in the urine, increasing to 3–8 mg /day at an intake of 60 mg, and to 12–30 mg /day at an intake of 90 mg (Kallner *et al.* 1979).

It is relatively easy to assess the state of body reserves of vitamin C by measuring the excretion after a test dose. A subject who is saturated will excrete more or less the whole of a test dose of 500 mg of ascorbate over 6 hours. A more precise method involves repeating the loading test daily until more or less complete recovery is achieved, thus giving an indication of how depleted the body stores were.

22.6.2 Blood concentrations of ascorbate

The plasma concentration of vitamin C falls relatively rapidly during experimental depletion studies, to undetectably low levels within 4 weeks of initiating a vitamin C-free diet, although clinical signs of scurvy may not develop for a further 3–4 months, and tissue concentrations of the vitamin may be as high as 50 per cent of saturation. In field studies and surveys, subjects with plasma ascorbate below 11 μmol /L are considered to be at risk of developing scurvy, while anyone with a plasma concentration below 6 μmol /L would be expected to show clinical signs (see Table 22.8).

The concentration of ascorbate in leukocytes is well correlated with the concentrations in other tissues, and falls more slowly than plasma concentration in depletion studies. The reference range of leukocyte ascorbate is 1.1–2.8 pmol /10^6 cells; a significant loss of leukocyte ascorbate coincides with the development of clear clinical signs of scurvy.

Without a differential white cell count, leukocyte ascorbate concentration cannot be considered to give a meaningful reflection of vitamin C status. The different types of leukocyte have different capacities to accumulate ascorbate (see Table 22.5). This means that a change in the proportion of granulocytes, platelets and mononuclear leukocytes will result in a change in the total concentration of ascorbate /10^6 cells, although there may well be no change in vitamin nutritional status. Stress, myocardial infarction, infection, burns, and surgical trauma all result in changes in leukocyte distribution, with an increase in the proportion of granulocytes, and hence an apparent change in leukocyte ascorbate. This has been misinterpreted to indicate an increased requirement for vitamin C in these conditions (Hume *et al.* 1977; Schorah *et al.* 1986).

22.7 Pharmacological uses and toxicity of vitamin C

Ascorbate enhances the intestinal absorption of inorganic iron, and therefore it is frequently prescribed together with iron supplements. It is also used when it is desired to acidify the urine, for example in conjunction with some antibiotics.

22.7.1 Cancer therapy and prevention

A number of studies have reported low ascorbate status in patients with advanced cancer—perhaps an unsurprising finding in seriously ill patients. However, there is also some evidence that a number of tumours can accumulate ascorbate at the expense of the host.

Cameron and Pauling (1974*a*, *b*) published a lengthy review of the supposed roles of ascorbate in enhancing host resistance to cancer, and suggested, on the basis of an uncontrolled open trial in terminally ill patients, that 10 g daily doses of vitamin C resulted in increased survival. In a controlled study with patients matched for age, sex, site, and stage of primary tumours and metastases, and for previous chemotherapy, Creagan *et al.* (1979) were unable to

demonstrate any beneficial effects of high dose ascorbic acid in the treatment of advanced cancer.

Ascorbate has some action *in vitro* in preventing the formation of nitrosamines, although it is doubtful if this is likely to be a useful effect in the presence of oxygen, or to have any beneficial effect in preventing human cancer (see section 22.4.4.2). Similarly, although ascorbate is an antioxidant, and is therefore perceived to provide protection against radical-induced carcinogenesis, it is also a pro-oxidant and source of oxygen radicals (see section 22.4.4.4). Again any beneficial effects remain to be demonstrated.

22.7.2 The common cold

High doses of vitamin C have been recommended for the prevention and treatment of the common cold, with some evidence that the vitamin reduces the duration of symptoms. However, the evidence from controlled trials is unconvincing. Chalmers (1975) reviewed 15 reports and considered that only 8 met the basic criteria of well-conducted scientific research. Assessment of these 8 reports gave no evidence of any beneficial effects. Similarly, Dykes and Meier (1975), reviewing only those reports which had been published in peer-reviewed journals, concluded that there was no evidence of any significant benefit.

22.7.3 Toxicity of vitamin C

Regardless of whether or not high intakes of ascorbate have any beneficial effects, large numbers of people habitually take between 1–5 g /day of vitamin C supplements (compared with reference intakes of 40–80 mg /day), and some take considerably more. There is little evidence of any significant toxicity from these high intakes, although there are a number of potential problems (Rivers 1987). Once the plasma concentration of ascorbate reaches the renal threshold, it is excreted more or less quantitatively with increasing intake, and there is no evidence that higher intakes increase the body pool above about 110 µmol/kg body weight.

Because ascorbate is largely absorbed by active transport, absorption is saturable, and a decreasing proportion of high doses is absorbed (see section 22.3.1). Unabsorbed ascorbate in the intestinal lumen is a substrate for bacterial fermentation, which may explain the diarrhoea and intestinal discomfort reported in some studies with high doses of the vitamin.

22.7.3.1 Oxalosis

Up to 5 per cent of the population are at risk from the development of renal oxalate stones. The risk is from both ingested oxalate and that formed endogenously, mainly from the metabolism of ascorbate and glycine. The process of stone formation is not well understood, and the concentration of oxalate in urine is not the main factor. People who form renal oxalate stones may well have a lower urine concentration of oxalate than people who do not.

Although some urinary oxalate arises from ascorbate, much of the oxalate that is found in urine after the ingestion of vitamin C may be the result of non-enzymic formation from ascorbate under alkaline conditions, occurring either in the bladder or after collection, and hence not a risk factor for renal stone formation (Chalmers *et al.* 1986).

Further reading

Bender, D.A. (1982). Vitamin C. In *Vitamins in Medicine*, Vol. 2, edn (ed. B. M.Barker and D.A. Bender), Chapter 2, pp. 1–68. Heinemann Medical Books, London.

Bender, D.A. (1992). Ascorbic acid (vitamin C). In *Nutritional Biochemistry of the Vitamins*, Chapter 13, pp. 360–93. Cambridge University Press.

Friedrich, W. (1988). Vitamin C. In *Vitamins*, Chapter 14, pp. 929–1002 Walter de Gruyter, Berlin.

Ginter, E. (1978). Marginal vitamin C deficiency, lipid metabolism and atherogenesis. *Advances in Lipid Research*, 16, 167–220.

Prockop, D.J., Kivirrikko, K.I., Turkman, L. and Guzman, N.A. (1979). The biosynthesis of collagen and its disorders. *New England Journal of Medicine*, 301, 13–23, 77–85.

Rose, R.C. (1988). Transport of ascorbic acid and other water-soluble vitamins. *Biochimica et Biophysica Acta*, 947, 335–66.

Sato, P. and Udenfriend, S. (1978). Studies on vitamin C related to the genetic basis of scurvy. *Vitamins and Hormones*, 36, 33–52.

Szent-György, A. (1963). Lost in the twentieth century. *Annual Review of Biochemistry*, 32, 1–15 .

Table 22.1: Reference Intakes for vitamin C

	US RDA (1989)	UK RNI (1991)	EU PRI (1993)
	mg	mg	mg
birth—6 m	30	25	-
7—12 m	35	25	20
1—3 y	40	30	25
4—6	45	30	25
7—10	45	30	30
males			
11—14	50	35	35
15—18	60	40	40
adult	60	40	45
females			
11—14	50	35	35
15—18	60	40	40
adult	60	40	45
pregnant	95	+10	55
lactating	90	+30	70

Source: National Research Council 1989; Department of Health 1991; Scientific Committee for Food 1993.

Table 22.2: Average intakes of vitamin C

(Apart from the SENECA study of the elderly, which involved 17 centres throughout Europe, all the studies quoted were in UK)

age	mean	males median	range[1]	mean	females median	range[1]	reference
1.5-2.5	48.2	36.9	10.2-158	48.2	36.9	10.2-158	Gregory *et al.* 1995
2.5-3.5	49.2	37.6	8.9-160	49.2	37.6	8.9-160	Gregory *et al.* 1995
3.5-4.5	50.8	38.4	9.0-183	45.9	38.7	9.6-113	Gregory *et al.* 1995
16-24	64.9	52.6	19.1-183.6	60.4	48.8	12.0-182.2	Gregory *et al.* 1990
25-34	69.7	59.3	21.2-171.8	55.9	48.5	11.8-141.2	Gregory *et al.* 1990
35-49	65.0	58.3	19.4-150.2	62.7	54.8	15.6-157.7	Gregory *et al.* 1990
50-64	66.5	60.2	17.7-151.2	67.6	58.8	17.9-169.0	Gregory *et al.* 1990
58-65	68	-	6-198	72	-	22-179	Davies and Holdsworth 1985
62-74	32.5	-	-	32.3	-	-	Lonergan *et al.* 1975
73-78[2]	-	101 (60-158)	28-315	-	97 (56-174)	31-317	Euronut SENECA Investigators 1991
75-90	32.3	-	-	29.4	-	-	Lonergan *et al.* 1975

(1) The range shown is the 2.5-97.5 centile for the studies of Gregory *et al.*, the 10-90 centile for the SENECA study, and the observed extreme range for the study of Davies and Holdsworth.
(2) Data were reported for 17 separate centres; the mean and extreme values of the published median values are shown, with the lowest 10th centile and highest 90th centile of those reported.

Table 22.3: Sources of vitamin C in the average British diet

	% of average intake
potatoes	16
other vegetables	19
fruit juice	18
fruit	17
salad vegetables	8
milk and milk products	5
meat	4
soft drinks	4
cereal products	3

Source: Gregory *et al.* 1990.

Table 22.4: Rich sources of vitamin C

	portion (g)	mg /portion
blackcurrants	80	160
oranges	250	125
orange juice	200	100
strawberries	100	60
grapefruit	140	56
melon	200	50
green peppers	45	45
sweet potato	150	38
loganberries	85	34
spinach	130	33
red currants	80	32
white currants	80	32
pineapple	125	31
Brussels sprouts	75	30
mangoes	100	30
satsumas	100	30
tangerines	100	30
turnips	120	30
gooseberries	70	28
potato chips	265	27
broccoli	75	26
swedes	120	24
spring greens	75	23
artichokes, globe	220	22
potatoes	140	21
avocados	130	20
leeks	125	20
lemons	25	20
okra	80	20
peas	75	20
raspberries	80	20
tomato juice	100	20
plantain, green	85	17
bilberries	80	16
blackberries	80	16
kidney	150	15
tomatoes	75	15
bananas	135	14
cauliflower	65	13
beans, broad	75	11
cabbage	75	11
nectarines	110	11
parsnips	110	11
rhubarb	100	10

Table 22.5: Vitamin C content of plasma and blood cells

	/10⁶ cells		/L packed cells	
	pmol	µg	µmol	µg
erythrocytes	3.9	0.7	43	7.5
platelets	30	5.3	1900	335
granulocytes	530	93	1200	211
mononuclear leukocytes	1370	241	3800	670
plasma, /L	23-57		4-10	

Source: from data reported by Evans *et al.* 1982; Hornig 1975.

Table 22.6: Vitamin C content of tissues

	μmol /kg	mg /kg
plasma	23-57	4-10
skeletal muscle	170-230	30-40
kidney	280-850	30-150
heart	280-850	50-150
brain	170-850	30-150
lung	400	70
thymus	570-850	100-150
liver	570-850	100-150
pancreas	570-850	100-150
lens of eye	1420-1760	250-310
adrenal gland	1700-2270	300-400
pituitary	2270-2840	400-500

Source: from data reported by Evans *et al.* 1982; Hornig 1975.

Table 22.7: Vitamin C dependent, 2-oxoglutarate-linked hydroxylases

aspartate -hydroxylase	EC 1.14.11.16
γ-butyrobetaine hydroxylase[1]	EC 1.14.11.1
p-hydroxyphenylpyruvate hydroxylase	EC 1.14.11.27
procollagen lysine hydroxylase	EC 1.14.11.4
procollagen proline 3-hydroxylase	EC 1.14.11.7
procollagen proline 4-hydroxylase	EC 1.14.11.2
pyrimidine deoxynucleotide dioxygenase	EC 1.14.11.3
thymidine dioxygenase	EC 1.14.11.10
thymine dioxygenase	EC 1.14.11.6
trimethyllysine hydroxylase[1]	EC 1.14.11.8

(1) Enzymes of carnitine synthesis, see section 23.5

Table 22.8: Plasma and leukocyte ascorbate concentrations as criteria of vitamin C nutritional status

		deficient	marginal	adequate
whole blood	mmol/L	< 17	17-28	> 28
	mg /L	< 3.0	3.0-5.0	> 5.0
plasma	mmol /L	< 11	11-17	> 17
	mg /L	< 2.0	2.0-3.0	> 3.0
leukocytes	pmol /10⁶ cells	< 1.1	1.1-2.8	> 2.8
	µg/10⁶ cells	< 0.2	0.2-0.5	> 0.5

Biotin, pantothenic acid and other organic compounds

In addition to the vitamins discussed in previous chapters, a number of compounds have clearly defined functions in the body. Two of them, biotin (vitamin H, see section 23.1) and pantothenic acid (see section 23.2), cannot be synthesized in the body, and are therefore dietary essentials. However, they are not nutritionally important, since they are sufficiently widespread in foods for deficiency to be more or less unknown, and there are no firm estimates of requirements.

A number of other compounds have essential functions in the body, but can be synthesized from common metabolic intermediates, and therefore, as far as is known, are not dietary essentials. Such compounds include: biopterin (section 23.4), carnitine (section 23.5), choline (section 23.6), inositol (section 23.7), pyrroloquinoline quinone (section 23.8), taurine (section 23.9), ubiquinone (section 23.10).

In addition to these compounds with clearly defined metabolic functions, a wide variety of compounds naturally present in foods, and especially in foods of plant origin, have potentially beneficial effects, although they are not nutrients. Collectively they are known as phytoceuticals—substances of plant origin with potential pharmaceutical action—or nutraceuticals. Such compounds include non-starch polysaccharides (dietary fibre, see section 7.3), glucosinolates and glycosides, many of which either inhibit the enzymes of phase I metabolism of foreign compounds (the reactions that activate many potential carcinogens) or induce the reactions leading to conjugation, and hence excretion, of foreign compounds (see section 7.6). Many of the terpenes that are found in the volatile (essential) oils of herbs and spices are potentially active as lipid-soluble antioxidants, as are many of the carotenoids that are not active as precursors of vitamin A (see section 13.1), and a variety of water-soluble compounds, including polyphenols, anthocyanins, and flavonoids (see section 23.3) also have antioxidant action. Equally, many of the non-nutrient compounds found in plant foods have adverse effects, acting as potential pro-oxidants, carcinogens or antimetabolites of vitamins; these are discussed in section 27.3.

A number of compounds were discovered during the early part of this century which were believed to be vitamins, because they were growth factors for experimental animals or micro-organisms. They were assigned vitamin nomenclature, shown in Table 23.1. Subsequent studies showed them either not to be dietary essentials, or to be compounds that had already been isolated under other names.

23.1 Biotin

Biotin was originally discovered as part of the complex called *bios*, which promoted the growth of yeast, and separately, as vitamin H, the protective or curative factor in 'egg white injury'—the disease caused in man and experimental animals by feeding diets containing large amounts of uncooked egg white. The glycoprotein avidin in uncooked egg white binds biotin with very high affinity. The vitamin is widely distributed in many foods. It is synthesized by intestinal flora, and in balance studies the total output of biotin in urine plus faeces is 3–6–fold greater than the intake, reflecting intestinal bacterial synthesis. It is not known to what extent this bacterial biotin is available to the host.

23.1.1 Biotin requirements

Dietary deficiency of biotin is unknown except in (extremely) rare people consuming large amounts of uncooked egg white. There is therefore little information concerning human biotin requirements, and no evidence on which to base recommendations. Average intakes are between 15–70 µg /day; such intakes are obviously adequate to prevent deficiency. Estimated safe and adequate levels of biotin intake are shown in Table 23.2, and average intakes in UK in Table 23.3.

The few early reports of human biotin deficiency are all of people who consumed large amounts of uncooked eggs, and therefore had a high intake of avidin, which binds biotin and renders it unavailable. They developed a fine scaly dermatitis and hair loss (alopecia). Histology of the skin showed an absence of sebaceous glands and atrophy of the hair follicles. Provision of biotin supplements of between 200–1000 μg /day resulted in cure of the skin lesions, and regrowth of hair, despite continuing the abnormal diet providing large amounts of avidin. There have been no studies of provision of modest doses of biotin to such patients, and none in which their high intake of uncooked eggs was not either replaced by an equivalent intake of cooked eggs (in which avidin has been denatured by heat, and the yolks of which are a good source of biotin) or continued unchanged, so there is no information from these case reports of the amounts of biotin required for normal health. More recently, similar signs of biotin deficiency have been observed in patients receiving total parenteral nutrition for prolonged periods, after major resection of the gut. The signs resolve following the provision of biotin, but again there have been no studies of the amounts of biotin required; intakes have ranged between 60–200 μg / day (Mock *et al.* 1985).

23.1.2 Absorption, metabolism, and functions of biotin

Most biotin in foods is present as biocytin (ε-aminobiotinyllysine), which is released on proteolysis, then hydrolysed by biotinidase in the pancreatic juice and intestinal mucosal secretions, to yield free biotin. The extent to which bound biotin in foods is biologically available is not known. The structures of biotin, biocytin, and carboxybiotin (the active metabolic intermediate) are shown in Fig. 23.1.

Free biotin is absorbed from the small intestine by sodium-dependent active transport. Biotin circulates in the bloodstream both free and bound to a serum glycoprotein which has biotinidase (EC 3.5.1.12) activity, catalysing the hydrolysis of biocytin. There is also some non-specific binding to albumin and globulins. The brush border of the kidney cortex has a sodium-biotin co-transport system similar to that in the intestinal mucosa, so providing for efficient resorption of free biotin filtered into the urine. It is only when this resorption mechanism is saturated that there is significant excretion of biotin.

Biotin enters tissues by a saturable transport system, and is then incorporated into biotin-dependent enzymes as the ε-amino-lysine peptide, biocytin.

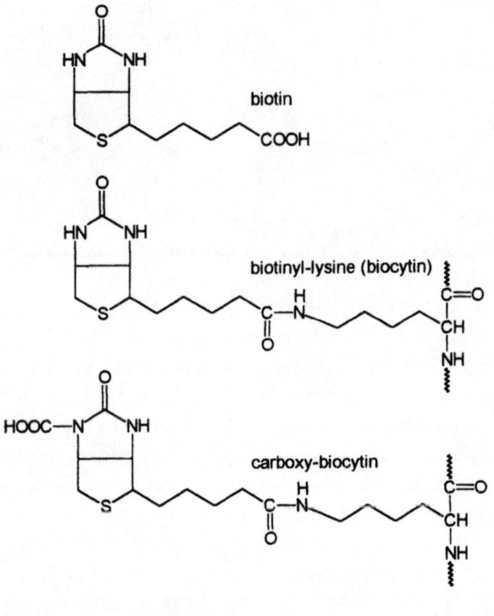

Figure 23.1 Biotin vitamers
Relative molecular masses (M_r): biotin 244.3, biocytin 372.5

Unlike other B vitamins, where concentrative uptake into tissues can be achieved by facilitated diffusion followed by metabolic trapping, the incorporation of biotin into enzymes is relatively slow, and cannot be considered part of the uptake process. On catabolism of the enzymes, biocytin is hydrolysed by biotinidase, permitting reutilization.

Biotin functions to transfer CO_2 in a small number of carboxylation reactions (see Table 23.4). The reactive intermediate is 1–N-carboxy-biocytin (see Fig. 23.1), formed from bicarbonate in an ATP-dependent reaction. A single holocarboxylase synthetase (EC 6.3.4.10) acts on the apo-enzymes of acetyl CoA carboxylase, pyruvate carboxylase, propionyl CoA carboxylase, and methylcrotonyl CoA carboxylase, to form the active holoenzymes from (inactive) apoenzymes and free biotin.

23.1.2.1 Glucose metabolism in biotin deficiency

The impairment of pyruvate carboxylase in biotin deficiency results in impaired gluconeogenesis (see Fig. 5.1). Additionally, biotin deficiency results in a lowering of the NADH:NAD ratio, and hence further reduction of gluconeogenesis by impairment of glyceraldehyde-3–phosphate dehydrogenase activity. Repletion of deficient animals results in restoration of the normal rate of gluconeogenesis when as little as 20 per cent of the control activity of pyruvate carboxylase has been achieved (Arinze and Mistry 1971). This impairment of gluconeogenesis may result in fatal hypoglycaemia in marginally biotin-deficient chicks subjected to a relatively minor metabolic stress.

Rather than the expected hypoglycaemia, biotin deficiency may sometimes be associated with hyperglycaemia. This seems to be due to reduction of hepatic glucokinase (EC 2.7.1.2) to less than half the normal activity. Biotin induces glucokinase independently of the effects of insulin, albeit by a similar mechanism, and also increases the activity of two other key enzymes of glycolysis, phosphofructokinase (EC 2.7.1.11) and pyruvate kinase (EC 2.7.1.40). This seems to be mediated by way of a cell-surface biotin receptor linked to guanylate cyclase (Dakshinamurti et al. 1970; Dakshinamurti and Chauhan 1994; Vesely et al. 1987).

23.1.2.2 Lipid metabolism in biotin deficiency

The skin lesions of biotin deficiency are similar to those seen in deficiency of essential fatty acids (see section 8.1.1.3), and serum linoleic acid is lower than normal in biotin deficient patients. In one patient with functional biotin deficiency due to multiple carboxylase deficiency, the alopecia and dermatitis responded to the administration of polyunsaturated fatty acids (Munnich et al. 1980), suggesting that these symptoms may be due to impairment of the elongation of polyunsaturated fatty acids as a result of reduced activity of acetyl CoA carboxylase. Tissue triacylglycerols from biotin deficient chickens contain a higher proportion of linoleic and γ-linolenic acids, and lower dihomo-γ-linoleate, than normal, regardless of the linoleic acid content of the diet.

The impairment of lipogenesis also affects the tissue fatty acid composition, with an increase in the proportion of palmitoleic acid, mainly at the expense of stearic acid, apparently as a result of increased fatty acid desaturase (EC 1.14.99.5) activity in biotin deficiency. While dietary protein and fat intake also affect tissue fatty acid composition, the ratio of palmitoleic:stearic acid may provide a useful index of biotin nutritional status in some circumstances.

Biotin deficiency also results in an increase in the normally small amounts of odd-chain fatty acids (mainly C15:0 and C17:0) in triacylglycerols, phospholipids and cholesterol esters. This is presumably a result of impaired activity of propionyl CoA carboxylase (Mock et al. 1988).

23.1.2.3 Inborn errors of metabolism affecting biotin-dependent enzymes

Congenital deficiencies of three of the four human biotin-dependent carboxylases have been reported.

1. Propionic acidaemia due to propionyl CoA carboxylase deficiency causes severe ketosis and acidosis, resulting in failure to thrive and mental retardation, and is generally fatal in infancy. Some reports of ketotic hyperglycinaemia may also, with hindsight, be attributed to propionyl CoA carboxylase deficiency.

2. Deficiency of pyruvate carboxylase does not cause the expected hypoglycaemia. Rather it seems that depletion of tissue pools of oxaloacetate results in impaired activity of citrate synthase, and hence a slowing of citric acid cycle activity, leading to accumulation of lactate, pyruvate and alanine, and also increased accumulation of acetyl CoA, resulting in ketosis. Affected infants have serious neurological problems, and rarely survive. A less severe variant of the disease is associated with low residual activity of pyruvate carboxylase.

3. Methylcrotonyl CoA carboxylase deficiency is the least severe of the carboxylase deficiencies. Maintenance on a low protein diet, to minimize the burden of leucine which must be catabolized, prevents the development of metabolic acidosis; at higher intakes of protein the affected infants become hypoglycaemic and comatose.

A number of patients have been reported with biochemical evidence of multiple biotin-dependent carboxylase deficiency, which responds to the administration of large doses of biotin, of the order of 10 mg /day. They have a scaly dermatitis and alopecia, as seen in biotin deficiency, and develop potentially life-threatening keto-acidosis and sometimes also hyperammonaemia, with mental retardation, delayed development and acute neurological problems. They also have high blood and urine concentrations of a number of abnormal organic acids (see Table 23.4). Doses of biotin of the order of 1 mg /day prevent clinical signs in most affected patients, but 10 mg / day or more is required to correct the organic aciduria.

There are two forms of biotin-responsive multiple carboxylase deficiency: a neonatal form which generally presents within the first 6 weeks of life, and a late-onset form, which develops about the third month of life. The underlying defect in neonatal multiple carboxylase deficiency is lack of holocarboxylase synthetase (Burri et al. 1981). The late-onset variant of multiple carboxylase deficiency is due to deficiency of biotinidase (Wolf and Feldman 1982).

Patients with holocarboxylase synthetase deficiency have a normal plasma concentration of biotin, and excrete normal amounts of biotin in the urine. Skin fibroblasts from these patients show extremely low activities of all four biotin-dependent carboxylases when they are cultured in media containing approximately physiological concentrations of biotin (of the order of 6 nmol /L). Culture in media providing higher concentrations of biotin (of the order of 100 nmol /L) results in normal activity of all four carboxylases. Addition of biotin to the culture medium results in a considerable increase in the activity of the carboxylases, even if new protein synthesis has been inhibited—the effect is obviously due to conversion of existing apo-enzymes to the active holo-enzymes.

Patients with multiple carboxylase deficiency due to biotinidase deficiency generally present later in life than those with holocarboxylase synthetase deficiency, and have a lower than normal blood concentration of biotin. Culture of fibroblasts in media containing low concentrations of biotin results in normal activities of carboxylases, and holocarboxylase synthetase activity is normal.

The problem in these patients is a functional deficiency of biotin, due both to their inability to release free biotin from dietary biocytin, and also to failure of the normal recovery of free biotin by biotinidase action on the biocytin released by proteolysis of biotin-containing enzymes. Normal intakes of biotin are inadequate to meet the requirements of these patients; the provision of pharmacological doses of free biotin provides an adequate amount to meet requirements without the need for reutilization. The delayed development of clinical and biochemical abnormalities is a result of the accumulation of biotin by the foetus; at birth the infant has more than adequate stores of the vitamin.

Biotinidase deficient patients have detectable amounts of biocytin in plasma and urine, and excrete larger than normal amounts of biotin, suggesting that biocytin may inhibit the renal resorption of biotin, as it inhibits intestinal active transport. Some patients show metabolic abnormalities despite near normal plasma concentrations of biotin, suggesting that biocytin may inhibit holocarboxylase synthetase.

23.2   Pantothenic acid

Pantothenic acid has a central role in energy-yielding metabolism as the functional moiety of coenzyme A, in the biosynthesis of fatty acids as the prosthetic group of acyl carrier protein, and through its role in CoA in the mitochondrial elongation of fatty acids,

the biosynthesis of steroids, porphyrins and acetylcholine, and in other acyl transfer reactions, including the post-synthetic acylation of proteolipids.

23.2.1 Pantothenic acid requirements and intake

Pantothenic acid is widely distributed in all foodstuffs; the name derives from the Greek for 'from everywhere', as opposed to other vitamins, which were originally isolated from individual especially rich sources. Since it is absorbed throughout the small intestine, it is possible that intestinal bacterial synthesis makes a contribution to pantothenic acid nutrition. As a result, deficiency has not been unequivocally reported in human beings except in specific depletion studies, which have generally used the antagonist ω-methyl pantothenic acid. Pantothenic acid deficiency was implicated in the burning foot syndrome (nutritional melalgia) seen in prisoners of war in south-east Asia, but was not confirmed; for obvious humanitarian reasons, sufferers were repleted with yeast extract as a source of all B vitamins. Estimated safe and adequate levels of intake are shown in Table 23.5, and average intakes in UK in Table 23.6.

23.2.2 Absorption, metabolism, and metabolic functions of pantothenic acid

Pantothenic acid is the peptide of pantoic acid and β-alanine (see Fig. 23.2). Free pantothenic acid and its sodium salt are chemically unstable, and therefore the usual pharmacological preparation is the calcium salt (calcium dipantothenate). The alcohol, pantothenol, is a synthetic compound which has biological activity because it is oxidized to pantothenic acid *in vivo*.

About 85 per cent of dietary pantothenic acid is as CoA or phosphopantetheine. In the intestinal lumen these are hydrolysed to pantetheine; intestinal mucosal cells have a high pantetheinase activity, and rapidly hydrolyse pantetheine to pantothenic acid. The intestinal absorption of pantothenic acid seems to be by simple diffusion, and occurs at a constant rate throughout the length of the small intestine (Shibata *et al.* 1983).

By contrast to intestinal uptake, tissues such as heart, muscle and liver have a sodium-dependent active uptake mechanism for pantothenic acid. The plasma concentration of pantothenic acid is of the order of 1 μmol /L while the K_m for transport is 10 μmol /L, so that transport is not saturated under normal conditions, and tissue uptake increases with the plasma concentration. The central nervous system

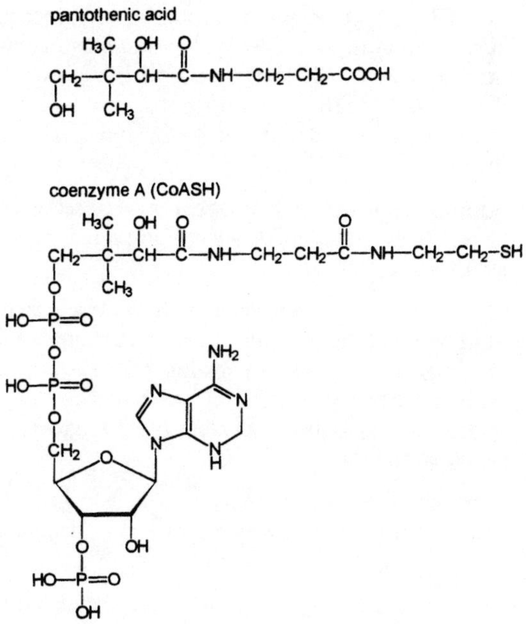

pantothenic acid

coenzyme A (CoASH)

Figure 23.2 Pantothenic acid and CoA
Relative molecular masses (M_r): pantothenic acid 219.2 (calcium dipantothenate 476.5), CoA 767.6

takes up pantothenic acid by facilitated diffusion rather than active transport, and, unlike other tissues, the availability of metabolic fuels has no effect on brain uptake of the vitamin (Spector 1986).

The first step in pantothenic acid utilization is phosphorylation. Pantothenate kinase (EC 2.7.1.33) is rate limiting, so that, unlike many vitamins which are accumulated by metabolic trapping, there can be significant accumulation of free pantothenic acid in tissues, and intracellular concentrations may be as high as 200–500 μmol/L.

23.2.2.1 The formation of CoA from pantothenic acid
All tissues are capable of forming CoA from pantothenic acid. Coenzyme A functions as the carrier of fatty acids, as thio-esters, in mitochondrial β-oxidation (see Fig. 5.3). The resultant two-carbon fragments, as acetyl CoA, then undergo oxidation in the citric acid cycle (see Fig. 5.2). CoA also functions as a carrier in the transfer of acetyl (and other fatty acyl) moieties in a variety of biosynthetic and catabolic reactions, including: steroidogenesis; long-chain fatty acid synthesis from palmitate in mitochondria, and endoplasmic reticulum; mono-unsaturation of palmitoyl CoA to palmitoleyl CoA (C16:1 ω9) and stearyl CoA to oleyl CoA (C18:1 ω9); elongation of

polyunsaturated fatty acids; acylation of serine, threonine and cysteine residues on proteolipids and the acetylation to form *N*-acetyl neuraminic acid.

Short chain fatty acyl CoA derivatives inhibit pantothenate kinase; in perfused rat hearts the addition of any of the major energy-yielding substrates (glucose, pyruvate, free fatty acids or 3–hydroxybutyrate) to the perfusion medium results in inhibition of pantothenate kinase and a reduced rate of CoA synthesis (Robishaw *et al.* 1982). *In vivo* studies show a similar reduction in the incorporation of pantothenic acid into CoA in the liver and heart of fed, compared with fasted, animals. These effects of fasting and feeding can be mimicked in isolated hepatocytes by the addition of insulin or glucagon, although in the perfused rat heart insulin only affects pantothenate kinase activity if glucose is also present in the perfusion medium, suggesting that the effect of the hormones is indirect: i.e. the result of increased intracellular concentrations of fatty acyl CoA, rather than any direct effect on the activity of the enzyme.

23.2.2.2 The formation of holo-acyl carrier protein (ACP)
Fatty acid synthesis (see Fig. 5.6) is catalysed by a cytosolic multi-enzyme complex in which the growing fatty acyl chain is bound by thio-ester linkage to an enzyme-bound 4′-phospho-pantetheine residue, rather than to free CoA, as in β-oxidation. This component of the fatty acid synthetase complex is the acyl carrier protein. Apo-acyl carrier protein is activated by a transferase, holo-ACP synthetase (EC 2.7.8.7), which transfers 4′-phosphopantetheine from CoA onto the hydroxyl group of a serine residue in the apo-protein. Acyl carrier protein is inactivated by a hydrolase which releases 4′-phosphopantetheine.

23.2.2.3 Catabolism of CoA and pantothenic acid
CoA is dephosphorylated by lysosomal acid phosphatase (EC 3.1.3.2), to dephospho-CoA, followed by pyrophosphatase action to release 4′-phosphopantetheine and 5′-AMP. CoA is also a substrate for direct pyrophosphatase action, at about 10 per cent of the rate of action on dephospho-CoA.

Phosphopantetheine, arising from either the catabolism of CoA or the inactivation of holo-ACP, can be reutilized for CoA synthesis. Alternatively, it may be dephosphorylated, again by a relatively unspecific phosphatase, to pantetheine, which is cleaved by pantetheinase, a specific amidase, to pantothenic acid and cysteamine. The resultant cysteamine may be an important precursor of taurine (see section 23.9). Pantetheinase is found in both liver and kidney. The kidney isoenzyme acts on both pantetheine and (at a lower rate) on phosphopantetheine, while the liver enzyme acts only on pantetheine. (Dupre *et al.* 1973; Wittwer *et al.* 1983).

Pantothenic acid is largely excreted unchanged. Some phosphopantetheine may also be excreted in the urine, and after the administration of [^{14}C]pantothenic acid some of the label may be recovered in exhaled CO_2. This is probably the result of intestinal bacterial metabolism, since many bacteria have a specific amidase which cleaves pantothenic acid to β-alanine and pantoic acid.

23.2.3 Pantothenic acid deficiency

Pantothenic acid deficiency in rats leads to a loss of fur colour—at one time pantothenic acid was known as the 'anti-grey hair factor'. There is no evidence that the normal greying of hair with age is related to pantothenic acid nutrition, nor that pantothenic acid supplements have any effect on hair colour. There is rapid depletion of adrenal corticosteroids, and reduced production of the steroids in isolated adrenal glands in response to stimulation with adrenocorticotrophic hormone (ACTH). This reflects the role of acetyl CoA in the synthesis of steroids; deficiency also results in atrophy of the seminiferous tubules of male rats and delayed sexual maturation in females. As deficiency progresses, there is enlargement and then congestion and haemorrhage of the adrenal cortex. In young animals, but not in adults, pantothenic acid deprivation eventually leads to necrosis of the adrenal cortex.

Prisoners of war in the Far East in the 1940s, who were severely malnourished, showed, among other signs and symptoms of vitamin deficiency diseases, a new condition of paraesthesia and severe pain in the feet and toes, which was called the burning foot syndrome or nutritional melalgia. Although it was tentatively attributed to pantothenic acid deficiency, no specific trials of pantothenic acid were carried out, rather the subjects were given yeast extract and other rich sources of all vitamins as part of an urgent programme of nutritional rehabilitation. There are no reports of neurological damage in deficient animals that could explain the burning foot syndrome.

Experimental pantothenic acid depletion, commonly together with the administration of ω-methyl pantothenic acid, results in the following signs and symptoms after 2–3 weeks.

1. Neuromotor disorders, including paraesthesia of the hands and feet, hyperactive deep tendon reflexes and muscle weakness. These can be explained by the role of acetyl CoA in the synthesis of the neurotransmitter acetyl choline (see section 23.6), and impaired formation of threonine acyl esters in myelin. Dysmyelination may explain the persistence and recurrence of neurological problems many years after nutritional rehabilitation in people who had suffered the burning foot syndrome.

2. Mental depression, which again may be related to either acetyl choline deficit or impaired myelin synthesis.

3. Gastrointestinal complaints, including severe vomiting and pain, with depressed gastric acid secretion in response to insulin and gastrin. As with the development of ulcers in deficient animals, this may reflect hypersensitivity to glucocorticoid stimulation.

4. Increased insulin sensitivity and a flattened glucose tolerance curve, which may reflect decreased antagonism by glucocorticoids.

5. Decreased serum cholesterol and decreased urinary excretion of 17–ketosteroids, reflecting the impairment of steroidogenesis.

6. Decreased acetylation of *p*-aminobenzoic acid, sulphonamides and other drugs, reflecting reduced availability of acetyl CoA for these reactions.

7. Increased susceptibility to upper respiratory tract infections, which presumably reflects the impairment of immune responses.

23.2.4 Assessment of pantothenic acid nutritional status

There are no functional tests of pantothenic acid nutritional status that are generally applicable. Some studies of depletion have followed the decline in the acetylation of *p*-aminobenzoic acid as an index of vitamin depletion, but this has not been developed as an index of nutritional adequacy.

Most of the pantothenic acid in blood (85–90 per cent) is as CoA in erythrocytes, with only a small amount of free pantothenic acid in plasma. On standing at room temperature there is considerable autolysis of CoA to free pantothenic acid. Because of this, most studies report whole blood total pantothenic acid after enzymic hydrolysis, rather than free pantothenic acid or red cell CoA. There is a wide range of individual variation; Sauberlich *et al.* (1974*a*) suggested that a whole blood total pantothenic acid below 4.5 μmol/L was indicative of inadequate intake. However, few studies have reported mean blood concentrations of pantothenic acid as high as

4.5 µmol /L in normal subjects. The mean value of 2.6 µmol /L shown in Table 23.7 is from a reported range of 1.0–8.7 µmol /L.

Urinary excretion of pantothenic acid mirrors intake, albeit with wide range of individual variation, and may provide a means of assessing status; adults consuming 5–7 mg /day excrete 2–7 mg (9–32 µmol) in the urine and 1–2 mg (4.5–9 µmol) in faeces. In subjects maintained on experimental diets providing 10 mg /day the urinary excretion is 4–7 mg (18–32 µmol) (Fry *et al.* 1976). Urinary excretion of less than 1 mg (4.5 µmol) of pantothenic acid /24 hours is considered to be abnormally low (Sauberlich *et al.* 1974*a*).

23.2.5 Pharmacological uses and toxicity of pantothenic acid

Blood levels of pantothenic acid have been reported to be low in patients with rheumatoid arthritis; some workers have reported apparently beneficial effects of supplementation, but these reports remain unconfirmed, and there are no established pharmacological uses of the vitamin.

Homopantothenic acid (pantoyl-γ-aminobutyric acid or 'hopanthate') has been reported to enhance cholinergic function in the central nervous system. It acts by binding to GABA receptors and stimulating the release of acetylcholine in the cerebral cortex and hippocampus, rather than by any direct effect on acetylcholine synthesis or cholinergic receptors. It appears to have some beneficial effect in senile dementia of the Alzheimer type, reducing loss of memory and cognitive impairment in some patients (Nakahiro *et al.* 1985).

Pantothenic acid has very low toxicity; intakes of up to 10 g of calcium pantothenate /day (compared with a normal dietary intake of 2–7 mg /day) have been given for up to 6 weeks with no apparent ill effects.

23.3 Bioflavonoids ('Vitamin P')

The existence of vitamin P was originally postulated by Szent-György in 1936, on the basis that extracts of paprika and lemon juice were more effective in the treatment of vascular fragility associated with vitamin C deficiency than was ascorbic acid (see section 22.5). The active substances were identified as flavonoids; the most studied are hesperitin, quercitin and the α-rhamnosyl-glucose (rutinose) glycoside of quercitin (see Fig. 23.3). Because they are biologically active, they are commonly called bioflavonoids. Cleavage of the heterocyclic ring yields chalcones, some of which are used as intense sweeteners (see Table 7.12). Most fruits and green leafy vegetables contain relatively large amounts of flavonoids; altogether some 2000 have been identified, and average intakes of flavonoids from a mixed diet are of the order of 1 g /day.

In experimental animals the bioflavonoids decrease the fragility of blood capillaries; the bioprocedure involves observation of the development of petechial haemorrhages after either suction or positive pressure applied to the skin. The two methods (positive and negative pressure) give different results, with little or no correlation (Munro *et al.* 1947). Although a number of studies have suggested that bioflavonoids have a pharmacological action in a number of conditions that may involve abnormal capillary fragility, this has generally been observed following intravenous administration; there is little evidence of any effect of oral bioflavonoids.

There is no evidence that the bioflavonoids are dietary essentials; indeed Clark and MacKay (1950) suggested that they are not absorbed from the gastrointestinal tract. If they have any useful action it is as antioxidants; oxidation of flavonoids may serve both to protect susceptible nutrients from damage in foods and the intestinal lumen, and also possibly act as

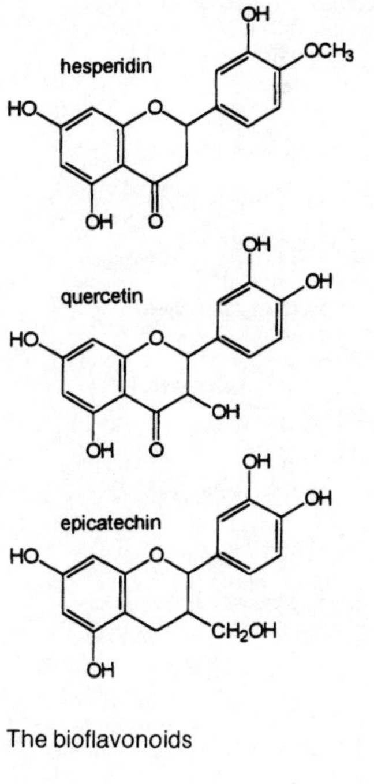

Figure 23.3 The bioflavonoids

antioxidants in plasma and tissues. Hertog *et al.* (1995) have shown that average intake of antioxidant flavonoids is inversely correlated with mortality from coronary heart disease, and have suggested that about 25 per cent of the variation in coronary heart disease in different countries may be accounted for by flavonoids. They showed no association of flavonoid intake with cancer or other causes of death.

23.4 Biopterin

Biopterin is the cofactor for a small number of mixed function oxidases: the aromatic amino acid hydroxylases (see section 23.4.1); alkyl glycerol mono-oxygenase (EC 1.14.16.5), which catalyses the cleavage of alkyl glycerol ethers; and arginine N-hydroxylase (nitric oxide synthase, see section 23.4.2). As shown in Fig. 23.4, the active form is tetrahydrobiopterin, which is oxidized to dihydrobiopterin in the reaction. Reduction back to tetrahydrobiopterin requires dihydrobiopterin reductase. Biopterin is not a dietary essential, since it can be synthesized from GTP.

23.4.1 Aromatic amino acid hydroxylases and atypical phenylketonuria

The same pool of tetrahydrobiopterin and the same dihydrobiopterin reductase are involved in the central nervous system in the hydroxylation of all three aromatic amino acids: phenylalanine (EC 1.14.14.1), tyrosine (EC 1.14.16.2) and tryptophan (EC 1.14.16.4). Classical phenylketonuria, which involves a defect of phenylalanine hydroxylase, responds well to dietary restriction of phenylalanine. There is an extremely rare atypical variant of phenylketonuria, which does not respond to dietary restriction. This condition involves either a defect in dihydrobiopterin reductase, or a failure of biopterin biosynthesis. In either case there are disturbances of phenylalanine, tyrosine and tryptophan metabolism, and deficits of catecholamines and 5–hydroxytryptamine, so that the neurological problem is more serious than in classical phenylketonuria.

There is little that can be done for patients who lack biopterin reductase, and are therefore unable to reduce dihydrobiopterin to the active form; tetrahydrobiopterin is chemically unstable, and is readily oxidized on exposure to oxygen. To date no useful synthetic analogues have been developed. For patients whose problem is an inability to synthesize biopterin treatment is simple, since dihydrobiopterin is chemically stable, and their condition can be controlled by administration of dihydrobiopterin, which, for them, has become a dietary essential.

23.4.2 Arginine N-hydroxylase (nitric oxide synthase) and nitric oxide formation

Nitric oxide (N=O) acts as an inter-cellular signalling agent. It is produced by vascular endothelial cells in

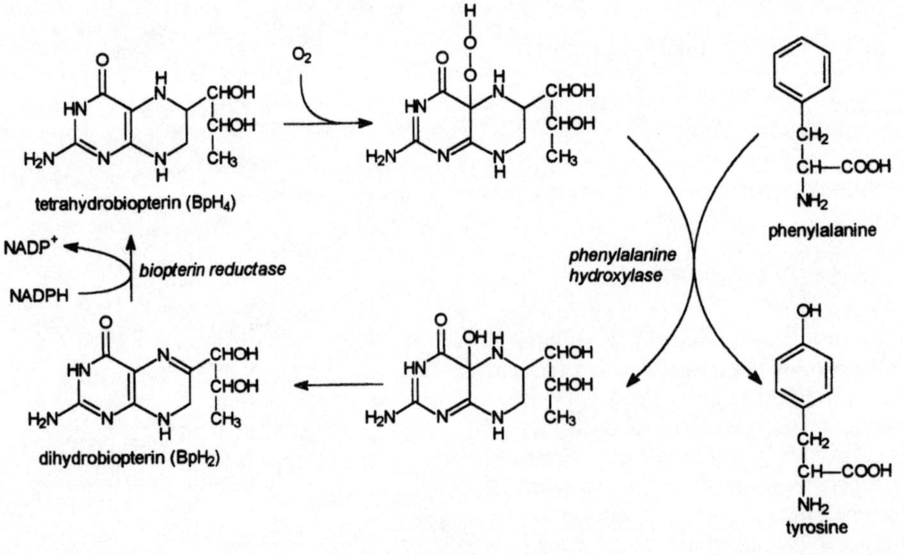

Figure 23.4 The role of biopterin in aromatic amino acid hydroxylases

response to a variety of physiological vasodilators, and causes relaxation of vascular smooth muscle—it is the endothelium-derived relaxation factor (EDRF). It activates a cytosolic guanylate cyclase in the smooth muscle cells, resulting in smooth muscle relaxation and hence vasodilatation as a result of reduced intracellular calcium in response to the increased concentration of cyclic GMP. This role of nitric oxide in stimulating guanylate cyclase explains the clinically useful vasodilatory action of nitroglycerine and aryl nitrites, which decompose *in vivo* to yield nitric oxide. Endothelium-derived nitric oxide also inhibits platelet aggregation, again acting by way of activation of guanylate cyclase.

Nitric oxide is formed from arginine in a variety of tissues, including the central nervous system, lung, macrophages and vascular endothelial cells. The reaction is a tetrahydrobiopterin-dependent *N*-hydroxylation catalysed by arginine *N*-hydroxylase (EC 1.14.13.99); *N*-hydroxyarginine then decomposes to citrulline and nitric oxide. The reaction also requires NADPH, and is assumed to follow the same reaction pathway as the hydroxylation of aromatic amino acids (see Fig. 23.4).

In the central nervous system, nitric oxide formation from arginine seems to be the immediate response of the glutamate-activated *N*-methyl-D-aspartate (NMDA) receptors. Again it acts intercellularly, being released from neurones and acting on neighbouring glial cells by stimulation of guanylate cyclase. These actions of nitric oxide are transient; activated macrophages continue to produce nitric oxide from arginine, in considerably higher concentrations, as a part of their cytotoxic action (Marletta *et al.* 1990; Tayeh and Marletta 1989).

23.5 Carnitine

Carnitine (3–hydroxy, 4–*N*-trimethylaminobutyric acid) has a central role in the transport of fatty acids across the mitochondrial membrane for β-oxidation (see Fig. 5.3); the major regulation of fatty acid oxidation is by control of carnitine acyltransferases (see section 23.5.2). It was originally isolated from Liebig's extract of meat in 1905, and later shown to be an essential nutrient (called vitamin B_T) for the mealworm, *Tenebrio molitor*, and some micro-organisms. Claims were made for effects in human beings, ranging from growth stimulation to the treatment of obesity, and a dimer was marketed under the name of bicarnesine, but there is no evidence of its efficacy.

23.5.1 Carnitine biosynthesis and metabolism

The synthesis of carnitine (see Fig. 23.5) involves the stepwise methylation of a protein-incorporated lysine residue at the expense of methionine, to yield a trimethyllysine residue. Free trimethyllysine is then released by proteolysis. It is not clear whether there is a specific precursor protein for the synthesis of carnitine, or whether methylation of lysine may occur in a variety of proteins. Both hydroxylations in the synthesis of carnitine from trimethyllysine are ascorbic acid dependent, 2–oxo-glutarate-linked, reactions (see section 22.4.3).

Tissues other than liver and skeletal muscle depend on active uptake from the blood-stream. The uptake of carnitine is stimulated by fasting, diabetes, glucagon and glucocorticoid hormones; tissues accumulate more carnitine at times when there will be an increased requirement for fatty acid oxidation. Tissues with high rates of fatty acid oxidation have high rates of carnitine turnover (e.g. liver carnitine has a half-life of 1.3 hours, heart 21 hours) while in tissues with low rates of fatty acid oxidation it has a longer half-life (e.g. brain 220 hours).

Deficiency of methionine or vitamin C may result in impaired synthesis of carnitine. In experimental animals, deficiency of lysine has little effect on plasma and tissue concentrations, but methionine deficiency can lead to carnitine depletion, and carnitine has a methionine-sparing effect in methionine deficient animals.

The total body content of carnitine is about 100 mmol, and about 5 per cent of this turns over daily. Plasma total carnitine is between 36–83 μmol /L in men (27–67 μmol /L free carnitine) and 28–75 μmol /L in women (21–59 μmol /L free carnitine). While both free carnitine and acyl carnitine esters are excreted in the urine, much is oxidized; the end-products in the urine are trimethylamine and trimethylamine oxide. It is not known whether the formation of these compounds is due to endogenous enzymes or intestinal bacterial metabolism of carnitine. Total urinary excretion of carnitine is between 300–530 μmol (men) or 200–320 μmol (women). Some 30–50 per cent of this is free carnitine; the remainder is a variety of acyl carnitine esters.

23.5.2 Metabolic functions of carnitine

Carnitine functions in the transport of long chain fatty acyl groups across the mitochondrial membrane. For the oxidation of fatty acyl CoA, or for mitochondrial elongation or desaturation of fatty acids, carnitine palmitoyl transferase 1 at the inner

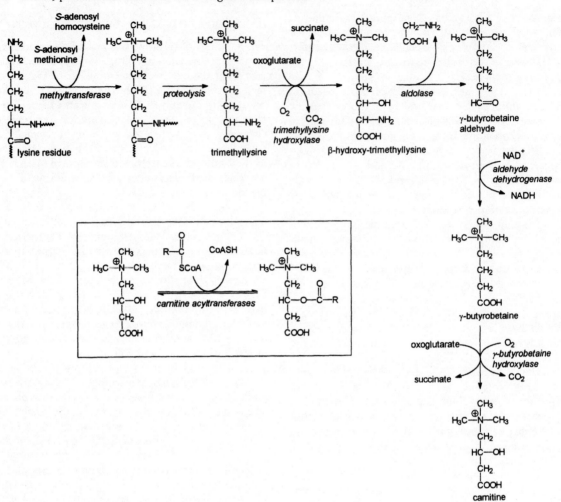

Figure 23.5 Carnitine biosynthesis
Trimethyllysine hydroxylase EC 1.14.11.8, butyrobetaine hydroxylase EC 1.14.11.1,

face of the outer membrane forms acyl carnitine from extra-mitochondrial acyl CoA, while at the inner face of the inner membrane carnitine palmitoyl transferase 2 forms acyl CoA derivatives from translocated acyl carnitine.

Carnitine palmitoyl transferase 1 is inhibited by malonyl CoA (the precursor for fatty acid synthesis, see Fig. 15.6), binding to the outer face of the outer mitochondrial membrane. Its activity thus controls the metabolic fate of acyl CoA—when fatty acids are being synthesized, and hence malonyl CoA concentrations are high, mitochondrial uptake of acyl CoA is inhibited, while when the concentration of malonyl CoA is low, and fatty acids are to be oxidized rather than synthesized, they are transported into the mitochondria for β-oxidation and ketogenesis.

There are three separate carnitine acyltransferases, named for their preferred substrates rather than for absolute specificity: carnitine acetyl transferase (EC 2.3.1.7), which forms short chain acyl carnitine esters; carnitine octanoyl transferase (EC 2.3.1.137), which forms medium chain acyl carnitine esters; and carnitine palmitoyl transferase (EC 2.3.1.21), which forms long chain acyl carnitine esters. The combined activities of these three enzymes results in a broad specificity for carnitine acylation, and a variety of acyl carnitine esters are excreted in the urine, including both esters of xenobiotics and a variety of esters in metabolic disorders associated with organic acid-aemias.

There is a significant increase in the urinary excretion of propionylcarnitine in vitamin B_{12} deficiency (see sections 21.7.1.1 and 21.8). The role of carnitine here seems to be as a means of detoxication and removal of acyl groups which cannot be further metabolized. Acyl carnitine esters other than acetyl carnitine are readily cleared at the kidney, while free carnitine and acetyl carnitine are reabsorbed until the plasma concentration exceeds the renal threshold. In this way carnitine seems to spare CoA (and hence pantothenic acid) by releasing the coenzyme from otherwise unmetabolizable esters which would trap the coenzyme, and hence cause functional pantothenic acid deficiency (see section 23.2).

23.5.3 The possible essentiality of carnitine

The average intake of carnitine by people eating a mixed diet is 100–300 mg /d; in strict vegetarians the intake may be only one tenth of this, yet plasma concentrations of carnitine are within the normal range of 30–80 μmol (5.2–13.3 mg) /L. Even in strict vegetarians, carnitine depletion is only seen together with general protein-energy malnutrition (and hence deficiency of methionine and lysine).

While endogenous synthesis of carnitine can meet normal metabolic demands, administration of the anticonvulsant valproic acid, which is excreted as the carnitine ester, or a variety of metabolic organic acidaemias which result in considerable excretion of acyl carnitine esters, can lead to carnitine depletion. This results in impaired β-oxidation of fatty acids and ketogenesis in the liver, and hence a non-ketotic hypoglycaemia, with elevated plasma non-esterified fatty acids and triglycerides. Because hepatocytes rely on fatty acid oxidation for their own energy-yielding metabolism in fasting, there may also be signs of liver dysfunction, with hyperammonaemia and encephalopathy. The administration of carnitine supplements in these conditions has a beneficial effect.

There are no known defects of carnitine synthesis in man, but a functional primary carnitine deficiency syndrome has been described; a defect of the membrane transport for carnitine into muscle, across the intestinal mucosa, and the renal tubular resorption mechanism.

Although carnitine is not generally nutritionally important, it may be required for premature infants, since they have an inadequate capacity to synthesize it. There is some evidence that full-term infants may also have a greater requirement for carnitine than can be met by endogenous synthesis; infants fed on carnitine-free soya milk formula have higher plasma concentrations of non-esterified fatty acids and triglycerides than those receiving carnitine supple-

ments. Carnitine depletion, with disturbed lipid metabolism has also been reported in adults maintained for prolonged periods on total parenteral nutrition.

There is some evidence that supplements of carnitine may increase the ability of muscle to oxidize fatty acids, and so increase physical work capacity, although other studies have shown no effect.

23.6 Choline

Choline is important as a base in phospholipids—both phosphatidylcholine (lecithin, see section 8.1.2) in all cell membranes and also sphingomyelin in the nervous system. In addition, acetylcholine is a transmitter in the central and parasympathetic nervous systems and at neuromuscular junctions. There is some evidence that the availability of choline may be limiting for the synthesis of acetylcholine in the central nervous system under some conditions, and supplements of phosphatidylcholine increase the rate of acetylcholine turnover. They have been reported to result in some improvement in cognitive function in patients with senile dementia, and have some beneficial effect in tardive dyskinesia.

In addition to being used as a trivial name for phosphatidylcholine, the name 'lecithin' is used for phospholipid fractions relatively rich in phosphatidylcholine, which are widely used as emulsifying agents in food manufacture (E-322). Such preparations typically contain some 40–80 per cent phosphatidylcholine, together with a variety of other phospholipids.

23.6.1 Biosynthesis and metabolism of choline

Phosphatidylcholine is synthesized by the pathway shown in Fig. 23.6, by decarboxylation of phosphatidylserine to phosphatidylethanolamine (cephalin) followed by methylation in which S-adenosylmethionine is the methyl donor to yield successively the relatively rare mono- and dimethyl derivatives, then phosphatidylcholine.

Free choline is released by the hydrolysis of dietary or endogenous phosphatidylcholine. Sequential removal of the fatty acids by phospholipase action results in the formation of lysolecithin (glycerophosphorylcholine), then hydrolysis to release choline. About 30 per cent of dietary phosphatidylcholine is absorbed intact into the lymphatic system; the remainder is hydrolysed to lysolecithin in the intestinal mucosa, and to free choline in the liver. Free choline in the diet is largely metabolized by

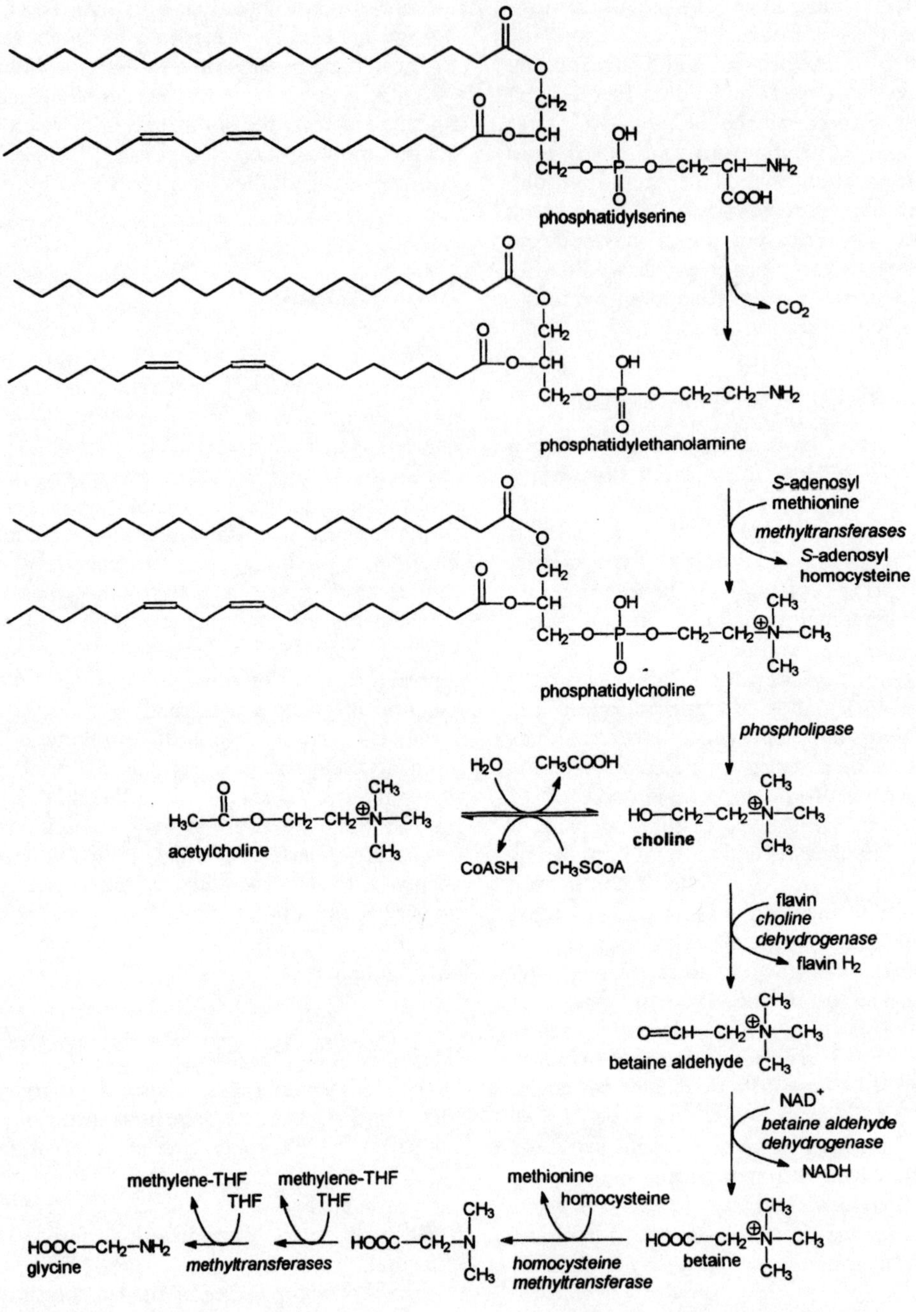

Figure 23.6 Choline biosynthesis and metabolism

intestinal bacteria, forming trimethylamine, which is absorbed and excreted in the urine. Only about 30 per cent of free choline is absorbed intact.

Choline can be used for synthesis of phosphatidyl-choline by reaction between CDP-choline and diacyl-glycerol, as a source of choline for the formation of

acetylcholine, or may be catabolized as shown in Fig. 23.6. Under normal conditions the major pathway of phosphatidylcholine synthesis is by the incorporation of preformed choline rather than methylation of phosphatidylethanolamine. The activities of the two pathways are regulated coordinately, so that increased choline availability reduces the methylation of phosphatidylethanolamine, while decreased availability of preformed choline results in increased *de novo* synthesis.

Choline catabolism involves two oxidations to form betaine (trimethylglycine), followed by three successive demethylations. The remethylation of homocysteine to methionine catalysed by the betaine-dependent methyltransferase (EC 2.1.1.5) can maintain adequate concentrations of methionine in tissues other than the central nervous system when the activity of methionine synthetase (EC 2.1.1.13) is impaired because of vitamin B_{12} deficiency (see section 21.7.2).

23.6.2 The possible essentiality of choline

In animals maintained on defined diets without added choline, the rate of endogenous synthesis may be inadequate to meet requirements. Deficiency of choline results in fatty infiltration of the liver, apparently as a result of impairment of the export of lipoproteins from hepatocytes; prolonged deficiency may result in cirrhosis. The kidney can also be affected, with tubular necrosis and interstitial haemorrhage, probably as a result of lysosomal membrane disruption. Choline deficiency is exacerbated by deficiency of methionine, folic acid or vitamin B_{12}, which impairs the capacity for *de novo* synthesis.

There is no evidence that choline is a dietary requirement for man, and no condition similar to the effects of choline deficiency in experimental animals has been reported in human beings. Since phosphatidylcholine is found in all biological membranes, dietary deficiency is unlikely to occur except when people are maintained on defined diets free from phospholipids. Plasma concentrations fall during long-term total parenteral nutrition, and it is possible that the impaired liver function seen in such patients is partly the result of choline depletion.

23.7 Inositol

Inositol is a hexahydric sugar alcohol; of the nine possible isomers, only *myo*-inositol has biological activity. Its main function is in phospholipids (see section 8.1.2); phosphatidylinositol constitutes some 5–10 per cent of the total membrane phospholipids. In addition to its structural role in membranes, phosphatidylinositol has a major function in the intracellular responses to peptide hormones and neurotransmitters, yielding two intracellular second messengers, inositol trisphosphate and diacylglycerol.

Plant foods contain relatively large amounts of inositol phosphates, including the hexaphosphate, phytic acid. Phytate chelates minerals such as calcium, zinc and magnesium, forming insoluble complexes which are not absorbed. However, both intestinal phosphatases and endogenous phosphatases (phytases, EC 3.1.3.8 and 3.1.3.26) in many foods dephosphorylate a significant proportion of dietary phytate, and the inositol released can be absorbed and utilized for phosphatidylinositol synthesis.

Inositol-1–phosphate is formed by isomerization of glucose-6–phosphate. The reaction is catalysed by *myo*-inositol-1–phosphate synthase (EC 5.5.1.4), which is an NAD-dependent enzyme, although the overall reaction does not involve a change in redox state. The reaction proceeds by way of oxidation of glucose-6–phosphate to the 5–oxo derivative, followed by and reduction to *myo*-inositol-1–phosphate. Phosphatidylinositol is formed by reaction between CDP-inositol and diacylglycerol. Most inositol is catabolized by oxidation to glucuronic acid.

23.7.1 Phosphatidylinositol in transmembrane signalling

As shown in Fig. 23.7, a proportion of the phosphatidylinositol in membranes undergoes two successive phosphorylations to yield phosphatidylinositol 4,5–bisphosphate. This is a substrate for hormone sensitive phospholipase C (EC 3.1.4.3), which is activated, by way of a guanine nucleotide binding protein regulated mechanism, in response to the binding of the hormone or neurotransmitter to the cell surface receptor. Phospholipase C cleaves phosphatidylinositol bisphosphate to release diacylglycerol and inositol 1,4,5–trisphosphate.

Inositol 1,4,5–trisphosphate causes an increase in the intracellular concentration of free calcium, by releasing calcium from intracellular storage, as a result of the opening of calcium pores in the endoplasmic reticulum membrane (and in muscle the sarcoplasmic reticulum membrane). By way of calmodulin, the increased intracellular free calcium then results in the activation of key enzymes which mediate the target tissue response to the hormone.

Inositol 1,4,5–trisphosphate can be inactivated in two ways:

(1) dephosphorylation to yield successively inositol 1,4–bisphosphate, inositol 4–phosphate and free inositol;

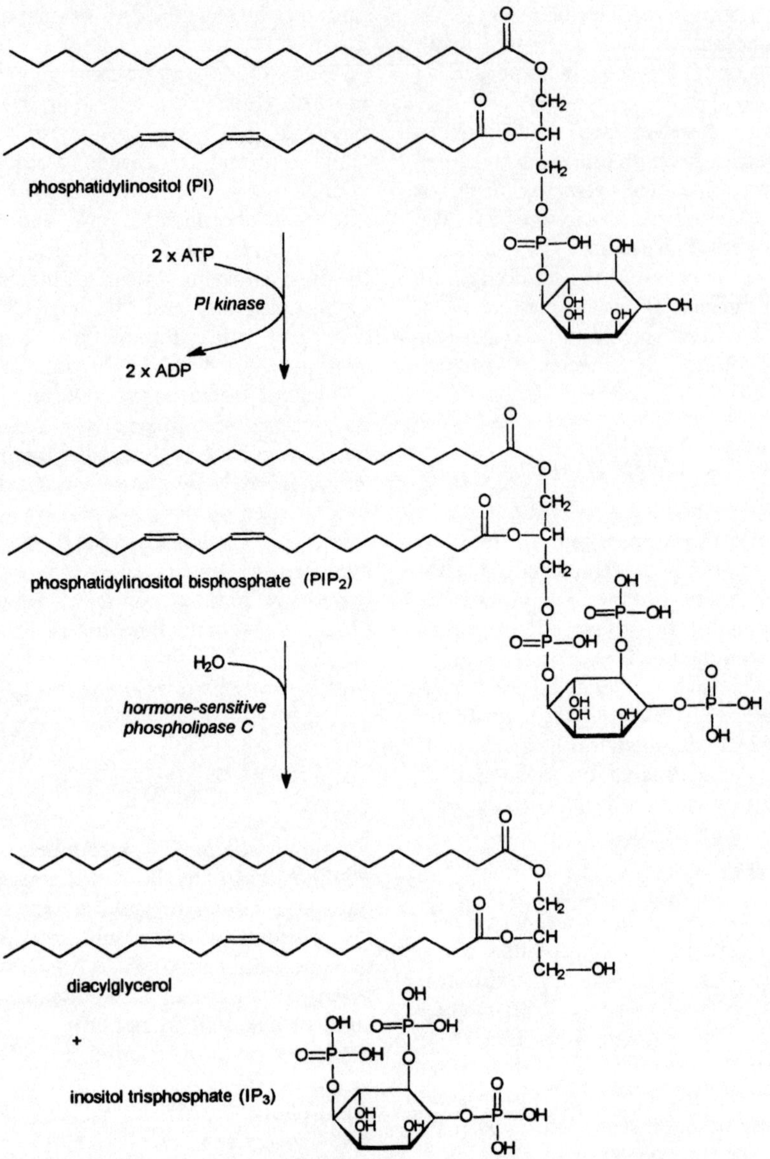

Figure 23.7 Phosphatidylinositol in transmembrane signalling

(2) Phosphorylation to inositol 1,3,4,5–tetrakisphosphate, followed by dephosphorylation to yield inositol 1,3,4–trisphosphate and successive dephosphorylations to yield free inositol.

Diacylglycerol activates protein kinase C (EC 2.7.1.123), which in turn phosphorylates serine, threonine and tyrosine residues in key regulatory enzymes, increasing or reducing their activity. In the presence of diacylglycerol, protein kinase C has a significantly higher affinity for calcium, which is the direct activator; diacylglycerol thus acts in concert with the increased intracellular free calcium resulting from inositol trisphosphate release.

23.7.2 The possible essentiality of inositol

There is no evidence that inositol is a dietary essential, since it is synthesized by all eukaryotic cells.

Infants may have a higher requirement than can be met by endogenous synthesis, and dietary inositol is a growth factor for the new-born mouse.

Untreated diabetics (see section 7.7.2) have high plasma concentrations of free inositol, and high urinary excretion of inositol, associated with relatively low intracellular concentrations of inositol, suggesting that elevated plasma glucose may inhibit the uptake of inositol. There is some evidence that impaired nerve conduction velocity in diabetic neuropathy in both patients and experimental animals is associated with low intracellular concentrations of inositol, and that inositol supplements improve nerve conduction velocity. However, high intracellular concentrations of inositol also impair nerve conduction velocity, and supplements may have a deleterious effect.

23.8 Pyrroloquinoline quinone (PQQ)

A number of enzymes that have been considered to be pyridoxal phosphate (vitamin B_6) dependent (see section 20.4) because they contain a carbonyl group that is essential to their catalytic activity, may contain pyrroloquinoline quinone (see Fig. 23.8) or another aromatic quinone, either as the sole reactive carbonyl compound or as well as pyridoxal phosphate. PQQ is known to be the cofactor for a number of dehydrogenases in Gram-negative micro-organisms (see Table 23.8). It has also been ascribed a role in a number of mammalian enzymes, including copper-dependent oxidases, where it also has a redox role, and some amino acid decarboxylases, which also contain pyridoxal phosphate.

Mammalian copper-dependent oxidases, including plasma amine oxidases and lysyl oxidase (which is involve in the cross-linking of collagen and elastin, see section 25.11.3) have long been known to contain a reactive carbonyl group which is essential for activity. While this was originally assumed to be pyridoxal phosphate, there is no evidence for its presence in these enzymes, and the apoenzymes cannot be reactivated with pyridoxal phosphate. On the basis of hydrazone formation, it has been suggested that these enzymes contain PQQ. The activity of lysyl oxidase falls in vitamin B_6 deficiency, and increases on repletion of deficient animals; if pyridoxal phosphate is not directly involved in the reaction mechanism, this suggests that it may be required for the post-synthetic modification of the precursor protein to form PQQ.

In bacteria, label from both glutamate and tyrosine is incorporated into PQQ. No intermediates in the pathway have been detected, and it seems likely that it is synthesized in a protein or peptide precursor by oxidation of a tyrosine residue to dihydroxyphenylalanine (dopa), followed by ring closure and condensation with glutamate to form a PQQ-peptide. Free PQQ arises as a result of proteolysis; however, there is no evidence that it can be incorporated into proteins. It is likely that PQQ in enzymes arises only as a result of post-synthetic modification, and therefore dietary PQQ would be useless.

PQQ has been reported to be present in a variety of foods. However, this may be the result of using a relatively unspecific redox cycling assay which may detect the presence of other redox active compounds, including ascorbate, riboflavin and pyridoxal phosphate. Using a specific assay based on activation of bacterial apo-glucose dehydrogenase (a PQQ-dependent enzyme), van der Meer *et al.* (1990) were unable to demonstrate PQQ in foods other than small amounts in vinegar and beer; *Acetobacter* spp. growing on ethanol excrete PQQ into the culture medium.

23.9 Taurine

Taurine was discovered in 1827 in ox bile, where it is conjugated with the bile acids in an amide linkage. It

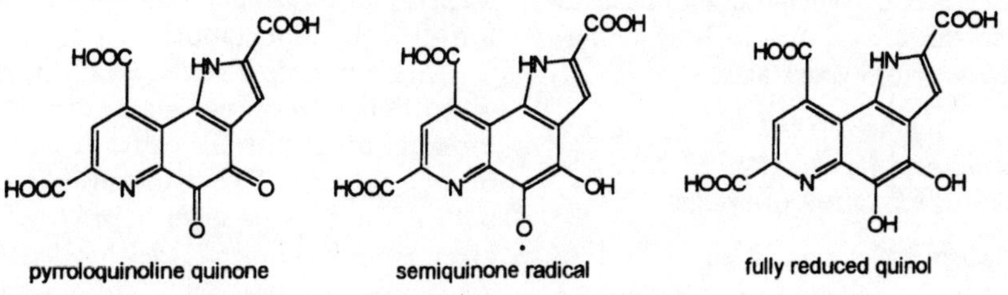

pyrroloquinoline quinone   semiquinone radical   fully reduced quinol

Figure 23.8 Pyrroloquinoline quinone
Relative molecular mass (M_r) = 331

was later shown to be a major excretory product of the sulphur amino acids methionine and cysteine. Until about 1976 it was assumed that it was a metabolic end-product whose only function was the conjugation of bile acids. In the rat taurine synthesis (mainly by way of cysteine sulphinic acid) accounts for some 70–85 per cent of total cysteine catabolism, and trans-sulphuration to cysteine is the major metabolic fate of methionine.

The discovery of retinal degeneration in kittens fed on casein diets with little pre-formed taurine, and its prevention by taurine supplements, and the occurrence of changes in the electrical activity of the retina in children maintained on long-term total parenteral nutrition without added taurine have shown that it has physiological functions, and have raised the question of whether or not it should be regarded as a dietary essential in man.

A major problem in attempting to determine the physiological functions of taurine, other than in bile acid conjugation, has been the difficulty of achieving significant changes in tissue levels. Under normal conditions there is careful regulation of the tissue content of taurine, something which in itself suggests that it is not a dietary essential, but is synthesized in the tissues where it is required.

23.9.1 Biosynthesis of taurine

As shown in Fig. 23.9, taurine is α-amino sulphonic acid (2–aminoethane sulphonic acid), and can be synthesized from cysteine by three pathways.

1. Oxidation to cysteine sulphinic acid, followed by decarboxylation to hypotaurine and oxidation to taurine. In most tissues it is the decarboxylation of cysteine sulphinic acid that is rate limiting for taurine synthesis, not the oxidation of cysteine.

2. Oxidation to cysteic acid, followed by decarboxylation to taurine. Cysteic acid and cysteine sulphinic acid decarboxylase activities occur in constant ratio in various tissues, and it is likely that both substrates are decarboxylated by the same enzyme. In general cysteine sulphinic acid is the preferred substrate and there is little formation of taurine by way of cysteic acid.

3. *S*-Oxidation of cysteamine released by the catabolism of pantothenic acid (see section 23.2.2.3) or formed by the decarboxylation of cysteine.

In addition to taurocholic acid in the bile, free taurine is excreted in the urine. At times of low intake or when synthesis is impaired, for example by vitamin B_6 deficiency, the renal tubular resorption of

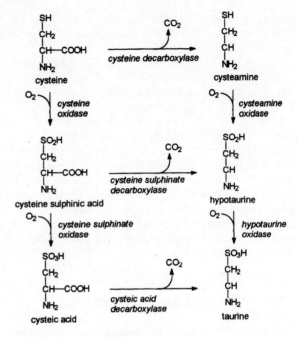

Figure 23.9 Taurine biosynthesis

taurine is increased, so reducing urinary losses. Feeding experimental animals on high taurine diets results in increased urinary excretion, but has little or no effect on endogenous synthesis.

23.9.2 Metabolic functions of taurine

23.9.2.1 Bile acid conjugation

In most species the bile acids arising from the oxidation of cholesterol (see section 8.2.3) may be conjugated with either taurine or glycine. Increased availability of taurine results in decreased glycine conjugation and an increase in biliary taurocholic acid. Conversely, glycine overload results in an increase in the plasma concentration of taurine, apparently as a result of increased glycocholic acid formation, and hence reduced utilization of taurine for bile acid conjugation.

Although supplements of taurine alter the ratio of taurocholic:glycocholic acids, they have no effect on the total output of bile salts, or on fat absorption in normal subjects. There is some evidence that patients with cystic fibrosis have improved fat absorption if given taurine supplements. This may be because taurine-conjugated bile acids are generally re-absorbed lower down the small intestine than glycine conjugates; in patients whose intestinal absorption is compromised, this may give a beneficial increase in the total length of intestinal tract available for fat absorption.

In addition to bile acid conjugation, a variety of other compounds may also be excreted as taurine conjugates, including retinoic acid (see section 13.2.3) and a number of xenobiotics.

23.9.2.2 Taurine deficiency and retinal degeneration in the kitten

Kittens maintained on a taurine-free diet show retinal degeneration. In the early stages, electroretinography shows changes similar to those seen in human retinitis pigmentosa. However, there is no evidence that retinitis pigmentosa is associated with taurine deficiency, and patients have normal plasma concentrations of the amino acid. Electron microscopy of the retinae of deficient kittens shows early disorientation of the cone photoreceptor outer segments, followed by extensive degeneration of both rod and cone outer segments. The function of taurine in the retina is unknown.

Patients maintained on long-term total parenteral nutrition without taurine (and also frequently without cysteine, because of the chemical instability of this amino acid in solution) show similar changes in the electroretinogram when the plasma concentration of taurine falls below about 30 μmol /L, compared with a reference range (in omnivores) of between 55–70 μmol /L.

23.9.2.3 Taurine in the central nervous system

There is a relatively high concentration of taurine in the central nervous system; higher than would be expected for a neurotransmitter, and without specific anatomical localization. It seems likely that it has a neuromodulatory role, either modifying responsiveness to other transmitters or suppressing the presynaptic release of neurotransmitters, rather than having a direct transmitter function in its own right. The concentration of taurine in the developing brain is some 3–4–fold higher than in the adult brain, and falls rapidly between birth and weaning. Unlike other amino acids, taurine is transported within axons to a greater extent in young animals than in adults.

The highest concentrations of taurine in the brain, and the greatest rates of axonal transport, occur prior to and during the process of synaptic development, suggesting that it may have a role in the development of the central nervous system and the post-natal development of synaptic connections. A variety of animal studies have shown that exogenous taurine has effects on the precisely scheduled processes of cellular proliferation, migration and differentiation in the development of the central nervous system.

23.9.2.4 Taurine and heart muscle

Cardiomyopathy is a major problem in taurine-deficient cats, and after prolonged deficiency there is a failure of contractility, leading to heart failure. Heart muscle concentrates taurine from the blood-stream, and the heart can synthesize taurine by oxidation of cysteamine, although not by the cysteine sulphinic acid decarboxylase pathway. Pharmacologically, taurine affects drug-induced cardiac arrhythmias by depressing the hyperirritability caused by loss of potassium—a digitalis-like action which suggests an effect on membrane permeability and ion flux, and perhaps especially on the maintenance of stable intracellular concentrations of calcium.

23.9.3 The possible essentiality of taurine

Taurine is a dietary essential in the cat. Kittens have a limited capacity for taurine synthesis from cysteine, and on a taurine free diet neither supplementary methionine nor cysteine will maintain normal plasma concentrations of taurine. The problem seems to be due to the existence of an alternative pathway of cysteine metabolism: reaction with mevalonic acid to yield felinine (3–hydroxy-1,1–dimethylpropyl)-cysteine, which is excreted in the urine. At the same time, the activity of cysteine sulphinic acid decarboxylase in cat liver is very low.

It is not known to what extent taurine may be a dietary essential for man. There is little cysteine sulphinic acid decarboxylase activity in human liver, and like the cat, loading doses of methionine and cysteine do not result in any significant increase in plasma taurine. This may be because cysteine sulphinic acid can also undergo transamination to β-sulphyryl pyruvate, which then loses sulphur dioxide non-enzymically to form pyruvate, so regulating the amount of taurine which is formed from cysteine. There is no evidence of the development of any taurine deficiency disease under normal conditions.

There are very few plant sources of taurine, and strict vegetarians have a very low intake of preformed taurine. Nevertheless, the plasma concentration of taurine in strict vegetarians is generally between 40–50 μmol /L, compared with concentrations between 55–70 μmol /L in omnivores.

In children undergoing long-term total parenteral nutrition without taurine supplements there are changes in the electroretinogram similar to those seen in the taurine-deficient cat, suggesting that at least in these children there is a requirement for some preformed taurine and that endogenous synthesis may be inadequate.

It has been suggested that pre-term infants may require a dietary source of preformed taurine; breast milk initially contains a high concentration of (about 300 µmol /L), and breast fed infants maintain a higher plasma concentration of taurine than those fed on formula without added taurine.

Although milk from Vegan mothers has a low concentration of taurine, and their infants have lower plasma concentrations and urinary excretion of taurine than the infants of omnivore mothers, there is no evidence that (full-term) infants of Vegan mothers show any signs of taurine deficiency.

23.10   Ubiquinone (coenzyme Q, 'Vitamin Q')

Ubiquinone is one of the electron carriers in mitochondria, and therefore has an essential function in all energy-yielding metabolism. The metabolically active coenzyme (coenzyme Q) has a ten isoprenyl-unit side chain, and is sometimes known as coenzyme Q_{10}. As shown in Fig. 23.10, it undergoes one-electron reduction to a semiquinone radical, and two-electron reduction to the quinol. In addition to its role in mitochondrial electron transport, ubiquinone may also have a general antioxidant role in membranes. Like vitamin E (see section 15.5.2), it can be anchored in membranes by the hydrophobic tail, with the reactive quinone group at the membrane surface.

Ubiquinone is readily synthesized in the body, and there is no evidence that it is a dietary essential, nor that supplements serve any useful purpose, although they may have non-specific antioxidant actions, and so spare vitamin E.

Further reading

Bender, D.A. (1992). Biotin (Vitamin H). In *Nutritional Biochemistry of the Vitamins*, Chapter 11, pp. 318–40. Cambridge University Press.

Bender, D.A. (1992). Pantothenic acid. In *Nutritional Biochemistry of the Vitamins*, Chapter 12, pp. 341–59 Cambridge University Press.

Bender, D.A. (1992). Compounds of doubtful nutritional status: taurine, carnitine, choline and inositol. In *Nutritional Biochemistry of the Vitamins*, Chapter 14, pp. 394–409 Cambridge University Press.

Berridge, M.J. (1987). Inositol trisphosphate and diacylglycerol: two interacting second messengers. *Annual Review of Biochemistry*, 56, 159–93.

Bieber, L.L. (1988). Carnitine. *Annual Review of Biochemistry*, 57, 261–283.

Bitsch, R., Toth-Dersi, A. and Hoetzl, D. (1985). Biotin deficiency and biotin supply. *Annals of the New York Academy of Sciences*, 447, 133–39.

Broquist, H.P. and Borum, P.R. (1982). Carnitine biosynthesis: nutritional implications. *Advances in Nutritional Research*, 4, 181–204.

Chesney, R.W. (1988). Taurine: is it required for infant nutrition? *Journal of Nutrition*, 118: 6–10.

Dakshinamurti, K. and Chauhan, J. (1989). Biotin. *Vitamins and Hormones*, 45, 337–84.

Dakshinamurti, K. and Chauhan, J. (1994). Biotin-binding proteins. In *Vitamin Receptors: Vitamins as Ligands in Cell Communication*, (ed K. Dakshinamurti), Chapter 8, pp. 200–49. Cambridge University Press.

Downes, C.P. (1989). The cellular functions of *myo*-inositol. *Biochemical Society Transactions*, 17, 2559–68.

Feller, A.G. and Rudman, D. (1988). Role of carnitine in human nutrition. *Journal of Nutrition*, 118, 541–7.

Friedrich, W. (1988). Biotin. In *Vitamins*, Chapter 11, pp. 735–806. Walter de Gruyter, Berlin.

Friedrich, W. (1988). Pantothenic acid. In *Vitamins*, Chapter 12, pp. 807–36 Walter de Gruyter, Berlin.

Hayes, K.C. (1988). Taurine nutrition. *Nutrition Research Reviews* 1, 99–113.

Hommes, F.A. (1986). Biotin. *World Review of Nutrition and Dietetics*, 48, 34–84.

Jeffery, D.M. (1982). Pantothenic acid. In *Vitamins in Medicine*, Vol. 2, 4th edn (ed B.M. Barker and D.A.

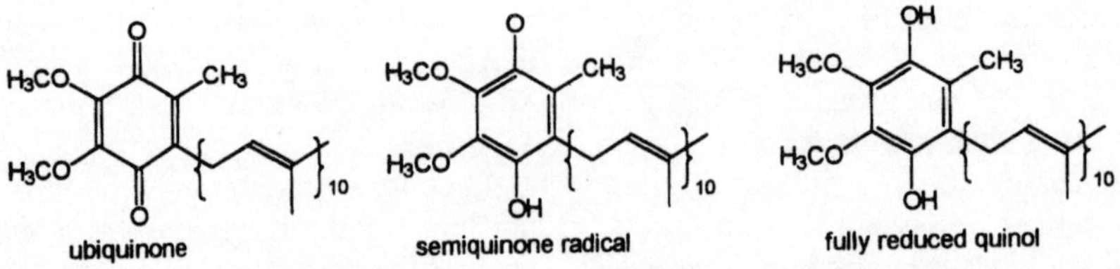

Figure 23.10 Ubiquinone (Coenzyme Q)

Bender), Chapter 2, pp. 69–91. Heinemann Medical Books, London.

Johnson, I.T., Williamson, G. and Musk, S.R.R. (1994). Anticarcinogenic factors in plant foods: implications for protetion against chemical carcinogenesis. *Nutrition Research Reviews*, 7, 175–204.

Rebouche, C.J. and Paulson, D.J (1986). Carnitine metabolism and function in humans. *Annual Review of Nutrition*, 6, 41–66.

Roth, K.S. (1981). Biotin in clinical medicine, a review. *American Journal of Clinical Nutrition*, 34, 1967–74.

Sturman, J.A. (1988). Taurine in development. *Journal of Nutrition*, 118, 1169–76.

Sweetman, L. and Nyhan, W.L. (1986). Inheritable biotin-treatable disorders and associated phenomena. *Annual Review of Nutrition*, 6, 317–43.

Zeisel, S.H. and Blusztajn, J.K. (1994). Choline and human nutrition. *Annual Review of Nutrition*, 14, 269–96.

Zeisel, S.H. (1981). Dietary choline: biochemistry physiology and pharmacology. *Annual Review of Nutrition*, 1, 95–121.

Table 23.1: Compounds at one time assigned vitamin nomenclature

B_3	Assigned to a compound which was probably pantothenic acid; incorrectly used for niacin.
B_4	Assigned to what was later identified as a mixture of arginine, glycine and cysteine.
B_5	Assigned to what was later assumed to be either vitamin B_6 or nicotinic acid, also used for pantothenic acid.
B_7	Never assigned.
B_8	Never assigned.
B_9	Never assigned.
B_{10}	Assigned to what was later identified as a mixture of folic acid and vitamin B_1.
B_{11}	Assigned to what was later identified as a mixture of folic acid and vitamin B_1.
B_{13}	Orotic acid—not a vitamin, but an intermediate in pyrimidine synthesis.
B_{14}	Assigned to a substance in urine which increases proliferation of bone marrow in culture.
B_{15}	Pangamic acid, no established vitamin function.
B_{16}	Never assigned.
B_{17}	Amygdalin or laetrile, a cyanogenic glycoside with no established vitamin function.
B_c	Obsolete name for folic acid.
B_p	Assigned to the 'anti-perosis' factor for chickens, can be replaced by choline and manganese.
B_T	Carnitine, a growth factor for the meal worm, but not a vitamin (see section 23.5)
B_W	Assigned to a factor which was probably biotin.
B_x	Obsolete name for *p*-aminobenzoic acid, required for folic acid synthesis in micro-organisms, not a vitamin. Also used at one time for pantothenic acid.
F	Essential fatty acids—not classified as vitamins.
G	Obsolete name for riboflavin.
H_3	Gerovital—novocaine (procaine hydrochloride), promoted without evidence as alleviating the symptoms of diseases associated with aging. Not recognised as a vitamin.
L	Factor in yeast claimed to promote lactation, not established as a vitamin.
M	Obsolete name for folic acid.
P	Bioflavonoids, pharmacologically active but not vitamins (see section 23.3).
PP	Obsolete name for niacin (pellagra-preventing vitamin).
Q	Ubiquinone (see section 23.10).
T	Assigned to a mixture of folic acid, vitamin B_{12} and nucleotides.
U	Methylsulphonium salts of methionine. May have pharmacological actions, but not a vitamin.

Table 23.2: Estimated safe and adequate levels of biotin intake

	US RDA (1989)	UK RNI (1991)	EU PRI (1993)
	µg	µg	µg
birth—6m	10	-	-
6m—1y	15	-	-
1—3	20	-	-
4—6	25	-	-
7—10	30	-	-
11—19	30-100	-	-
adults	30-100	10-200	15-100

Source: National Research Council 1989; Department of Health 1991; Scientific Committee for Food 1993.

Table 23.3: Average intakes of biotin (µg/day) in UK

age	males			females		
	mean	median	95% range	mean	median	95% range
1.5-2.5	17.1	16.0	6.3-33.3	17.1	16.0	6.3-33.3
2.5-3.5	17.0	15.9	7.3-32.5	17.0	15.9	7.3-32.5
3.5-4.5	17.7	17.2	7.5-33.2	16.8	15.9	7.0-32.7
16-24	34.6	33.5	12.8-64.9	23.7	23.6	8.1-42.6
25-34	40.2	39.1	15.7-70.6	26.6	24.9	8.3-56.7
35-49	40.8	39.3	16.2-72.1	31.4	28.6	11.4-69.5
50-64	38.6	37.4	14.1-67.4	28.8	27.1	11.0-51.1

Source: from data reported by Gregory *et al.* 1990; 1995.

Table 23.4: Biotin-dependent enzymes

enzyme	EC number	pathway	abnormal urinary acids in deficiency or multiple carboxylase deficiency
acetyl CoA carboxylase	6.4.1.2	fatty acid synthesis	2-ethyl-3-hydroxyhexanoic, 2-ethyl-hexanedioic
methylcrotonyl CoA carboxylase	6.4.1.4	leucine catabolism	3-methylcrotonyl, 3-hydroxyisovaleric, 3-methylcrotonylglycine
propionyl CoA carboxylase	6.4.1.3	isoleucine, valine, methionine, threonine, cholesterol catabolism	propionic, 3-hydroxypropionic, propionylglycine, methylcitric, tiglic, tiglylglycine, 2-methyl-3-hydroxybutyric, lactic
pyruvate carboxylase	6.4.1.1	gluconeogenesis	lactic, pyruvic, alanine

Table 23.5: Estimated safe and adequate levels of pantothenic acid intake

	US RDA (1989)	UK RNI (1991)	EU PRI (1993)
	mg	mg	mg
birth—6m	2	1.7	-
6m—1y	3	1.7	-
1—3	3	-	-
4—6	3-4	-	-
7—10	4-5	-	-
11—19	4-7	-	-
adults	4-7	3-7	3-12

Source: National Research Council 1989; Department of Health 1991; Scientific Committee for Food 1993.

Table 23.6: Average intakes of pantothenic acid (mg /day) in UK

age	males			females		
	mean	median	95% range	mean	median	95% range
1.5-2.5	2.7	2.6	1.2-4.8	2.7	2.6	1.2-4.8
2.5-3.5	2.7	2.6	1.4-4.8	2.7	2.6	1.4-4.8
3.5-4.5	2.8	2.7	1.4-4.6	2.7	2.6	1.4-4.5
16-24	6.3	6.0	2.7-11.7	4.4	4.3	2.1-7.4
25-34	6.4	6.1	3.3-10.5	4.5	4.5	2.0-7.5
35-49	6.4	6.2	2.9-10.4	4.7	4.5	2.5-8.2
50-64	6.1	5.8	3.2-10.2	4.4	4.3	2.1-7.0

Source: from data reported by Gregory *et al.* 1990, 1995.

Table 23.7: Blood concentrations and urine excretion of panthothenic acid

total pantothenic acid		
whole blood	0.7-4.5 µmol /L	140-980 µg /L
plasma	0.4-1.4 µmol /L	90-310 µg /L
erythrocytes	4.5-6.7 µmol /L	1000-1500 µg /L
coenzyme A		
erythrocytes	13 µmol /L	9.7 µg /L
platelets	80-140 µmol /g protein	60-110 µg /g protein
urine pantothenic acid		
	12-22 µmol /24h	2.7-4.9 mg /24h
	0.8-1.6 mmol /mol creatinine	1.6-3.0 mg /g creatinine

Source: Modified from Bender 1992.

Table 23.8: Enzymes known or believed to contain pyrroloquinolinequinone (PQQ)

	EC number
alcohol dehydrogenase	1.1.99.8
aldehyde dehydrogenase	1.2.99.3
choline dehydrogenase	1.1.99.1
glycerol dehydrogenase	1.1.99.22
lysine oxidase	1.4.3.14

24

Iron

Iron deficiency is probably the most common nutritional problem; WHO estimates that world-wide some 2.15×10^9 people (approximately one-third of the world's population) suffer from iron deficiency. Table 24.1 shows the numbers affected in different regions.

The total body content of iron is about 800–1040 mmol (45–60 mg)/kg body weight in men, and 630–730 mmol (35–41 mg) in women. The distribution of this iron in metabolically active and storage pools is shown in Table 24.2. Men have considerable iron reserves (equivalent to up to 50 per cent of the functional body pool), and as discussed in section 24.5 are potentially at risk of iron overload. By contrast, women have low reserves of iron (from almost none to 16 per cent of the functional pool) and, as discussed in section 24.4 are at considerable risk of iron deficiency.

24.1   Metabolic functions of iron

Iron has two main functions in the body.

1. In the oxygen-transporting proteins, haemoglobin in erythrocytes and myoglobin in muscle, where it is present as the tetrapyrrole chelate, haem (see Fig. 24.1). Fully oxygenated haemoglobin carries 4 mol of oxygen—1.39 mL of oxygen /g.

2. In a variety of enzymes catalysing oxidation and reduction reactions, where it may be present as haem (e.g. in cytochromes) or a variety of non-haem-iron proteins in which the iron is bound to the protein by sulphydryl bridges from cysteine residues.

In haemoglobin and myoglobin the iron is present as Fe^{2+}, and does not undergo oxidation when transporting oxygen. Indeed oxidation of the iron of haemoglobin to Fe^{3+} results in loss of its oxygen

transporting ability—methaemoglobinaemia. This oxidation of haemoglobin occurs to a small extent all the time (normally about 1 per cent of circulating haemoglobin is present as methaemoglobin), and erythrocytes contain a variety of enzymes that reduce methaemoglobin back to the active Fe^{2+} form.

In the cytochromes and other haem enzymes, and in non-haem iron proteins, the iron acts as a single electron carrier in oxidation and reduction reactions, cycling between Fe^{2+} and Fe^{3+}.

As shown in Table 24.2, some 82 per cent of total functional body pool of iron is in the oxygen carrying protein of the red blood cells, haemoglobin. A further 12 per cent is in the muscle oxygen transport protein, myoglobin, slightly more in males than females because of the greater proportion of muscle in males than females (see Tables 2.9 and 2.10). The remaining 5 per cent is in the various iron-dependent enzymes.

Haemoglobin is a tetrameric protein, consisting, in the adult, of two α- and two β-globin chains (haemoglobin A). The chains show cooperativity in the binding of oxygen, so that it has a high affinity to take up oxygen under conditions of high oxygen tension (i.e. in the lungs) and a low affinity for oxygen, so that it gives it up readily, under conditions of low oxygen tension, as in muscle and other tissues. The affinity of haemoglobin for oxygen at low oxygen tension is further reduced by low pH, as occurs in exercising muscle. Myoglobin is a monomeric protein, with a higher affinity for oxygen than that of haemoglobin under the conditions that exist in muscle.

Foetal haemoglobin (haemoglobin F) has a higher affinity for oxygen than normal adult haemoglobin, consisting of two α- and two γ-globin chains. Shortly before birth the synthesis of the β-globin chain begins to replace that of γ-globin, and by the age of 7 months more than 90 per cent of the infant's haemoglobin is haemoglobin A.

24.2 Iron losses, intakes and requirements

As with other minerals, it is relatively simple to estimate physiological iron requirements, by measurement of the obligatory losses from the body. Total body iron loss can be measured by following the dilution by dietary iron of the long-lived radioactive isotope ^{55}Fe given by intravenous injection. Such studies show a loss of 0.25 μmol (14 μg)/kg body weight/day for men, or a total of about 1 mg/day for an adult (Charlton *et al*. 1980).

24.2.1 Intakes and sources of iron

It is difficult to translate the requirement to replace the physiological loss of 0.25 μmol/kg body weight into an appropriate level of intake, because of the low and variable availability of dietary iron. On average only about 10 per cent of dietary iron is absorbed, with a range between 5–15 per cent (see section 24.2.3). Table 24.3 shows average intakes of iron, Table 24.4 the proportion of average iron intakes provided by different foods, and Table 24.5 those foods that are rich sources of iron.

24.2.2 Iron losses

There is no active excretion of iron in urine or faeces; iron is only lost in shed epithelial cells (skin, intestinal mucosa, urinary tract) and hair. Although bile contains a significant amount of iron, resulting from haemoglobin breakdown (see section 24.33.2), and about 1 mg /day is secreted in bile, most of this is reabsorbed in the small intestine, and little endogenous iron reaches the faeces from bile. Faeces also contains a large amount of unabsorbed dietary iron, both that which remains in the intestinal lumen, and also that which is absorbed into epithelial cells, but then remains in those cells, being lost into the lumen when the cells are shed at the tip of the villus (see section 24.2.3)

Some 30–40 per cent of endogenous iron loss is in the faeces; urinary loss of iron is variously estimated as 0.1–3.3 mg /day, mainly in shed epithelial cells of the urinary tract, although urinary iron increases considerably if iron-chelating drugs are given (see section 24.5).

The remaining iron loss is in shed skin cells, hair and sweat. The iron content of cell-free sweat is about 0.36 μmol (20 μg)/L. Normal sweat volume is about 0.5 L/day, rising some 20–fold under extreme conditions, so it is unlikely that sweat losses of iron will be significant, even under tropical conditions (Brune *et al*. 1986). Furthermore, the iron content of sweat falls with falling total body iron reserves.

For women, in addition to the basal loss of 0.25 μmol/kg body weight, there is a considerable loss of iron in menstruation. Menstrual blood losses are relatively constant from one period to another, but show a very wide range of individual variation. The distribution of menstrual losses is not statistically normal, but skewed, with a large 'tail' of women with very high losses. Because of this, it is conventional to consider the 90th or 95th centile as defining the reference intake, rather than the 97.5th centile, as for other nutrients (see section 4.1). Oral contraceptive agents reduce menstrual blood losses by 50 per cent, while intra-uterine contraceptive devices double the loss. Daily amounts of absorbed iron to meet maintenance turnover and replace menstrual losses are shown in Table 24.6; adolescent girls have a higher iron requirement than menstruating women, despite a lower menstrual blood loss, because of the requirement for iron for growth.

Very large amounts of iron can be lost as a result of blood loss. Haemoglobin contains 3.4 mg iron /g; at 150 g haemoglobin /L of blood, loss of 100 mL of blood will be a loss of 50 mg iron; even a standard 10 mL blood sample will represent a loss of 5 mg of iron, and donation of 450 mL of blood is a loss of 225 mg iron. A common cause of iron deficiency is occult intestinal bleeding, associated with either gastrointestinal disease or intestinal parasites that cause bleeding, such as hookworm (*Ancylostoma duodenale*)—severe hookworm infestation can lead to loss of up to 250 mL of blood per day. Conversely, repeated blood transfusion (e.g. for the treatment of sickle cell disease and thalassaemia) commonly leads to the development of iron overload (see section 24.5).

24.2.3 Iron absorption

There are two intestinal mechanisms for iron absorption—one for haem iron in meat and a separate mechanism for inorganic (ferrous) iron. Although meat, and therefore haem, only accounts for some 25 per cent of average iron intake (see Table 24.4), the absorption of haem is considerably more efficient than that of inorganic iron; up to 25 per cent of haem iron is absorbed, while only 5–10 per cent or less of inorganic iron is absorbed.

Haem from the hydrolysis of haemoglobin and myoglobin is taken up into duodenal mucosal cells, where it is cleaved by haem oxygenase (EC 1.14.99.3), yielding free iron, which binds to ferritin intracellularly, and bilirubin (see Fig. 24.2 and section 24.3.3.2).

Inorganic iron is only absorbed in the ferrous (Fe^{2+}) oxidation state; therefore reducing compounds such as ascorbate present in the gut lumen at the same time as iron enhance its absorption (see section 22.4.4.1). Uptake of inorganic iron into the intestinal mucosal cell is carrier-mediated, but not active, transport; iron will only accumulate in the cell as long as there is free apo-ferritin to bind it and shift the equilibrium of the passive uptake system. Once ferritin in the mucosal cell is saturated with iron, no more will be taken up from the intestinal lumen, unless there is a very high luminal concentration of iron salts, or in the presence of alcohol, which stimulates iron uptake (see section 24.5).

Iron will only be transferred across the basolateral membrane of the mucosal cell into the circulation if there is free apo-transferrin in plasma; once transferrin is more or less saturated, iron will not leave the mucosal cell, but will remain bound to ferritin until the cell is shed at the tip of the villus.

Iron deficiency commonly develops after gastrectomy. It is likely that gastric acid enhances the release of iron from complexes in foods, and the acid environment stabilizes Fe^{2+}. It is also postulated that a proteoglycan secreted in gastric juice is important for iron binding and intestinal absorption, although there is little evidence for this.

24.2.3.1 Dietary factors affecting iron absorption

The biological availability of iron from foods differs widely, with 5 per cent or less of the iron in some foods being absorbed (Hallberg 1982; Bothwell *et al.* 1989). Table 24.7 shows the relative availability of iron in various foods, as determined by feeding isotopically labelled foods in single test meals.

In addition to the innate biological availability of the iron in individual foods, a number of compounds present in foods interact with the iron present in other foods, and may increase or decrease its absorption (see Table 24.8). Reducing compounds, which maintain inorganic iron in the Fe^{2+} state, and various organic acids (including citric acid and various amino acids), which chelate iron, enhance its absorption considerably. As discussed in section 22.4.4.1, it has been argued that intakes of vitamin C considerably greater than those required to meet requirements may be desirable to enhance iron absorption. The iron in alcoholic beverages is also highly available, and it is likely that alcohol stimulates iron absorption, although the mechanism is unclear.

The presence of fish and meat in a meal enhances the absorption of both inorganic and haem iron; this does not seem to be solely a result of hydrolysis to amino acids, and no satisfactory mechanism has been advanced to account for this. Hallberg and Rossander-Hultén (1991) quote absorption of 20–23 per cent of iron from a meal containing a relatively large amount of meat and vegetables, and as little as 5–12 per cent from a vegetarian diet.

A number of dietary factors inhibit the absorption of inorganic iron, including egg and soya proteins and a variety of polyphenols (those found in tea and coffee are especially important). Phytate (inositol hexaphosphate) is also reported to impair iron absorption by forming insoluble salts in the intestinal lumen, but this seems to require the presence of some forms of non-starch polysaccharide (see section 7.3) as well as phytate; under experimental conditions the iron from iron phytate fed alone is biologically available.

Calcium inhibits the absorption of both haem and non-haem iron, apparently by inhibiting the transport of iron across the mucosal cell into the bloodstream. This effect is seen not only with relatively large supplements of calcium (as are recommended for protection against osteoporosis, see section 14.1.1), but also with more moderate amounts of calcium normally present in a meal—for example the calcium in a glass of milk taken with a meal will reduce iron absorption significantly (Hallberg *et al.* 1992).

24.2.3.2 The effect of iron nutritional status on iron absorption

Overall, only about 10 per cent of dietary iron is absorbed by subjects with good iron status. However, this increases significantly in iron deficiency. Hallberg and Rossander-Hultén (1991) quote a range from 5 per cent absorption in iron-replete subjects to nearly 30 per cent in deficiency. They state that the dietary iron requirement to maintain a body reserve of 300 mg of iron (the maximum normally occurring in women, see Table 24.2) is twice that required to prevent the development of deficiency.

Part of the mechanism for this increased efficiency of iron absorption in deficiency is that there will be greater transport across the basolateral mucosal cell membrane, since plasma transferrin will be less saturated than in replete subjects. There is also adaptation of the intestinal haem oxygenase, with greater activity in iron deficiency and a fall in activity on iron repletion (Raffin *et al.* 1974). In addition, subjects with a lower iron status will have more apo-transferrin in plasma, and will therefore be able to take up a greater proportion of dietary iron from the intestinal mucosal cell into the plasma.

24.2.4 Reference intakes of iron

Because of the skewed distribution of menstrual losses of iron, reference intakes for women are usually based on meeting the requirement of the 95th centile, rather than the 97.5th centile, as for other nutrients (see section 4.1). Table 24.9 shows the US, UK and EU reference intakes. These are largely based on the FAO (1988) estimates of requirements; the EU expert committee was able to incorporate the more recently available information on menstrual iron losses (Hallberg and Rossander-Hultén 1991). This committee set two population reference intakes for women of child-bearing age, to meet the 90th and 95th centiles of menstrual losses respectively, and also proposed separate labelling reference values for iron for men and women (see Table 4.10). It is acknowledged that the reference intakes for women of child-bearing age are higher than can be met from foods, and supplements of iron are probably necessary for the 10–25 per cent of women with high menstrual losses.

Pregnancy and lactation might also be considered as significant causes of blood loss, since the mother has to provide the 12 mmol (680 mg) of iron of the foetus and placenta, and then approximately 5–6 μmol (0.25–0.54 mg) /day through 3 months of lactation. However, since menstruation ceases in pregnancy and lactation, the saving on menstrual blood losses probably meets the iron requirement of the foetus and suckling infant. As shown in Table 24.9 the US RDA includes an additional allowance of iron in pregnancy and lactation, while the UK and EU reference intakes do not.

24.3   Iron metabolism

Ferrous ions in free solution will react with hydrogen peroxide, forming the hydroxyl radical; the resultant ferric ion can be reduced back to the ferrous ion by non-enzymic reaction with ascorbate (see section 22.4.4):

$$Fe^{2+} + H_2O_2 \rightarrow Fe^{3+} + {}^{\bullet}OH + OH^-$$

$$Fe^{3+} + ascorbate \rightarrow Fe^{2+} + monodehydroascorbate.$$

There is thus the potential for the generation of significant amounts of hydroxyl radicals, and significant depletion of vitamin C, when iron ions occur in free solution in body fluids; this is a major part of the pathology of iron overload (see section 24.5).

Under normal conditions, there is little or no free iron in solution. In plasma it is more or less completely bound to transferrin, and in tissues that which is not incorporated into haem or non-haem iron proteins is bound to one of two iron storage proteins, ferritin and haemosiderin (see Fig. 24.1).

24.3.1 Transferrin

Transferrin (also known as siderophilin) is a relatively small glycoprotein (M_r 80 000), one of the β-globulins, which circulates as a dimer, with two iron binding sites per dimer, although it is rare for both sites to be occupied. In addition to minimizing the risk of hydroxyl radical generation by binding iron, it also has antibacterial actions, since it prevents the uptake of iron by invading micro-organisms. Transferrin has a relatively short half-life in plasma (of the order of 8–10 days), and as well as changing in response to both iron nutritional status (increasing in deficiency and falling in iron overload), its synthesis is markedly affected by protein-energy malnutrition (see section 12.2). It is also one of the acute phase response proteins (see section 10.8.4.2), falling in response to trauma and infection. There is a marked diurnal variation, and total serum iron may vary two-fold through the day.

The extent to which transferrin is saturated with iron provides a sensitive index of iron nutritional status, reflecting the pool of iron that is available and being transported between storage sites (the reticuloendothelial system) and utilization (mainly in erythropoietic cells of bone marrow, see section 24.3.3.1). Determination of the ratio of plasma iron concentration:total iron binding capacity permits calculation of the fractional saturation of transferrin; see Table 24.10.

24.3.2 Ferritin and haemosiderin

Ferritin and haemosiderin are the two main iron storage proteins in liver, spleen, and bone marrow. Ferritin is globulin protein which forms a hollow sphere of 24 subunits surrounding a central core of ferric hydroxide-ferric phosphate complex; it may contain up to 20 per cent iron, or about 2500 atoms of iron per molecule.

Haemosiderin is an ill-defined complex of hydrated iron oxide with various organic constituents, containing up to 35 per cent iron. It arises by partial enzymic hydrolysis of ferritin in lysosomes. At normal levels of iron in liver and spleen (around 9 μmol (500 μg) /g tissue), ferritin is the predominant storage protein, and there is little or no haemosiderin;

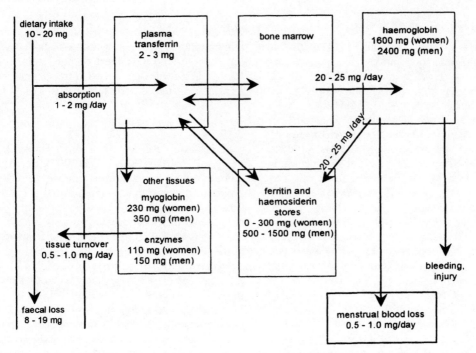

Figure 24.1 Daily iron turnover

as the level increases above 18 µmol /g tissue, the proportion of haemosiderin increases.

Ferritin also occurs in plasma; its function is unclear, but the concentration (readily measured by immunological methods) reflects total iron reserves in the body. Each 1 µg /L serum ferritin corresponds to 0.14–0.18 mmol (8–10 mg) of storage iron. Serum ferritin provides a more sensitive index of iron nutritional status than does transferrin saturation, reflecting the underlying state of body reserves rather than the amounts of iron available for transport between tissues. Unlike transferrin, a low serum ferritin concentration seems to reflect only depletion of body iron stores; serum ferritin below 12 µg /L gives no indication of the severity of deficiency

24.3.3 Red blood cell turnover

Red blood cells are formed in bone marrow, and have an average life in the circulation of 120 days (range 74–153). The mean red cell count is 5.4 x 10^{12} /L blood in men and 4.8 x 10^{12} in women; the daily production of erythrocytes is of the order of 3 x 10^9 /kg body weight /day. This represents a daily turnover of some 6 g of haemoglobin, or 0.9 mmol (20 mg) of iron.

24.3.3.1 Erythropoiesis

The process of red cell formation (erythropoiesis) takes place in the red bone marrow of the spongy bone of the cranium, ribs, sternum, bodies of the vertebra and proximal epiphyses of the humerus and femur. Stem cells (haemocytoblasts) undergo differentiation to yield proethryoblasts, then erythroblasts, in which haemoglobin synthesis is maximal. The late erythroblast expels its nucleus, becoming a reticulocyte. Reticulocytes pass from the bone marrow into the bloodstream, and there undergo further maturation over a period of 1–2 days to become mature erythrocytes. Normally between 1–1.5 per cent of circulating red cells are reticulocytes, which are larger than mature erythrocytes, do not yet have their full complement of haemoglobin, and retain some mitochondria and ribosomes. The proportion of reticulocytes is higher in new-born infants (see Table 24.13), and increases in iron deficiency.

Under normal conditions the processes of erythropoiesis and red cell destruction occur at the same rate; when there is a modest degree of tissue hypoxia (due to either a reduced number of red cells (anaemia) or moving to high altitude), the kidney secretes additional amounts of the hormone erythropoietin, which stimulates the differentiation of haemocytoblasts, and hence increased erythropoiesis.

24.3.3.2 Erythrocyte destruction

As erythrocytes age, the cell membrane becomes modified, and the senescent cells are recognized and dealt with by fixed mononuclear phagocytes in the spleen, liver and bone marrow. After phagocytosis, haemoglobin is catabolized, with the release of haem. The porphyrin ring of haem is cleaved by haem oxygenase (EC 1.14.99.3) to form biliverdin, which circulates in plasma to the liver, where it is reduced to bilirubin, conjugated with glucuronic acid and excreted in the bile (see Fig. 24.2). It is failure to metabolize and excrete bilirubin in liver failure or obstruction of the bile duct that leads to the development of jaundice. The iron that is released is salvaged by binding to ferritin.

A proportion of the bilirubin diglucuronide in the intestinal lumen is hydrolysed to free bilirubin by intestinal bacteria, and reduced to urobilinogen. Some of this is further metabolized by intestinal bacteria to yield stercobilin, and some is absorbed, undergoing metabolism in the kidney to yield urobilin, which is excreted in the urine.

About 10 per cent of daily erythrocyte breakdown is intravascular, with the release into the circulation of 0.6 mg haemoglobin. This dissociates into α-β dimers, which are bound by plasma haptoglobins, and free haem, which is bound by plasma haemopexin. This binding to relatively large proteins prevents renal filtration of the haem, and loss into the urine of the 2 mg of iron released by intravascular haemolysis.

Haemoglobinuria only develops when the rate of intravascular haemolysis is abnormally high, exceeding the capacity of haptoglobin. The normal range of haptoglobin, expressed as the total haemoglobin binding capacity, is 0.4–1.4 g /L blood. Both haptoglobin and haemopexin are positive acute phase proteins (see section 10.8.4.2), with increased synthesis in response to trauma and infection.

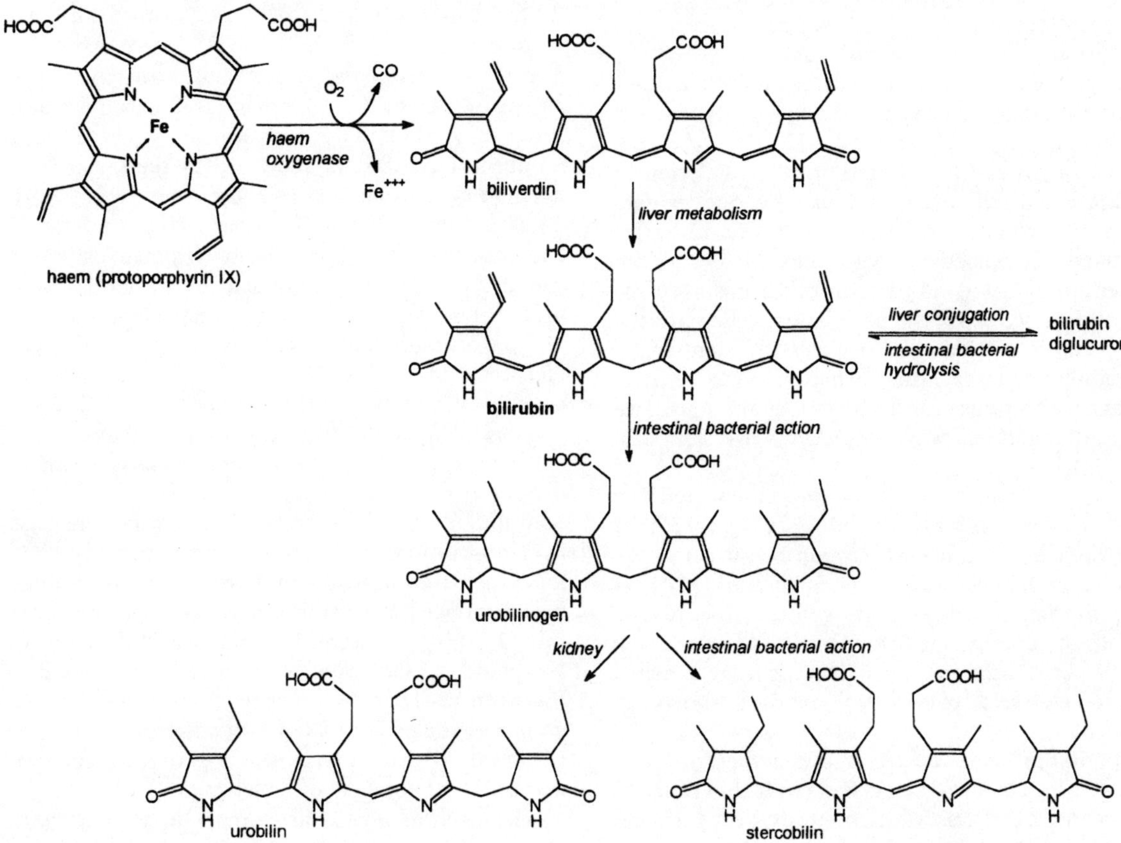

Figure 24.2 Haem catabolism and the bile pigments
Haem oxygenase EC 1.14.99.3

24.4 Iron deficiency anaemia

Anaemia is insufficiency of haemoglobin in the circulation, leading to impaired ability to transport oxygen to tissues. The clinical signs of anaemia include a significant impairment of work capacity, listlessness, persistent tiredness, shortness of breath, palpitations, headache, dizziness and irritability. Far and away the most important cause of anaemia is iron deficiency, due to inadequate intake and / or excessive losses. Iron deficiency anaemia is microcytic (the erythrocytes are smaller than normal) and hypochromic (there is a reduced amount of haemoglobin per erythrocyte, as well as reduced erythrocyte number and size). Before the mean cell volume is significantly lower than normal, there is an increase in the variance of red cell diameter, determined as the red cell distribution width (RDW)—a value > 16 per cent indicates early microcytosis.

Hypochromic anaemia can also develop (rarely) in cases of vitamin B_6 deficiency (see section 20.5), as a result of impaired synthesis of haem, or vitamin C deficiency (see section 22.5.1), because of its role in iron absorption. Haemolytic anaemia, due to increased red cell fragility and increased intravascular haemolysis, may occur with deficiency of vitamins E (see section 15.6) or C (see section 22.5.1), and megaloblastic anaemia (the release into the circulation of immature red cell precursors) may be due to deficiency of vitamin B_{12} or folate (see section 21.8.1).

Anaemia is defined as a whole blood haemoglobin concentration below 85 per cent of the mean for the appropriate sector of the population. Alternatively, the proportional volume of red cells after centrifugation of a blood sample (the haematocrit) can be used. Normal mean values for haemoglobin and haematocrit, and values indicative of anaemia are shown in Table 24.11.

In the last trimester of normal pregnancy there is a greater increase in plasma volume (by up to 55 per cent) than in red cell mass (by up to 30 per cent), resulting in apparent mild anaemia and a lower haematocrit than in non-pregnant women. More precise diagnostic criteria, which permit differentiation between iron deficiency and this apparent anaemia due to increased plasma volume, are shown in Table 24.12.

In addition to the effects on the mother, anaemia during pregnancy is associated with lower birth weight, increased risk of prematurity and perinatal mortality. Iron deficient infants and children have impaired psychomotor development and cognitive skills, as a result of impairment of brain development

(Dallman 1989). Even moderate iron depletion, with more or less normal haemoglobin, is associated with reduced T-lymphocyte numbers and impaired bactericidal activity of leukocytes, resulting in increased susceptibility to infection.

A significant proportion of women of child-bearing age suffer from iron deficiency; on the basis of the threshold haemoglobin concentrations shown in Table 24.10, anaemia occurs in some 10–15 per cent of women of child-bearing age in developed countries, and in 20–30 per cent of pregnant women. If the more sensitive criterion of low plasma ferritin (see Tables 24.13 and 24.14) is used to indicate inadequate iron reserves, then 25–30 per cent of women of child-bearing age are inadequately supplied with iron in developed countries. In Britain one in twelve of children aged between 1-4 years is anaemic (haemoglobin < 110 g /L) and 20 per cent have plasma ferritin < 10 µg /L (Gregory *et al.* 1995).

24.5 Iron overload (haemochromatosis)

There is no physiological mechanism for removal of excess iron from the body, and although the major problem world-wide is iron deficiency, there are a number of conditions under which there can be a dangerous accumulation of body iron reserves, leading to accumulation of abnormally large amounts of haemosiderin in tissues (haemochromatosis). This can lead to enlargement of the liver, the development of diabetes, hypogonadism, extremely painful inflammation of joints and potentially fatal heart disease. Herbert (1987) notes that while 1 in 500 adult men in developed countries suffers from iron deficiency, twice as many suffer from haemochromatosis.

The main cause of haemochromatosis is excessive dietary iron intake, especially associated with the consumption of alcoholic beverages, which increase iron absorption. Two groups are commonly cited here: the Bantu of southern Africa, whose traditional beer is brewed in (rusty) iron vessels (and may contain 15–120 mg iron /L), and heavy drinkers of Normandy cider, which is extremely rich in iron (between 10–16 mg /L). Young children in developed countries are also at risk of iron overload, as a result of mistaking iron supplements for sweets, and consuming large numbers of tablets.

Haemochromatosis also occurs in patients with sickle cell trait and thalassaemia, who receive frequent blood transfusions; the iron arising from breakdown of the transfused red cells is stored in the usual way, leading to a very considerable accumulation of iron.

There are only two methods available for treatment of haemochromatosis.

1. Venesection—the removal of some 500 mL of blood per week. While this will be effective for those whose iron overload is the result of excessive intake, or rare genetic defects of the regulation of synthesis, it is hardly appropriate for those who receive blood transfusions for the control of sickle cell disease or thalassaemia.

2. Administration of chelating compounds, such as desferrioxamine, which form soluble iron chelates that are small enough to be filtered in the kidney,

so gradually depleting the body of its excessive iron burden.

Further reading

Baynes, R.D. and Rothwell, T.H. (1990). Iron deficiency. *Annual Review of Nutrition*, 10, 133–48.

Cook, J. D., Baynes, R.D. and Skikne, B.S. (1992). Iron deficiency and the measurement of iron status. *Nutrition Research Reviews*, 5, 189–202.

Dallman, P.R. (1986). Biochemical basis for the manifestation of iron deficiency. *Annual Review of Nutrition*, 6, 13–40.

Hallberg, L. (1981). Bioavailability of dietary iron in man. *Annual Review of Nutrition*, 1, 123–47.

Table 24.1: Number of people suffering from iron deficiency

	millions
Western Pacific	1058
SE Asia	616
Africa	206
Eastern Mediterranean	149
Americas	94
Europe	27
total	2150

Source: WHO 1995.

Table 24.2: Total body iron content /kg body weight

	man		woman	
	μmol	mg	μmol	mg
haemoglobin	570	32	520	29
myoglobin	84	4.7	75	4.2
haem and non-haem enzymes	35	2.0	35	2.0
transferrin-bound	0.7	0.04	0.7	0.04
ferritin + haemosiderin (storage)	120-360	6.7-20	0-100	0-5.5
ratio, storage : functional	0.17-0.52		0-0.16	

Table 24.3: Average intakes of iron (mg /day)

(Apart from the SENECA study of the elderly, which involved 17 centres throughout Europe, all the studies quoted were in UK)

age	males			females			reference
	mean	median	range[1]	mean	median	range[1]	
1.5-2.5	4.9	4.7	2.4-9.2	4.9	4.7	2.4-9.2	Gregory *et al.* 1995
2.5-3.5	5.4	5.3	2.6-9.1	5.4	5.3	2.6-9.1	Gregory *et al.* 1995
3.5-4.5	6.1	5.9	3.1-10.4	5.6	55	3.0-9.1	Gregory *et al.* 1995
16-24	12.6	12.4	5.4-23.0	9.8	9.1	4.3-17.5	Gregory *et al.* 1990
25-34	13.8	13.2	6.8-25.9	10.2	9.4	4.5-19.1	Gregory *et al.* 1990
35-49	14.2	13.3	6.9-25.7	11.0	10.2	4.9-25.6	Gregory *et al.* 1990
50-64	13.9	13.7	6.2-26.3	10.6	10.1	5.6-21.1	Gregory *et al.* 1990
58-65	13.6	-	7.3-24.4	11.0	-	4.6-23.0	Davies and Holdsworth 1985
62-74	11.7	-	-	9.0	-	-	Lonergan *et al.* 1975
73-78[2]	-	13.6 (9.7-16.0)	2.8-25.5	-	10.7 (7.5-13.0)	4.6-21.0	Euronut SENECA Investigators 1991
75-90	10.7	-	-	8.1	-	-	Lonergan *et al.* 1975

(1) The range shown is the 2.5-97.5 centile for the studies of Gregory *et al.*, the 10-90 centile for the SENECA study, and the observed extreme range for the study of Davies and Holdsworth.

(2) Data were reported for 17 separate centres; the mean and extreme values of the published median values are shown, with the lowest 10th centile and highest 90th centile of those reported.

Table 24.4: Major sources of iron in average British diets

	% of average intake
white bread[1]	9
other bread	10
breakfast cereals[1]	10
other cereal products	13
eggs	4
milk and milk products	2
beef and veal	7
liver	3
other meat	13
fish	2
vegetables	15
fruit and nuts	2
confectionery	2
beverages	4

(1) White flour for bread making is fortified with iron in UK,
as are many breakfast cereals
Source: Gregory *et al.* 1990.

Table 24.5: Rich sources of iron

	portion (g)	mg /portion
black pudding	80	16
cockles	50	13
hare	150	12
kidney	150	12
liver	150	12
venison	150	12
mussels	150	9
beans, red kidney	100	7
goose	150	7
sardines canned in tomato	150	7
beef	150	5
cooked chickpeas	150	5
spinach	130	5
duck	150	4
lentils, mung beans (dahl)	150	4
oatmeal	100	4
sardines canned in oil	150	4
beans, haricot	100	3
bloater	150	3
chocolate, plain	125	3
cider	650	3
hamburger	100	3
lamb	150	3
leeks	125	3
pilchards in tomato sauce	100	3
shrimps	150	3
avocados	130	2
bacon joint	150	2
bread, wholemeal or brown	70	2
chocolate, milk	125	2
coconut	75	2
crab	175	2
dogfish	150	2
herring	150	2
mackerel	150	2
pork	150	2
prawns	150	2
rabbit	150	2
scampi	150	2
skate	150	2
trout	150	2
tuna	150	2
veal	150	2
whiting	150	2

Table 24.6: Amounts of absorbed iron required for maintenance and to replace menstrual losses in women

| | adult women | | | | | | adolescent girls | |
| | no contraception | | oral contraceptives | | intra-uterine device | | no contraception | |
centile	mg/d	μmol/d	mg/d	μmol/d	mg/d	μmol/d	mg/d	μmol/d
50	1.36	24	1.11	20	1.82	32.5	1.73	31
75	1.74	31	1.31	23.5	2.58	46	2.11	37
90	2.27	41	1.59	28.5	3.64	65	2.65	47
95	2.84	51	1.89	33.5	4.78	85.5	3.21	57.5

Source: from data reported by Hallberg and Rossander-Hultén 1991.

Table 24.7: Relative biological availability of iron in foods

	low availability	mg /portion	moderate availability	mg /portion	high availability	mg /portion
cereals	maize	1	maize flour	1.4 mg/100g		
	oats	4	white flour	2.0 mg/100g		
	rice	< 0.1				
	whole wheat flour	4 mg/100g				
fruits	apples	0.2	melon	1	guava	< 0.1
	avocado	2	mango	1	lemons	0.1
	bananas	1	pineapple	1	oranges	1
	grapes	0.2			pawpaw	< 0.1
	peaches	0.3				
	pears	< 0.1				
	plums	0.3				
	rhubarb	0.4				
	strawberries	1				
vegetables	aubergine	0.2	carrots	0.2	tomatoes	0.3
	butterbeans	1	potatoes	1	beetroot	0.16
	broad beans	1			cabbage	1
	lentils	4			cauliflower	0.3
	spinach	5			turnip	0.5
nuts	almonds	1				
	brazil nuts	1				
	coconut	2				
	walnuts	1				
	peanuts	1				
protein foods	egg	1			fish	
	soya flour	7 mg/100g			meat	see Table 24.5
					poultry	

Classification of biological availability as reported by Bothwell *et al.* 1989.

Table 24.8: Factors affecting iron absoprtion

inhibition	enhancement
calcium[1]	ascorbic acid
dietary fibre	alcohol
oxalates	organic acids
phosphates	amino acids
phytates	meat protein
polyphenols	
soya protein	
egg protein	

(1) High intakes of calcium inhibit absorption of haem and non-haem iron; other factors shown here affect only the absorption of non-haem iron.

Table 24.9: Reference intakes of iron

	US RDA (1989)	UK RNI (1991)		EU PRI (1993)
	mg	mol	mg	mg
birth-3 m	6	30	1.7	-
3-6 m	6	80	4.3	-
7-9 m	10	140	7.8	6
9m-1y	10	140	7.8	6
1-3 y	10	120	6.9	4
4-6	10	110	6.1	4
7-10	10	160	8.7	6
males				
11-14	12	200	11.3	10
15-18	12	200	11.3	13
19-24	10	160	8.7	9
25-50	10	160	8.7	9
> 50	10	160	8.7	-
females				
11-14	15	260	14.8	18-22
15-18	15	260	14.8	17-21
19-24	15	260	14.8	16-20
25-50	15	260	14.8	16-20
> 50	10	160	8.7	8
pregnant	30	-	-	-
lactating	15	-	-	10

The UK reference intakes are calculated in molar terms; UK and EU figures make no recommendation for any increment in pregnancy.
Where two figures are shown for the EU PRI, the lower figure is to meet the 90th centile, and the higher the 95th centile, of requirements.
Source: National Research Council 1989; Department of Health 1991; Scientific Committee for Food 1993.

Table 24.10: Serum iron, total iron binding capacity and transferrrin saturation in various conditions

	serum iron				TIBC				fractional saturation
	μg/dL		μmol/L		μg/dL		μmol/L		
	mean	range	mean	range	mean	range	mean	range	
normal adults	127	67-191	22.7	67-191	333	253-416	59.6	45-74	0.35 ± 10
iron deficiency anaemia	32	0-78	5.7	0-14	482	204-705	86.3	36-126	< 0.16
late pregnancy	94	22-185	16.8	4-33	532	373-712	95.3	67-127	0.18
haemochromatosis	250	191-290	44.7	34-52	262	205-330	46.9	37-59	0.4-1.0
infection	47	30-72	8.4	5-13	260	182-270	46.6	33-48	0.18
chronic inflammatory disease	-	20-50	-	3.5-9	< 260	-	< 46	-	0.1-0.25

Source: from data reported by Underwood 1977.

Table 24.11: Whole blood haemoglobin concentrations and haemotocrit values indicative of anaemia (for people living at or near sea level).

	haemoglobin (g/L)		haematocrit[1]	
	normal	anaemia	normal	anaemia
children 0.5-6 y	130	< 110	-	-
6-14 y	140	< 120	-	-
adult men	153	< 130	> 0.44	< 0.38
adult women	140	< 120	> 0.33	< 0.32
pregnant women	130	< 110	-	< 0.31

(1) Haematocrit is the proportional volume of packed cells after centrifugation of a blood sample.

Table 24.12: Diagnostic criteria for iron deficiency

		diagnostic range
storage iron	bone marrow examination	not detectable
	total iron binding capacity	> 400 µg/dL (> 72 µmol/L)
	serum ferritin	< 20 µg/L
functional iron	transferrin saturation	< 0.16
	erythrocyte protoporphyrin IX[1]	> 1.2 µmol /L red cells
	mean cell volume	< 80 fL
	serum transferrin receptor	> 9 mg/L
	haemoglobin	< 130 g/L (men), < 120 g/L (women)

(1) Red cell protoporphyrin IX is also elevated in lead poisoning.
Source: from data reported by Cook and Skikne 1989.

Table 24.13: Reference ranges for red cell parameters

	red cell count x 10^{12} /L	haematocrit	whole blood haemoglobin g/L	mean corpuscular haemoglobin (MCH), pg	mean cell volume (mcv) fL	reticulocytes %
new-born infants	4.0-5.6	0.44-0.62	136-196	32-39	106	2-6
3 m old	3.2-4.5	0.32-0.44	95-125	24-34	-	-
1 y old	3.6-5.0	0.36-0.44	110-130	23-31	70-86	0-2
2-6 y old	-	0.34-0.40	110-140	-	74-87	0-2
6-12 y old	4.2-5.2	0.37-0.44	115-148	24-30	77-91	0-2
males 12-18	-	0.38-0.48	130-160	-	78-88	0-2
adult males	4.5-6.5	0.40-0.54	135-180	27-32	76-94	0-2
females 12-18	-	0.36-0.46	120-160	-	78-88	0-2
adult females	3.9-5.6	0.36-0.46	115-160	26-31	76-94	0-2
post-menopausal	4.3-6.0	0.40-0.48	130-160	27-32	83-95	0-2

Source: from data reported by Dallman 1977; Eastham and Slade 1992; Firkin *et al.* 1989; Hall and Malia 1991.

Table 24.14: Iron deficiency and overload

	iron overload	reference range	iron depletion	iron deficient	microcytic anaemia
reticulo-endothelial marrow iron	> 4	2-3	< 1	0	0
total iron binding capacity (μmol /L)	< 53	59 ± 5	65	70	73
plasma ferritin (μg /L)	> 300	100 ± 60	20	10	< 10
iron absorption %	> 15	5-10	10-15	10-20	10-20
plasma iron (μmol /L)	> 31	20.5 ± 0.9	20	< 10	< 7
transferrin saturation %	> 60	35 ± 15	30	< 15	< 15
sideroblasts %	40-60	40-60	40-60	< 10	< 10
protoporphyrin IX[1] μmol /L rbc	0.5	0.5	0.5	1.8	3.6

(1) Red cell protoporphyrin IX is also elevated in lead poisoning.

Source: Herbert 1987.

25

Mineral nutrition

Any mineral for which a metabolic or physiological function has been determined is, by definition, a dietary essential. The various functions of minerals include forming the mineral of the skeleton (a structural role), membrane function (trans-membrane ion gradients), prosthetic groups of enzymes (probably one-third of all enzymes require a metal ion or a metal-derived prosthetic group), and metabolic and cell regulation and hormone action. In addition, a number of minerals are known to be dietary essentials, but as yet no metabolic functions have been defined, and some minerals have (beneficial) effects in the body, but these are probably pharmacological actions rather than reflecting a true essential function and dietary requirement. In Table 25.1 the minerals are listed under these functions; some have more than one function, and appear under more than one heading. Table 25.2 shows the total body content, and Table 25.3 the plasma concentrations, of minerals.

Estimation of physiological mineral requirements is, in principle, simpler than estimation of requirements for vitamins, since balance studies are simpler to conduct for individual elements than for organic compounds which may be excreted as a variety of metabolites. For many of the minerals discussed in this chapter, and for iron (see Chapter 24), calcium and phosphate (see sections 14.1 and 14.2) and selenium (see section 15.1.2), this is true. However, for other minerals the amounts required are extremely small, and dietary deficiency is virtually unknown; the small amounts present in water and plant foods are (more than) adequate to meet requirements. For these minerals there are no estimates of requirement or reference intakes, but simply ranges, based on observed intakes, that are obviously safe and adequate. In such cases requirements are probably considerably lower than these ranges of safe intakes. For some minerals that are known to be dietary essentials it is not possible to quote even ranges of safe and adequate intakes.

Determination of mineral balance is complicated by the fact that many minerals are lost from the body not only in urine, but also by other routes.

1. Secretion into the bile, so that it is difficult to differentiate between endogenous losses and unabsorbed dietary intake. In general, cationic minerals such as zinc, manganese and copper are excreted largely in the bile, while anionic minerals such as chromium, molybdenum and iodine are excreted largely by the kidneys.

2. In sweat, so that losses are difficult to measure and vary with environmental temperature.

3. In shed skin cells, hair and nails.

The accumulation of minerals in hair and nails has been used to assess both the adequacy or otherwise of body reserves, and possible toxic accumulation. In some cases this provides useful information, while in others either the hair content is unrelated to status or, as in the case of zinc (see section 25.26.3), exogenous sources confound the interpretation of results.

Table 25.4 gives estimated intakes of various minerals, and the proportions lost in urine, faeces, sweat, and hair and nails. Menstrual blood loss is an important loss of iron and zinc in women.

A major problem in attempting to define nutritional requirements for minerals is that of biological availability and efficiency of absorption. For many minerals, the proportion of dietary intake that is absorbed varies with the state of the body's reserves of the mineral, partly as a result of the presence or absence of free binding proteins in the intestinal mucosa, and apo-transport proteins in the bloodstream.

The biological availability of minerals depends on a number of factors.

1. The chemical form and oxidation state of the mineral in the food, or under the conditions prevailing in the intestinal lumen.

2. The presence in the intestinal lumen of antagonistic ligands such as carbonate, oxalate, phosphate, phytate, and tannate ions, and polyphenols, which form insoluble salts or complexes with many minerals, fatty acids that form insoluble calcium and magnesium soaps, and some forms of dietary fibre, which bind mineral salts.

3. The presence on the intestinal lumen of facilitatory ligands such as ascorbate, carboxylic acids, amino acids, phosphatidic acid, and some sugars, which form soluble chelates that are readily absorbed.

4. The presence in the intestinal lumen of competing metal ions; the major deleterious interactions between minerals are shown in Table 25.5.

The mineral content of plant foods is especially variable, depending not only on variety, but also, to a very considerable extent, on the growth conditions and the availability of minerals from the soil. Therefore in many cases data on minerals in tables of food composition must be regarded as being very approximate.

25.1 The major electrolytes: sodium, potassium and chloride

The major cation in extracellular fluid is sodium, while the major intracellular cation is potassium; the major anion in all body fluids is chloride. For a discussion of total body potassium as an index of cell fat-free mass, see section 2.2.1.3. Reference ranges for plasma electrolytes are shown in Table 25.3. Maintenance of sodium balance is essential for control of the volume and osmotic pressure of extracellular fluid and acid–base balance, as well as the electrophysiological activity of nerve and muscle membranes, and active transport across cell membranes.

The excitability of cell membranes is due to active, ATP-dependent pumping of Na^+ ions out of the cell, and K^+ ions inwards—the sodium-potassium pump (Na^+-K^+ ATPase, EC 3.6.1.37). The electrical activity of nerves is the result of rapid entry of Na^+ ions, and efflux of K^+, leading to transient depolarization of the nerve membrane. Sodium that has been pumped out of cells in exchange for hydrogen ions (the sodium pump) can re-enter together with substrates (sodium-dependent co-transport, see section 6.2) or in exchange for products and waste material being exported from the cell (sodium-dependent counter-transport).

The regulation of plasma and tissue concentrations of sodium and potassium depends on control of their excretion. Sodium losses are controlled by varying the rate of resorption of sodium ions from the glomerular filtrate, while potassium losses are controlled by varying the rate of potassium secretion in the renal tubules. The ability to conserve sodium is considerably greater than the ability to conserve potassium; in times of deficiency sodium losses may be less than 1 mmol (23 mg)/day, while potassium losses cannot be reduced below 5–15 mmol (600–1800 mg)/day. Potassium depletion may occur in starvation, while sodium depletion is unlikely unless there is significant loss in sweat.

The mineralocorticoid hormone aldosterone, secreted by the adrenal cortex, stimulates the resorption of sodium, by increasing the activity of the Na^+-K^+ pump, so as sodium is retained, potassium will be lost. In turn, aldosterone secretion is regulated by angiotensin II and adrenocorticotrophic hormone (ACTH).

Angiotensinogen is an inactive peptide precursor, secreted by the liver; it is cleaved to angiotensin I by the enzyme renin (EC 3.4.23.15), which is secreted by the kidney in response to a fall in either plasma sodium or blood pressure. Angiotensin I is inactive, and is activated to angiotensin II by a further peptidase, which is located in the blood vessels of the lungs (angiotensin converting enzyme, EC 3.4.15.1). Angiotensin II is the active hormone which stimulates the synthesis and secretion of aldosterone, and the release of ACTH and antidiuretic hormone (ADH) from the pituitary. ADH acts to increase water resorption in the distal kidney tubules.

The 95 per cent range of sodium intakes in UK (based on determination of urinary sodium excretion) is 65–240 mmol (1.5–5.6 g)/day in men and 50–160 mmol (1.1–3.7 g) in women (Gregory *et al.* 1990)—considerably above the minimum levels of intake at which adults can maintain sodium balance (10–20 mmol (230–460 mg)/day). Sanchez-Castillo *et al.* (1987) labelled table salt with lithium chloride, and estimated that 10 per cent of sodium intake was from the sodium naturally present in foods, 15 per cent from that added in cooking and at the table, and 75 per cent from salt added in manufacture and processing.

In most countries, the problem is not one of inadequate sodium intake to meet requirements, but rather one of sodium intake sufficiently in excess of requirements that it poses a health hazard. There is excellent epidemiological evidence that in some individuals high intakes of sodium are associated with the development of (clinically significant) hypertension, which in turn is a risk factor for coronary thrombosis and stroke. Equally, patients with hypertension benefit from severe restriction of sodium intake. The benefits for the population as a whole of a more modest restriction of sodium intake are less clear, but it is estimated that 10 per cent of the population are salt sensitive, and are at risk of developing hypertension as a result of excessive sodium intake (Intersalt Cooperative Research Group 1988).

Potassium depletion elevates blood pressure, even in normotensive subjects, and potassium-depleted subjects become salt sensitive. Therefore as well as sodium intake, the ratio of sodium:potassium in the diet is an important factor. Acute hyperkalaemia, associated with an intake of about 450 mmol (18 g) of potassium in an adult, can prove fatal because it may cause cardiac arrest.

Estimates of requirements for sodium, potassium and chloride are shown in Table 25.6. The US Recommended Dietary Allowances publication (National Research Council 1989) gives no figures for RDA for these minerals, but notes that the requirement of 22 mmol (500 mg) sodium for adults is substantially exceeded by usual diets, and on the basis of the evidence linking sodium intake and hypertension recommends that sodium intake be limited to no more than 100 mmol (2.4 g) /day (equivalent to 6 g of table salt). There is also a note that although the adult requirement for potassium is 50 mmol (2 g)/day, a desirable level of intake for reduction of the risk of hypertension is 90 mmol (3.5 g)/day. The European Union Population Reference Intakes publication (Scientific Committee for Foods 1993) quoted an acceptable range of intakes of sodium (for adults) as being 25–150 mmol (575–3500 mg)/day. The UK Reference Intakes for sodium and potassium, and the EU Population Reference Intakes for potassium, are shown in Table 25.7.

25.2 Aluminium

Aluminium is the third most abundant element in the earth's crust, but because of its low solubility little is present in most foods. It is more soluble in acid media; indeed one of the problems associated with acid rain is that plants absorb toxic amounts of aluminium from acid soil water. Significant amounts of aluminium may dissolve from aluminium cooking vessels and cans containing acid foods and beverages. However, much of this will be precipitated in the alkaline conditions of the small intestine, and as little as 0.4 μmol (10 μg) of the 0.4–0.8 mmol (10–20 mg) aluminium in average diets is absorbed (Powell and Thompson 1993).

Studies with radioactive ^{26}Al given intravenously show that most is excreted in the urine within a few days. However, 5–10 per cent was retained in the body, only being lost with a very long half-time, suggesting that aluminium can accumulate in the body, and especially in the liver and skeleton (Priest 1993).

Considerable amounts of aluminium are absorbed from the dialysis fluid by patients undergoing routine haemodialysis for kidney failure. Aluminium intoxication is a factor in the aetiology of dialysis dementia, metabolic bone disease and microcytic anaemia. The mechanism by which aluminium causes bone mineral loss is not clear, but *in vitro* it reduces the proliferation of osteoblasts; aluminium also inhibits the secretion of parathyroid hormone, and may inhibit calcidiol 1–hydroxylase (see section 14.3.2.2). Aluminium also causes hypercalciuria, but this seems to be the result of reduced uptake of calcium into bone, rather than the cause (Klein 1995).

Aluminium has similar coordination chemistry to iron, and it will bind to both transferrin and ferritin (see section 24.3). Ferritin has 7 binding sites for iron/molecule; when it contains 1 mol aluminium / mol of protein it is insoluble and unable to bind iron in the usual way. There is some evidence that aluminium loading of ferritin leads to increased free iron ions in tissues, and hence increased oxygen radical damage (see section 24.5). Loss of normal iron reserves by precipitation of ferritin presumably explains the development of microcytic anaemia in dialysis patients (Joshi 1990).

There is no evidence that aluminium is an aetiological factor in Alzheimer's disease; although the abnormal neurofibrillar tangles that characterize this condition have been reported to contain aluminium, there is no difference in aluminium content between brain tissue from affected patients and controls. Although some epidemiological studies have suggested an association between high levels of aluminium in drinking water and increased incidence of Alzheimer's disease, others fail to show such an association. Experimentally, aluminium salts induce the formation of neurofilamentous inclusions in the central nervous system, but these, and those that develop in dialysis dementia, differ from those seen in Alzheimer's disease (Priest 1993; Rowan 1993).

25.3 Antimony

Antimony is not known to be a dietary essential, and has no known function in the body. About 15 per cent of the intake of 2–10 µmol (0.25–1.25 mg)/day is absorbed, and accumulates in liver, kidney, skin and adrenals; toxic effects include gastrointestinal symptoms and respiratory depression.

25.4 Arsenic

Arsenic-deficient animals suffer growth retardation, impaired fertility, altered protein synthesis and elevated plasma uric acid. There is, however, no evidence that it is essential for human beings, and no metabolic function has been described. It is well known as a toxic mineral; there is no evidence that even shellfish, which can accumulate relatively large amounts from industrial effluent, provide a toxic hazard to human beings. Average intakes are considerably greater than those required to prevent the development of deficiency signs in experimental animals.

Most arsenic is excreted in the urine, mainly as dimethylarsenic acid (cacodylic acid), and a considerable amount accumulates in the hair and nails.

25.5 Boron

The average intake of boron is 140–370 µmol (1.5–4 mg) /day. Dietary borates are well absorbed (> 90 per cent), and rapidly excreted in the urine. Tissue concentrations are of the order of 9–20 µmol (0.1–0.2 µg) /g, and several-fold higher in bone. There is no evidence of essentiality, or any physiological function, of boron in human or animal metabolism, although it is well-established as an essential mineral in plants.

Boron-deficient animals suffer growth retardation and bone abnormalities, including elevated serum alkaline phosphatase (EC 3.1.3.1). There is some evidence of effects of boron on the actions of calcitriol and oestrogens and a role has been suggested in cell membrane function and transmembrane signalling. Boron supplements have been shown to reduce urinary excretion of calcium, magnesium and phosphate in post-menopausal women (Nielsen 1987, 1991), but the results have not been confirmed in other studies, and there is no evidence to suggest that boron supplements may be beneficial in the treatment of prevention of post-menopausal osteoporosis (see section 14.5).

25.6 Bromine

There is no evidence that bromine serves any physiological function in plants or animals. Bromide exchanges with chloride in tissues to a considerable extent, and it is accumulated in the thyroid gland in iodine deficiency (see section 25.14.4), although it is not utilized. It has been suggested that bromide depletion results in insomnia in patients undergoing renal dialysis; however bromides have long been used as hypnotics, and this may represent a pharmacological rather than physiological action.

25.7 Cadmium

There is evidence that animals maintained on highly purified diets develop muscle weakness and mitochondrial abnormalities if not provided with cadmium. The enzyme carnosinase (EC 3.4.13.20), which hydrolyses the dipeptide carnosine (β-alanyl-histidine) is a cadmium-dependent metallo-enzyme. However, cadmium toxicity is of greater concern; the WHO recommended upper limit of habitual cadmium intake is 500–630 nmol (57–71 µg)/day, compared with an estimated intake (in USA) of 180–360 nmol (20–40 µg)/day. About 5 per cent of dietary cadmium is absorbed, increasing in iron deficiency and inhibited by copper and zinc, suggesting a common absorption mechanism.

Only a very small fraction of the body content of cadmium is excreted, and the total body content increases with age. Most accumulates in the kidneys, where it has a long half-life (of the order of 18–30 years), and causes damage to the proximal tubules where small proteins are resorbed. Early cadmium poisoning can be detected by the urinary excretion of detectable amounts of β_2-microglobulin; as the kidney burden of cadmium increases, so there is irreversible damage and significant proteinuria. Cadmium toxicity may also lead to the development of a painful osteomalacia, known by its Japanese name of *itai-itai* disease.

25.8 Caesium

There is no evidence that caesium has any function in the body; the radioactive isotope ^{137}Cs has a half-life of 30 years, and is accumulated in muscle, so that meat from animals grazing on contaminated pasture is unfit for consumption, because of the radiation hazard.

25.9 Chromium

The body content of chromium is of the order of 0.4–0.8 µmol (20–40 µg)/kg, falling rapidly post-natally, and decreasing steadily throughout adult life. Less than 1 per cent of a test dose of chromium (Cr^{3+}) salts is absorbed; in plasma it is transported bound to the iron-binding protein transferrin (see 24.3.1), and to a lesser extent albumin. Most chromium excretion is in the urine, although a small amount is excreted in bile and sweat. Urinary excretion of chromium increases markedly after administration of either insulin or a glucose load.

There are few reliable data on the chromium content of foods; falsely high values result from contamination of samples by chromium-containing stainless steel blenders and other implements, as well as contamination from particulate chromium in the air. Average intakes of chromium are between 0.2–1.3 µmol (10–60 µg)/day.

Patients maintained on long-term total parenteral nutrition without any source of chromium develop impaired glucose tolerance (see section 7.7.2), which responds (relatively slowly) to the administration of chromium salts, and more rapidly to organic chromium complexes in such sources as yeast extract.

Chromium deficiency may be a factor in the impairment of glucose tolerance and glucose utilization in children suffering from protein-energy malnutrition (see section 12.2); a number of studies have demonstrated improved glucose tolerance after administration of inorganic chromium salts (chromium chloride) to malnourished children. Some adequately nourished elderly people with impaired glucose tolerance or frank diabetes show an improvement after the administration of chromium salts, although the majority show no response. In those who do respond there is an increase in plasma chromium, suggesting that there may have been some degree of chromium depletion. There is inadequate evidence to make any recommendations concerning chromium intakes for people with impaired glucose tolerance or diabetes (Glinsmann and Mertz 1966; Levine *et al.* 1968).

25.9.1 Glucose tolerance factor

The organic chromium complex isolated from yeast has been called the glucose tolerance factor (GTF); *in vitro*, partially purified preparations greatly increase the uptake and utilization of glucose by adipose tissue incubated with insulin. The mechanism of this enhancement of insulin responsiveness is not known, but GTF binds to the α-amino groups, and possibly ε-amino groups of lysine, in insulin, resulting in enhanced binding to cell-surface receptors (Evans *et al.* 1973).

Early studies of GTF suggested that it was a nicotinic acid chelate of trivalent chromium (Cr^{3+}), and synthetic chromium-nicotinic acid complexes do indeed enhance insulin action in isolated adipose tissue. However, in experimental animals the synthetic chromium-nicotinic acid complex does not have the same tissue distribution as injected chromium chloride. The greater biological activity of organic chromium complexes, such as those found in yeast, may be the result of their greater absorption; up to 10–25 per cent, compared with less than 1 per cent for inorganic chromium salts (Mertz 1974).

A variety of different organic complexes containing chromium chelated to various amino acids and small peptides, as well as nicotinic acid, have been shown to possess GTF activity *in vitro*; suggesting that it may not be a single compound. Growing yeast in presence of relatively high concentrations of chromium salts leads to increased formation of organic complexes with GTF activity, suggesting that this may represent a mechanism for detoxication of chromium in the yeast.

Estimated safe and adequate levels of chromium intake are shown in Table 25.8.

25.9.2 Chromium toxicity

Trivalent chromium salts have low toxicity; no adverse effects have been observed in experimental animals fed diets containing 2 mmol (100 mg) /kg diet. By contrast, hexavalent chromium salts (chromates, CrO_4^{2-}) are very toxic, both by ingestion and by inhalation. Industrial exposure to chromate-containing dust is associated with increased incidence of lung cancer, and ingestion of chromates leads to liver and kidney necrosis.

Chromates are potent oxidizing agents both *in vitro* and *in vivo*, and result (indirectly) in oxidative damage to DNA, and hence carcinogenesis. Tissue necrosis may be the result of inhibition of mitochondrial activity by chromate, which both oxidizes NADH directly (hence short-circuiting normal electron transport) and also inhibits a number of key mitochondrial enzymes at relatively low concentrations (Wetterhahn and Hamilton 1989; Ryberg and Alexander 1990).

25.10   Cobalt

The importance of cobalt in ruminant nutrition has been known for many years. The established role of cobalt in mammalian metabolism is in vitamin B_{12} (see section 21.5). Therefore, apart from ruminants, whose intestinal flora can synthesize vitamin B_{12} that is subsequently available to the host, there is no evidence that inorganic cobalt is a dietary requirement. Cobalt deficiency in ruminants is, apparently, vitamin B_{12} deficiency, and can be treated by injection of the vitamin or dietary cobalt.

Although deficiency of cobalt *per se* is unknown, it is presumably an essential mineral in its own right, since methionyl aminopeptidase (EC 3.4.11.18), the enzyme which catalyses the removal of the amino terminal methionine from most nascent peptides on the ribosome, has two cobalt atoms in its catalytic site. A number of other aminopeptidases are also cobalt metallo-enzymes, and there is some evidence that phosphoprotein phosphatase (EC3.1.3.16) is a cobalt metallo-enzyme.

Inorganic cobalt salts are well absorbed; balance studies suggest that between 20–95 per cent of the dietary intake is absorbed. The absorption increases in iron deficiency, and there is mutual competition between test doses of inorganic iron and cobalt, suggesting that they share the same mechanism for intestinal uptake (see section 24.2.3).

Inorganic cobalt salts stimulate erythropoeisis; however, the amounts required to have any significant effect are within the toxic range, and thyroid hyperplasia, and congestive heart failure may occur. During the 1950s and 1960s, cobalt salts were used as an additive in brewing, to maintain the head on beer. In Belgium, Canada, and the USA there were outbreaks of cardiac failure, with pericardial effusion and low cardiac output, among heavy beer drinkers. The problem was attributed to cobalt toxicity, possibly together with high alcohol consumption, and perhaps thiamin deficiency (Kesteloot *et al.* 1968), since the levels of cobalt intake were very considerably lower than those previously associated with toxicity.

25.11   Copper

In addition to classical nutritional studies, a great deal has been learnt about copper metabolism, and the effects of both deficiency and excess, from two rare inborn errors of metabolism: Menkes' steely (or kinky) hair syndrome, in which there is defective intestinal absorption of copper, and defective tissue uptake, leading to severe functional copper deficiency, and Wilson's disease, in which there is defective excretion of copper in bile, leading to abnormal tissue accumulation.

25.11.1 Intakes and sources of copper

The reference intakes for copper shown in Table 25.9 are based on a limited number of studies showing that balance can be maintained on intakes around 20 μmol (1.2 mg)/day, and copper-responsive metabolic abnormalities have been observed in subjects maintained on intakes of 11–16 μmol (0.7–1.0 mg) /day. In addition to the food sources shown in Table 25.10, significant amounts can be obtained from drinking water where there is copper plumbing, especially with soft water. Average daily intakes of copper in UK are 25 μmol (1.6 mg) for men (range 12–54 μmol) and 19 μmol (1.2 mg) for women (range 9–44 μmol) (Gregory *et al.* 1990).

25.11.2 Absorption, metabolism, and excretion of copper

Copper is absorbed by carrier-mediated uptake into duodenal mucosal cells, followed by binding to the protein metallothionein (see section 25.26.1). The genetic defect in Menkes' steely hair syndrome appears to involve a copper-dependent ATPase, suggesting that copper is either taken into the mucosal cell, or transported from the mucosal cell into the plasma, by an active process. Normally about 30 per cent of dietary copper is absorbed; there is some evidence that the proportion absorbed increases in deficiency.

Zinc in excess of normal levels of intake (see section 25.26) significantly impairs the absorption of copper; two mechanisms have been proposed to explain this.

1. Both ions compete for the same binding protein in the intestinal mucosa.

2. Zinc induces synthesis of increased amounts of metallothionein in mucosal cells, leading to increased intracellular retention of copper and failure of transport from the mucosal cell into plasma.

Calcium supplements (see sections 14.1.1 and 24.2.3.1) may also impair copper absorption, by increasing the pH of the intestinal contents, and so rendering copper salts less soluble.

Newly absorbed copper is bound to serum albumin and the high affinity transport protein transcuprein. Some is also present in plasma as amino acid chelates. After absorption it accumulates in the liver, and is then released into the circulation bound to ceruloplasmin.

More than 80 per cent of plasma copper is bound to ceruloplasmin (EC 1.16.3.1), an α_2-globulin that contains 6 copper atoms /mol. Ceruloplasmin both serves as a copper transport protein and also has two oxidase activities:

(1) amine oxidase, which is of unknown importance;

(2) ferri-oxidase, which is important in the mobilization of iron reserves (see section 24.3.2).

Copper is taken up by tissues by binding to what is probably the same copper-binding metallothionein as occurs in the intestinal mucosa, since in patients who lack this protein (Menkes' steely hair syndrome), tissue uptake of copper is also impaired, and intravenous administration of copper has no beneficial effect.

The body content of copper is about 11 μmol (720 μg), or 277 nmol (1.7 μg) /g fat-free tissue in adults, and 2.5–3–fold higher in new-born infants. The tissue distribution of copper is shown in Table 25.11.

Copper balance is maintained almost entirely by excretion in the bile. Normally less than 5 per cent of absorbed copper is excreted in urine (although the proportion increases considerably in biliary obstruction). The copper secreted in bile is not biologically available for reabsorption, and there is no enterohepatic circulation. The chemical form of this copper has not been identified; it may be present either as partially degraded ceruloplasmin or chelated to bilirubin (see section 24.3.3.2).

25.11.3 Metabolic functions of copper and signs of deficiency

The main copper-dependent enzymes are shown in Table 24.12.

Copper deficiency (either dietary deficiency, which is extremely rare, or the functional deficiency of Menkes' steely hair syndrome) leads to what appears to be iron-deficiency anaemia, a hypochromic microcytic anaemia, which does not respond to iron therapy, and occurs despite adequate iron reserves (see section 24.4). The cause of this functional iron deficiency is impaired ferri-oxidase activity of ceruloplasmin, which catalyses the oxidation of Fe^{2+} in ferritin to Fe^{3+}, permitting its transfer onto transferrin (see section 24.3).

The importance of ceruloplasmin in iron metabolism has been demonstrated by two reports of patients with a genetic total lack of ceruloplasmin— in addition to neurological damage, the affected subjects showed apparent iron deficiency anaemia together with haemochromatosis (iron overload, see section 24.5, Danks 1995). Ceruloplasmin also catalyses the oxidation of manganese $Mn^{2+} \rightarrow Mn^{3+}$, permitting this ion also to be carried by transferrin (see section 25.16).

The signs for which Menkes' steely hair syndrome is named, the abnormal texture and pigmentation of the hair, can be attributed to two copper-dependent enzymes: thiol oxidase, which is responsible for the oxidation of the sulphydryl groups of cysteine to form disulphide bridges in proteins, and tyrosinase, which is responsible for the oxidation of tyrosine to form melanin. Similar changes in the texture of wool occur in copper-deficient sheep. As a result of impaired formation of disulphide bridges, hair contains an abnormally high proportion of free sulphydryl groups in copper deficiency.

Serious neurological damage, a demyelinating encephalopathy leading to ataxia, also occurs in copper deficiency. Part of the problem may be due to either impaired synthesis of catecholamines (noradrenaline and adrenaline) as a result of reduced activity of dopamine β-hydroxylase, or impaired inactivation of neurotransmitter amines as a result of impaired amine oxidase activity. Impaired energy-yielding metabolism as a result of reduced activity of cytochrome oxidase may also be an important factor; in experimental copper deficiency there is characteristic swelling of mitochondria in metabolically active tissues.

Copper deficiency leads to abnormal fragility of bones, similar to the bone defects seen in scurvy (see section 22.5), and, in severe cases, to loss of elasticity of elastin, and aortic aneurysms. The cause of both is defective cross-linking in collagen (leading to impaired bone mineralization, see section 14.3.3.3) and elastin. The cross-links in these two connective tissue proteins are formed by oxidation of the ε-amino group of a lysine residue to an aldehyde (allysine, α-aminoadipic-δ-semialdehyde), followed, in the case of collagen, by reaction of the aldehyde with the ε-amino group of another lysine residue to form dehydrolysinonorleucine (see Fig. 25.1).

Hydroxylysine undergoes similar oxidation to hydroxy-allysine (α-amino-γ-hydroxyadipic-δ-semialdehyde), which forms a Schiff base with lysine to yield hydroxy-dehydrolysinonorleucine. In elastin, the cross-links are formed by reaction between three allysine residues and one lysine, with four chains linked by the formation of desmosine or isodesmo-

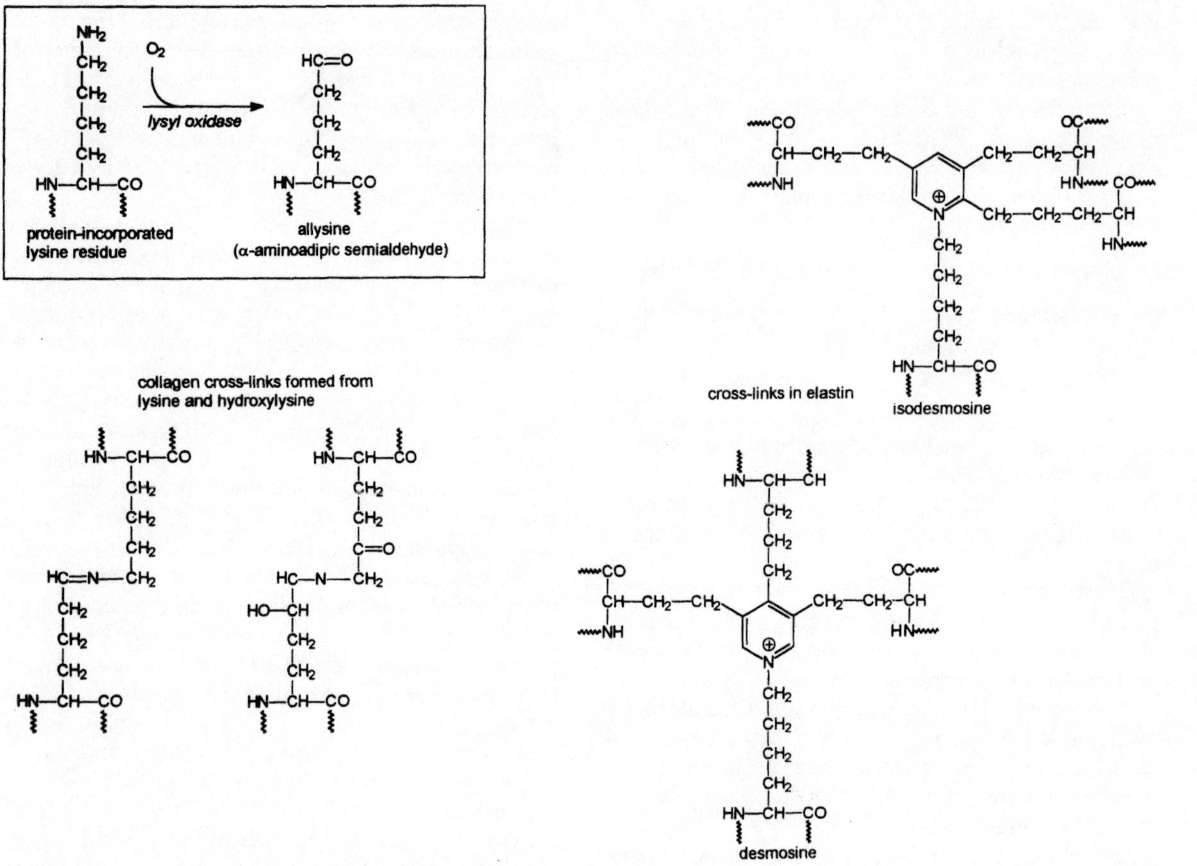

Figure 25.1 The reaction of lysyl oxidase and cross-links in collagen and elastin
Lysyl oxidase EC 1.4.3.13

sine. Measurement of the excretion of the collagen cross-link compounds in urine may provide useful information on the development of osteoporosis (see section 14.5).

Lysyl oxidase, the enzyme that catalyses this oxidation of lysine to allysine, is a copper-dependent enzyme, and its activity is severely impaired in copper deficiency. The enzyme is also inhibited by β-aminopropionitrile, one of the toxins in the sweet pea (*Lathyrus vulgaris*). Lathyrism, sometimes fatal as a result of aortic rupture, is a relatively common problem in drought-stricken areas, where lathyrus peas, which are especially drought resistant, may be the only source of food available. The enzyme contains a catalytic carbonyl group which is believed to be pyrroloquinoline quinone (see section 23.8).

Superoxide dismutase catalyses the dismutation of the superoxide radical to yield hydrogen peroxide:

$$\cdot O_2^- + \cdot O_2^- + 2\,H^+ \rightarrow H_2O_2$$

It is thus an important part of the body's protection against oxygen radical damage. The cytosolic superoxide dismutase is a copper- and zinc-dependent metallo-enzyme; the erythrocyte enzyme is sometimes known as erythrocuprein. Copper deficiency is associated with increased radical damage to tissue lipids, and increased serum low-density lipoprotein (see section 8.3), implying increased risk of atherosclerosis and cancer (Strain 1994). As discussed in section 12.4, copper and zinc deficiency, superimposed on protein-energy malnutrition, leading to reduced activity of superoxide dismutase, have been implicated in the aetiology of kwashiorkor

25.11.4 Copper toxicity

Intake of gram amounts of copper salts can lead to acute intoxication, and hazardous amounts may be ingested from acidic foods that have been in prolonged contact with metallic copper. The symptoms of acute copper poisoning include a metallic taste in the mouth, excessive salivation (ptyalism, or sialorrhea), nausea, vomiting, epigastric burning, gastrointestinal bleeding, and diarrhoea. There may also be haemolysis, hepatic necrosis, tachycardia, convulsions, and coma.

Free copper ions in solution are a major source of oxygen radicals, independent of the presence of superoxide or peroxide. Indeed, copper solutions are used to prepare oxidized low density lipoprotein *in vitro* for experimental studies. Under normal conditions there is little free copper in tissues; most is bound to ceruloplasmin, transcuprein or metallothionein, although a significant proportion of plasma copper is present as soluble amino acid chelates, rather than bound to proteins. However, under conditions of chronic copper overload, there will be an increase in free copper, and increased oxygen radical damage to lipids.

Chronic copper intoxication is a result of the failure of copper excretion, rather than excessive intake—as noted above (section 24.11.2) copper balance is controlled by excretion in the bile. Defects of copper excretion, as occur in Wilson's disease (hepatolenticular degeneration), primary biliary cirrhosis, Indian childhood cirrhosis, and extra-hepatic biliary atresia, lead to a considerable accumulation of copper in the liver (3–50 μmol /g dry weight of tissue, compared with a normal range of 0.3–0.8 μmol /g dry weight), and result in the development of cirrhosis. Especially in Wilson's disease, which is also associated with impaired synthesis of ceruloplasmin, there is also accumulation of copper in the brain (resulting in neurological symptoms), kidneys, and cornea (resulting in corneal degeneration and blindness). Treatment of copper overload is by administration of penicillamine, to chelate tissue stores of copper and permit its excretion in the urine.

25.11.5 Indices of copper status

Measurement of plasma, serum or whole blood copper does not give useful information on copper nutritional status. Most plasma copper is in ceruloplasmin, which is a positive acute phase protein (see section 10.8.4.2), increasing 2–3–fold in chronic' inflammatory disease, and acute and chronic infection. As shown in Table 25.13, there is also an age-related increase in plasma copper, due to an increase in ceruloplasmin, and women have higher plasma concentrations of copper and ceruloplasmin than men. Oral contraceptive steroids, menopausal hormone replacement therapy, and pregnancy also increase ceruloplasmin and copper concentrations markedly. At the time of delivery, plasma copper may be 2–2.5–fold higher than in non-pregnant women of the same age.

The enzymic activity of ceruloplasmin is reduced in experimental copper deficiency, while the total plasma content of ceruloplasmin (as measured immunologically) is unaffected; Milne (1994) suggests that the ratio of enzymically determined:immunologically determined ceruloplasmin may provide a useful index of copper nutrition. Other potential indices of copper status are the erythrocyte superoxide dismutase activity and the activity of cytochrome oxidase in platelets or mononuclear leukocytes. Mean values for these are shown in Table 25.14; there is, as yet, inadequate information from which to construct useful reference ranges and threshold levels that would indicate inadequate copper status.

The hair content of copper, unlike some minerals, is not useful as an index of either inadequate status or copper intoxication; it is neither significantly lower than normal in infants with nutritional deficiency or patients with Menkes' steely hair syndrome, nor significantly elevated in patients suffering from Wilson's disease.

25.12 Fluoride

Fluorine and its ion, fluoride, are not essential, since animals raised on fluoride-deficient diets show no impairment of growth or reproduction over several generations. It is, however, of considerable nutritional interest since a large amount accumulates in bone, forming fluoro-apatite by reaction with hydroxyapatite, which increases the strength and hardness of bone mineral. It also accumulates in dental enamel, and adequate levels of fluoride intake are associated with resistance to dental caries.

The dietary intake of fluoride is extremely variable, depending to a great extent on the fluoride content of drinking water. Natural levels of fluoride in drinking water in most countries range between 10–135 μmol (0.2–2.6 mg) /L, although levels as high as 625 μmol (12 mg) /L have been reported in parts of China, India and Africa, where fluorosis is a common problem. Drinking water containing 130 μmol (2.5 mg) /L fluoride causes dental fluorosis—permanent discoloured patches (mottling) of the teeth. At higher levels of intake, skeletal fluorosis develops—changes in the long bones, with thickening of the cortical areas, and calcification of ligaments and tendons, leading eventually to osteolysis and irreversible skeletal rigidity.

Where drinking water contains negligible amounts of fluoride, the diet provides some 16 nmol (0.3 mg) fluoride /day, and the use of fluoride-containing toothpaste may add up to 100 nmol (2 mg) /day to intake. Safe and adequate levels of fluoride intake are shown in Table 25.25.

The main beneficial effect of fluoride intake on dental caries is seen when the level in drinking water is between 35–60 nmol (0.7–1.2 mg) /L—of the order of 1 ppm; fluoride is added to drinking water in many countries to achieve this level. Where fluoride is not added to water, dietary supplements of fluoride are generally recommended, especially for children, to minimize dental decay. The American Dental Association recommends 0.25 mg /day up to age 2, 0.5 mg /day from age 2–3, and 1 mg /day from age 3–13. However, Pendrys and Stamm (1990) suggested, on the basis of an increase in the incidence of dental fluorosis, that the recommendation for children over the age of 3 is too high, especially in view of the widespread (almost universal) use of fluoride-containing toothpastes. They noted that in areas where fluoride was added to water there had been a 33 per cent increase in the prevalence of dental fluorosis, while in areas where fluoride was not added to water, but supplements were recommended, there had been a 10-fold increase in fluorosis.

There is epidemiological evidence that the incidence of osteoporosis (see section 14.5) is lower in areas where the fluoride intake is high, and fluoride supplements have been tested as both prophylactic and therapeutic treatments of osteoporosis. The results are unclear, and it is not possible to make any recommendations for fluoride intake other than those concerned with reducing dental caries; Gruber and Baylink (1991) concluded that fluoride cannot be recommended for general use in the treatment of osteoporosis.

In addition to the chronic toxicity of fluorosis, fluoride is potentially acutely toxic; at millimolar concentrations it inhibits glycolysis (by inhibition of enolase, EC 4.2.1.11), and stimulates the activity of adenylate cyclase (EC 4.6.1.1), thus increasing intracellular concentrations of cyclic AMP, and potentially disrupting normal metabolic regulation.

25.13   Germanium

There is no evidence that germanium is essential, nor that its consumption confers any benefits. Normal intakes of about 14 μmol (1 mg) /day are excreted rapidly, but there is evidence that consumption of supplements of the order of 0.7–3.4 mmol (50–250 mg) /day cause kidney damage (Matsusaka *et al.* 1988). There is insufficient information to establish safe maximum levels of intake.

25.14   Iodine

Iodine deficiency is a major problem of public health nutrition, affecting some 200 million people worldwide, especially in inland areas over limestone, where the soil content of iodine is extremely low, and hence locally grown crops contain little. In parts of the Andes and Himalayas the incidence of iodine deficiency goitre may be 20–30 per cent, and in some areas may approach 100 per cent. Deficiency also occurs in lowland areas, especially where the soil is acid and water-logged, so that plants are unable to take up much of the iodine that is present. Table 25.16 shows the estimated prevalence of iodine deficiency diseases in developing countries; in addition, deficiency still occurs in other regions, and would be considerably more serious were it not for public health policies of adding iodine (as iodate) to salt or bread, either statutorily or voluntarily.

25.14.1 Iodine intakes and requirements

Intakes of iodine between 0.8–1.2 μmol (100–150 μg) /day are adequate to prevent the development of iodine deficiency disease; in areas where there are relatively large amounts of goitrogens in the diet (see section 7.6), the intake should be between 1.6–2.4 mol (200–300 μg) /day. Foods that are especially rich in goitrogens include cassava, groundnuts and brassicas. The amounts eaten in western countries are not considered to pose any added risk of developing functional iodine deficiency. Reference intakes of iodine are shown in Table 25.17, and rich sources in Table 25.18.

25.14.2 Absorption and metabolism of iodine

Inorganic iodine is readily absorbed in the small intestine, as iodide ions, but probably only 50 per cent of the iodine present in organic compounds in foods is absorbed. The total body content of iodine is 120–160 μmol (15–20 mg), of which 70–80 per cent is accumulated by the thyroid gland. Once requirements for thyroid hormone synthesis have been met, the thyroid does not accumulate more iodide, and excess is excreted in the urine.

The thyroid has an active iodide pump, which is stimulated by the pituitary thyroid-stimulating hormone, thyrotropin, and hence increases in activity in iodine deficiency. Thiocyanate (SCN⁻), formed by the metabolism of cyanide, competes with iodide for uptake, and when present in the diet can be a precipitating factor in the development of goitre (see section 25.14.4).

Within the thyroid, iodide diffuses into the colloid space in the follicles, where it is oxidized to elemental iodine (I_2). As shown in Fig. 25.2, the enzyme iodinase (peroxidase, EC 1.11.1.8) catalyses the iodination of tyrosine residues in the protein thyroglobulin, forming mono-iodo and then di-iodotyrosine residues. The same enzyme then catalyses the transfer of a di-iodophenyl group from one di-iodotyrosine residue onto another, forming protein-incorporated thyroxine, and small amounts of tri-iodothyronine when one of the residues is mono-iodotyrosine. Although one-third of the 140 tyrosine residues in thyrogloblin are iodinated, only four are involved in the coupling reaction, those at positions 5, 2555, 2569, and 2748.

Iodinated thyroglobulin is then taken up into the thyroid cells from the colloid, and undergoes proteolysis to release thyroxine (T_4) and small amounts of tri-iodothyronine (T_3). The hormones are released from the thyroid under stimulation by thyrotropin; in turn, circulating T_4 regulates the secretion of thyrotropin. Free iodotyrosine is de-iodinated in the thyroid, and the iodine re-utilized. Under normal conditions, the amount of iodinated thyroglobulin in the colloid of the gland is sufficient to meet hormone secretion requirements for about 100 days.

Various glucosinolates and other compounds found naturally in foods (see section 7.6 and Table 7.13) are goitrogenic; they act by inhibiting the iodination of tyrosine, and especially the iodination of mono-iodotyrosine to di-iodotyrosine. Both naturally occurring and synthetic goitrogens are used in the treatment of thyrotoxicosis (over-activity of the thyroid).

Thyroxine (T_4) and tri-iodothyronine (T_3) circulate bound to the thyroid-binding globulin, transthyr-

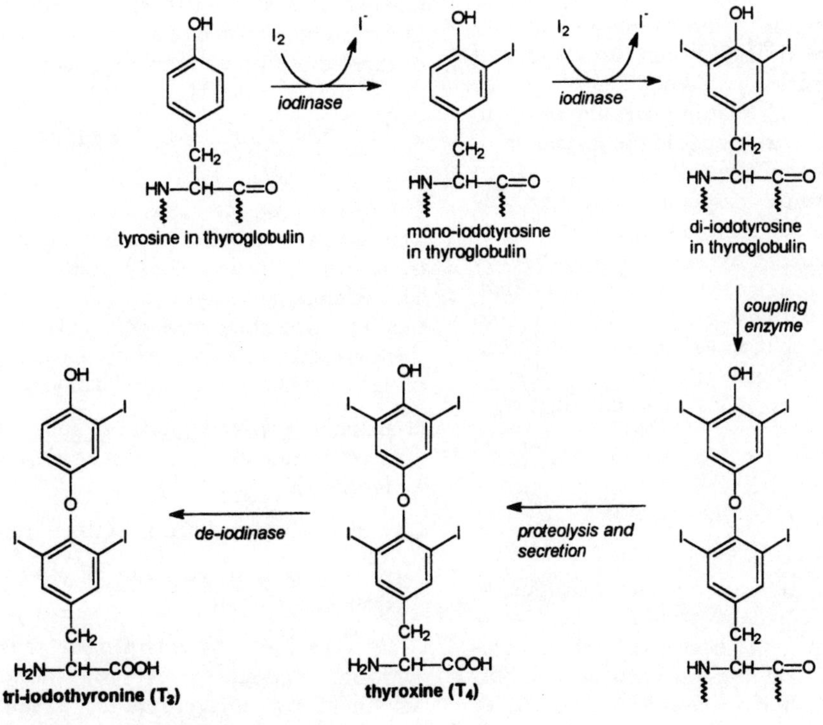

Figure 25.2 The synthesis of thyroid hormones
Iodinase (peroxidase) EC 1.11.1.8, thyroxine deiodinase EC 3.8.1.4

etin, which forms a 1:1 complex with retinol binding protein (see section 13.5.2). Both hormones are taken up by liver, kidney and target tissues; thyroxine undergoes de-iodination to T_3, which is the active hormone.

There are two thyroxine 5'-deiodinases (EC 3.8.1.4) which catalyse the outer ring de-iodination of T_4 to yield active T_3 (3,3',5–tri-iodothyronine).

1. Deiodinase I in liver and kidney is the main source of T_3 in the circulation. Deiodinase I also occurs in the thyroid gland; some T_3 is released by the thyroid. It is a selenoprotein, with selenocysteine at the catalytic site (see section 15.4.1).

2. Deiodinase II is found in brown adipose tissue, the central nervous system, and pituitary. This enzyme is responsible for the local formation of T_3 within target tissues. It is not selenium dependent.

Thyroxine may also undergo inner-ring deiodination to produce biologically inactive reverse-T_3 (3,3',5'-tri-iodothyronine). Further deiodination of reverse-T_3 is catalysed by both types I and II deiodinase. The iodine released from hormone catabolism is either excreted in urine or taken up by the thyroid for re-utilization.

The role of selenium in formation of active T_3 means that selenium deficiency may be a cause of functional iodine deficiency, although unless iodine is also deficient it is likely that the selenium-independent type II deiodinase will result in the formation of (marginally) adequate amounts of T_3.

Normally, the pituitary responds to increased circulating T_4 by reduced synthesis and secretion of thyrotropin, thus reducing the stimulation of thyroid iodine uptake and hormone synthesis. Selenium deficiency is associated with elevated circulating T_4 and high levels of thyrotropin; in the absence of intracellular formation of T_3, the pituitary is unable to respond to increased circulating T_4 in the usual way.

25.14.3 Thyroid hormone receptors and functions

Tri-iodothyronine is a nuclear-acting hormone; it binds to a nuclear receptor protein, and after dimerization and activation, the hormone-receptor complex binds to a hormone response element on DNA, regulating transcription of one or more genes. The T_3 receptor is one of the steroid hormone receptor superfamily of zinc finger proteins (see section 25.26.1),

similar to the calcitriol (see section 14.3.3.1) and retinoid (see section 13.3.3) receptors.

There are at least two T_3 receptor genes, α and β, and alternative splicing of the mRNA for both genes means that there are four different T_3 receptor proteins: $\alpha 1$, $\alpha 2$, $\beta 1$, and $\beta 2$. The $\beta 2$ receptor is limited to the brain, while the other receptors are found in all tissues, although the amounts of each receptor differ not only from tissue to tissue, but also with the stage of development. The different receptors can form both homo-dimers and also hetero-dimers with other T_3 receptor proteins and with various retinoid receptors (see section 13.3.3), so that there are multiple possible T_3-receptor complexes, capable of binding to different hormone response elements on different genes.

Only a few of the genes whose expression is modulated by T_3 have yet been identified: in cardiac and skeletal muscle, it increases the expression of both the fast and slow calcium ATPases, while in the heart it increases expression of myosin heavy chain α and decreases that of heavy chain β protein. In liver and adipose tissue it increases expression of the genes for malate dehydrogenase, glucose-6–phosphate dehydrogenase and fatty acid synthetase, while in the pituitary it represses the gene for thyrotropin. It also increases expression of thermogenin in brown adipose tissue, suggesting a mechanism for the increased metabolic rate and heat output in response to thyroid hormone stimulation (Brent 1994).

25.14.4 Iodine deficiency diseases

25.14.4.1 Endemic goitre

The pituitary responds to a low circulating concentration of T_4 by increased secretion of thyrotropin. This stimulates not only iodide uptake into the thyroid, but also enlargement of the gland. In mild cases the thyroid may not be visibly enlarged. Three grades of visible enlargement can be defined.

(1) palpably enlarged (grade 1a) and visible when the neck is extended and the head is thrown back (grade 1b);

(2) visible when the head is in the normal position;

(3) so grossly enlarged as to be clearly visible at a distance of 10 m.

In some cases the enlargement of the thyroid is sufficient to permit normal production of T_4 from a marginal iodine intake, resulting in normal circulating concentrations of the hormone—euthyroid goitre. More usually, however, despite the enlargement of the thyroid, the iodine supply is inadequate to meet requirements for T_4 synthesis, and the result is hypothyroidism—low circulating concentrations of T_4 and T_3.

Hypothyroidism (myxoedema) is characterized by a low metabolic rate, low body temperature, dull mental apathy, a 'moon-faced' appearance, and weight gain. Iodine-deficient children have lower school achievement and lower IQ than those with adequate iodine status.

The goitrogens naturally present in foods have not been shown to cause development of goitre in people receiving an adequate intake of iodine, but are certainly a precipitating factor when iodine intake is marginal.

25.14.4.2 Endemic (goitrous) cretinism

The effects of iodine deficiency in pregnancy are disastrous for the developing foetus; there is severe impairment of brain development, leading to cretinism. There are disorders of gait and other neurological signs that reflect damage to the cerebral cortex and basal ganglia; deafness, mutism, and squint are common, and all affected children are severely intellectually impaired.

When the infant's iodine intake post-natally is not too severely deficient, it may show euthyroid goitre, and suffer only the neurological and intellectual signs of the condition—this is sometimes known as neurological cretinism. By contrast, if the infant's postnatal iodine intake is severely deficient, then it will suffer from hypothyroidism, with marked retardation of growth and puberty—myxoedematous cretinism. In addition, those who suffer from myxoedematous cretinism have atrophy of the thyroid, rather than the hyperplasia that is seen in those cretins who develop euthyroid goitre. The cause of this thyroid atrophy is unclear; the infants are born with functioning thyroid tissue. Possible contributing factors include concomitant selenium deficiency and high intakes of thiocyanates and other goitrogens (Boyages 1993; Thilly *et al.* 1993). The role of selenium deficiency in thyroid atrophy, as opposed to failure of T_3 formation, is probably due to lack of selenium-dependent glutathione peroxidase in the gland. Oxidation of iodide to iodine is achieved by reaction with hydrogen peroxide generated in the thyroid gland; excess peroxide not removed by glutathione peroxidase will cause tissue necrosis (Dumont *et al.* 1994).

25.14.4.3 Hyperthyroidism

When patients with hypothyroid or euthyroid goitre are given adequate intakes of iodine (as for example when iodine supplementation programmes are initiated), a significant proportion of those over the age of about 40 will develop signs of hyperthyroidism (thyrotoxicosis). Hyperthyroid patients have a high metabolic rate, high body temperature, and lose weight on normal energy intakes; characteristically their eyes are protuberant (exophthalmus). Similar exophthalmic goitre develops in patients with enhanced stimulation of the thyroid by thyrotropin (sometimes as a result of auto-immune disease) despite adequate iodine intake—this is Grave's disease or Basedow's syndrome. It may be treated surgically, or, more commonly, by administration of synthetic goitrogens to decrease the activity of the gland.

25.14.5 Assessment of iodine nutritional status

Iodine status can be assessed by measurement of urinary excretion of iodine; under 390 nmol (50 µg) /g creatinine (3.5 µmol /mol creatinine) indicates deficiency. Alternatively, circulating concentrations of thyroid hormones can be measured. The original method was measurement of protein-bound iodine in plasma, since this is, effectively, a measure of circulating T_3 and T_4 bound to transthyretin, or the butanol-extractable iodine, which measures organic iodine compounds. More precise assessment of status depends on measurement by immunoassay or cellular bio-assay of T_4, T_3, reverse T_3, and thyrotropin. Normal circulating T_4 is about 100 nmol (80 µg) /L, and T_3 1.8 nmol (1.2 µg) /L.

Such sophisticated techniques are neither feasible nor necessary in regions of endemic goitre. Here the extent of the problem can be assessed by the prevalence of goitre.

1. An area is classified as suffering from mild iodine deficiency when the prevalence of goitre in schoolchildren is between 5–20 per cent, and mean urine excretion of iodine is > 50 µg /g creatinine.

2. Moderate iodine deficiency is defined as prevalence of goitre up to 30 per cent, some hypothyroidism and median iodine excretion between 25–50 µg /g creatinine.

3. Severe iodine deficiency is indicated by a prevalence of goitre > 30 per cent and endemic cretinism between 1–10 per cent; median iodine excretion is < 25 µg /g creatinine.

25.14.6 Prevention of iodine deficiency

In industrialized countries where iodine deficiency is a problem, disease can be prevented by iodization of a dietary staple. The first such measure was in Switzerland, in 1900, when chocolate was used as the vehicle, in order to target the enrichment at children. More commonly, salt is enriched with sodium iodate (which is less volatile than iodide). In some countries only iodized salt is sold, in others it is optionally available in areas of risk. In Australia and the Netherlands, by law bread is made with iodized salt.

Such measures are unlikely to be effective in less developed remote regions of the world, and here prevention depends on intermittent administration of iodized oil, given either by intramuscular injection or orally. Iodine will add across carbon–carbon double bonds in unsaturated fatty acids (indeed, the early chemical method of estimating the degree of unsaturation of a fat was by measurement of its iodine number—the amount of iodine taken up by 1 g of the oil). Iodized poppyseed oil contains 38 per cent iodine by weight, so that 1 mL provides 3.8 mmol (480 mg) iodine, sufficient to maintain an adult in an adequate state of iodine nutrition for 3–5 years when given by injection and 1–2 years when given by mouth.

Boyages (1993) suggests that in areas of mild iodine deficiency, provision of salt iodized to a level of 10–25 mg iodate /kg will suffice, while in areas of moderate iodine deficiency either salt iodized to a level of 25–40 mg /kg or iodized oil should be used. In areas of severe iodine deficiency iodized oil is required for adequate prevention.

25.24.7 Other causes of thyroid disease

Apart from iodine deficiency there are many other causes of thyroid dysfunction; some 5 per cent of the population of developed countries are estimated to suffer from hypo- or hyperthyroidism as a result of infection, auto-immune disease, hormonal imbalance, tumours, or hereditary disease.

25.15   Lithium

Lithium has no known physiological function; lithium carbonate and other salts are used in the treatment of bipolar manic-depressive illness, with doses ranging between 5–60 mmol (0.25–2.5 g) lithium carbonate /day. The therapeutic effect is presumed to be due to alterations in the sensitivity or responsiveness of neurotransmitter receptors.

There is a narrow therapeutic window between the dose at which lithium salts have their beneficial effect and the level at which (potentially fatal) signs of intoxication develop. Acute lithium toxicity leads to tremor, ataxia, nystagmus, renal impairment and convulsions; there is some evidence that long-term use of lithium salts may led to the development of histological and functional changes in the kidney.

25.16   Magnesium

Intakes of magnesium are between 5–20 mmol (120–500 mg) /day, of which 30–50 per cent is absorbed, mainly by active transport; the proportion absorbed decreases with increasing intake. There is no competition with calcium for absorption, and although there is some evidence that calcitriol is involved in magnesium absorption, the effect is considerably less marked than that on calcium absorption (see section 14.3.3.2). About 25 per cent of the absorbed magnesium is secreted into the intestinal lumen in digestive secretions, but is largely reabsorbed; magnesium balance is maintained by regulation of urinary excretion. Excretion is enhanced by thyroid hormones, acidosis, aldosterone and depletion of phosphate and potassium. Calcitonin, glucagon and parathyroid hormone all increase the resorption of magnesium from the glomerular filtrate.

The body content of magnesium is about 1 mol (24 g), of which 60–65 per cent is in bone mineral, 27 per cent in muscle and 6 per cent in other tissues. Some 20–30 per cent of bone magnesium is freely exchangeable with plasma magnesium, acting as a buffer to maintain plasma concentrations, while the non-exchangeable bone magnesium remains constant even when magnesium intakes are inadequate to maintain balance. About 1 per cent is in extracellular fluids, and the normal plasma concentration is 1.5–1.9 mmol/L, of which half is present as free ions, one-third bound to albumin and the remainder present in a variety of complexes with ions such as citrate.

In muscle and other soft tissues the main function of magnesium is to stabilize the structure of ATP, being chelated by the phosphate groups; about 80 per cent of total intracellular magnesium is chelated by ATP. The true substrate for ATP-utilizing enzymes is in fact the magnesium-ATP complex. Total intracellular magnesium is around 10 mmol/L, of which only 0.4–1.0 mmol/L is free in the cytosol, the remainder being bound to ATP, membranes and proteins, or inside mitochondria (where the concentration is between 25–40 mmol/L).

Magnesium also plays a role in neuromuscular transmission, being required for potassium transport and calcium channel activity. Deficiency leads to increased muscle irritability, cardiac arrhythmias, and tetany. It causes relaxation of vascular smooth muscle, and thus has the opposite effect to that of calcium ions on blood pressure; low intakes and excessive renal loss of magnesium have been associated with elevated blood pressure.

Reference intakes for magnesium are shown in Table 25.19. It is widely distributed in foods, and dietary deficiency would appear unlikely. Nevertheless, hypomagnesaemia is not uncommon, occurring in up to 10 per cent of hospital patients in some studies, and a considerably higher proportion of those in intensive care units. Kidney disease, metabolic acidosis and diuresis all lead to increased magnesium loss, while persistent diarrhoea will impair absorption.

Hypomagnesaemia (serum concentration < 1.5 mmol /L) is associated with hypokalaemia; there is loss of intracellular potassium, together with failure to reabsorb potassium in the kidney. Administration of potassium alone does not correct the hypokalaemia; magnesium is also required. This presumably reflects the need of the Na^+-K^+ pump for magnesium-ATP. Hypomagnesaemia is also accompanied by hypocalcaemia; here the effect seems to be on the secretion of parathyroid hormone; injection of magnesium salts leads to increased secretion. Although the mechanism by which magnesium modulates parathyroid hormone secretion is unclear, it is likely that it reflects the requirement for magnesium-ATP as a substrate for adenylate cyclase; parathyroid hormone secretion is cAMP dependent.

The simplest way of assessing magnesium status is by measurement of serum magnesium. More sensitive assessment, and detection of subjects at risk of developing hypomagnesaemia because of depleted body reserves, is possible by determining the proportion of a test dose that is retained in the body. Normally some 15 per cent of an infused magnesium load of 0.2 mmol /kg body weight is retained, while hypomagnesaemic subjects retain 85 per cent, and those at risk of deficiency around 50 per cent (Ryzen *et al.* 1985). However, in subjects with hypomagnesaemia due to kidney disease or diuresis, urinary losses will continue, making interpretation of the loading test impossible.

Toxicity, as may occur in patients with renal failure who are treated with magnesium supplements, can lead to hypotension, central nervous system depression, decreased deep tendon reflexes, anaesthesia and even paralysis. If plasma magnesium rises above 9 mmol /L there may be decreased respiration, marked muscle weakness and possibly cardiac arrest; in such cases intravenous calcium infusion antagonizes the effects of magnesium intoxication.

25.17 Manganese

The total body content of manganese is 180–360 μmol (10–20 mg), with a biological half-life of 3–10 weeks. Intakes are about 35–70 μmol (2–4 mg) /day, although intakes as high 150 μmol (8 mg) have been reported; 2–5 per cent of the intake is absorbed. Absorption is enhanced by chelation by histidine and citrate, and by alcohol, and inhibited by calcium, cobalt and iron. It is transported in plasma bound to transferrin, and there is some evidence that manganese shares the same intestinal uptake system as iron and cobalt (Sandström 1992). Most absorbed manganese is excreted in the bile and pancreatic juice, with little or none in urine. Bile duct obstruction leads to increased excretion in pancreatic juice.

Manganese functions as the prosthetic group of a small number of metallo-proteins, including acetyl CoA (EC 6.4.1.2) and pyruvate (EC 6.4.1.1) carboxylases (key enzymes in, respectively, fatty acid synthesis and gluconeogenesis), the mitochondrial isoenzyme of superoxide dismutase (EC 1.15.1.1), and arginase (EC 3.5.3.1). It is also involved in the regulation of activity of a wide variety of enzymes, including hydroxylases, kinases, phosphatases, decarboxylases and some dehydrogenases and peptidases, as well as regulation of the activity of a number of neurotransmitter receptors. It is difficult to be certain whether this represents a true requirement for manganese or not, since studies in deficient animals suggest that for many of these regulatory roles magnesium can substitute for manganese. Magnesium can substitute for manganese in pyruvate carboxylase, with little or no apparent effect on the catalytic activity of the enzyme (Scrutton *et al.* 1972). At least three enzymes are only partially maintained by magnesium: phosphoenolpyruvate carboxykinase (EC 4.1.1.32, a key enzyme in gluconeogenesis), farnesyl pyrophosphate synthetase (EC 2.5.1.10, a key enzyme in cholesterol synthesis) and a number of glycosyltransferases involved in glycosaminoglucan synthesis. Vitamin K epoxidase (EC 1.14.99.20, see section 16.4) is also dependent on manganese activation.

Estimated safe and adequate levels of manganese intake are shown in Table 25.20. In experimental animals, manganese deficiency results in hypocholesterolaemia as a result of impaired activity of farnesyl pyrophosphate synthetase, and, more importantly, defective growth of endochondral bone, as a result of impaired connective tissue formation, which is presumably the result of impaired vitamin K metabolism.

Orally, manganese salts have little toxicity. However, inhalation of manganese oxide as a result of industrial exposure, can lead to a psychotic disease, and later the development of a condition clinically indistinguishable from Parkinson's disease, with slow degeneration of dopaminergic neurones in the substantia nigra. Although the mechanism of this manganese neurotoxicity has not been established, it is likely that it is due to redox cycling between manganese ions and the catecholamines, leading to the formation of oxygen radicals.

25.18   Mercury

Mercury is not an essential mineral, and is neurotoxic. Inorganic mercury toxicity is mainly the result of industrial exposure to vapour, while potentially hazardous amounts of organic mercury complexes (especially methyl mercury) can enter the food chain as a result of accumulation in marine sediment, or the use of mercury-containing seed dressings. Average intakes are 10 nmol (2.5 μg) /day, and most foods contain less than 20 nmol (5 μg) /kg. Tuna and other fish may contain up to 5 μmol (1 mg) /kg. There was an outbreak of methyl mercury poisoning around Minimata Bay in Japan in the 1950s, as a result of industrial pollution, locally raised shellfish contained up to 145 μmol (30 mg) /kg, and intakes were estimated as 15 μmol (3 mg) /day.

25.19   Molybdenum

The intake of molybdenum is around 3 μmol (300 μg) /day. It is readily absorbed as molybdate (MoO_4^{2-}), although sulphate competes with molybdate for intestinal absorption, and, more importantly, for resorption in the renal tubule, so that high sulphate excretion can lead to increased urinary loss of molybdenum.

Molybdenum is required for three human enzymes: xanthine (EC 1.1.1.204), aldehyde (EC 1.2.3.1), and sulphite (EC 1.8.3.1) oxidases. In all three it is present as a pterin-like cofactor, molybdopterin (see Fig. 25.3). The pathway of molybdopterin synthesis has been elucidated in micro-organisms, where it is formed from GTP by the action of GTP cyclohydrolase—the same pathway as occurs in human tissues for the synthesis of biopterin (see sec-

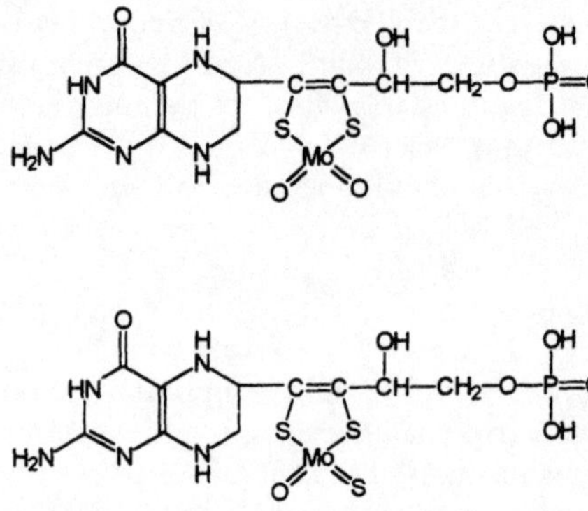

Figure 25.3 The molybdenum-derived coenzymes

tion 23.4). However, in human beings with genetic defects of biopterin synthesis (so-called malignant, or unresponsive, phenylketonuria, see section 23.4.1.), there is no evidence of molybdopterin deficiency, and no impairment of the molybdopterin-dependent enzymes. It is not known whether human beings are capable of *de novo* synthesis of molybdopterin or not, although it seems likely, since patients receiving long-term total parenteral nutrition are able to utilize inorganic molybdate.

Estimated safe and adequate levels of molybdenum intake are shown in Table 25.21. High intakes can impair the absorption of copper as a result of the formation of unavailable copper molybdate and thiomolybdates; this is unlikely to be a problem of human nutrition, but can lead to copper deficiency in animals grazing on molybdate-rich pasture.

25.20   Nickel

Intakes of nickel are between 5–10 μmol (0.3–0.6 mg) /day, of which 3–10 per cent is absorbed. Most nickel excretion is in urine (60 per cent), although there is a significant amount in bile and sweat.

No clear function has been defined for nickel in mammalian metabolism, although a number of plant and bacterial enzymes are known to be nickel metallo-proteins. Deficiency results in decreased activity of lactate, glucose-6–phosphate, isocitrate, malate, and glutamate dehydrogenases, suggesting a role in energy-yielding metabolism, and pancreatic amylase. There are also ultrastructural changes in the cell in nickel deficiency, including disorganization of the endoplasmic reticulum and nucleus, and mitochondrial swelling.

A nickel-binding protein, nickeloplasmin, has been isolated from human plasma; its function is unknown.

25.21 Silicon

Apart from oxygen, silicon is the most abundant element in the biosphere. It is a dietary essential for the growth and development of experimental animals, and deficiency leads to abnormalities of bone development. Most tissues in the adult contain between 0.7–1.5 μmol (20–40 mg) silicon /kg, with slightly more in the lungs (about 2 μmol /kg) and a very much higher concentration in lymph nodes, up to 18–21 μmol /kg), associated with the presence of grains of quartz. In other tissues, silicon is present as silanoate incorporated into mucopolysaccharides of connective tissue, forming -O-Si-O- and -O-Si-O-Si-O- bridges between carbohydrate moieties, and contributing to the strength of connective tissue.

Silicon in foods occurs as monosilicic acid, solid silica and silanoates in pectin and connective tissue; little is known of the absorption or metabolism of dietary silicon compounds, but urinary output of silicon dioxide, which increases with increasing silicon intake, represents no more than about 4 per cent of total intake. The quartz grains in lymph nodes are believed to come from crystals in plants, which are small enough to be absorbed intact.

In young animals, silicon is localized in the actively growing areas of bone, and the concentration rises with that of calcium as mineralization proceeds, falling later as mature hydroxyapatite is formed (Carlisle 1970).

There is no information on which to base estimates of silicon requirements, and little reliable information on the silicon content of foods—significant amounts can dissolve from glass equipment during sample preparation. The ubiquitous distribution of silicon means that dietary deficiency is unlikely; average intake has been estimated as around 35 μmol (1 mg) /day. There is some evidence that atherosclerosis is associated with a low content of silicon in the connective tissue of the arterial wall, and it has been suggested that a deficiency of silicon may be a factor in the development of atherosclerosis—a suggestion that is confounded by the fact that the major sources of silicon are plant foods that are rich in non-starch polysaccharides, which themselves have potentially protective actions (see section 7.3.2).

25.22 Strontium

There is no evidence that strontium is an essential mineral; average intakes are between 10–30 μmol (1–3 mg) /day, and the total body content is about 3.7 mmol (320 mg), almost entirely in bone mineral. At normal levels of intake there is no evidence of toxicity. However, strontium salts have been used to treat lead poisoning in children (it displaces lead from bones, aiding its elimination from the body); at the doses used there is inhibition of calcidiol 25-hydroxylase, leading to strontium-induced, vitamin D-resistant rickets (see section 14.4.1). The radioactive isotope ^{90}Sr, with a half-life of 29 years, is dispersed in fallout from nuclear explosions; it poses a significant health hazard, since it behaves metabolically like calcium, and is concentrated in bones.

25.23 Sulphur

Organic sulphates are involved in proteoglycans of the extracellular matrix, and sulphation is a mechanism of inactivation or detoxication of some phenolic compounds. There is no evidence of any requirement for inorganic sulphate intake; the sulphate that is required for these sulphation reactions is derived from the sulphur oxidation of the amino acid cysteine. Intakes of sulphate in excess of 20 μmol/day exceed the absorptive capacity of the small intestine, and may be reduced to hydrogen sulphide by colonic bacteria.

25.24 Tin

Studies of animals maintained under extremely stringent conditions have demonstrated an absolute requirement for tin for normal growth (Schwarz 1974), but no physiological function has been described. Intakes are extremely variable, between 8–300 μmol (1–38 mg) /day; most is obtained from acid foods in tin cans, but little of this is absorbed. Excretion is in the bile, and toxicity from food sources is unknown. Organic tin compounds are readily absorbed and retained in the body, leading to toxicity, but this is the result of industrial exposure rather than from foods.

25.25 Vanadium

Little is known about average intakes of vanadium; it is estimated that between 5–10 per cent of dietary intake is absorbed. Root crops and pulses contain about 20 pmol (1 ng) vanadium /g, and meats about 200 pmol (10 ng) /g; the highest concentrations are found in oils and fats. There is homeostatic control over the body content of vanadium, so that, unlike metals such as aluminium, lead and cadmium, it does not accumulate with age; most is excreted in the urine.

Vanadium is essential for growth, bone development, and fertility in experimental animals. No vanadium-dependent enzymes have been identified in animals, but it may have a role in thyroid hormone synthesis; vanadate is oxidized to pervanadate in the presence of hydrogen peroxide; pervanadate then oxidizes iodide to elemental iodine (see section 25.14.2). The chemical similarity of vanadate and phosphate means that vanadate accumulates at sites of bone mineralization, and there is some evidence that it may stimulate osteoblast activity (Nielsen 1991).

Vanadate also activates, or potentiates the stimulation of, tyrosine kinases involved in hormone action, and *in vitro* it can mimic the effects of insulin on adipose tissue, although there is no evidence that this is a significant effect at physiological levels of vanadate (Duckworth *et al.* 1988).

Vanadate ions inhibit the Na^+-K^+ ATPase (the sodium pump, EC 3.6.1.37), Ca^{2+} ATPase of muscle (the calcium pump), and the proton pump of gastric mucosa (see section 6.1.2) at physiological concentrations. Because of the inhibition of the sodium pump, intravenous vanadate acts as a potent diuretic, since there is considerable impairment of the normal recovery of sodium from the glomerular filtrate (see section 25.1). The converse of this is that vanadium deficiency may explain the retention of sodium and water leading to oedema in protein-energy malnutrition (see section 12.4); Golden and Golden (1981) reported that in children with kwashiorkor, circulating concentrations of vanadium were about 60 per cent of those seen in adequately nourished children.

Despite its potent actions on ion transport, vanadate has low toxicity; cell membranes have an NADH-dependent vanadate reductase, which reduces vanadate ($VO_4{}^{3-}$) to vanadyl (VO^{2+}) which has little or no activity.

25.26 Zinc

Zinc occurs in wide variety of enzymes; it may have a role in the catalytic site, a structural role (e.g. in the copper-zinc-dependent cytoplasmic superoxide dismutase (EC 1.15.1.1), alkaline phosphatase (EC 3.1.3.1) and alcohol dehydrogenase (EC 1.1.1.1), where it also has a role in the catalytic site), or a regulatory role (e.g. in fructose-1,6–bisphosphatase (EC 3.1.3.11), where it also has a structural role). In the nuclear-acting hormone receptors it has a structural role. Zinc is also required to form insulin hexamer crystals in pancreatic β-cells prior to secretion; impaired insulin secretion and glucose tolerance are associated with inadequate zinc nutrition. It also has a role in the maintenance of the native structure of RNA and DNA.

Reference intakes for zinc are shown in Table 25.22, and rich sources in Table 25.23.

25.26.1 Absorption and metabolism of zinc

Studies of children suffering from acrodermatitis enteropathica have suggested that an endogenous ligand is necessary for intestinal absorption of zinc. Acrodermatitis enteropathica is a lethal autosomal recessive condition that develops during the first few months after weaning from breast feeding. There is a progressive dermatitis, with conjunctivitis, photophobia and corneal opacity, severe gastro-intestinal disturbance and neurological signs; the patients have retarded growth and hypogonadism. The condition is associated with a failure of zinc absorption and extremely low plasma and tissue concentrations of zinc.

The underlying defect in acrodermatitis enteropathica appears to be a failure to synthesize or secrete a zinc-binding ligand that is normally secreted in pancreatic juice. This ligand has been tentatively identified as picolinic acid, a metabolite of tryptophan, although other zinc-binding ligands have been identified in both pancreatic juice and human milk; cows' milk does not contain zinc-binding ligands (Hahn and Evans 1973; Evans and Johnson 1980; Hurley *et al.* 1977).

The total body content of zinc is about 45 mmol (3 g), of which 60 per cent is in muscle, 20–30 per cent in bone, 8 per cent in skin and hair and 4–6 per cent in liver. Daily intakes are around 150–200 μmol (9–12 mg), of which about one-third is absorbed. The main excretion is through the gut; a relatively large amount of zinc (15–30 μmol (1–2 mg) /day) is secreted by the pancreas. Urinary excretion is relatively small, but a considerable amount is also lost in sweat, which contains 15–20 µmol (0.85–1.45 mg) / L. Indeed, severe nutritional deficiency has been reported only among people living in tropical and subtropical climates.

Plasma zinc is between 11–19 mmol /L; 80–85 per cent is bound to albumin, 15 per cent to α_2-macroglobulin, less than 2 per cent to retinol-binding protein (see section 13.2.4) and only 1–2 per cent is present as free ions. The α_2-macroglobulin-bound zinc remains more or less constant in deficiency; the main change is in albumin-bound zinc. Elevated plasma concentrations (20–40 µmol/L) are seen in renal dialysis patients, as a result of absorption of zinc from the dialysis fluid, and in cases of intravascular haemolysis, or rare cases of acute zinc poisoning.

Metallothionein is a low molecular weight protein, with an unusually high cysteine content (30–40 per cent of its 60 amino acids), which binds 7 metal ions per molecule. The metal bound may be zinc, cadmium, or copper. It has been suggested that the main function of metallothionein is in the regulation of whole body zinc metabolism; it binds zinc tightly, but has a short half-life. Zinc-metallothionein will both donate zinc ions to apo-metalloenzymes and also remove zinc from metalloenzymes. Expression of the metallothionein gene is modified by glucocorticoids, glucagon, oestrogens, catecholamines, interferon, interleukin I, and zinc. It may also be involved in the detoxication of metals such as cadmium (see section 25.7), copper (see section 25.11.4), and mercury; it was originally discovered as a cadmium-binding protein.

The receptors for nuclear acting hormones, including the steroids, thyroid hormone (see section 25.14.3), retinoids (see section 13.3.3) and calcitriol (see section 14.3.3.1), have a common structure, which has been termed a zinc finger. There are two finger-like projections of the protein, which bind to, and interact with, hormone-response elements on DNA to modulate gene expression. Each finger is stabilized by a zinc ion, chelated by four cysteine residues. Experimental zinc depletion leads to considerably reduced sensitivity of target tissues to steroid hormone action (Bunce and Vessal 1987).

Bettger and O'Dell (1993) suggested that zinc both has structural role in cell membranes and is important in trans-membrane signal transduction. Zinc is lost from plasma membranes early in experimental deficiency, and this results in loss of sensitivity to signal transduction.

Zinc also has a role in protection against oxygen radical damage. It is an essential (structural) component of cytoplasmic superoxide dismutase (EC 1.15.1.1). Zinc ions will bind to sulphydryl groups in proteins, thus protecting them against oxidation, and, at least *in vitro*, it reduces the non-enzymic formation of hydroxyl and superoxide radicals by iron in the presence of oxygen (Bray and Bettger 1990).

25.26.2 Zinc deficiency

Zinc deficiency was first reported in Iran, and then later in Egypt (Prasad *et al.* 1961, 1963). The subjects were young men with iron-deficiency anaemia who were severely stunted in growth and despite being aged between 16–18 were prepubertal, with testicular atrophy. All had diets that were based very largely on unleavened bread and beans. The Iranian subjects, but not those in Egypt, also showed marked hepatosplenomegaly. Treatment with iron and zinc led to resolution of the anaemia and hepatosplenomegaly, and normal growth and development, with development of secondary sexual characteristics within a few months.

Zinc deficiency has since been reported from a number of centres; in all cases the subjects live on a diet based very largely on unrefined cereals (and hence a high intake of fibre and phytate). All reports have been from tropical and subtropical regions, suggesting that high zinc losses in sweat may be a precipitating factor when intake and availability are low. Zinc depletion also occurs in association with heavy alcohol consumption. Although urinary excretion is not normally a major route of zinc loss, it is greatly increased by alcohol consumption.

Even relatively mild zinc deficiency leads to impairment of the sense of taste (hypogeusia, see section 6.1.1.1,); repletion of deficient subjects with zinc leads to normalization of taste acuity (Ruz *et al.* 1992). There is no evidence that the normal blunting of the sense of taste with increasing age is associated with zinc depletion, nor that it will response to zinc supplements.

There is also evidence that wound healing is impaired in moderate zinc deficiency, and a number of studies have shown that in subjects with low zinc status healing is improved by administration of zinc supplements. In subjects with adequate zinc status, supplements have no effect on wound healing.

Deficiency is associated with impaired cell-mediated immunity; the thymus-specific hormone thymulin, which binds to high affinity receptors in T-cells, is zinc dependent, and in deficiency a zinc-free apo-peptide with no biological activity circulates in plasma; it can be activated *in vitro* by addition of zinc (Prasad *et al.* 1988).

Zinc deficiency occurs in association with sickle cell disease; like nutritionally zinc-deficient subjects, the affected patients are of short stature, and have delayed onset of puberty and hypogonadism. They also show impaired wound healing. Zinc supplements lead to increased growth, normal development and improvement in wound healing. It is likely that the continuing haemolysis associated with sickle cell disease results in a considerable loss of zinc from the body; more than can be replaced from the diet (Prasad *et al.* 1975).

25.26.3 Indices of zinc nutritional status

Cases of clear zinc deficiency are associated with plasma concentrations below 6 μmol /L, compared with a reference range of 11–19 μmol /L; interpretation of marginal plasma concentrations, between 7–10 μmol /L, is difficult, since there are changes in circulating zinc in response to acute infection, pregnancy, administration of oestrogens and hypoalbuminaemia, as well as inadequate zinc intake. More importantly, the plasma concentration can be maintained within the normal range even in severe deficiency, as a result of breakdown of muscle tissue (Aggett 1991). The concentration of zinc in serum is about 16 per cent higher than that in plasma, as a result of zinc liberated from platelets during clotting.

The reference range of erythrocyte zinc is 200 ± 50 μmol /L red blood cells or 30–60 μmol /g haemoglobin, mainly associated with carbonic anhydrase (EC 4.2.1.1). However, it does not fall significantly even in severe zinc depletion, and therefore does not provide a useful index of zinc status. There is no evidence that erythrocyte carbonic anhydrase activity is sensitive to zinc status. Leukocyte zinc is difficult to interpret, without a differential white cell count, since neutrophils have a lower zinc content than mononuclear or other polymorphonuclear leukocytes (Delves 1985; Goode *et al.* 1989). Thompson (1991) suggested that in the absence of any other useful indices of zinc status, the concentration in polymorphonuclear leukocytes is the most useful. Table 25.24 shows reference ranges for zinc concentrations in biological fluids.

Plasma concentrations of metallothionein may prove to be a useful index of zinc status; in experimental animals this protein responds to changes in zinc status, but not to non-nutritional factors that affect the total plasma zinc concentration. However, it is subject to diurnal variation, and is affected by iron nutritional status (Thompson 1991).

The zinc content of hair and nails has been proposed as an index of status. Hair zinc is unreliable, since many shampoos contain relatively large amounts of zinc, and this can be adsorbed onto the hair, yielding falsely high values. Furthermore, in both experimental animals and severely malnourished children there is a paradoxical increase in hair zinc with depletion, as a result of impaired hair growth. Fingernail zinc is presumably subject to the same problem. Toenail zinc is also unhelpful; as noted above, sweat contains a relatively high concentration of zinc, and the soles of the feet are especially rich in sweat glands. Lavis *et al.* (1986) showed that there is a gradient of zinc in toenails from the germinal matrix to the distal end, and on the great toe also from the exterior to interior surface, reflecting the regions most exposed to sweat.

The activities of a number of zinc-dependent enzymes in plasma reflect zinc status in depletion / repletion studies: alkaline phosphatase (EC 3.1.3.1), lactate dehydrogenase (EC 1.1.1.27), and ribonucleases. However, the plasma levels of all of these enzymes are subject to changes unrelated to zinc nutritional status. The activity of copper-zinc-dependent superoxide dismutase in erythrocytes does not change with zinc status. Erythrocyte membrane alkaline phosphatase and membrane zinc fall significantly in experimental zinc depletion (Ruz *et al.* 1992).

Prasad *et al.* (1988) have suggested that activation of serum thymulin by zinc added *in vitro* may provide useful information of zinc nutritional status, but this seems not to have been developed further.

25.26.4 Zinc toxicity

Zinc has low toxicity, and does not accumulate in the body. Acute intoxication may occur as a result ingestion of relatively large amounts of zinc salts, leading to drowsiness and lethargy, as well as nausea and vomiting. Ingestion of more than about 2 g of zinc sulphate leads to vomiting, and indeed it has been recommended as an emetic.

Habitually high intakes of zinc may well compromise copper nutrition, since there is competition between these two minerals for absorption (see section 25.11.2).

Further reading

al-Ghamdi, S.M., Cameron, E.C. and Sutton, R.A. (1994). Magnesium deficiency: pathophysiologic and clinical overview. *American Journal of Kidney Diseases*, **24**, 737–52.

Baynes, R.D. and Bothwell, T.H. (1990). Iron deficiency. *Annual Review of Nutrition*, 10, 133–48.

Boyages, S.C. (1993). Clinical review 49: iodine deficiency disorders. *Journal of Clinical Endocrinology and Metabolism*, 77, 587– 91.

Bremner, I. and Beattie, J.H. (1990). Metallothionein and the trace minerals. *Annual Review of Nutrition*, 10, 63–83.

Dafnis, E. and Sabatini, S. (1994). Biochemistry and pathophysiology of vanadium. *Nephron*, 67, 133–43.

Danks, D.M. (1988). Copper deficiency in humans. *Annual Review of Nutrition*, 8, 235–57.

Danks, D.M. (1995). Disorders of copper transport. *The Metabolic and Molecular Bases of Inherited Disease*, Vol II (ed. C.R. Scriver, A.L. Beaudet, W.S. Sly, and D. Valle), Chapter 68, pp. 2211–35. McGraw-Hill, New York.

Delange, F. (1994). The disorders induced by iodine deficiency. *Thyroid*, 4, 107–28.

French, R.J. and Jones, P.J. (1993). Role of vanadium in nutrition: metabolism, essentiality and dietary considerations. *Life Science*, 52, 339–46.

Hetzel, B.S. and Dunn, J.T. (1989). The iodine deficiency disorders. *Annual Review of Nutrition*, 9, 21–38.

Hetzel, B.S., Potter B.J. and Dullberg, E.M. (1990). The iodine deficiency disorders: nature, pathogenesis and epidemiology. *World Review of Nutrition and Dietetics*, 62, 59–119.

Jandhyala, B.S. and Hom, G.J. (1983). Minireview: physiological and pharmacological properties of vanadium. *Life Science*, 33, 1325–40.

McLean, R.M. (1994). Magnesium and its therapeutic uses: a review. *American Journal of Medicine*, 96, 63–76.

Mertz, W. (1993). Chromium in human nutrition: a review. *Journal of Nutrition*, 123, 626–33.

Nielsen, F.H. (1984). Ultratrace elements in nutrition. *Annual Review of Nutrition*, 4, 21–41.

Nielsen, F.H. (1991). Nutritional requirements for boron, silicon, vanadium, nickel and arsenic: current knowledge and speculation. *FASEB Journal*, 5, 2661–7.

Offenbacher, E.G. and Pi-Sunyer, F.X. (1988). Chromium in human nutrition. *Annual Review of Nutrition*, 8, 543–63.

Prasad, A.S. (1978). *Trace Elements and Iron in Human Metabolism*. Wiley, Chichester.

Prasad, A.S. (1988). Clinical, endocrinological and biochemical effects of zinc deficiency. *Clinics in Endocrinology and Metabolism*, 14, 567–89.

Prasad, A.S. (1991). Discovery of human zinc deficiency and studies in an experimental human model. *American Journal of Clinical Nutrition*, 53, 403–12.

Rajagopalan, K.V. (1988). Molybdenum: an essential trace element in human nutrition. *Annual Review of Nutrition*, 8, 401–27.

Rude, R.K. (1993). Magnesium metabolism and deficiency. *Endocrinology and Metabolism Clinics of North America*, 22(2), 377–95.

Strain, J.J. (1994). Newer aspects of micronutrients in chronic disease: copper. *Proceedings of the Nutrition Society*, 53, 583–98.

Underwood, E.J. (1977). *Trace Elements in Human and Animal Nutrition*, 4th edn. Academic Press, New York.

Wedler, F.C. (1993). Biological significance of manganese in mammalian systems. *Progress in Medicinal Chemistry*, 30, 89–133.

Table 25.1: Classification of minerals by function

(Several minerals have more than one function, and hence appear under more than one category)

structural function
    calcium, magnesium, phosphate, silicon, fluoride
membrane function
    sodium, potassium
prosthetic groups in enzymes
    cadmium, cobalt, copper, iron, manganese,
    molybdenum, selenium, zinc
regulatory role or role in hormone action
    calcium, chromium, iodine, magnesium, manganese,
    sodium, potassium, vanadium, zinc
other metabolic functions
    magnesium
known to be essential, but function unknown
    nickel, tin
not established as essential, but have effects in the body
    fluoride, lithium
minerals of uncertain status
    arsenic, boron, bromine
occur in foods and known to be toxic in excess
    aluminium, arsenic, antimony, boron, bromine, cadmium,
    caesium, germanium, lead, mercury, silver, strontium

Table 25.2: Body content of minerals

essential minerals

	atomic mass	mol	g
calcium	40.08	25	1000
phosphorus	30.9738	25	770
sodium	22.9898	4.35	100
potassium	39.102	3.58	140
chlorine	35.453	2.67	95
magnesium	24.312	0.78	19
		mmol	mg
fluorine	18.9984	136	2600
iron	55.847	75	4200
zinc	65.37	35	2300
cobalt	58.9332	25	1500
		μmol	mg
chromium	51.996	126	66
copper	63.54	11	72
vanadium	50.942	3.5	180
manganese	54.938	2.2	120
selenium	78.96	1.7	130
tin	118.69	1.4	170
iodine	126.9044	1.0	130
nickel	58.71	0.017	1.0
molybdenum	95.94	0.010	1.0

minerals not known to be essential

	atomic mass	mmol	mg
rubidium	85.47	7955	680
strontium	87.62	3652	320
bromine	79.909	2500	200
aluminium	26.9	2260	61
lead	207.19	580	120
titanium	47.90	188	9
lithium	6.939	97	670
cadmium	112.40	45	500
boron	10.811	18	200
caesium	132.9	11	150
beryllium	90.122	4	36
bismuth	208.98	1	210
silver	107.87	0.7	79

Source: from data reported by Snyder *et al.* 1975.

Table 25.3: Plasma concentrations of minerals and electrolytes

	mmol /L	mg /L
sodium	132-151	3030-3470
potassium	3.4-5.2	130-200
chloride	100-110	3545-3790
phosphate	2	96
bicarbonate	21-29	1470-2030
	µmol/L	µg /L
aluminium	4-29	110-780
barium	0.2-0.6	25-80
cadmium	0.02-0.11	2.3-12
cobalt	0.003-0.105	0.2-6.2
chromium	0.038-0.38	2-20
copper	15-25	970-1640
iron	15-33	870-1870
iodine	0.35-0.79	45-100
lithium	1.2-3.9	8-27
manganese	0.009-0.11	0.5-6
molybdenum	0.06-0.28	6-27
nickel	0.14-10	8-580
lead	0.08-0.63	16-130
selenium	0.3-4.1	100-325
silicon	90-360	2500-10000
zinc	10-28	670-1830
fluoride	0.4-1.9	7-36

Table 25.4: Estimates of intake of minerals and routes of loss

	intake		% of output in:			
	µmol	mg	urine	faeces	sweat	hair / nails
minerals known or believed to be essential						
cadmium	1.3	0.15	67	33	-	-
calcium	27 450	1100	17	69	14	-
chlorine	147 000	5200	83	1	15	-
chromium	2.9	0.15	46	73	0.7	0.4
cobalt	5	0.3	68	30	1	1
copper	55	3.5	1	79	9	-
fluorine	95	1.8	56	8	36	-
iodine	1.6	0.2	86	10	3	1
iron (male)	290	16	1.6	95	3	-
iron (female)	215	12	1.6	89	4	-
magnesium (male)	14 000	340	38	62	0.4	-
magnesium (female)	11 000	270	40	59	0.6	-
manganese	67	3.7	0.8	98	1	-
molybdenum	3.1	0.3	52	41	7	-
nickel	6.8	0.4	3	92	5	0.25
phosphorus	45 000	1400	64	36	-	-
potassium	84 000	3300	85	11	4	-
selenium	1.9	0.15	33	13	53	0.2
silicon	700	20	49	49	-	1.3
sodium	192 000	4400	75	2	20	-
tin	34	4	0.5	87	12	-
vanadium	40	2	0.7	99	-	-
zinc	200	13	4	89	6	0.2
minerals not known to be essential						
aluminium	1700	45	0.8	97	2	-
antimony	410	50	80	18	-	2
arsenic	13	1	6	94	-	-
barium	5.5	0.75	6	84	1	9
beryllium	1330	12	8	91	-	-
bismuth	95	20	8	92	-	-
boron	120	1.3	79	21	-	-
bromine	90	7.5	96	0.1	2.6	-
germanium	20	1.5	92	8	-	-
lead	2.2	0.45	10	68	15	7
lithium	290	2.0	40	60	-	-
mercury	0.08	0.016	-	92	-	7
niobium	6.7	0.62	58	42	-	-
rubidium	26	2.2	84	13	2	-
silver	0.7	0.07	13	86	0.6	1
strontium	22	1.9	18	81	1	-
sulphur	29,000	940	80	14	3	3
tellurium	4.7	0.6	83	16	-	-
thallium	0.01	0.0015	33	67	-	-
thorium	0.01	0.003	3	97	-	-
titanium	18	0.85	39	61	-	-
zirconium	46	4.2	4	96	-	-

Source: from data reported by Snyder *et al.* 1975.

Table 25.5 Deleterious interactions between minerals

essential mineral	antagonism by	site of antagonism
calcium	phosphate	kidney
chromium	iron (haemochromatosis)	plasma
copper	cadmium	kidney, liver, intestinal mucosa
	iron, nickel	liver
	zinc	kidney, liver, plasma, intestinal mucosa
	calcium	intestinal mucosa
fluoride	aluminium	bone
iron	calcium	intestinal mucosa
	copper, cadmium	erythrocyte
	zinc	intestinal mucosa, erythrocyte
magnesium	calcium, phosphate	bone
phosphate	aluminium	bone, ? other tissues
	iron(haemochromatosis)	intestinal mucosa
selenium	cadmium, mercury, silver	liver, kidney
zinc	copper, cadmium	liver

Table 25.6: Estimated requirements for sodium, potassium and chloride

	sodium		potassium		chloride	
	mg /d	mmol /d	mg /d	mmol /d	mg /d	mmol /d
0-5 m	120	5.2	500	12.8	180	5.1
6-11 m	200	8.7	700	17.9	300	8.5
1 y	225	9.8	1000	25.6	350	9.9
2-5 y	300	13.0	1400	35.8	500	14.1
6-9 y	400	17.4	1600	40.9	600	16.9
10-18 y	500	21.7	2000	51.1	750	21.2
> 18 y	500	21.7	2000	51.1	750	21.2

Source: National Research Council 1989.

Table 25.7: Dietary Reference Values for sodium and potassium

	Lower Reference Nutrient Intake[1]				Reference Nutrient Intake[1]				Population Reference Intake[2]	
	sodium		potassium		sodium		potassium		potassium	
	mg /d	mmol /d	mg /d	mmol /d	mg /d	mmol /d	mg /d	mmol /d	mg /d	mmol /d
0-3 m	140	6	400	10	210	9	800	20	-	-
4-6 m	140	6	400	10	280	12	850	22	-	-
7-9 m	200	9	400	10	320	14	700	18	800	20
10-12 m	200	9	450	12	350	15	700	18	800	20
1-3 y	200	9	450	12	500	22	800	20	800	20
4-6 y	280	12	600	15	700	30	1100	28	1100	28
7-10 y	350	15	950	24	1200	50	2000	50	2000	50
11-14 y	160	20	1600	40	1600	70	3100	80	3100	80
> 15 y	575	25	2000	50	1600	70	3500	90	3100	80

Source: (1) Department of Health 1991; (2) Scientific Committee for Food 1993.

Table 25.8: Safe and adequate levels of chromium intake

	μmol /day	μg /day
birth—6 m	10-40	0.2-0.8
7—12 m	20-60	0.4-1.2
1—3 y	20-80	0.4-1.5
4—6	30-120	0.6-2.3
7—10	50-200	1.0-3.8
11—24	50-200	1.0-3.8
adults	50-200	1.0-3.8

Source: National Research Council 1989.

Table 25.9 Reference intakes of copper

	US RDA[1] (1989)		UK RNI (1991)		EU PRI (1993)	
	mg	μmol	mg	μmol	mg	μmol
birth—6 m	0.4-0.6	6.3-9.4	0.3	4.7	-	-
7—12 m	0.6-0.7	9.4-11	0.3	4.7	0.3	4.7
1—3 y	0.7-1.0	11-15.7	0.4	6.3	0.4	6.3
4—6	1.0-1.5	15.7-23.6	0.6	9.4	0.6	9.4
7—10	1.0-2.0	15.7-31.4	0.7	11.0	0.7	11.0
11—14	1.5-2.5	23.6-39.3	0.8	12.6	0.8	12.6
15—18	1.5-2.5	23.6-39.3	1.0	15.7	1.0	15.7
19—24	1.5-2.5	23.6-39.3	1.2	18.9	1.1	17.3
adults	1.5-3.0	23.6-47.2	1.2	18.9	1.1	17.3
pregnant	-	-	-	-	-	-
lactating	-	-	+0.3	+4.7	1.4	22.0

(1) US figure is for safe and adequate range of intakes
Source: National Research Council 1989; Department of Health 1991; Scientific Committee for Food 1993.

Table 25.10: Rich sources of copper

	portion (g)	mg /portion
crab	175	8.40
liver	150	3.75
lobster	150	2.55
chocolate, plain	125	2.13
prawns	150	1.05
kidney	150	0.99
mussels	150	0.72
mung beans (dahl)	150	0.70
beans, red kidney	100	0.68
venison	150	0.54
lentils	150	0.50
oatmeal	100	0.49
duck	150	0.47
Brazil nuts	25	0.44
chickpeas	150	0.42
coconut	75	0.42
beer	500	0.40
beef	150	0.38
chocolate, milk	125	0.38
pork	150	0.38
potato	260	0.37
mushrooms	50	0.36
sardines canned in tomato	150	0.34
walnuts	25	0.34
scampi	150	0.33
black pudding	80	0.30
salmon	150	0.30
tuna	150	0.30
lamb	150	0.28
mackerel	150	0.28
sardines canned in oil	150	0.28
almonds	25	0.25
avocados	130	0.25
hamburger	100	0.25
peanuts	25	0.25
Barcelona nuts	25	0.24
broad beans	75	0.24
gammon	150	0.23
goose	150	0.23
shrimps	150	0.23
turkey	150	0.23
kipper	150	0.21
rice	165	0.21
sweet potato	150	0.21
cider	500	0.20
dried currants	25	0.20
dogfish	150	0.19
ham	85	0.19
pilchards in tomato sauce	100	0.19
pork	150	0.19
bread, wholemeal	70	0.18
chicken	150	0.18
herring	150	0.18
chestnuts	75	0.17
grapes	140	0.17
bacon	150	0.16

Table 25.10 (Cont'd)

	portion (g)	mg /portion
beans, haricot	100	0.16
herring	150	0.16
lemon sole	150	0.15
pasta	150	0.15
semolina	100	0.15
bananas	135	0.14
cockles	50	0.14
peanuts	25	0.14
pineapple	125	0.14
tripe	150	0.14

Table 25.11: Tissue copper

	nmol /g wet weight
liver	230
brain	90
lung	35
kidney	33
ovary	19
testis	12
muscle	11

Source: from data reported by Hamilton *et al.* 1992.

Table 25.12: Copper-dependent enzymes

enzyme	EC number	function	effects of copper deficiency
ceruloplasmin	1.16.3.1	copper transport, iron metabolism, diamine oxidase	impaired mobilization of iron reserves
cytochrome oxidase	1.9.3.1	terminal electron transport enzyme in mitochondria	impaired energy-yielding metabolism
diamine oxidase	1.4.3.6	inactivation of amines	unknown
dopamine β-hydroxylase	1.14.17.1	catecholamine synthesis	reduced noradrenaline and adrenaline formation
lysyl oxidase	1.4.3.13	collagen and elastin cross-links	abnormal collagen and elastin
superoxide dismutase	1.15.1.1	anti-oxidant; removal of superoxide radicals	increased oxygen radical damage
thiol oxidase	1.8.3.2	formation of disulphide bridges in proteins	hair abnormalities
tyrosinase	1.14.18.1	melanin synthesis	poor hair pigmentation

Table 25.13: Mean normal values for indices of copper nutritional status.

age	plasma Cu μmol/L	enzymic mg/L	ceruloplasmin immunological mg/L	enzymic / immunological	erythrocyte SOD[1] U/g Hb	cytochrome oxidase platelets U/10^9 cells	mononuclear leukocytes U/10^6 cells
men							
20-29	12.2	408	266	1.56	3240	2.75	0.33
30-39	12.0	416	296	1.49	3080	2.94	0.31
40-49	13.5	442	337	1.31	3010	3.52	0.40
50-59	13.7	441	310	1.43	3170	3.89	0.35
60-69	14.2	470	284	1.70	2990	4.92	0.43
> 70	14.0	485	332	1.51	2900	4.51	0.45
women							
20-29	15.9	503	330	1.53	2840	2.36	0.27
30-39	15.5	516	314	1.66	3170	2.75	0.36
40-49	16.8	519	359	1.48	2944	3.08	0.35
50-59	17.0	516	370	1.44	3327	3.88	0.38
60-69	17.9	559	354	1.60	3910	4.56	0.37
> 70	16.6	470	368	1.29	2840	3.65	0.39
women + oral contraceptives							
20-29	21.2	612	371	1.71	3380	2.87	0.32
30-39	25.3	744	525	1.42	2890	3.87	0.39
women + hormone replacement therapy							
50-59	19.2	593	384	1.57	2840	3.54	0.42

(1) SOD = superoxide dismutase (EC 1.15.1.1)
Source: Milne DB and Johnson PE 1993.

Table 25.14: Reference values for indices of copper status

concentration of copper in

plasma or serum	13-22 μmol /L
whole blood	13-22 μmol /L
erythrocytes	4.8-20.8 μmol /L
leukocytes	4.1-36.8 pmol /10^6 cells
urine	0.1-1.0 μmol /24h
sweat	0.9-25 μmol /24h
saliva	0.74-1.95 μmol /L
hair	0.24-0.40 μmol /g
liver	79-111 nmol /g
serum ceruloplasmin	2-4 μmol /L
urinary hydroxylysine	11.2-15.6 μmol /d

Source: from data reported by Arnaud 1993.

Table 25.15: Safe and adequate levels of fluoride intake

	μmol /day	mg /day
birth—6 m	5-25	0.1-0.5
7—12 m	10-50	0.2-1.0
1—3	25-80	0.5-1.5
4—6	50-130	1.0-2.5
7—10	80-130	1.5-2.5
11—24	80-130	1.5-2.5
adults	80-210	1.5-4.0

Source: National Research Council 1989.

Table 25.16: Prevalence of iodine deficiency

	at risk	millions of people with goitre	with cretinism
Africa	227	39	0.5
Latin America	60	30	0.3
Southeast Asia	280	100	4.0
Asia	400	30	0.9
Eastern Mediterranean	33	12	-
Total	1000	211	5.7

Table 25.17: Reference intakes for iodine

	US RDA (1989) μg	US RDA (1989) μmol	UK RNI (1991) μg	UK RNI (1991) μmol	EU PRI (1993) μg	EU PRI (1993) mol
birth—3 m	40	0.32	50	0.39	-	-
3—6 m	40	0.32	60	0.47	-	-
7—12 m	50	0.39	60	0.47	50	0.39
1—3 y	70	0.55	70	0.55	70	0.55
4—6	90	0.71	100	0.79	90	0.71
7—10	120	0.95	110	0.87	100	0.79
11—14	150	1.18	130	1.02	120	0.95
15—18	150	1.18	140	1.10	130	1.02
adults	150	1.18	140	1.10	130	1.02
pregnant	175	1.38	-	-	130	1.02
lactating	200	1.58	-	-	160	1.26

Source: National Research Council 1989; Department of Health 1991; Scientific Committee for Food 1993.

Table 25.18: Rich sources of iodine

	portion (g)	μg /portion
mackerel	150	255
mussels	150	180
cod	150	165
kipper	150	107
whiting	150	100
yoghourt	150	95
milk	560	86
cockles	50	80
fish fingers	75	75
pilchards in tomato sauce	100	64
scampi	150	62
herring	150	48
beer	560	45
lemon sole	150	42
plaice	150	42
prawns	150	42
egg	70	37
sardines canned in oil	150	35
trout	150	24
kidney	150	23
liver	150	22
tuna	150	21
bacon	150	18
cheese	40	18
potato chips	265	13

Table 25.19: Reference intakes of magnesium

| | US RDA (1989) | | UK RNI (1991) | |
	mg	mmol	mg	mmol
birth—3 m	40	1.6	55	2.3
3—6 m	40	1.6	60	2.5
7—9 m	60	2.5	75	3.1
9m—1 y	60	2.5	80	3.3
1—3 y	80	3.3	85	3.5
4—6	120	4.9	120	4.9
7—10	170	7.0	200	8.2
males				
11—14	270	11.1	280	11.5
15—18	400	16.5	300	12.3
19—24	350	14.4	300	12.3
25—50	350	14.4	300	12.3
> 50	350	14.4	300	12.3
females				
11—14	280	11.5	280	11.5
15—18	300	12.3	300	12.3
19—24	280	11.5	270	11.1
25—50	280	11.5	270	11.1
> 50	280	11.5	270	11.1
pregnant	320	13.2	-	-
lactating	355	14.6	+ 50	+ 2.1

The European Union Scientific Committee for Food (1993) quotes an acceptable range for adults of 150-500 mg (6-21 mmol)
Source: National Research Council 1989; Department of Health 1991.

Table 25.20: Safe and adequate levels of manganese intake

	mg/day	μmol /day
birth—6m	0.3-0.6	5.5-10.9
7—12 m	0.6-0.7	10.9-12.7
1—3	0.7-1.0	12.7-18.2
4—6	1.0-1.5	18.2-27.3
7—10	1.0-2.0	18.2-36.4
11—24	1.5-2.5	27.3-45.5
adults	1.5-3.0	27.3-54.6

The European Union Scientific Committee for Food (1993) quotes an acceptable range for adults of 1-10 mg (18-180 μmol)
UK safe level of intakes: adults 1.4 mg (25 μmol), infants and children 16 μg (0.1 mol).
Source: National Research Council 1989.

Table 25.21 Safe and adequate levels of molybdenum intake

	μg/day	μmol/day
birth—6m	15-30	0.15-0.30
7—12 m	20-40	0.21-0.42
1—3	25-50	0.26-0.52
4—6	30-75	0.31-0.78
7—10	50-150	0.52-1.56
11—24	75-250	0.78-2.6
adults	75-250	0.78-2.6

Source: National Research Council 1989.

Table 25.22: Reference intakes of zinc

| | US RDA (1989) | | UK RNI (1991) | | EU PRI (1993) | |
	mg	μmol	mg	μmol	mg	μmol
birth—6 m	5	75	4	60	-	-
7—9 m	5	75	5	75	4	60
9m—1 y	5	75	5	75	4	60
1—3 y	10	150	5	75	4	60
4—6	10	150	6.5	100	6	90
7—10	10	150	7	110	7	110
males						
11—14	15	230	9	140	9	140
15—24	15	230	9.5	145	9	140
adults	15	230	9.5	145	9.5	145
females						
11—14	12	180	9	140	9	140
15—24	12	180	7	110	9	140
adults	12	180	7	110	7	110
pregnant	15	230	-	-	7	110
lactating	19	290	+ 0.3	+ 5	12	180

Source: National Research Council 1989; Department of Health 1991; Scientific Committee for Food 1993.

Table 25.23: Rich sources of zinc

	portion (g)	mg /portion
crab	175	9.63
beef	150	9.45
lamb	150	6.45
liver	150	6.00
venison	150	5.85
kidney	150	4.50
sardines canned in oil	150	4.50
pork	150	4.35
veal	150	4.20
gammon	150	4.05
mung beans (dahl)	150	4.05
sardines canned in tomato	150	4.05
duck	150	3.90
goose	150	3.90
bacon joint	150	3.60
turkey	150	3.60
oatmeal	100	3.30
hamburger	100	3.20
mussels	150	3.15
beans, red kidney	100	3.00
lobster	150	2.70
rabbit	150	2.55
prawns	150	2.40
chicken	150	2.25
tripe	150	2.25
milk	560	2.24
cheese, Parmesan	40	2.12
lentils	150	2.10
barley	100	2.00
ham	85	1.95
kipper	150	1.95
chickpeas	150	1.80
shrimps	150	1.65
tuna	150	1.65
wheat bran	10	1.62
pilchards in tomato sauce	100	1.60
potato chips	265	1.59
bacon rashers	85	1.36
salmon	150	1.35
bread, wholemeal	70	1.26
rice, boiled	165	1.15
cheese, soft (camembert)	40	1.08
Brazil nuts	25	1.05
lemon sole	150	1.05
skate	150	1.05
yoghourt	150	1.05
beans, baked	200	1.00

Table 25.24: Reference ranges of zinc in biological fluids

plasma zinc	9-22 μmol /L
erythrocyte zinc	200 $\pm$ 50 μmol /L
urinary zinc	4.6-9.2 μmol /24h
mixed leukocytes	0.76 nmol /mg dry cells
	75-120 pmol /10^6 cells
lymphocytes	1.85 $\pm$ 0.32 nmol /mg protein
mononuclear leukocytes	180 $\pm$ 30 pmol /10^6 cells
	2.58 $\pm$ 0.65 nmol /mg protein
polymorphonuclear leukocytes	120 $\pm$ 2 pmol /10^6 cells
	1.26 $\pm$ 0.32 nmol /mg protein
platelets	30-60 μmol/10^6 cells
	0.76-3.8 mmol /L blood
saliva (total)	150 $\pm$ 10 nmol /L
saliva sediment	1.8 μmol /g

Source: from data reported by Aggett 1991; Aggett and Favier 1993.

Food processing

26.1 Traditional methods of food processing

Man the hunter-gatherer lived on what he could find—molluscs, fish, seals, wild grain, nuts, berries, tubers, leaves, insects and their grubs, birds and their eggs, and such animals as were available. He roamed from one area to another seeking and hunting food and had no need to store it; storage became necessary between harvests only when people settled in one place and cultivated crops and herded animals. The first crops were wheat and barley; grains have been found in Palestine dating from 8000 BC. The wild variety of wheat was Emmer wheat from which the range of modern varieties was developed. Bread made from wheat has been dated around 5000 BC in the Nile Valley (2000 BC in England). Domestication of animals dates back to 8000 BC for cows, 6000 BC for sheep, goats and swine.

The beginning of urbanization around 1000 BC required food supplies from outside the community, and massive increases in agricultural production, transport and food preservation came with the growth of large cities during the eighteenth century, allowing transport from regions where food was plentiful.

The oldest processed food known is bulgur—Turkish and Persian for bruised grain—also called ala, borghul, cracked wheat and American rice. Wheat is soaked, cooked and dried, then lightly milled to remove the outer bran and cracked. It is still a common food, often in soup or in place of rice, in the Middle East.

In more recent years the convenience of partially or fully prepared foods and meals together with market competition have brought about a vast expansion in processing. Table 26.1 shows the chronology of the introduction of new foods, Table 26.2 the chronology of introduction of methods of food processing, Table 26.3 milestones in the distribution of foods and Table 26.4 milestones in food legislation.

26.1.1. Preservation

Many foods are edible for only a very short time, such as fruits and vegetables, others for somewhat longer but all are subject to deterioration by enzymes present in the food, by oxidation by air, and by the growth of bacteria, yeasts and fungi on the food. Micro-organisms can render the food not only unpalatable (see Table 26.9) but in many instances harmful through the growth of pathogens and the production of toxins (see sections 27.5 and 27.6).

Deterioration is slowed by reducing the temperature and largely inhibited by freezing to temperatures as low as -18°C or, in some instances -30°C.

Enzymic action can be prevented by heat destruction. The growth of micro-organisms can be prevented by (1) heat destruction (sterilization) so long as the food is protected from subsequent contamination (e.g. in bottles, cans or sealed plastic containers); (2) removal of water (dehydration) or the osmotic effect of added sugar or partial dehydration with the addition of osmotic substances (as in intermediate moisture foods); (3) the formation of acid or alcohol by fermentation; (4) the addition of chemical preservatives such as salt, sulphur dioxide, vinegar, etc. (see section 26.2.2). Smoking helps to dry the outer parts of the food and deposits chemicals with a preservative action as well as adding flavour.

These methods have been used for some thousands of years, long before there was any scientific explanation of the processes. For example, centuries ago along the north-west coast of North America both dried and smoked salmon were common; in many regions of the world meat was preserved by drying, salting and embedding in fat (described in ancient Egyptian writings); milk was converted into cheese and yogurt. Sausages were preserved by drying, salting, smoking and fermentation before 2000 BC; figs, grapes and dates are described in the bible; smoking is said to have been practised by early cavemen in Europe.

The preservative effects of cooling were recognized long ago when communities stored root crops and legumes in cool cellars, and preservation by chilling with ice was carried out by the ancient Romans.

Methods of preservation differed in various regions depending on the climate and the availability of materials. For example in the West Indies where salt was scarce, meat was preserved by drying in the sun and smoking over a fire of green wood resting on a wooden frame—a boucan—a process termed boucanning.

The preservation of meat by drying has a long history exemplified by xarqui (charqui) in Brazil, biltong in South Africa, akutok (caribou meat) of the Eskimos, and pemmican, a mixture of powdered dried meat and fat made by the American prairie Indians. In Scandinavia, in contrast to the tropics, it was found that even in a cold climate foods could be dried by the wind.

Milk was preserved traditionally by making cheese and by fermentation to products such as yogurt and a range of drinks in which the lactose was fermented to acid or alcohol which serves as a preservative, e.g. busa (Turkestan), cieddu (Italy), dadhi (India), kefir (Balkans), daboo (Iraq), tako (Hungary), kumiss (Russian steppes), laban zabadi (Egypt), mazum (Armenia), taette (N Europe), mafi (S Africa), skyr (Iceland), nasy (Iran), crowdies (Scotland). These were made from milk of various species: mare, cow, buffalo, goat, camel, sometimes with additions such as rice, palm sugar, spices, etc.

Part of the milk, the fat, could be preserved by conversion to butter. It was relatively recently shown that in the process there is a change of phase (inversion) from small fat globules suspended in an aqueous medium to small water droplets trapped in a fatty phase and so unavailable to micro-organisms. The addition of salt prolongs the shelf life.

26.1.1.1 Salting

Salt has been used as a preservative since at least 3500 BC when fish and fowl were dried and salted in China, but was probably used long before that. Meat has been traditionally preserved with salt, both by dry curing where the meat is covered with powdered salt, and brining, where the food is immersed in salt solution. Salt inhibits the growth of most spoilage organisms when the concentration in the aqueous phase is greater than 4 per cent; it functions as a complete preservative at 17 per cent but the product would be unpalatable. With the addition of nitrite, meat can be preserved with salt concentrations between 2.5 and 5 per cent. This has the effect of preserving the food by inhibiting the growth of pathogens, particularly *Clostridium botulinum*, while salt-tolerant bacteria develop, at the same time producing a desirable red colour and also flavour. Nitrate is converted into nitrite by the salt-tolerant bacteria and the consequent nitric oxide combines with the muscle pigment, myoglobin, to form nitrosomyoglobin, which is stabilized to form nitrosohaemochromogen when the meat is cooked. Nitrite reacts with amines present in foods to form nitrosamines (see section 27.4.4), which are carcinogenic in animals, so there is a tendency to reduce the amount of nitrite in the cure in some countries and to add ascorbic acid (vitamin C, see Chapter 22) which inhibits the formation of nitrosamines, as well as preventing rancidity by acting as an antioxidant.

Although curing has traditionally been used for preservation, the process results in a wide range of products such as bacon, ham, sausages, with numerous variants, which are wanted as foods in their own right.

26.1.1.2 Acids

The growth of micro-organisms is inhibited by acids, either by addition or by fermentation of the sugars present naturally in the food (fermentation). Acids such as acetic, citric, lactic, tartaric, glycolic and phosphoric are in use; the process of fermentation was known to the ancients without knowledge of the underlying science. Historically, failure of heat sterilization in some instances is now known to be due to insufficient acidity, when micro-organisms are less readily destroyed.

Sauerkraut, fermented cabbage, was known to the Romans; the use of moulds as in the preparation of sofu, tofu and tempeh from soya beans dates back at least to 2000 BC in the Far East; similarly fish sauces such as nuoc-mam in Vietnam, nampla in Burma, are essentially hydrolysates of fish in which the added salt prevents the growth of pathogens.

26.1.1.3 The addition of chemical preservatives

Preservation by the addition of chemicals—benzoic acid, specified antibiotics, antioxidants—is often regarded as a modern process but sulphur dioxide, salt, sugar and vinegar have been used traditionally, as have spices (see section 26.2.2).

In Egypt as far back as 1500 BC must seed (named after its capacity to preserve must) was used as a preservative, and other spices were used as long ago as 2700 BC.

26.1.1.4 Temperature control

Modern refrigeration dates back little more than a century, but food was chilled with ice in 1100 BC.

Centuries before ice-making equipment was developed, ice was harvested from lakes in winter and stored under sawdust or peat or in caves, until required during the summer months.

The modern process of freeze-drying, whereby water sublimes in high vacuum from solid to vapour stage without melting in between, was carried out in France in 1906 (lyophilization) but a similar process was practised by pre-Columbian Indians in Peru and Bolivia. Potatoes were crushed and subjected to night frosts; daytime sunshine melted the ice and water was squeezed out. Several repetitions resulted in dried potato—chuno—which could be stored for long periods. Similarly reindeer meat was freeze-dried by the Lapps of northern Scandinavia, stockfish in Norway and meat in Tibet.

In recent years, as more details of the chemistry and physics of foodstuffs have become known, and driven by market competition, new methods of processing, as well as improvements of established methods, have been developed.

26.1.2 New methods of food processing

With the development of food science and technology in the twentieth century, new methods of processing, as distinct from modifications and improvements of traditional methods, have been and still are being developed.

26.1.2.1 Ionizing Radiation

While the method is not new—it was suggested in 1896, one year after the discovery of X rays—its application to foods is recent and is still limited. X rays and gamma rays from radioactive isotopes or the linear accelerator kill micro-organisms (or reduce the number of pathogenic and spoilage organisms) and insects, inhibit sprouting of potatoes and delay ripening of some fruits.

A French patent was taken out for the preservation of food by irradiation in 1930 (Wust) which was followed by intensive research on the safety of such treatment. Joint Expert Committees of the United Nations (JECFI 1979, 1977) concluded that certain foods irradiated for specific purposes and within certain dose limits were unconditionally safe for human consumption. A subsequent report (JECFI 1981) concluded that doses up to 10 kGy posed no toxicological hazard and introduced no special nutritional problems.

Complete bacterial sterilization requires doses up to 50 kGy; doses to achieve specific objectives are shown in Table 26.5. Since 1963 various countries

have given approval to use specified doses on certain foods but to date the process is not widely used.

26.1.2.2 Ultra-high Temperature Sterilization

Products such as milk have long been heat treated either to pasteurize, i.e. destroy pathogens, or sterilize, i.e. destroy all micro-organisms. Pasteurization has been in use in some towns since 1880 and more generally since 1920. Raw milk will keep for 24 hours at room temperature; pasteurized milk will keep for a few days. Sterilized milk will keep for several months but the original method had the disadvantage that the product developed a cooked flavour, became discoloured and some 50 per cent of the vitamin C and 30 per cent of the thiamin were destroyed.

When it was shown that a 10°C rise in temperature multiplied the effect on biological material (organisms) by a factor of 10, compared with a factor of 2 for chemical reactions, sterilization was carried out at a higher temperature for a shorter time; thus:

(1) pasteurization of milk (holder method) 63–65°C for 30 min;

(2) flash pasteurization 74°C for a few seconds;

(3) sterilization in bottle 105–112°C for 20–30 min;

(4) high-temperature short-time (HTST) 71°C for 15 sec;

(5) ultra-high temperature (UHT) 140°C for 2 sec.

Thermization is heating to a lesser extent than pasteurization (60–66°C for 5–10 sec) which destroys most psychrophilic organisms that grow in refrigerated milk, and which produce damaging lipases and proteases; thermized milk will keep for 4 days at 4°C without changes in proteins and is used by some cheese makers.

26.1.2.3 Ohmic heating

The objective of limiting damage to appearance, texture, nutrients, and palatability has led to a variety of methods of heating such as the use of higher temperatures for a shorter time, pasteurization, indirect heating, steaming, etc. A more recent development, applicable to food products containing particles and liquid, is ohmic heating, in which heat is developed by passing an electric current through the food or mixture. This process has the advantage of better retention of flavour and nutrients.

26.1.2.4 High pressure treatment

Pressures up to 1000–6000 atmospheres alter the physical structure of large molecules (as in foods).

The process, which originated in Japan, maintains colour, flavour, and nutrients in fruits and juices.

26.1.2.5 Inter-esterification

Hydrogenation of oils to produce fats useful in margarines and for baking leads to the formation of *trans*-fatty acids (see section 8.1.1.2) which have been implicated in coronary heart disease. The amounts of *trans*-fatty acids can be reduced if hydrogenation is partially replaced by inter-esterification. This is a heat process in which there is an exchange of fatty acids between the glycerol molecules of the fat resulting in some degree of hardening. While there is no clear evidence that *trans*-fatty acids are harmful (see section 8.1.1.2.1) this is considered to be a sensible precaution.

26.1.2.6 Biotechnology

Biotechnology is the application of biological processes to make useful products—foods, chemicals and medicines—and includes fermentation as used traditionally for the preparation of cheese, yogurt, bread, beer, wine, vinegar. Modern biotechnology, also called genetic engineering or genetic modification, is the newest of all processes but biotechnology is also the oldest method of plant and animal breeding, practised by man since the beginning of agriculture. For thousands of years farmers have selected 'better' plants and animals and bred from them to produce, eventually, improved varieties. Modern biotechnology is a rapid way of producing the required varieties compared with the very slow hit-and-miss process of selection. It consists of identifying the particular gene that governs the required trait, its extraction, multiplication and insertion into the organism— or blocking an undesirable trait. It is thus possible to produce plants that are resistant to disease, drought, frost, or pests, or are tolerant of herbicides so that weeds can be destroyed while the food plant survives, also richer in specified nutrients and with extended shelf-life. Animals can be developed that resist diseases, produce less fatty meat, grow faster, and have increased fertility.

So far as food processing is concerned 'modern' biotechnology can lead to the production of raw materials more suited to specific purposes of food processing such as starch consisting of 100 per cent amylopectin (see section 7.1.1.3), enzymes for specific functions (see Table 26.11), improved yeasts for both bread-making and brewing, the production of a substitute for animal rennet (chymosin) in cheese-making, and a vast range of other purposes. It is thus another of the modern developments of traditional food processing where new knowledge provides an understanding of the scientific principles and permits better control of the process.

26.2   Food additives

An additive is any substance not normally regarded as a food that is added to foods as an aid in manufacturing or processing, or to improve the keeping properties, flavour, colour, texture, appearance, or stability of the food, or as a convenience to the consumer. Additives may be synthetic compounds, naturally occurring compounds extracted from natural sources, or synthesized to resemble the natural products in all respects (nature-identical). Technically and legally the term excludes vitamins, minerals and other nutrients added to enrich or restore nutritional value. Herbs, spices, hops, salt, sugar, yeast, protein hydrolysates, air and water are also excluded from the definition of additives; they are considered as ingredients.

The overall functions of additives can be classified as follows (see also Table 26.6).

1. To preserve foods, i.e. to prevent growth of microorganisms, and to protect fats from oxidation (antioxidants).

2. To affect the texture or consistency—emulsifiers, stabilizers, thickeners, gelling agents.

3. To modify appearance and taste (colours and flavours).

4. As processing aids, and to improve the food in some specific way (e.g. anti-spattering agents in frying oils, polyphosphates to hold water and fat in meat products, anti-caking agents to prevent powders from clogging).

5. To enable ingredient modifications to suit health needs (e.g. products low in fat, or sugar, high in fibre, etc).

About 3 750 food additives are used, of which 3 500 are flavours, and of these 250 are artificial. These figures may be compared with the several hundred non-nutritive substances found in foods such as meat or a fruit or a vegetable.

An example of the extremely wide range of properties of additives is given in Table 26.3 which lists the various additives that can be used in baking. These affect crumb structure, softness of crumb and shelf-life, and loaf volume, and include oxidizing and reducing agents and emulsifiers in addition to sugars, enzymes and inorganic salts. While it is possible to make bread and cakes domestically without any of these, commercial production demands a consistent product despite the variability of the raw materials and many of the additives in use are required for this purpose.

26.2.1 Permitted additives

Only additives that have been tested and not demonstrated to be hazardous (see section 26.2.9) may be used, and they must usually be declared on the label, together with the ingredients (see section 4.3). Within the European Union additives may be declared either by name or by the number on the list of permitted additives (the 'E-number'). The EU list of permitted additives (amended with effect from January 1996) is shown in Table 26.8.

Some additives are permitted only in specified foods. The maximum amounts that may be added are controlled by law in the case of some additives (and the amount of the same additive permitted in different foods may differ). For other additives there is no regulation of the amount that may be added; EU legislation uses the term *quantum satis* for such additives, while US legislation suggests the limitation is a matter of Good Manufacturing Practice (GMP)—the intensity of colour or flavour, or effects on the texture and other properties of the product will determine upper limits of the use of such additives.

26.2.2 Preservatives

Every food (apart from pure, crystalline sucrose) will deteriorate; some such as vegetables and fruits after a few days, others such as cereals and some root crops after a few months. Deterioration takes place through the action of enzymes naturally present in the food, and by dehydration and oxidation, but most importantly through the growth of bacteria, moulds, and yeasts (see Table 26.9), which not only damage the food but can cause disease (see section 27.6). All these processes can be delayed by cooling or freezing, by destruction or inhibition of enzymes by brief heat treatment (blanching), and by destruction of microorganisms by heat. Relatively brief heat treatment (pasteurization) may destroy specific pathogenic organisms, but not those that may cause further deterioration; sterilization (the destruction of all microorganisms) requires lengthier heat treatment and higher temperatures, or irradiation. Obviously, pasteurized and sterilized foods must be protected from further contamination.

A range of chemicals will also serve to preserve food, by inhibiting the growth of micro-organisms, including sugar, salt, acids, smoke, nitrite, sulphite, benzoate, etc. Many of these methods—salting, smoking, air-drying, fermenting—are traditional, and modern techniques are often modifications of traditional methods, using controlled conditions and sophisticated equipment. The list of chemical preservatives has been extended over the years and includes a small number of antibiotics that are permitted for specific foods. Table 26.10 lists the major preservatives, and the foods in which they are commonly used.

26.2.3 Antioxidants

The deterioration of fats and oils takes place by two processes, hydrolysis and oxidation. Hydrolysis is a reaction between water and the triacylglycerols to form free fatty acids and mono- and diglycerides. It takes place mostly at the high temperatures of frying and, apart from unpleasant flavours of the free fatty acids and their breakdown products, results in poor quality of the fats for frying purposes. Hydrolysis cannot be prevented by the use of antioxidants or other additives but only by good manufacturing practice.

Hydrolysis can also proceed at lower temperatures, catalysed by lipases naturally present in the food, which can cause deterioration during storage; the enzymes can be destroyed by heat.

Oxidation leads to rancidity and occurs during processing and storage. The extent of oxidation largely depends on the degree of unsaturation of the fatty acids of the triacylglycerols (see section 8.1.1). Oxygen radicals, generated by reaction with metal ions, heat, or light, attack unsaturated bonds in fatty acids, leading to a chain reaction (see section 15.5.1), and the production of lipid peroxides, which then decompose to aldehydes, ketones and acids which have rancid flavours.

Antioxidants for fats and oils function by interfering with the formation of free radicals and the propagation of the chain reaction, not as oxygen scavengers. They include some 20 compounds ranging from butylated hydroxyanisole (BHA) through a number of gallates to two vitamins, ascorbic acid and tocopherols—used as antioxidants rather than for nutritional purposes. Table 26.11 lists the major antioxidants and the foods in which they are used.

Tocopherols (vitamin E) occur in many vegetable oils as natural antioxidants; as discussed in section 15.2, the vitamers of tocopherol have different vitamin activity; as antioxidants *in vitro* γ- and δ-tocopherol are the most effective, although *in vivo* α-tocopherol has the highest vitamin activity.

Antioxidants are added to fats and oils intended for frying and baking and to nut, meat and fish products, and breadspreads, and may be included in packaging materials. They are also useful in protecting foods such as dried cereals, where, although the amount of fat is small it is highly unsaturated.

26.2.4 Colours

Colour, although by no means essential in food and drinks, is important in the perception of flavour, so colours, originally all of natural origin, have been added to foods and drinks for centuries. Additional pigments have become available since the discovery of dye synthesis in 1856; because they are often much more intense than natural colours, they may be preferred to natural extracts because they are needed in much smaller amounts, as well as, sometimes, being more stable to heat and light.

Colouring materials may be used to ensure uniformity since basic foodstuffs can vary seasonally and from batch to batch. For example, Citrus red no 2 is specifically permitted in USA only for colouring the skins of citrus fruits, because some tree-ripened oranges may have patches of discoloration on the skin, which diminish the visual appeal of the fruit. The natural colour of some foods is partially bleached or otherwise changed during processing or storage, and colours may be added to restore the original appearance.

In USA, colours are considered in two groups.

1. Certifiable colours for food use (see Table 26.12). These are synthetic dyes; each batch must be tested and certified by the manufacturers and the US Food and Drug Administration as conforming to standards of purity. Seven such compounds are permitted for use in food, drugs and cosmetics, and are known as FD and C colours. Six of these are also on the EU list of permitted additives.

2. Colours exempt from certification (see Table 26.13). These are natural extracts, or chemically synthesized nature-identical compounds, for which batch analysis is not required by law.

26.2.5 Flavours

The flavours of foods are obviously of outstanding importance to their appeal. Made-up products such as sugar-fat desserts need flavouring, and added flavours may be needed to replace processing losses, as well as to standardize foods that vary seasonally, as is the case with colours.

Flavours fall into three groups: those extracted from natural sources which comprise some 93 per cent of the total used, those synthesized in the laboratory to be identical with these (nature-identical), and those that do not occur in nature and are purely synthetic.

The number of flavouring substances used is about 3500 out of a total of 3750 additives in general use. Very few of these have been tested for safety and it would be quite impossible to examine all of them through the full procedures employed for food additives in general. However, since so many are of natural origin (or nature-identical) and are regularly consumed in so many natural foods, and have been for centuries, it is likely that most, if not all, can be Generally Regarded as Safe (see section 26.2.9.1)

Essential oils are derived from plant materials, herbs and spices. They occur in small oil sacs (as is obvious in citrus peel oils) but they bear no chemical relation to edible oils (triacylglycerols, see section 8.1.1). They are used for flavouring, particularly of soft drinks.

26.2.6 Emulsifiers and stabilizers

Emulsifiers allow aqueous and fatty phases in foods to mix, and are consequently known also as surface-active agents or surfactants. They include in the molecule both hydrophilic and hydrophobic groupings, so part is attracted towards the water and part towards the oil, making emulsions of oil-in-water such as milk, cream, mayonnaise, ice cream, and water-in-oil such as butter and margarine. Free fatty acids, mono- and diacylglycerols and phospholipids (see section 8.1.2) are widely used as emulsifying agents.

Emulsifiers also allow interaction between ingredients such as starch and proteins, modify the crystallization of fats, and function as antistaling agents in baked products, by complexing with the soluble amylose component of starch (see section 7.1.1.3), and reduce the stickiness of products such as instant dried potato.

Emulsifiers containing saturated fatty acids are useful as whipping agents in cake mixes and instant desserts, because they stabilize aqueous foams, while those with unsaturated fatty acids serve as antifoaming agents.

Stabilizers may be required to maintain emulsions; they function largely by increasing the viscosity of the mixture so reducing the movements of the dispersed particles which could lead to their coalescence. In some instances they are of additional value in food preparations for their effect on the viscosity of the product and so its texture.

Stabilizers include compounds of high molecular weight such as proteins and complex carbohydrates such as starches, pectins, gums and alginates.

26.2.7 pH control

The relative acidity or alkalinity of a system can have a marked influence on the changes that occur in foods during processing and preparation. In most foods the pH lies between 4 and 7, alkaline foods being rare. In pickles of various types the pH can lie well outside this range—high acidity serves to preserve the product and to provide the strong flavours. In specialized products such as a Norwegian preserved herring, the product is strongly alkaline.

Acidity has effects on the swelling of starch granules which is modified by the presence of sucrose and fats.

A large number of acids occur naturally in foods and their synthetic equivalents (nature-identical) are used to control the acidity of foods (see Table 26.14).

26.2.8 Enzymes

Enzymes are used extensively in various food processes and although not strictly additives are classed as such in many countries. Some enzymic processes, such as brewing of beer and vinegar, making wine, cheese, and yogurt have been practised for centuries. This was long before enzymes were recognized, extracted and characterized; the enzymes involved are naturally present in micro-organisms in or on foods (such as yeast on grapes) or are present in the environment.

Tenderization of meat has long been practised in some communities, for example by wrapping meat in pawpaw leaves (a source of papain) or treating with pineapple juice (a source of bromelain).

Modern developments include isolation of purified enzymes from animal, plant, bacterial, or fungal sources, and, increasingly, production of enzymes modified for specific purposes by genetic manipulation of micro-organisms. In some cases immobilization of enzymes on an inert support permits more precise control over the reaction than is possible with addition of the enzyme (or micro-organism) to a bulk foodstuff.

A major advantage of using enzymes to carry out reactions is that they are specific for both the substrate(s) acted on and the reaction catalysed (see Tables 29.7 and 29.8 for the classification of enzymes). Enzymes act at temperatures between 20–50°C, so, unlike many chemical reactions, do not require high temperatures, which will affect the flavour and other properties of the finished product. Furthermore, there is little or no residue from an enzyme-catalysed reaction (for example, acid hydrolysis of a protein requires neutralization of the excess acid afterwards, and acid hydrolysates are therefore, of necessity, high in salt).

The enzymes commonly used in food processing, and their principal sources, are shown in Table 26.15; not all of these enzymes are permitted in all countries.

26.2.9 Safety

The use of additives is controlled in all countries. Safety is the prime requirement but it must also be shown that there is a need for the additive under consideration (technical or economic or social).

Methods of testing for safety have been developed and extended over the years and the full procedure (see Table 26.16) can take as long as three years and is consequently extremely expensive. Preliminary studies such as consideration of the chemical structure of the compound, and hence prediction of likely hazards, and mutagenicity testing in micro-organisms, may eliminate a potential additive at an early stage. Otherwise the tests are continued until the toxicologist is satisfied that he can recommend its use under the conditions and in amounts specified. The principle is that the amount of the substance permitted must be considered safe to consume for a lifetime.

26.2.9.1 GRAS (Generally Regarded As Safe)
Many food additives were in use before safety testing was developed; when legislation was first introduced it was operated on a banned list (i.e. compounds were permitted unless they were banned because of evidence of harm) rather than, as nowadays, on a permitted list (with evidence of safety). With the technical resources available, even on a world-wide basis, full-scale systematic testing of all additives used is impossible. Many substances are accepted under the classification of GRAS (Generally Regarded As Safe).

Such substances include those whose metabolic pathway has been established and the end-products of which are known to be substances that are normal metabolic intermediates, e.g. lactic and pyruvic acids which are products of carbohydrate metabolism, derivatives of amino acids which are intermediates in their metabolism, and the products of fat digestion and partial digestion (fatty acids, mono- and diacylglycerols). Apart from naturally occurring toxins (see section 27.3), substances that are present in significant quantities in foods that have been eaten by man for many years may be GRAS, although traditional use is no guarantee of safety.

29.2.9.2 Testing procedure

Assuming that a substance is not shown to be mutagenic (and hence potentially carcinogenic) in bacterial testing or in tests with human cells in culture, it will proceed to toxicity testing, which is in three phases.

1. Acute toxicity testing. The acute toxicity of a compound is generally expressed as the single dose that kills half of the experimental animals—the LD_{50}. Acute toxicity testing also permits identification of the principal target organ(s) of the substance under test. Assuming that the LD_{50} is sufficiently greater than likely intakes, the substance proceeds to the next phase of testing.

2. Short term toxicity testing. Animals are fed diets containing various (subtoxic) levels of the substance, usually for 90 days. During this period they are investigated for any abnormalities of blood and urine chemistry, and behaviour, and at the end of the study they undergo a complete pathological and chemical examination of all organs and tissues. This will detect cumulative toxicity and carcinogenicity. Assuming that the substance has negligible cumulative toxicity at likely levels of intake, and is not carcinogenic, it proceeds to the next phase of testing.

3. Chronic toxicity testing, extending over a complete reproductive cycle. This will detect any teratogenic effects (effects on the embryo *in utero*), as well as any effects on fertility and reproduction. Chronic tests are carried out on several species of animals; rats, mice and hamsters are commonly used, with other species when considered necessary, so as to allow for possible species differences in the metabolism and toxicity of the test compound.

At a sufficiently high dosage everything, including common foods, has some detrimental effect; the aim of the tests is to determine the highest level of intake that has no detectable effect. This is termed the maximum no-effect level (NEL), and provides the basis for calculation of acceptable levels of intake. Two safety factors are used when considering the NEL: it is divided by 10 to allow for possible differences between man and the test species, and by a second factor of ten to allow for individual variation. This then becomes the acceptable daily intake, ADI—one-

hundredth of the highest dose that has no detectable effect in test animals. Compounds for which no evidence of hazard can be detected at any dose that has been tested are classified as 'ADI not stated'

The amount of an additive that is legally permitted may be limited and the use of some is restricted to specified foods.

WHO suggests that no additives should be used in foods intended for infants under three months of age because their detoxication mechanisms and kidney function are not fully developed. However, if there is any potential risk, such as from rancidity of fats, then the foods may be protected with antioxidants such as vitamins E and C.

26.3   Effect of food processing on nutrients

Nutritional changes take place during food processing (which includes domestic cooking), the extent varying with the type of food, the process, the degree of control exercized, and with the particular factory plant or domestic appliance involved. As discussed below, in some instances processing improves nutritive value.

Fresh, raw plant foods vary in their nutrient content, especially the micronutrients, with cultivar, soil, time and method of application of fertilizers, climate, state of maturity of the crop, time of harvesting, and severity of handling after harvesting. Nutrients in animal foods vary with breed, feed and husbandry, although generally to a lesser extent than do plant foods. The diet particularly affects nutrients that can be stored in the body, e.g. retinol in liver and egg yolk.

The literature includes many contradictory reports of the changes associated with food processing, for example the effect of microwave cooking has been variously reported as being superior to, inferior to, and the same as that of conventional methods. Such contradictions may be explained by the use of different samples of the named food, differences in analytical procedures, the use of laboratory model systems versus foods, but some contradictions cannot be explained.

The wide range of nutrients in foods reaching the consumer was shown in a large survey of 27000 packages of foods from 150 freezing plants in USA analysed between 1953 and 1954 (Burger *et al.* 1956). The history of the samples was not identified, since the project was intended to ascertain the nutrient content of products available to the consumer. In

20 samples of spinach, vitamin C ranged between 8–45 mg /100 g; in 28 samples of sprouts it was 70–105 mg; in 15 samples of broccoli the range of carotene was 0.8–2.7 mg; in 32 samples of Lima beans niacin ranged between 0.9–1.7 mg; in 18 samples of asparagus thiamin was 0.12–0.23 mg; in 8 samples of rhubarb sodium was 0.9–12.8 mg /100 g.

Such differences indicate the unreliability of depending on average food composition tables when attempting to assess the intake of micronutrients of individuals. As regards methods of analysis, those for vitamins in particular have evolved over the years and some used in earlier (and not so early) publications are now regarded as unreliable.

Variations between cultivars may affect the retention of nutrients during processing. A trial on 15 cultivars grown in the same area and examined in the same laboratory showed an enormous variation in the retention of vitamin C. Samples were blanched, and canned at two temperatures, 124°C for 8 min or 116°C for 25 min (Marchesini *et al.* 1975). Vitamin C can be destroyed and / or lost into the blanching water and the water in the can; part is converted into the biologically active dehydroascorbic acid (see section 22.2). One cultivar lost virtually all the vitamin C at 124°C, both in the beans and the brine; at the lower temperature half the ascorbate and one-quarter of the dehydroascorbate were lost. Another cultivar lost only a quarter of the ascorbate and a quarter of the dehydroascorbate at 124°C; at the lower temperature it lost more ascorbate (half), but less dehydroascorbate (one-fifth). Such large differences between cultivars show the difficulties in the way of reaching generalized conclusions about a particular food.

Among the unexplained differences, Bender (1958) found that losses of vitamin C from replicated samples of fruit juice preparations stored under identical conditions ranged between 16 and 24 per cent; under another set of conditions between 33 and 55 per cent. He reported that others had found similar differences between replicated samples. Further examples of variations in findings reported from a single laboratory, using established analytical procedures, were reported by Mikkelsen *et al.* (1984) with meat products. Four types of meat products based on pork and veal were stored at -24°C and -12°C for one year and analysed for B vitamins every two months. The figures were very erratic; thus for pork loin stored at -24°C, retention of thiamin was 80, 40, 70, 80 and 50 per cent. At -12°C the results were somewhat more regular—85, 110, 90, 105, and 85 per cent. The authors state that it is difficult to explain such fluctuations, and their results show how difficult it is to draw firm conclusions.

While generalizations may be made from the stabilities of individual nutrients—some are heat labile, water-soluble nutrients will be lost in wet processes, some are damaged under acid or alkaline conditions—it would seem that each particular product subjected to the individual factory and cooking process must be examined individually. Tables of vitamin losses on cooking listed in standard publications indicate losses ranging from zero to as much as 70 per cent.

26.3.1 Nutrient losses in food processing

26.3.1.1 Intentional losses
A specific example of intentional losses in food processing is the milling of cereals: a large proportion of the vitamins and minerals is lost with the bran and germ when wheat is milled to white flour (see Table 26.17) and when whole rice is milled to white, polished rice (see Table 26.18). Such losses must be regarded as intentional because it is the refined product that is required.

Intentional losses are similarly incurred when oil is pressed from the seed or nut and the residue used as animal feed, when fish is eviscerated and filleted, and when the outer leaves of vegetables are discarded.

26.3.1.2 Inevitable losses
Losses take place when the process includes heating or water treatment. Even under the most carefully controlled laboratory conditions any wet process will leach out part of the water-soluble nutrients, particularly the B vitamins and vitamin C, together with lesser (and less important) amounts of mineral salts, protein and even carbohydrate. Heat-labile nutrients, by definition, will be damaged.

Extraction losses will depend on the volume-to-surface-area ratio of the food and will therefore be much greater in foods that are finely chopped before processing. They can be reduced by limiting the volume of water in blanching processes, by re-using the water and by using steam or hot gases rather than hot water. There is little detailed information available on such modern processes.

The blanching of fruits and vegetables that is necessary before drying, canning, and freezing causes considerable loss. In general, the freezing process itself causes very little or no loss, and the nutrients are often quite stable during several months frozen storage but the finished product is lower in water-soluble vitamins than the raw material. Since the process is mostly carried out on fruits and vegetables, the major damage is to vitamin C and folate.

26.3.1.3 Factory and domestic cooking losses

The inevitable losses into processing water mean that losses of a similar type must occur during cooking, which means, in turn, that home cooking must be included as a food process. This consideration leads logically to the principle that many factory losses are in place of, not additional to, losses that would take place in the home. This is because many processed foods are partly cooked—frozen and dried foods have been partly cooked during the preliminary blanching process, or completely cooked if canned or bottled. The former would require less cooking at home and the latter would require only heating, or no further treatment at all.

Consequently it is incomplete and may be misleading to discuss losses in the factory without considering the losses that would take place, or as indicated, would not take place, in the home; comparisons must be made of foods on the plate, as eaten. When factory processes are to be compared with home cooking, or comparisons are made between different processes, it is the nutrient content available to the consumer that is important, not the difference between the raw material and the finished product.

Table 26.19 shows the loss of vitamin C on cooking fresh and frozen peas. Freezing and freeze-drying involve some loss of vitamin C and there is a further loss on completing the cooking in the home. The total loss, however, differs very little from cooking the raw food in one stage. This comparison was made in the laboratory under controlled conditions of 'home cooking' and it is likely that uncontrolled home cooking would inflict a greater loss of vitamin C.

Table 26.20 shows that peas that have been canned or air-dried, two processes generally regarded as being destructive of vitamin C, may be little worse than freezing and freeze-drying or, indeed, than peas cooked under controlled conditions in one step.

It should be noted that it is possible to find examples in the literature (e.g. Table 26.21), where different processes do cause greater differences in vitamin C loss than those shown in Table 26.20—an example of the different results from similar laboratories. Furthermore, as discussed above, different samples of the same type of food can behave in different ways.

26.3.1.4 The freshness of raw materials

The term 'fresh' is often applied to raw foods to distinguish them from processed products. The description, however, is open to different interpretations epitomized by the terms 'garden fresh' and 'market fresh'. Garden fresh describes food immediately after harvesting when labile nutrients would be at their maximum value. In fact the one nutrient that undergoes loss immediately after harvesting is vitamin C, due to destruction by the enzyme, ascorbic acid oxidase (EC 1.10.3.3). This is present in the plant tissue physically separated from the vitamin. When the fruit or vegetable is bruised or the leaf wilts, damage to the cell walls allows access of the enzyme to its substrate. To a lesser extent, folate is also lost early after harvesting.

The losses of vitamin C that occur after harvesting can be very rapid. One study on kale reported that the loss due to wilting was 1.5 per cent per hour, totalling some 30 per cent in one day. Table 26.22 shows the loss of vitamin C from green leaves in a market in Nigeria; very little remained by the close of the market, although the leaves had been gathered freshly that day. Table 26.23 shows that home-prepared dishes can lose vitamin C very rapidly, so any process that halts such a loss is likely to be beneficial, even if the process itself causes some destruction.

'Market fresh' foods that have been several days in transit and storage will have lost a considerable proportion of the vitamin C before preparation and consumption. The factory usually obtains its raw materials 'garden fresh' and so starts with foods of higher vitamin C content than does the housewife. No true comparisons can be made because of the enormous variability of results in the laboratory and in the factory, and because there are few figures available for the domestic products.

Other foods such as fish and meat are obtained by the manufacturer in fresher state than is available to the housewife but the nutrients are stable in the raw food for the periods of time under discussion, so while eating quality may be affected there is no change in nutritional quality.

26.3.1.5 Losses of vitamins

The two major causes of loss of nutrients are heat damage and extraction into the processing water. Proteins, fats, carbohydrates, mineral salts, and several of the vitamins are relatively stable to heat. Vitamin C and folate are oxidized in air, accelerated by heat (and by iron and traces of copper) and thiamin is unstable to heat. Vitamin A is stable at temperatures around boiling point and damaged only at frying temperatures (and also by oxidized fats). Vitamin B_6 and riboflavin are stable to heat, as are many other vitamins. Therefore, processing losses involve mainly vitamin C, folate and thiamin.

Some part of the water-soluble nutrients, including B vitamins and vitamin C, is inevitably leached into the processing water in amounts depending on the surface area. However, the main dietary sources of

B vitamins are cereals and meat, which are not usually subjected to the type of treatment that permits leaching. Cereals are mostly processed by heat alone, as in baking; the juices expressed from meat during cooking and processing do contain several of the B vitamins but since they are usually consumed with the meat there is no loss apart from the heat-labile thiamin. Vegetables, which do lose a considerable proportion of vitamin C into the cooking water, contain only small amounts of the other water-soluble vitamins.

Destruction of vitamin C by ascorbate oxidase can be prevented if the enzyme is denatured by heat. Birch *et al.* (1974) found that during cooking two processes were occurring simultaneously: breakdown of the cell structure, allowing the enzyme to come into contact with the vitamin, and destruction of the enzyme. For garden peas they found that the point of maximum cell disruption and minimum rate of enzyme inactivation, i.e. the greatest loss of vitamin, was at 50°C. Good cooking practice recommends that vegetables should be put into boiling water to achieve rapid destruction of the enzyme, although this cannot prevent leaching into the water.

It was common practice at one time to use the loss of vitamin C as an index of overall reduction in nutritional value, but this is misleading. Foods can lose a great deal of their vitamin C and still retain most, if not all, of the other nutrients. In modern catering research vitamin C content is often used as an index of palatability, being simpler and more rapid than tasting panels—foods that have been stored hot lose vitamin C and palatability at the same time.

26.3.1.6 The importance of the food in the diet as a whole
While there may be nutritional damage, it may not be of any consequence. Damage to foods eaten in small amounts, or which make an unimportant contribution to the diet, is of little consequence. The converse of this statement is that foods that supply exceptionally large amounts of a nutrient can also suffer damage without any consequence. Those who drink fruit juices in quantity will obtain several hundred milligrams of vitamin C daily, possibly 10–50 times the reference intake, so even if half of it were destroyed it would have no nutritional effect.

The role of the food in the diet as a whole is illustrated by data obtained from canned meals prepared for the Dutch Army (see Table 26.24). Here the vitamin A was severely damaged in canning and completely lost after 18 months storage. However, since the initial content was only about 16 µg, which is about 2 per cent of the reference intake, the food would have been an unimportant source of this vitamin even if it

had all been conserved. Of the thiamin 50 per cent was destroyed by canning and 75 per cent after storage, but the food still contained about 7 times the reference intake, so this loss was also unimportant.

Table 26.24 shows the results of one of the few investigations reporting the effects of storage after processing; most studies report the effect of the process alone and consequently provide limited information on the nutritional quality of the food as it will be available to consumers.

Another example of the importance of the food in the diet is provided by breakfast cereals. Table 26.25 shows the fall in the quality of protein (see section 10.7) when the cereal has been exposed to the high temperatures and pressures required for 'explosion puffing'. This appears to be a considerable loss in nutritive value but viewed against the perspective of the total diet it is insignificant. A 30 g portion of cereal will provide approximately 3 g of protein and if the quality is reduced by one-third, this can be regarded as effectively a fall of one-third in the amount of the protein, which is 1 g. Since average daily intakes are between 75–100 g (see Table 10.13) this is clearly of no importance whatever. Furthermore, the effect is due to a reduction in available lysine. When milk, with a relative surplus of lysine, is added, this more than compensates for the fall in lysine; the quality of the protein in a mixture of heat-damaged cereal and milk will differ little from that of undamaged cereal and milk.

Another example is that of white rice, which for nearly a century was the cause of beriberi in the Far East (see section 17.5). The introduction of steam-powered mills resulted in more effective removal of the germ than had been achieved by traditional hand-milling with consequent loss of a very considerable part of the B vitamins (see Table 26.20). The loss of thiamin in milling has become of much less consequence only because other foods have become more available and supply the missing thiamin. It makes no significant difference to the mixed Western diet whether the small amount of rice that is consumed is white or brown.

26.3.1.7 Vulnerable groups of the population
Infants may be reliant on the product of a single manufacturer and so could be at risk while an adult, who consumes a variety of foods, would be unaffected. Similarly, people living on restricted diets, as do some elderly and certain socially incompetent individuals, could be at risk.

This is illustrated by the damage to vitamin B_6 caused in an infant formula milk treated by a new process in 1954 (see section 20.2.1.2). Before that time it had not been demonstrated that vitamin B_6 was essential to human beings. The processing of the milk resulted in 72 cases of infant convulsions, found to be due to vitamin B_6 deficiency.

Another example which was a potential, rather than a real, problem arose when instant potato powder was reintroduced onto the market in Great Britain in the early 1960s. Some brands were almost devoid of vitamin C and others had low levels. Since the British population at that time relied on potatoes for 30 per cent of its average vitamin C intake, and 50 per cent in winter (but see Table 22.3), this could have become a major public health problem. Later, the manufacturers added vitamin C to a higher level than is present in the fresh potato, so demonstrating that it is possible for a manufactured product to have a higher nutrient content than the traditional food.

22.3.1.8 Nutritional damage versus advantages of processing

Even when there is clear evidence of nutritional damage the loss must be weighed against the advantages. The balance will vary as the following examples demonstrate.

Pasteurization of milk results in the loss of about 25 per cent of the vitamin C and about 10 per cent of several of the B vitamins (see Table 26.26). This treatment, however, provides safe milk and clearly the benefit outweighs the nutritional damage. Less clear is the benefit of using sulphur dioxide as a preservative of comminuted meat products as practised in Great Britain (but in few other countries). This treatment results in destruction of the thiamin within 48 hours (see section 17.5.7) and the advantage is mainly economic in that such foods have a longer shelf life. However, there is also the advantage of protection from infection.

A third example shows less benefit. Ready-peeled and ready-chipped potatoes are protected from enzymic browning by treatment with sulphite, with some consequent loss of thiamin. Not only is there some immediate loss of thiamin, but the subsequent loss on frying the chipped potatoes is greater than from the untreated potato. Since potatoes supply about 17 per cent of the total thiamin intake in western Europe (see Table 17.3) such a loss may be considered to outweigh the advantages.

Another illustration of loss versus advantage is the very severe destruction of protein and B vitamins on the surface of roasted meat when the 'only' advantage is the development of flavour. Here, however, the surface area of the meat is so small relative to the whole that the loss is quite insignificant. A parallel example is the loss of available lysine (Gorback and Regula 1964) and of thiamin (Farrer 1955; Downs and Meckel 1943) when bread is toasted—this amounts to about 10–30 per cent of the thiamin and a similar loss of available lysine—again 'merely' for preferred flavour, but again this does not seem to have any nutritional significance. Nevertheless these examples indicate possible nutritional problems in some communities where individuals may be either marginally adequately supplied with the nutrient in question or heavily reliant on the damaged food.

22.3.1.9 Factory versus home

The question of interest to the consumer is whether the processed food is nutritionally 'as good as' the comparable product prepared at home. There can be no simple answer to such a question since it will vary with the food, the process, and the relative skills of the factory processor and the home cook.

Firstly, large-scale factory processes generally cannot reach the overall qualities that can be achieved by a skilled cook on the small scale. At the same time it is more likely that the average quality of foods from a factory under control of a food technologist would be consistently of a higher standard than reached by some housewives.

Secondly, there are not many instances where direct comparisons can be made. Manufactured foods include dried milk powder, cheese, margarine, prepared breakfast cereals, dessert mixtures, and certain types of canned products such as beans, none of which has a domestic parallel—they are foods that the housewife does not produce at home from her own starting materials.

Types of foods that can be purchased from the manufacturer or prepared at home include fruit preserves, salad dressings, meat pies, fish cakes, and a range of flour confectionery, including bread. Here there will often be a difference in the ingredients. The housewife is likely to include more fruit in her preserves, use eggs in the preparation of salad creams, include more meat in a meat pie and more fish in a fish cake, and so on.

Products intended for a mass market at competitive prices can rarely contain as much of the expensive ingredients as the housewife includes, and fillers and substitutes are used. This means that they could be inferior in eating quality and / or in nutritional quality, but this is not necessarily so. Each instance would have to be examined separately.

For example, while it may appear likely that the protein content and quality of a meat pie will be higher if it contains more meat, this is not necessarily so. Meat contains about 20 per cent protein while cereal filler contains 10 per cent, so that products containing differing ratios of these two do not differ very much. As regards protein quality (see section 10.7.1), there is a relative surplus of lysine in the meat to compensate for the relative shortage in the cereal, and a relative surplus of the sulphur amino acids in cereals which can compensate for the relative shortage in the meat—so that the quality of the protein of the mixture could even be higher than that of a product consisting of meat alone. Similarly a fish cake made largely from fish may not be superior to the cheaper commercial product diluted with cereal and potato flour.

Finally, between harvests, the comparison is often not between processed food and the fresh (unprocessed) food but between the processed product and none at all.

26.3.2 Nutritional gains in food processing

26.3.2.1 Increased food availability
Man has preserved food for centuries by methods such as smoking, air-drying and pickling on a domestic scale, but the recent developments of canning, chilling, freezing and controlled drying together with the enormous developments of traditional methods of preservation have resulted in Western supermarket shelves being filled with a vast variety of foods from many countries throughout the year. Hence the major nutritional benefit of processing is the increased availability of food. The solution to many of the problems of food shortages in developing countries (see section 12.1.3), apart from buying power, lies in the preservation of food, much of which is lost after harvesting.

Processing also converts relatively unpalatable raw materials into attractive foods and allows the possibility of upgrading of waste materials into edible foods. Examples of converting unpalatable materials include the removal of toxic substances, the blending of unpromising materials into attractive products ranging from chocolate to flour confectionery and breakfast cereals, and the flavouring and texturizing of relatively tasteless raw materials as is effected during spinning and extrusion processes.

Upgrading of waste includes conversion of slaughter-house waste and fishhouse waste into reformed meat and fish products, the extraction of protein from leaves and the use of single cell protein and fungal mycelia. All these types of processing make a major contribution to nutrition since a nutritionally good diet depends largely on a varied supply.

26.3.2.2 Increased nutritional quality
Most cereals contain relatively large amounts of niacin but it is present in the bound state, as niacytin, which is largely unavailable (see section 19.1.1). Many authorities consequently exclude the niacin content of cereals from calculations of average intakes. However, the niacin is liberated by heat and by alkali, hence baking, especially in the presence of alkaline baking powder, will liberate variable amounts, depending on the temperature, time of treatment and pH. This is a clear example of nutritional improvement through processing.

Along similar lines is the formation of niacin from trigonelline in coffee beans during roasting. The beverage contains sufficient niacin to supply about 20 per cent of the reference intake in one cup, so that it is an extremely good source of this vitamin—produced during the processing stage.

A number of phenolic substances in plants have marked antithiamin activity as a result of oxidation by the enzyme polyphenol oxidase (EC 1.10.3.1) also present in the food (see section 17.5.7). Since the enzyme is denatured by heat, proper processing prevents this.

Dry legumes in the raw state may be toxic because of the presence of lectins (see section 27.3.5), inhibitors of proteolytic enzymes (see section 27.2.1) and cyanogenic glycosides (see section 7.6) and their proteins are often of low nutritional quality (see section 10.7). Adequate heating both destroys these toxins and in some instances, see Table 26.27, increases the protein quality. Dry legumes are seldom eaten unprocessed but when they are (after preliminary soaking) they cause considerable health problems (see section 27.3.5). While domestic cooking is perfectly adequate to obviate this problem, there have been outbreaks of food poisoning from inadequately cooked legumes which could not occur from factory-canned beans simply because the latter require heat treatment adequate to sterilize and this, at the same time, destroys the offending lectins.

26.3.2.3 Nutrient enrichment and fortification
The general procedure of nutrient fortification can be included among the nutritional improvements effected through processing.

In many countries margarine is enriched with vitamins A and D levels higher than found in average samples of butter; white bread has restored to it some of the B vitamins and iron lost in the milling process; foods such as chocolate and salt are iodized in regions where dietary iodine deficiency poses a public health problem (see section 25.14.6); in some countries vitamin A is added to salt, sugar and mono-sodium glutamate to overcome widespread deficiency (see section 13.4.1), and iron is added to many foods in an attempt to prevent iron-deficiency anaemia (see section 24.4).

Apart from such public health measures, often imposed by regulations, many manufactured foods are voluntarily enriched with nutrients including iron, fluoride and extra protein. Even if such enrichment is carried out primarily for sales appeal, it does add to the nutrient intake and must be included among the benefits of processing.

26.3.2.4 The use of nutrients as processing aids

Vitamins C and E are widely used as antioxidants and as preservatives. It is recommended by the World Health Organization that no additives should be used in baby foods, since the infant's poorly developed detoxication systems are often unable to metabolize substances that are perfectly harmless to the older child and the mature adult, but problems can arise from oxidation of fats which might render infant foods harmful. In that case vitamins C and E, not only harmless but beneficial, may be used.

Vitamin C is widely used as a processing aid. For example, the browning of fruits and vegetables is caused by the enzyme polyphenol oxidase (EC 1.10.3.1), which converts o-diphenols to quinones in the presence of oxygen. In addition to the loss of visual appeal, the quinones can initiate radical-generating reactions in the presence of metal ions. While the enzyme can be inactivated by heat, unwanted flavours sometimes develop; the enzyme can be inhibited by adding ascorbic acid. Relatively large amounts (150–200 mg /L of fruit juice) are used and two-thirds of this may remain after processing and storage, so making a major contribution to the diet. Ascorbic acid is also added to frozen and canned fruit, frozen fish (at the rate of 1 g /kg), for pickling olives in brine, and as an antioxidant in oils and fats. The amount left after processing and storage varies.

It is used in concentrations of 20–40 mg /L as an oxygen acceptor to prevent changes in colour and flavour in beer, and is sometimes added to wine at a rate of 50–100 mg /L to preserve taste and colour, and to prevent turbidity arising from the precipitation of ferric phosphate by converting it to the more stable ferrous salt.

Ascorbic acid accelerates the curing process of meat by acting as a reducing agent, reducing the met-myoglobin of the meat to myoglobin so that it reacts with the nitric oxide present from the pickling salts and aids even and more rapid colour development. Of much greater importance is the role of vitamin C in blocking the formation of possible carcinogenic nitrosamines formed in the pickling process (see section 22.4.2.2). Here it is essential that some of the vitamin C survives the process and it has been found even after frying of bacon. The presence of vitamin C in processed meats is of considerable nutritional importance to people who do not consume fruits and vegetables. Ascorbic acid is also used in bread processing—the Chorleywood process—but this is completely destroyed during baking.

Canning of some fruits and vegetables leads to a several-fold increase in the availability of iron (see section 24.2.3.1), apparently as a result of both the addition of acidulants and antioxidants and also the loss of tannins and other inhibitors of absorption with the discarding of the skin and outer layers.

Further reading

Bender, A.E. (1978). *Food Processing and Nutrition.* Academic Press, London.

Department of Health and Social Security (1982). *In vitro tests: Guidelines for the testing of chemicals for toxicity,* Report on Health and Social Subjects No 28. HMSO, London.

Gibson, G.G. and Walker, R. (1985). *Food Toxicology: Real or Imaginary Problems,* Taylor and Francis, London.

Institute of Food Science and Technology (1987). *Food Additives: the Professional and Scientific Approach.* Institute of Food Science and Technology, London.

Millstone, E. (1986). *Food Additives: taking the lid off what we really eat.* Penguin, London.

Ministry of Agriculture, Fisheries and Food (1976). *Food Quality and Safety: a Century of Progress.* HMSO, London.

Wheelock, V. (1986). *Food Additives in Perspective.* Food Policy Research Unit, University of Bradford.

WHO Food Additives Series: *Toxicological evaluation of certain food additives and contaminants,* International Programme on Chemical Safety. WHO, Geneva. Annual publication series.

Table 26.1: Chronology of the introduction of new foods

7000 BC	Wheat cultivated (Euphrates Valley)
6500 BC	Rye known, Asia Minor
3000 BC	Soya beans known, China
3000 BC	Rice known, India
325 BC	Sugar known in India
100 AD	Potato cultivated
7th Century	Sugar cane introduced into Europe
1456	Shipment of sugar from Madeira to England
1506	Tomatoes introduced into UK from S America
1650s	Coffee introduced into UK
1657	Tea brought to UK (according to legend accidentally discovered by Chinese Emperor Shen Nung 2700 BC)
1660	Ice cream (and frozen fruit juices; P. Coltello, Florence, Italy)
1762	Sandwich 'invented' (Earl of Sandwich)
1780	Ice cream sold in New York
1809	Vegetarianism (UK)
1810	Sugar beet factory (Benjamin Delessert, France)
1810	Canned vegetables
1811	Discovery of starch sugars (Kirchhoff)
1847	Solid 'eating' chocolate
1853	Potato crisps (chips—Chef George Crum, USA) in response to complaints of 'too thick' chips.
1856	Canned milk (Gail Borden, USA)
1869	Margarine (Hippolyte Mege Mouries, France)
1870	Bananas introduced from Jamaica to USA (Z D Baker)
1876	Milk chocolate (Switzerland)
1879	Accidental discovery of sweetener, saccharin (Fahlberg and Remsen) (Commercial production 1894, Germany)
1880	First convenience food—fish and chips (John Rouse of Oldham, UK)
1884	Powdered soups (Switzerland)
1884	Coca-Cola produced as a tonic (Dr John Pemberton, pharmacist in Atlanta, Georgia, USA)
1889	Hamburgers (Hamburg steaks) introduced into USA by German immigrants
1891	Canned beans (USA)
1890s	Peanut butter 'invented' by housewives of Missouri (USA)
1900	Liquid coffee extract (Camp coffee)
1925	Canned pet foods
1930	Sliced bread introduced from USA to UK
1931	Birds Eye frozen peas introduced to American market
1935	BMA proposes Basic Healthy Diet at 5s 10½d (29p); Ministry of Health reduces this to 4s 8d (24p)
1937	Powdered coffee (Hans Morgenthaler, Switzerland)
1938	Frozen foods on British market (Birds Eye)
1938	Instant coffee (Nestlé)
1939	National wheatmeal loaf introduced into UK (until 1953)
1941	Introduction of All Bran breakfast cereal (Kelloggs)
1942	All margarine fortified with vitamins A and D (UK)
1942	Calcium carbonate added to bread in UK
1955	Introduction of fish fingers into UK (Birds Eye)
1965	Introduction of Ultra heat treated milk (UHT, Long Life Milk)

Table 26.2: Chronology of the introduction of methods of food processing

20 000 BC	Breeding of animals
15 000—10 000 BC	Development of agriculture—Neolithic Age—change from nomadic life to food production
7,000 BC	Man aquired reliable firemaking techniques
4000 BC	Drying, fermenting, milling
2000 BC	Pickling, curing
400 BC	Alembic to distil fresh water from sea water (Aristotle)
1276	First whiskey distillery, Ireland
1680	Autoclave (Papin's Digester—D Papin, France)
1685	Antonie van Leeuwenhoek developed microscope and described micro-organisms (Holland)
1747	Sucrose extracted from sugar beet (Germany)
1799	Concentration of fruit juices by freezing (J C Georges, apothecary, Sweden)
1804	Variety of foods sterilized in bottles (trials started 1803, book published 1810 ; Nicholas Appert, confectioner, France)
1805	Start of ice trade (Frederick Tudor, New England, USA)
1807	Fruit bottled 'without sugar' (Thomas Saddington, UK)
1810	Patent for foods sterilized in tinned canisters (Peter Durand and Augustus de Heine, UK) Commercial production Bryan Donkin, John Hall and John Gamble (UK)
1812	Canning introduced into USA, (Thomas Kennet, UK and William Underwood UK)
1830	Modern 'Coffey' still (Aeneas Coffey)
1834	Patent for refrigeration plant (Jacob Perkins, American in UK)
1861	Heat destroys microbes—pasteurization (Louis Pasteur, France)
1864	Louis Pasteur demonstrated omnipresence of bacteria and role in putrefaction, and destruction by heat
1870	Patent for steam-heated autoclave to sterilize canned foods (Albert Fryer, UK)
1870	Patent for globe-stoppered glass bottle (Hiram Codd)
1872	Henry Tate built Liverpool Sugar Refinery
1875	Joseph Rank rented his first mill
1877	Invention of centrifugal cream separator (Gustav de Laval, Sweden)
1887	Hydrogenation of oils with nickel catalyst (Sabatier and Senderens)
1900	Pasteurization commercially employed
1902	Hardening of oils by hydrogenation (W Norman, Germany)
1906	Freeze-drying (Arsene d'Arsonaval)
1912	Maillard reaction named (Louis-Camille Maillard, France, see section 27.4.1)
1913	Home refrigerator (F Bordas, France)
1922	Iodized salt in Switzerland (see section 25.14.6)
1929	Plate freezer developed by Clarence Birdseye (USA)
1937	Lacquered tin can introduced
1937	Britain's first frozen food—asparagus (Smedley's)
1940	First commercially successful aseptic canning plant (C O Ball, USA)
1941	Introduction in UK of boron compounds and sulphur dioxide as preservatives for meat products
1944	Infra-red radiation technology used to dehydrate foods
1945	Application of freeze-drying to foods
1952	First commercially operated HTST pasteurizing plant (APV, J Lyons)
1961	Chorleywood Bread Process
1970	Aseptic Packaging
1980	Modified Atmosphere Packaging
1994	Widget for canned draught beer

Table 26.3: Milestones in food distribution

1815	First biscuit factory (Carlisle, UK)
1826	Tea retailed in sealed packets under proprietary name (John Horniman UK)
1851	Complete dinners in cans—Great Exhibition, UK, (J Chevet, France)
1871	Multiple retail food shops (Thomas Lipton, Scotland)
1871	JJ Sainsbury opened retail dairy
1877	First trans-ocean shipment of chilled meat (Carre's refrigeration plant) Buenos Aires to Marseilles in 'Le Frigorifique' (6 months at -17°C)
1879	First refrigerated shipment of meat to UK (SS Strathleven, Sydney November 29th 1879—London Feb 2 1880)
1905	Tea sold in infusible bags
1951	Introduction of Tetra Pak
1952	First teabag in UK (Tetley—J Lyons)
1953	First nationally-branded loaf in UK (Wonderloaf—Spillers)
1956	Introduction in UK of supermarkets

Table 26.4: Milestones in food legislation

1266	The Assize of Bread, laws controlling quality of bread and ale (England)
1730	Tea Act (no oak leaves permitted in tea, UK)
1758	Bread Act (no sand, ashes or sawdust permitted in bread (UK)
1785	Food Adulteration Law, Massachusetts, USA.
1820	'Treatise on the Adulteration of Foods and Culinary Poisons' (FC Accum, UK)
1855	'Food and its Adulterations' (A H Hassall, UK)
1860	First general food laws—Adulteration of Food and Drugs Act (UK) amended 1872, 1875
1865	All sailors under British flag required to receive a daily ration of lime juice
1906	First National Food and Drugs Law USA
1922	Low Temperature Research Station of the Food Investigation Board of the Department of Scientific and Industrial Research in Cambridge (UK)
1928	(Consolidating) Food and Drugs (Adulteration) Act (UK)
1933	End of Alcohol Prohibition in USA
1938	Federal Food, Drug and Cosmetic Act, USA
1939	First edition of The Composition of Foods, RA McCance and EM Widdowson (UK)
1941	First publication of Recommended Dietary Allowances (USA)
1942	All margarine fortified with vitamins A and D in UK
1947	Establishment of UK Food Standards Committee
1954	UK Food and Drugs Act puts onus on food manufacturers on use of colours
1990	Nutrition Labelling and Education Act (USA)

Table 26.5: Doses of radiation required for food preservation

	dose (kGy)
Inhibition of sprouting	0.05-0.115
Delayed ripening	0.2-1.0
Kill insects	0.2-1.0
Reduction of microbiological load	0.5-5.0
Elimination of non-sporulating bacteria	3-10
Bacteriological sterility	50

Table 26.6: Types of food additives

	number permitted
Preservatives	14
Antioxidants	14
Colours	47
Humectants	-
Flavours	3500
Flour improvers and processing aids (lubricants, anti-caking agents, etc)	-
Emulsifiers and stabilizers	56
Solvents	9
Sweeteners	12
pH regulation	-

Table 26.7: Additives used in flour confectionery and baked goods

Additive	E-number[1]	function
Acesulfame K	950	sweetener
Agar	406	stabilizer, thickener
Ammonium bicarbonate	503	raising agent
Ammonium chloride, sulphate	-	yeast nutrient
β-Amylase (EC 3.2.1.2)	-	converts starch to glucose, aids fermentation
Ascorbic acid	300	processing aid
Aspartame	951	sweetener
Azodicarbonamide (ADA)	927a	oxidant, processing aid
Butylated hydroxyanisole (BHA)	320	antioxidant, retards rancidity
Butylated hydroxytoluene (BHT)	321	antioxidant, retards rancidity
Calcium bromate	-	oxidant, processing aid
Calcium carbonate	170	enrichment, buffering
Calcium caseinate	-	enrichment
Calcium iodate	-	oxidant, processing aid
Calcium peroxide	-	oxidant, processing aid
Calcium propionate	282	preservative, retards mould growth
Calcium stearoyl lactylate	482	dough strengthener, texture improver
Calcium sulphate	516	enrichment
Caramel	150	colour
Carob bean	410	stabilizer, thickener
Carageenan	407	stabilizer, thickener
Cellulose gum	-	stabilizer, thickener
Citric acid	330	antioxidant, retards rancidity
Cream of tartar	336	leavening agent
L-Cysteine	920	reducing agent, dough improver
Diacetyl tartaric esters of mono- and diglycerides (DATEM)	472	emulsifier
Ethoxylated mono- and diglycerides	-	dough strengthener, texture improver
Gelatin	-	stabilizer, thickener
Iron	-	enrichment
Lecithin	322	emulsifier
Malt, malted barley flour	-	source of β-amylase (EC 3.2.1.2), converts starch to glucose, aids fermentation
Mono- and diglycerides	471	emulsifier and crumb softener, retards staling
Monocalcium phosphate	341	leavening agent, dough conditioner
Niacin	375	enrichment
Pectin	440	stabilizer, thickener
Polydextrose	1200	low-calorie carbohydrate, bulking agent
Polyglycerol esters	475	emulsifier and crumb softener, retards staling
Polysorbate 60, 65	435-6	emulsifier, retards staling, aids whipping
Potassium bromate	-	oxidant, processing aid
Potassium sorbate	202	preservative, retards mould growth
Propylene glycol mono-esters	-	emulsifier and crumb softener, retards staling
Propyl gallate	310	antioxidant, retards rancidity
Protease	-	enzyme softens protein, processing aid
Riboflavin	101	enrichment
Sodium acid pyrophosphate	339	leavening agent
Sodium alginate	401	stabilizer, thickener
Sodium benzoate	211	preservative, retards mould growth
Sodium bicarbonate	500	leavening agent
Sodium bisulphite, metabisulphite	222-223	dough conditioner, processing aid
Sodium caseinate	-	enrichment
Sodium diacetate	262	preservative, retards mould growth
Sodium propionate	281	preservative, retards mould growth
Sodium stearoyl lactate	481	dough strengthener, texture improver

Table 26.7: (Cont'd)

Additive	E-number[1]	function
Sorbic acid	200	preservative, retards mould growth, reducing agent, processing aid
Sorbitan monostearate	491	emulsifier and crumb softener, retards staling
Starch, corn starch	-	thickener
Sucrose polyesters	473	emulsifier
Succinylated monoglycerides	-	dough strengthener, texture improver
TBHQ	-	antioxidant, retards rancidity
Thiamin (mononitrate)	-	enrichment
Vinegar	-	acidification, mould retardation
Wheat gluten	-	wheat protein concentrate

(1) See Table 26.8

Table 26.8: Food additives permitted within the European Union

Colouring materials

Yellow and orange colours

E-100	Curcumin
E-101	Riboflavin, riboflavin phosphate (vitamin B$_2$)
E-102	Tartrazine (= FD and C Yellow no 6)
E-104	Quinoline yellow
E-110	Sunset yellow FCF or orange yellow S (= FD and C Yellow no 6)

Red colours

E-120	Cochineal or carminic acid
E-122	Carmoisine or azorubine
E-123	Amaranth
E-124	Ponceau 4R or cochineal red A
E-127	Erythrosine BS (= FD and C Red no 3)
E-128	Red 2G
E-129	Allura red (= FD and C Red no 40)

Blue colours

E-131	Patent blue V
E-132	Indigo carmine or indigotine (= FD and C Blue no 2)
E-133	Brilliant blue FCF (= FD and C Blue no 1)

Green colours

E-140	(i) Chlorophylls, (ii) chlorophyllins
E-141	Copper complexes of (i) chlorophylls, (ii) chlorophyllins
E-142	Green S or acid brilliant green BS

Brown and black colours

E-150a	Plain caramel
E-150b	Caustic sulphite caramel
E-150c	Ammonia caramel
E150d	Sulphite ammonia caramel
E-151	Black PN or brilliant black BN
E-153	Carbon black or vegetable carbon (charcoal)
E-154	Brown FK
E-155	Brown HT (Chocolate brown HT)

Derivatives of carotene

E-160(a)	(i) Mixed carotenes, (ii) β-carotene
E-160(b)	Annatto, bixin, norbixin
E-160(c)	Paprika extract, capsanthin or capsorubin
E-160(d)	Lycopene
E-160(e)	β-apo-8'-carotenal (vitamin A active)
E-160(f)	Ethyl ester of β-apo-8'-carotenoic acid

Other plant colours

E-161(b)	Lutein
E-161(g)	Canthaxanthin
E-162	Beetroot red or betanin
E-163	Anthocyanins

Inorganic compounds used as colours

E-170	(i) Calcium carbonate (chalk), (ii) calcium hydrogen carbonate
E-171	Titanium dioxide
E-172	Iron oxides and hydroxides
E-173	Aluminium
E-174	Silver
E-175	Gold
E-180	Pigment rubine or lithol rubine BK

Table 26.8: (Cont'd)

Preservatives

Sorbic acid and its salts

E-200	Sorbic acid
E-202	Potassium sorbate
E-203	Calcium sorbate

Benzoic acid and its salts

E-210	Benzoic acid
E-211	Sodium benzoate
E-212	Potassium benzoate
E-213	Calcium benzoate
E-214	Ethyl *p*-hydroxybenzoate
E-215	Ethyl *p*-hydroxybenzoate sodium salt
E-216	Propyl *p*-hydroxybenzoate
E-217	Propyl *p*-hydroxybenzoate sodium salt
E-218	Methyl *p*-hydroxybenzoate
E-219	Methyl *p*-hydroxybenzoate sodium salt

Sulphur dioxide and its salts

E-220	Sulphur dioxide
E-221	Sodium sulphite
E-222	Sodium hydrogen sulphite
E-223	Sodium metabisulphite
E-224	Potassium metabisulphite
E-226	Calcium sulphite
E-227	Calcium hydrogen sulphite
E-228	Potassium hydrogen sulphite

Biphenyl and its derivatives

E-230	Biphenyl or diphenyl (for surface treatment of citrus fruits)
E-231	Orthophenylphenol (2-hydroxybiphenyl) (for surface treatment of citrus fruits)
E-232	Sodium orthophenylphenol (sodium biphenyl-2-yl oxide)

Other preservatives

E-233	2-(Thiazol-4-yl) benzimidazole (thiobendazole) (for surface treatment of citrus fruits and bananas)
E-234	Nisin
E-235	Natamycin (NATA) (for surface treatment of cheeses and dried cured sausages)
E-239	Hexamethylene tetramine (hexamine)
E-242	Dimethyl dicarbonate
E-912	Montan acid esters (for surface treatment of citrus fruits)
E-914	Oxidized polyethylene wax (for surface treatment of citrus fruits)

Pickling salts

E-249	Potassium nitrite
E-250	Sodium nitrite
E-251	Sodium nitrate
E-252	Potassium nitrate (saltpetre)

Acids and their salts

E-260	Acetic acid
E-261	Potassium acetate
E-262	(i) Sodium acetate, (ii) sodium hydrogen acetate (sodium diacetate)
E-263	Calcium acetate
E-270	Lactic acid

Table 26.8: (Cont'd)

Acids and their salts (Cont'd)
E-280   Propionic acid
E-281   Sodium propionate
E-282   Calcium propionate
E-283   Potassium propionate
E-284   Boric acid (as preservative in caviare)
E-285   Sodium tetraborate (borax) (as preservative in caviare)
E-290   Carbon dioxide
E-296   Malic acid
E-297   Fumaric acid
Antioxidants
Vitamin C and derivatives
E-300   L-Ascorbic acid (vitamin C)
E-301   Sodium-L-ascorbate
E-302   Calcium-L-ascorbate
E-304   (i) Ascorbyl palmitate, (ii) ascorbyl stearate
E-315   Erythorbic acid (*iso*-ascorbic acid, see section 22.2)
E-316   Sodium erythorbate (sodium *iso*-ascorbate)
Vitamin E
E-306   Natural extracts rich in tocopherols
E-307   Synthetic α-tocopherol
E-308   Synthetic γ-tocopherol
E-309   Synthetic δ-tocopherol
Other antioxidants
E-310   Propyl gallate
E-311   Octyl gallate
E-312   Dodecyl gallate
E-320   Butylated hydroxyanisole (BHA)
E-321   Butylated hydroxytoluene (BHT)
E-322   Lecithins
More acids and their salts
Salts of lactic acid (E270)
E-325   Sodium lactate
E-326   Potassium lactate
E-327   Calcium lactate
E-585   Ferrous lactate
Citric acid, its salts and esters
E-330   Citric acid
E-331   (i) Monosodium citrate, (ii) disodium citrate, (iii) trisodium citrate
E-332   (i) Monopotassium citrate, (ii) dipotassium citrate, (iii) tripotassium citrate
E-333   (i) Monocalcium citrate, (ii) dicalcium citrate, (iii) tricalcium citrate
E-1505   Triethyl citrate
Tartaric acid and its salts
E-334   L(+)Tartaric acid
E-335   (i) Monosodium tartrate, (ii) disodium tartrate
E-336   (i) Monopotassium tartrate (cream of tartar), (ii) dipotassium tartrate
E-337   Sodium potassium tartrate
Phosphoric acid and its salts
E-338   Phosphoric acid
E-339   (i) Monosodium phosphate, (ii) disodium phosphate, (iii) trisodium phosphate

Table 26.8: (Cont'd)

Phosphoric acid and its salts
E-340   (i) Monopotassium phosphate, (ii) dipotassium phosphate, (iii) tripotassium phosphate
E-341   (i) Monocalcium phosphate, (ii) dicalcium phosphate, (iii) tricalcium phosphate
E-450   Diphosphates: (i) disodium diphosphate, (ii) trisodium diphosphate, (iii) tetrasodium diphosphate, (iv) dipotassium diphosphate, (v) tetrapotassium diphosphate, (vi) dicalcium diphosphate, (vii) calcium dihydrogen diphosphate
E-451   Triphosphates: (i) pentasodium triphosphate, (ii) pentapotassium triphosphate
E-452   Polyphosphates: (i) sodium polyphosphate, (ii) potassium polyphosphate, (iii) sodium calcium polyphosphate, (iv) calcium polyphosphate
E-540   Dicalcium diphosphate
E-541   Sodium aluminium phosphate, acidic
E-542   Edible bone phosphates (bone meal, used as anticaking agent)
E-544   Calcium polyphosphates (used as anticaking agent)
E-545   Ammonium polyphosphates (used as anticaking agent)
Salts of malic acid (E-296)
E-350   Sodium malate
E-351   Potassium malate
E-352   Calcium malate
Other acids and their salts
E-353   Metatartaric acid
E-354   Calcium tartrate
E-355   Adipic acid
E-356   Sodium adipate
E-357   Potassium adipate
E-363   Succinic acid
E-370   1,4-Heptonolactone
E-375   Nicotinic acid
E-380   Triammonium citrate
E-381   Ammonium ferric citrate
E-385   Calcium disodium EDTA
Emulsifiers and stabilizers
Alginates
E-400   Alginic acid
E-401   Sodium alginate
E-402   Potassium alginate
E-403   Ammonium alginate
E-404   Calcium alginate
E-405   Propane-1,2-diol alginate
Other plant gums
E-406   Agar
E-407   Carrageenan
E-410   Locust bean gum (carob gum)
E-412   Guar gum
E-413   Tragacanth
E-414   Gum acacia (gum Arabic)
E-415   Xanthan gum
E-416   Karaya gum

Table 26.8: (Cont'd)

Other plant gums (Cont'd)
E-417   Tara gums
E-418   Gellan gums

Fatty acid derivatives
E-431   polyoxyethylene (40) stearate
E-432   polyoxyethylene (20) sorbitan monolaurate
           (Polysorbate 20)
E-433   polyoxyethylene (20) sorbitan mono-oleate
           (Polysorbate 80)
E-434   polyoxyethylene (20) sorbitan monopalmitate
           (Polysorbate 40)
E-435   polyoxyethylene (20) sorbitan monostearate
           (Polysorbate 60)
E-436   polyoxyethylene (20) sorbitan tristearate
           (Polysorbate 65)

Pectin and derivatives
E-440   (i) Pectin, (ii) amidated pectin

Other compounds
E-442   Ammonium phosphatides
E-444   Sucrose acetate isobutyrate
E-445   Glycerol esters of wood rosins

Cellulose and derivatives
E-460   (i) Microcrystalline cellulose, (ii) powdered
           cellulose
E-461   Methyl cellulose
E-463   Hydroxypropyl cellulose
E-464   Hydroxypropylmethyl cellulose
E-465   Ethylmethyl cellulose
E-466   Carboxymethylcellulose, sodium
           carboxymethylcellulose

Salts or esters of fatty acids.
E-470a   Sodium, potassium and calcium salts of fatty
           acids
E-470b   Magnesium salts of fatty acids
E-471   Mono-and di-glycerides of fatty acids
E-472a   Acetic acid esters of mono- and diglycerides of
           fatty acids
E-472b   Lactic acid esters of mono- and diglycerides of
           fatty acids
E-472c   Citric acid esters of mono- and diglycerides of
           fatty acids
E-472d   Tartaric acid esters of mono- and diglycerides
           of fatty acids
E-472e   Mono- and diacetyl tartaric esters of mono-
           and diglycerides of fatty acids
E-472f   Mixed acetic and tartaric acid esters of mono-
           and diglycerides of fatty acids
E-473   Sucrose esters of fatty acids
E-474   Sucroglycerides
E-475   Polyglycerol esters of fatty acids
E-476   Polyglycerol esters of polycondensed esters of
           castor oil (polyglycerol polyricinoleate)
E-477   Propane-1,2-diol esters of fatty acids
E-479b   Thermally oxidized soya bean oil interacted
           with mono- and diglycerides of fatty acids
E-481   Sodium stearoyl-2-lactylate
E-482   Calcium stearoyl-2-lactylate

Table 26.8: (Cont'd)

Salts or esters of fatty acids. (Cont'd)
E-483   Stearyl tartrate
E-491   Sorbitan monostearate
E-492   Sorbitan tristearate
E-493   Sorbitan monolaurate
E-494   Sorbitan mono-oleate
E-495   Sorbitan monopalmitate
E-1518   Glyceryl triacetate (triacetin)

Acids and salts used for special purposes
Carbonates
E-500   (i) Sodium carbonate, (ii) sodium bicarbonate
           (sodium hydrogen carbonate), (iii) sodium
           sesquicarbonate
E-501   (i) Potassium carbonate, (ii) potassium
           bicarbonate (potassium hydrogen carbonate)
E-503   (i) Ammonium carbonate, (ii) ammonium
           hydrogen carbonate
E-504   (i) Magnesium carbonate, (ii) magnesium
           hydrogen carbonate (magnesium hydroxide
           carbonate)

Hydrochloric acid and its salts
E-507   Hydrochloric acid
E-508   Potassium chloride
E-509   Calcium chloride
E-510   Ammonium chloride
E-511   Magnesium chloride
E-512   Stannous chloride

Sulphuric acid and its salts
E-513   Sulphuric acid
E-514   (i) Sodium sulphate, (ii) sodium hydrogen
           sulphate
E-515   (i) Potassium sulphate, (ii) potassium hydrogen
           sulphate
E-516   Calcium sulphate
E-517   Ammonium sulphate
E-518   Magnesium sulphate
E-520   Aluminium sulphate
E-521   Aluminium sodium sulphate
E-522   Aluminium potassium sulphate
E-523   Aluminium ammonium sulphate

Alkalis
E-524   Sodium hydroxide
E-525   Potassium hydroxide
E-526   Calcium hydroxide
E-527   Ammonium hydroxide
E-528   Magnesium hydroxide
E-529   Calcium oxide
E-530   Magnesium oxide

Other salts
E-535   Sodium ferrocyanide
E-536   Potassium ferrocyanide
E-538   Calcium ferrocyanide
E-540   Dicalcium diphosphate
E-541   Sodium aluminium phosphate, acidic

Compounds used as anti-caking agents, and other uses
E-542   Edible bone phosphate (bone meal)
E-544   Calcium polyphosphates

Table 26.8: (Cont'd)

Compounds used as anti-caking agents, and other uses
E-545   Ammonium polyphosphates
Silicon salts
E-551   Silicon dioxide (silica)
E-552   Calcium silicate
E-553a   (i) Magnesium silicate, (ii) magnesium trisilicate
E-533b   talc
E-554   Sodium aluminium silicate
E-555   Potassium aluminium silicate
E-556   Calcium aluminium silicate
Other compounds
E-558   Bentonite
E-559   Kaolin (aluminium silicate)
E-570   Fatty acids
E-574   Gluconic acid
E-575   Glucono-δ-lactone
E-576   Sodium gluconate
E-577   Potassium gluconate
E-578   Calcium gluconate
E-579   Ferrous gluconate
E-585   Ferrous lactate
Compounds used as flavour enhancers
E-620   L-Glutamic acid
E-621   Monosodium glutamate (MSG)
E-622   Monopotassium glutamate
E-623   Calcium diglutamate
E-624   Monoammonium glutamate
E-625   Magnesium diglutamate
E-626   Guanylic acid
E-627   Disodium guanylate
E-628   Dipotassium guanylate
E-629   Calcium guanylate
E-630   Inosinic acid
E-631   Disodium inosinate
E-632   Dipotassium inosinate
E-633   Calcium inosinate
E-634   Calcium 5′-ribonucleotides
E-635   Disodium 5′-ribonucleotides
E-636   Maltol
E-637   Ethyl maltol
E-640   Glycine and its sodium salt
E-900   Dimethylpolysiloxane
Compounds used as glazing agents
E-901   Beeswax
E-902   Candelilla wax
E-903   Carnauba wax
E-904   Shellac
E-912   Montan acid esters
E-914   Oxidized polyethylene wax
Compounds used to treat flour
E-920   L-Cysteine hydrochloride
E-925   Chlorine
E-926   Chlorine dioxide
Propellant gases
E-938   Argon
E-939   Helium
E-941   Nitrogen

Table 26.8: (Cont'd)

Propellant gases (Cont'd)
E-942   Nitrous oxide
E-948   Oxygen
Sweeteners and sugar alcohols (see also Table 7.12)
E-420   (i) Sorbitol, (ii) sorbitol syrup
E-421   Mannitol
E-422   Glycerol
E-927a   Azodicarbonamide
E-927b   Carbamide
E-950   Acesulfame K
E-951   Aspartame
E-952   Cyclamic acid and its sodium and calcium salts
E-953   Isomalt
E-954   Saccharin and its sodium, potassium and
             calcium salts
E-957   Thaumatin
E-959   Neohesperidine dichalcone
E-965   (i) Maltitol, (ii) maltitol syrup
E-966   Lactitol
E-967   Xylitol
Miscellaneous compounds
E-999   Quillaia extract
E-1105   Lysozyme (EC 3.2.1.17)
E-1200   Polydextrose
E-1201   Polyvinyl pyrrolidone
E-1202   Polyvinyl polypyrrolidone
E-1505   Triethyl citrate
E-1518   Glyceryl triacetate (triacetin)
Modified starches
E-1404   Oxidized starch
E-1410   Monostarch phosphate
E-1412   Distarch phosphate
E-1413   Phosphated distarch phosphate
E-1414   Acetylated distarch phosphate
E-1420   Acetylated starch
E-1422   Acetylated starch adipate
E-1440   Hydroxypropyl starch
E-1442   Hydroxypropyl distarch phosphate
E-1450   Starch sodium octanoyl succinate

Table 26.9: Micro-organisms associated with spoilage of foods

food	spoilage	organisms
bacon	putrefaction	*Clostridium sporogenes*
beer	slimes, gassing	*Saccharomyces lactis; S. fragilis*
bread	ropey	*Rhizopus oryzae*
bread	sourness	*Bacillus mesentericus*
butter	free fatty acids	*Cladosporium suaveolens*
cereals	musty / mouldy flavour	*Penicillium glaucum; Serratia marcescens*
cheese	mouldy	*Penicillum glaucum; P. expansum; Monilia sitophila*
cream	rancidity, free fatty acids	*Streptococcus cremoris; Oidium lactis*
cucumber	sourness	*Bacillus polymyxa*
fish	putrefaction	*Achromobacter* spp.; *Pseudomonas* spp.; *Flavobacterium* spp.; *Micrococcus* spp.; *Proteus* spp.; *Sarcina* spp.; *Bacillus* spp.
fruit	souring, bitterness, soft rot	*Streptomyces faecalis; Byssochamys fulva; Penicillium* spp.
fruit juice	alcohol	yeasts
fruit juice concentrate	slime formation	*Leuconostoc* spp.
fruit juice, canned fruit	acidification, carbon dioxide	*Lactobacillus* spp.; *Acetobacter* spp.
fruit, bottled	alcohol, butyric acid	*Osmophilic yeasts; Clostridium* spp.
ham	greening	*Lactobacillus viridiscens*
lard	free fatty acids	*Paecilyomyces aureocinnamonium*
margarine	rancidity, ketones	*Clostridium butyri; Candida lipolytica*
meat	degradation of elastin	*Clostridium histolyticum*
meat	liquefaction of collagen	*Clostridium welchii*
meat	putrefaction	*Aeromonas* spp.; *Achromobacter* spp.; *Proteus* spp.; *Pseudomonas* spp.
meat	surface slime	*Clostridium perfringens*
milk	coagulation	*Bacillus subtilis*
milk	off-flavours, rancidity	*Bacillus cereus; Pseudomonas putrefaciens; P. ichthyosmia; Proteus vulgaris; Streptococcus liquefaciens; S. lactis.*
milk	souring	*Lactobacillus* spp.; *Streptococcus lactis*
oats	bitterness	*Aspergillus restrictus*
oil, coconut	ketones	*Margarinomyces bubaki*
oil, corn	free fatty acids	*Aspergillus tamarii*
oil, cottonseed	rancidity	*Lactosaprophiticus* spp.
oil, olive	rancidity	*Aspergillus repens*
oil, rapeseed	rancidity	*Aspergillus niger*
poultry	putrefaction, bone taint	*Clostridium* spp.; *Pseudomonas fluorescens; Vibrio costocolus; Micrococcus* spp.
sauerkraut	slimes	*Lactobacillus plantarum*
vinegar and pickles	slime	*Monilia acetobutans*
wheat	soapiness	*Paecilomyces variotii*
wine	acetic acid	*Acetobacter* spp.; *Acetomonas* spp.

Table 26.10: Major uses of preservatives

	E-number[1]	major uses
Sulphites	220-228	wines, beer, sausages, jam, fruit drinks, dried fruits
Benzoates	210-213	beer, fruit pulps, soft drinks
Nitrates and nitrites	249-252	cured meat products
Propionic acid	280-283	bread, cakes, dried fruits
Sorbic acid	200-219	snack meals, bread, cakes, Xmas pudding
Acetic acid	260-263	flour confectionery, dried fruits
Thiobendazole, biphenyl	230-234	skin of fruits

(1) See Table 26.8

Table 26.11: Major uses of antioxidants

	E-number[1]	major uses
Gallates	310-312	butter, essential oils, edible oils
Butylated hydroxyanisole (BHA)	320	dried cream, dried cheese, essential oils, edible oils, potato powder
Butylated hydroxytoluene (BHT)	321	dried cream, dried cheese, essential oils, edible oils, potato powder
Diphenylamine	-	apples, pears
Ethoxyquin	-	apples, pears
Tocopherols (vitamin E)	306-309	widespread
Ascorbic acid (vitamin C)	300-316	widespread

(1) See Table 26.8

Table 26.12: Certifiable colours for food use in USA
(Synthetic colours for which each batch is tested and certified by manufacturers and FDA)

name	common name	EU equivalent	hue
FD & C blue no 1	brilliant blue FCF	E-133	bright blue
FD & C blue no 2	indigotine	E-132	royal blue
FD & C green no 3	fast green FCF	-	sea green
FD & C red no 40	allura red AC	E-129	orange-red
FD & C red no 3	erythrosine	E-127	cherry red
FD & C yellow no 5	tartrazine	E-102	lemon yellow
FD & C yellow no 6	sunset yellow	E-110	orange
Citrus red no 2	for use on skins of citrus fruits only		

(FD & C = permitted for food, drug and cosmetic uses).

Table 26.13: Colours permitted in USA and exempt from certification
(Natural colours and synthesized natural compounds)

Annatto extract	E-160b
β-Apo-8 -carotenal[1]	E-160e
β-Carotene	E-160a
Beet powder	(E-162)
Canthaxanthin	E-161g
Caramel colour	E-150a-d
Carrot oil	-
Cochineal extract (carmine)	E-120
Cottonseed flour, toasted, partially defatted, cooked	-
Ferrous gluconate[1]	E-579
Fruit juice	-
Grape colour extract[1]	-
Grape skin extract (enocianina)[1]	-
Paprika , paprika oleoresin	E-160c
Riboflavin (vitamin B$_2$)	E-101
Saffron	-
Titanium dioxide[1]	E-171
Turmeric, turmeric oleoresin	-
Vegetable juice	-

(1) Restricted to specific uses.

Table 26.14: Naturally occurring food acids.

		major sources
Monocarboxylic acids	formic	grapes
	acetic	grapes, dates
	butyric	grapes
	para-sorbic	*Sorbus* spp.
Hydroxy-monocarboxylic acids	glycolic	apples, pears, bananas
	glyceric	green fruits
Mono-carboxylic oxo-acids	pyruvic	common in many fruits
	glyoxylic	unripe grapes, apples
Dicarboxylic acids	oxalic	rhubarb, spinach, bananas
	succinic	many fruits and vegetables
	fumaric	vegetables, green apples
	oxaloacetic	traces in many fruits
	2-oxoglutaric	traces in many fruits and vegetables
Hydroxy-dicarboxylic acids	malic	apples, bananas, grapes, rhubarb, plums, pears
	tartaric	grapes, avocadoes
	citramalic	citrus fruits, apple peel
Tricarboxylic acids	citric	common in many fruits, tomatoes, berries
	isocitric	traces in blackberries
	aconitic	traces in grapes
Aromatic acids	benzoic	cranberries, cloudberries
	salicylic	*Ribes, Fragaria, Rubes* spp.
	shikimic	gooseberries, blackberries, quince, elderberries
	quinic	apples, gooseberries, blackberries, elderberries
	chlorogenic	blueberries, peaches, plums, cherries, potatoes
Sugar-derived acids	saccharic	pineapples
	mucic	eleocarpus fruits
	galacturonic	plums, apples

Table 26.15: Enzymes permitted for food use in UK, USA and Canada.

(Not all of these enzymes, and not from all sources, are permitted in all three countries)

Enzyme	EC number	source(s)
acid proteinase (incl pepsin and chymosin)	-	animal gastric mucosa, *Mucor miehi, M. pusillus*
α-amylase	3.2.1.1	animal pancreas, *Aspergillus niger, A, oryzae, Bacillus licheniformis, B. stearothermophilus, B. subtilis, Rhizopus oryzae*
β-amylase	3.2.1.2	barley malt.
bromelain	3.4.22.32, 3.4.22.33	*Ananas bractetus, A. comosus*
catalase	1.11.1.6	bovine liver, *Aspergillus niger, Micrococcus lysodeikticus*
cellulase	3.2.1.4	*Aspergillus niger, Trichoderma viride*
chymosin (rennet)	3.4.23.4	ruminant abomasum
dextranase	3.2.1.11	*Penicillium funiculosum, P. lilacinum*
endothia carboxyl proteinase	-	*Endothia parasitica*
esterase / lipase	-	*Mucor miehei, Bacillus licheniformis, Aspergillus niger, Bacillus subtilis, Ficus* spp.
ficin (ficain)	3.4.22.3	*Ficus* spp.
α-galactosidase	3.2.1.22	*Morteirella vinaceae*
β-glucanase	3.2.1.6, 3.2.1.39	*Aspergillus niger, Bacillus subtilis*
glucose isomerase	-	*Streptomyces rubiginosus, Actinoplanes missouriensis, Streptomyces olivaceaus, S. olivochromogenes, Bacillus coagulans, Arthrobacter globiformis, Streptomyces murinus*
glucose oxidase	1.1.3.4	*Aspergillus niger*
hemicellulase	-	*Bacillus subtilis*
invertase	3.2.1.26	*Saccharomyces cerevisiae*
lactase	3.2.1.23	*Aspergillus niger, A. oryzae, Kluyveromyces fragilis, Candida pseudotropicalis, Saccharomyces* spp.
laminarinase	3.2.1.39	*Aspergillus niger, Bacillus subtilis, Penicillium emersonii*
lipase	3.1.1.3	animal gastric mucosa, pancreas, *Aspergillus niger, A. oryzae*
lipoxidase	1.13.11.13	*Glycine max*
maltase	3.2.1.20	*Aspergillus niger, A. oryzae, Rhizopus oryzae, R. niveus, R. delemar, Mulitplici sporus*
milk clotting enzyme	-	*Endothea parasitica, Bacillus cereus, Mucor pusillus, M. miehei*
neutral proteinase	-	*Aspergillus oryzae, Bacillus subtilis*
pancreatin	-	animal pancreas
papain / chymopapain	3.4.22.2 / 3.4.22.6	*Carica papaya*
pectin esterase (pectinase)	3.2.1.11, 3.2.1.15	*Aspergillus niger, Rhizopus oryzae*
pectin lyase	4.2.2.10	*Aspergillus niger*
pectosanase	-	*Aspergillus niger*
pepsin	3.4.23.1-3	animal gastric mucosa
polygalacturonase	3.2.1.15, 3.2.1.67	*Aspergillus niger*
protease	-	*Aspergillus niger, A. oryzae, Bacillus subtilis*
pullulanase	3.2.1.41	*Klebsiella aerogenes*
serine protease (incl trypsin)	-	animal pancreas, *Bacillus licheniformis, Streptomyces fradiae*
trypsin	3.4.21.4	animal pancreas

Source: from data reported by Smith 1991.

Table 26.16: Steps in safety assessment of food additives.

Chemical structure
Specification (purity)
In vitro mutagenicity testing
Acute toxicity and target organs
Metabolism
Short-term toxicity (90 day test)
Chronic toxicity (life-time tests, carcinogenicity)
Reproductive toxicity / teratogenicity
Calculation of likely exposure, risk / benefit analysis

Table 26.17: Losses of nutrients in milling of wheat

	100% extraction /100 g	85% extraction /100 g	% remaining	72% extraction /100 g	% remaining
protein (g)	13.2	12.8	97	11.3	86
dietary fibre (g)	9.6	7.5	78	3.0	31
thiamin (mg)	0.46	0.30	65	0.10	22
riboflavin (mg)	0.08	0.06	75	0.030	38
niacin (mg)	5.6	1.7	30	0.7	12
folate (μg)	57	51	89	31	54
pantothenate (mg)	0.8	0.4	50	0.3	38
iron (mg)	4.0	2.5	63	1.5	38
zinc (mg)	3.0	2.4	80	0.9	30

Source: from data reported by Paul and Southgate 1978.

Table 26.18: Vitamin content of rice

	brown rice mg /100 g	milled mg /100 g	% remaining	bran mg /100 g	polishings mg /100 g	germ mg /100 g
thiamin	0.34	0.07	21	2.26	1.84	6.5
riboflavin	0.05	0.03	60	0.25	0.18	0.5
niacin	4.7	1.6	34	30	28	3.3
vitamin B_6	1.0	0.45	45	2.5	2.0	1.6
pantothenate	1.5	0.75	50	2.8	3.3	3.0
folate	0.02	0.02	100	0.15	0.19	0.43

Source: from data reported by Morriscu 1974.

Table 26.19: Loss of vitamin C from fresh and frozen peas on cooking

fresh	% loss	frozen	% loss
boil 6.3 min (1.1 min to reach boiling point)	40	blanch 3 min	11
		boil 3 min	30
total loss	40		41

Source: from data reported by Robertson and Sissons 1966.

Table 26.20: Percentage losses of vitamin C from peas on processing and cooking

fresh	loss	frozen	loss	canned	loss	air-dried	loss	freeze-dried	loss
-	-	blanching	25	blanching	30	blanching	25	blanching	25
-	-	freezing	0	canning	7	drying	30	drying	5
-	-	thawing	4	-	-	-	-	-	-
cooking	56	cooking	32	heating	27	cooking	20	cooking	35
total loss	56		61		64		75		65

Source: from data reported by Mapson 1956.

Table 26.21: Vitamin C content of peas after cooking

	fresh variety 1	variety 2	frozen	canned	air-dried	freeze-dried
min boiled	10	10	3.5	brought to boil	15	2
water (x vol of food)	1.2	1.2	1.0	0	23.6	12.3
vitamin C (mg /100 g)	16.4	18.5	14.0	9.2	11.3	15.8

Source: from data reported by Robertson and Sissons 1966.

Table 26.22: Loss of vitamin C from freshly-harvested green leaves in the market

time after harvesting (h)	% lost
2	5-18
4	10-30
8	35-60
10	38-66
24	90

Source: from data reported by Fafunso and Bassir 1976.

Table 26.24: Vitamin losses after canning and storing whole meals

	initial content	% loss after canning	after storage 1.5 y	3 y	5 y
vitamin A	16.5 µg	50	100	100	100
vitamin E	80 mg	0	0	50	50
thiamin	9 mg	50	75	75	75
riboflavin	6 mg	0	0	0	0
niacin	110 mg	10	20	20	20
vitamin B_6	5 mg	0	0	0	0
vitamin B_{12}	18 µg	0	0	0	0
folate	14 µg	0	0	0	0
pantothenate	21 mg	25	50	50	50
inositol	26 mg	0	0	0	0
choline	27 mg	0	0	0	0

Source: from data reported by Hellendoorn et al. 1971.

Table 26.23: Percentage loss of vitamin C on cutting fresh vegetables

	cucumber	cabbage	tomato
immediate loss	22	7	0
after 1 h	35	12	4
after 3 h	49	20	6

Table 26.25: Heat damage to protein of oat preparations

	PER[1]
drum dried (boiled 15 min, dried 15 sec at 130°C)	1.6
rolled oats	1.5
oven exploded (cooked 1-2 min under pressure, dried 1-2 min at 200°C)	1.6
preparation of oats, corn and rye (boiled, dried, heated at 190-232°C 52-62 min under pressure, exploded)	0.5
puffed oats (5 min at 122°C, live steam under pressure at 198°C for 2 min, then puffed)	0.3

(1) PER = Protein Efficiency Ratio, see section 10.7.2.
Source: from data reported by Stewart et al. 1943.

Table 26.26: Percentage losses of vitamins from milk during heat treatment

	thiamin	vitamin B_6	vitamin B_{12}	folate	vitamin C
pasteurized	< 10	< 10	< 10	< 10	< 25
sterilized in bottle, old method	35	50	90	50	90
sterilized in bottle, new method	20	20	20	30	60
UHT sterilized	< 10	< 10	< 10	< 10	< 25
evaporated	20	40	80	25	60
sweetened-condensed	10	< 10	30	25	25

Source: from data reported by Porter and Thompson 1976.

Table 26.27: Effects of home cooking of beans

	protein (g/100 g)	fat (g/100 g)	available lysine (mg /g protein)	PER[1]
raw	24.6	1.9	5.83	0
cooked	24.9	0.7	6.30	1.24
strained	24.0	0.6	6.35	1.43
fried	17.8	13.3	5.17	0.87

(1) PER = Protein Efficiency Ratio, see section 10.7.2.
Source: from data reported by Bressani and Elias 1972.

Adverse reactions to food

Apart from the presence of toxic substances, adverse reactions to food fall into several categories depending on the cause and the mechanism of the reaction. There are two main classes, food intolerance and food aversion. The former is defined as a reproducible, unpleasant reaction to a specific food or food ingredient that is not psychologically based and occurs even when the food is disguised. Food aversion is psychologically based and reactions do not occur when the food is disguised.

Food intolerance may be due to the following:

(1) allergic reactions involving the immune system;

(2) symptoms similar to allergic reactions which do not involve the immune system and are caused by histamine-containing foods such as fish, yeast extracts and fermented products such as cheese and wine, or by foods that stimulate the release of histamine;

(3) inborn errors of metabolism such as enzyme deficiencies e.g. alactasia (see section 7.2.1), phenylketonuria (see section 10.10), and favism (see sections 27.3.4 and 7.7.1);

(4) irritation of the digestive tract by substances such as spices or alcohol;

(5) pharmacological effects due to caffeine, sulphur dioxide, monosodium glutamate, etc.;

(6) fermentation of unabsorbed food in the lower bowel, e.g. diarrhoea caused by high intakes of bulk sweeteners such as sorbitol and xylitol (see section 7.2).

In addition, adverse effects of foods include the following:

(1) poisoning as a result of accidental contamination with harmful substances (see Table 27.1);

(2) toxins naturally present in foods (see section 27.3);

(3) formation of harmful substances during processing (e.g. effects of heat, acid, or alkali, see section 27.4);

(4) poisoning due to the presence of micro-organisms or the toxins they produce (see section 27.5).

27.1 Allergy

The term allergy is popularly used to refer to almost any type of adverse reaction, to both food and environment, but is correctly applied only when the immune system is involved. Many substances in the environment can cause allergy; food and food ingredients form only a small part of these allergens. Exposure to the harmful agent, the antigen, can be via the gastrointestinal tract, by skin contact, or by inhalation of the dust from a food. Many physiological reactions may be involved, as shown in Table 27.2.

The difficulty of diagnosis is largely due to the variable times taken for clinical symptoms to appear, ranging from immediately after exposure to the allergen to several hours or even days. Symptoms appear at a second and subsequent exposures after the subject has been sensitized at the first exposure.

27.1.1 The immune system

The immune system protects the body from foreign materials including bacteria, viruses, fungi, pollens and parasites by producing specific antibodies. The offending substances, termed antigens, are commonly proteins or complex carbohydrates attached to proteins. The immune system has four components: B-lymphocytes (named after the organ, Bursa of Fabricius, found in animals although not in man), together with T-lymphocytes (thymus-derived), phagocytes, and a system of proteins termed 'complement'.

The B-lymphocytes produce the antibodies which include five types of immunoglobulins—Ig A, D, G, M, and, especially important in regard to allergy, IgE. They bind specifically both to the antigen and to white blood cells. IgE molecules have 40 000 to 400 000 binding sites, which accounts for their high degree of specificity. Lymphocytes are white blood cells which form the main constituents of lymphoid tissues and circulate in the blood and lymph throughout the body.

The thymus and bone marrow are primary lymphoid organs; secondary lymphoid organs include spleen, tonsils, appendix, lymph nodes, lymph glands of liver and various parts of the gastrointestinal tract.

Food allergy appears to be an aberration of the immune system whereby ordinary food ingredients that are normally quite harmless are regarded by the system as harmful foreign bodies. The antibodies react specifically with the foreign substances and then phagocytic cells (macrophages, neutrophils, basophils and eosinophils) engulf and digest the antigen-antibody complex. The complement system comprises a number of plasma proteins that react together to release histamine, causing swelling of the membranes and cells and enhancing phagocytosis, and so give rise to the allergic reaction.

The immediate reaction to eating the harmful food is believed to involve IgE (immunoglobulin E), occurring within an hour. When the IgE cells are sensitized to the antigen they attach themselves to specialized cells, mast cells, in the skin, eyes, nose, mouth, respiratory tract and intestines and trap the antigen and cause release of chemicals into the surrounding tissues (mast cells occur rarely in the blood where they are termed basophils). Histamine is one of the most important of these and the swelling in the tissues and the contraction of muscles in the bronchi give rise to the sneezing and coughing—hence the use of antihistamines in treatment.

Allergic reactions can be classified into four types, ranging from anaphylaxis (immediate reaction) to type 4, delayed reaction (see Table 27.3). The term 'masked allergy' is used when only minor symptoms arise from a food eaten regularly, but when it has been avoided for a few days and then ingested there can be a violent reaction. The release of histamine and prostaglandins without participation of the immune system gives rise to symptoms resembling allergy; it occurs particularly in children who later outgrow their sensitivity to histamine.

27.1.2 Prevalence of food allergies

Adverse reactions to food are not new—Hippocrates (460–360 BC) said 'a particular food or change of diet makes some unfortunate individuals ill'—but they have only recently received recognition as an important problem. Even health professionals have been slow to accept that a number of common clinical disorders can be caused by food. With the types of adverse reactions to food listed above it is difficult to diagnose true allergy as distinct from other forms of intolerance. The only reliable procedure is a detailed dietary history, followed by a limited diet restricted to foods of low allergenicity (see Table 27.4) until clinical signs disappear. Then the suspected foods are introduced without the subject knowing (blind test) until the culprit reveals itself. This procedure must be repeated, some authorities recommend two repeats, to ensure that the food or foods responsible have been correctly identified. The only treatment is for the subject to avoid the particular food and, in the instance of anaphylaxis, have appropriate treatment immediately available.

Many people believe that they are allergic to a particular food, but only a small proportion of them have been tested properly. The risk of incorrect self-diagnosis is the unnecessary restriction of the diet, which may have adverse nutritional consequences. The problem is aggravated by the publicity that has been given to commercial offers of unreliable methods of diagnosis. The imprecision of diagnostic criteria adds to the difficulties of assessing the prevalence of food intolerance.

The commonest causes of allergy are milk, egg, wheat, soya and their derivatives, cocoa, the antioxidants BHA and BHT (butylated hydroxyanisole and butylated hydroxytoluene), the preservatives sulphur dioxide and benzoate, the flavour-enhancer glutamate and azo colours. Table 27.5 lists some of the commonest causes identified by patients attending allergy clinics.

The difficulty in obtaining reliable figures is illustrated by two postal surveys carried out in the United Kingdom, one to ascertain allergy to food additives and the second to natural foods (Young *et al.* 1987, 1994). 7.4 per cent of respondents believed themselves to be allergic to food additives, but this was reduced to 0.01–0.23 per cent in a subgroup subjected to a double-blind allergen challenge trial. In the second survey, dealing with natural foods, 20.4 per cent of the population group considered themselves allergic—a figure that was reduced to 2.9–3.6 per cent when tested, although limitations of the method suggest that the true figure may be considerably higher. A population survey in The Netherlands similarly showed that while some 15 per cent of the population group considered themselves to be allergic to foods this could be confirmed in only one-fifth of them.

While true allergic reactions are associated with circulating antibodies (IgE), and a positive skin prick test to the food in question, false positives can occur as well as false negatives and tests can remain positive after the clinical problems have been resolved. The only reliable procedure is a direct test seeking clinical improvement when the suspect food is withdrawn, confirmed by repeated challenges with the food.

Immediate sensitivity or anaphylaxis, Type 1 allergy, renders dietary challenge procedures potentially dangerous. When the responsible food has been eliminated from the diet and then re-introduced (i.e. a challenge) there can be a violent reaction. Hence challenges should be carried out under medical supervision when remedial measures can be undertaken. The likelihood of such a reaction may be indicated by a positive clinical history, together with a clearly positive prick skin test and the demonstration of the presence of IgE antibodies.

27.1.3. Food intolerance in children

Figures for intolerance in children quoted in the literature range between 0.3 and 20 per cent (Royal College of Physicians 1984). Young babies can absorb larger amounts of intact proteins than can adults (see section 10.3); at the same time there is a low level of circulating IgA, which has an inhibitory effect on the absorption of macromolecules. Absorption of intact proteins leads to production of antibodies even in the absence of any symptoms.

Before 4 months of age there is an additional problem because the kidneys may not be sufficiently developed to deal with high concentrations of solutes present in weaning foods, and the secretion of digestive enzymes and the absorptive capacity of the intestine may not be adequately developed. Early weaning onto foods such as cow's milk, cereals and egg and their products can therefore give rise to problems. It is suggested that many bouts of colic common in babies may be due to cow's milk.

Intolerance to cow's milk occurs in about 2 per cent of infants, decreasing with age. The primary allergens are casein, α-lactalbumin and β-lactoglobulin. The symptoms include anaphylaxis, eczema, urticaria, angio-oedema, vomiting, diarrhoea, and failure to thrive.

Symptoms may appear immediately the food has been eaten, i.e. IgE mediated, or more slowly when other mechanisms are involved. The reaction may be due to damage of the intestinal mucosa following, for example, a bout of gastroenteritis. Substitutes for cow's milk include soya preparations but many patients allergic to cow's milk are also allergic to soya. Goat's milk is sometimes, but not always, tolerated. The only preparations regarded as suitable are those based on hydrolysed milk or alternatives such as comminuted chicken or beef serum. Hypoallergenic foods are defined in US as those which, within 95 per cent confidence limits, do not cause allergy in 90 per cent of patients shown to be allergic to the parent food.

The UK Department of Health (1994) recommended weaning practice based on good nutrition and the formation of good eating habits, which at the same time minimize allergy. Thus no solid foods before 4 months; unmodified cow's milk should not be given as a main drink before 12 months, although milk products such as yoghurts, custard and cheese sauce can be introduced at 4 months, and cow's milk can be given with cereals at 6 months. It is suggested that suitable first weaning foods should include non-wheat cereals, pureed potatoes, fruits and vegetables; at 6–9 months meat, fish, eggs, all cereals, and pulses may be included. No added salt is necessary and sugars should be limited.

Where there is a family history of allergic disease, the advice is that breast feeding should be prolonged (breast milk contains high levels of IgA which protect the immature gut wall) and the introduction of potentially allergenic foods—wheat, cow's milk, eggs, fish—should be delayed beyond 6 months.

When small children are put on a parent-selected diet in response to self-diagnosis of allergy, many foods may be banned, resulting in relative deficiencies of protein, energy, calcium, iron, riboflavin and/or folate. Since the average 2 year old child obtains about 50 per cent of the protein intake, 25 per cent of the energy, and 100 per cent of the riboflavin and calcium from 570 mL (1 pint) of milk obvious problems can arise if milk products are removed from the diet.

27.1.4 Coeliac disease

Coeliac disease is an inherited condition, an allergic reaction to the gliadin fraction of gluten, one of the major proteins of wheat, rye, barley and oats. There is damage to the intestinal mucosa, leading to failure of fat absorption, and hence steattorrhoea—pale fatty faeces. There is also commonly secondary deficiency of lactase (see section 7.2.1), as a result of the mucosal damage. Elimination of the offending cereals leads to recovery of normal intestinal function. Rice and maize are generally tolerated, but even small amounts of gluten can lead to an acute reaction—coeliac shock. As a result of the previous intestinal damage, allergic reactions to other foods are more common in treated coeliac patients than in the population at large.

27.1.5 Data banks

In UK a data bank of foods free from the ten ingredients that are most important in causing food intolerance has been compiled by the UK food industry, the Royal College of Physicians, The British Dietetic Association and the Leatherhead Food Research Association (see Table 27.6); to ensure proper supervision, this is restricted to hospital physicians and State Registered Dietitians. A similar data bank exists in The Netherlands and one is being compiled in EU.

27.1.6 Food processing

The problem of food allergy is not easily solved by simply omitting the offending ingredients from the diet, since allergens can arise after processing and storage. For example, fungi and mites and their faeces are significant causes of intolerance. Mites infest a wide variety of stored products—cereals, milk powder, cheese, dried fruit, even sugar—and can cause asthma or dermatitis in food handlers. Packers of dried mushrooms have been found to have respiratory problems, and asthma can arise from soybeans and papain during packaging.

Histamine poisoning gives rise to symptoms similar to those seen in cases of allergy, yet this is a normal constituent of fermented foods such as cheese, fermented sausages, and sauerkraut. It is formed from the amino acid histidine and the amount is greatly increased if *Proteus morganii* proliferates. It is possible that tyramine (derived from tyrosine) in very mature cheeses, and phenyethylamine (derived from phenylalanine) in chocolate may have similar effects. Observations are complicated by the effects of heat processing or cooking since some of the responsible agents are modified. For example chlorogenic acid in oranges and coffee is destroyed by heat; some individuals who react to boiled egg have been shown to tolerate egg in cakes; it is not clear whether this is because of the smaller amounts or the fact that the egg has been more strongly heated in baking.

Very small amounts of allergens have been reported to cause clinical problems. For example problems have arisen from the small amount of maize allergens in corn syrup, the small amounts included in Scotch whiskey when corn liquor is added to make the product resemble Bourbon; the traces of animal charcoal remaining after purification of sucrose from sugar cane, and the minute amounts of groundnut protein in cold-pressed arachis oil. Breast milk can cause a rash in babies when the mother has eaten foods such as chocolate, eggs, wheat, or milk. Many medicines contain colours and preservatives which may be allergenic; many orange, red, green and yellow tablets contain azo dyes; even toothpastes, vitamin preparations and antibiotics may be coloured or preserved with substances that are allergenic to some individuals.

Foods are usually classed into biological families (see Chapter 28), but may also be classed into biochemical families, as shown in Table 27.7; foods in the same biochemical family contain similar antigens.

27.1.7 Hyperactivity (hyperkinesis)

Hyperactivity in children is a difficult and controversial diagnosis—sustained activity, impulsiveness, aggressiveness, inability to concentrate—that was originally blamed on salicylates in foods, then on added colours, and then all types of food additives (Feingold 1975). However, subsequent properly controlled trials have failed to confirm claims for a high incidence of hyperactivity caused by diet although it is possible that a small proportion of children may suffer hyperactivity as a result of allergic or chemical response to substances such as histamine, tyramine, phenylethylamine, caffeine, monosodium glutamate, tartrazine, or benzoate (National Advisory Committee 1980; Egger *et al.* 1985).

27.2   Antinutrients in foods

Many foods contain harmful substances but most of these are either destroyed in traditional cooking or are present in amounts small enough to be dealt with by the body's various detoxicating systems. We rarely know what levels are tolerable, whether regular consumption of small quantities poses a hazard to health, whether some individuals are more sensitive than others, what environmental factors depress detoxifying ability, and how much of the suspected substances is being ingested.

Some toxic substances give rise to clear-cut cases of damage, such as cyanide in cassava, tetrodontin in puffer fish, favism from broad beans (see section

27.3.4), and toxins in shellfish (see section 27.5.2). Many foods contain substances that destroy or reduce the availability of nutrients but are themselves mostly destroyed by heat. The antinutrients may be classed as

(1) enzyme inhibitors;

(2) antimetabolites of vitamins and minerals;

(3) mineral-binding agents (phytates, oxalates);

(3) toxins.

27.2.1 Protease inhibitors

Peptides that inhibit the protein digestive enzymes, trypsin, chymotrypsin, elastase, and carboxypeptidase (see section 10.3.1) are widespread in many legumes, cereals (oat, barley and maize) as well as Brussels sprouts, onions, beetroot and other fruits and vegetables (see Table 27.8). Many of these also inhibit fungal, bacterial and insect proteases, suggesting that they serve a protective function in the plants.

Inhibitors of both trypsin and chymotrypsin are present in wheat and finger millet, and in a number of seeds and leaves. Since these are proteins, they are denatured and inactivated by adequate cooking, but even when vegetables are eaten raw there is no evidence of any deleterious effects on human beings. One of the few legumes eaten raw is the peanut (*Arachis hypogaea*) which contains inhibitors of trypsin and chymotrypsin but there do not seem to be any reports of harm. Harmful effects do arise in animals fed on unusually large quantities of some of these foods eaten raw, such as cabbage and kale; legumes and oilseed cake are heat treated but not always adequately.

Several types of enzyme inhibitors have been found in legumes and those of soya beans have been examined in depth. The general picture is that unless destroyed by heat the inhibitors stimulate the pancreas to excessive secretion which results in its enlargement. The inhibitors are relatively rich in sulphur amino acids but these are not available so that the protein quality is lower than expected from amino acid analysis. When heated the sulphur amino acids become available and the quality improves. However, it has been shown that antitryptic preparations still retard growth in rodents when the protein has been predigested (Westfall *et al.* 1948; De Muelenaere 1964) and inhibit proteolytic activity in chicks. Kakade *et al.* (1973) showed that 40 per cent of the pancreatic hypertrophy was accounted for by trypsin inhibitors and 60 per cent of the hypertrophy and

growth retardation was due to resistance to attack by digestive enzymes. Two types of protease inhibitors are present, those of high M_r, approximately 20 000 (Kunitz inhibitors) and those with M_r around 6000 (Bowman-Birk inhibitors). The binding sites for the inhibition of trypsin and chymotrypsin are independent.

The mechanism of pancreatic enlargement is not clear; possibilities include the following:

1. Stimulation by humoral agents released through the action of the inhibitor on the gastrointestinal tract.

2. Failure of the negative feedback mechanism by which trypsin and chymotrypsin normally suppress further secretion of pancreatic enzymes.

3. Increased conversion of methionine in the pancreas.

Species differences have been explained on the basis of relative pancreatic size (Kakade *et al.* 1976). Species with pancreatic weight exceeding 0.3 per cent of total body weight (mouse, rat, chicken) develop pancreatic hypertrophy, while those with lower pancreatic weight (dog, pig, calf, human being) do not. The effects demonstrated in animals require much larger intakes of the foodstuffs than are usually consumed by human beings.

27.2.2 Amylase inhibitors

Wheat contains a group of inhibitors of pancreatic and salivary amylases (EC 3.2.1.1), as well as the bacterial and insect enzymes. Although these inhibitors are inactivated by heat they have been detected in the centre of loaves of bread and in some wheat-based breakfast cereals. It is not known whether they pose any problems.

Anti-amylases extracted from kidney beans have been marketed as acarbose, claimed to act as a 'starch-blocker', in the mistaken belief that it reduces the digestion of starch *in vivo* and so is helpful in weight-reduction (see section 11.4). While the overall energy yield of starch, due to small intestinal digestion and colonic fermentation, is unaffected by acarbose, it does have an effect on the rate at which starch is hydrolysed. It also inhibits intestinal mucosal glucosidases, and hence delays the absorption of sucrose. Acarbose lowers post-prandial plasma glucose, and is sometimes used as an adjunct to the treatment of non-insulin-dependent diabetes mellitus (see section 7.7.2), since it improves glycaemic control (Balfour and McTavish 1993).

27.2.3 Tannins (polyphenols)

Tannins are present in tea, coffee and cocoa, in beans, especially broad beans (*Vicia faba*) and in sorghum, where the concentration is reflected in the colour. They have been shown to cause growth depression in experimental animals and to reduce protein quality (presumably by combining with part of the protein and rendering it resistant to digestion) but there is no evidence of any problem in human nutrition. In some communities, e.g. parts of India, tea is given to very young children without evidence of harm.

27.2.4 Antivitamins

These fall into three classes.

1 Substances chemically similar to vitamins that are competitive inhibitors of vitamin metabolism and utilization (e.g. pyridoxyllysine, formed by reaction between vitamin B_6 and lysine in proteins, see section 20.2.1.2).

2. Compounds that complex with, or chemically modify the vitamin.

3. Enzymes that destroy vitamin activity.

Avidin, a protein in egg-white, binds biotin and renders it unavailable; it is denatured by heat, and cooked egg is a good source of biotin. Dietary deficiency of biotin has been reported only in very rare cases where abnormally large amounts of uncooked egg-white were consumed (see section 23.1).

Antithiamin compounds have been found in a variety of plants, including *Allium* spp., ragi, mung beans, rice bran, beets, Brussels sprouts, and some berries. Caffeic acid (3,4–dihydroxycinnamic acid) in bracken fern causes 'blind staggers' in horses and cattle since it inactivates thiamin. Similar effects have been observed with other *o*-dihydroxyphenols, including catechol. The presence of these compounds in tea and coffee poses at least a potential problem. Somogyi and Nageli (1976) found a reduction in urinary excretion of thiamin and a fall in blood thiamin concentration after drinking 1 L of coffee over a 3 hour period. It has been reported that drinking tea and chewing tea leaves reduces thiamin status as shown by the transketolase activation test (see section 17.6.4) but there is no evidence of deficiency as a result of normal levels of intake (Vimokesant *et al.* 1974).

Thiaminases, enzymes which catalyse the cleavage of thiamin to inactive fragments, are found in fish, shellfish, ferns, bacteria, yeasts, and fungi. Some of the products of enzymic cleavage of thiamin may have further antithiamin metabolic activity, and some also have anti-vitamin B_6 metabolic activity. The high prevalence of thiamin deficiency in southeast Asia is at least partially attributable to the consumption of fermented fish, in which most, if not all, of the thiamin has been destroyed by thiaminase action.

Most plants, which are the main source of dietary vitamin C, contain ascorbate oxidase; as discussed in section 26.3.1.4, there is a considerable loss of vitamin C as leafy vegetables wilt, when the enzyme is released from intracellular vacuoles.

27.2.5 Goitrogens

There is a great disparity in the prevalence of goitre in several adjacent communities around the world, despite the same low intake of dietary iodine as measured by urinary excretion—in many instances a tenfold difference. Goitre can even occur in regions where iodine intake is apparently adequate and this is attributed to the presence of goitrogens in the diet. These are mostly glucosinolates (see Table 7.13), which are hydrolysed to isothiocyanates and oxazolidine-2–thiones, which inhibit the iodination of tyrosine and the coupling process in the synthesis of thyroxine; their action is not relieved by the administration of iodine (see section 25.14.4).

Goitrogens are common in members of the Brassica and Cruciferae families of vegetables, in leaves, stems, roots and seeds, the amounts varying with the cultivar and growing conditions. Much may be leached into the cooking water, but even in foods eaten raw there is usually insufficient to affect human beings. A survey in Great Britain indicated an average intake of 76 mg of glucosinolinates—46 mg from raw and 29 mg from cooked vegetables, with individual intakes up to 200 mg (Fenwick and Heaney 1983; Sones *et al.* 1984). In some areas in Czechoslovakia, Yugoslavia, and Sicily, where iodine intake is marginal, the consumption of vegetables is associated with increased incidence of goitre (Michajlovskij and Langer 1959; Michajlovskij *et al.* 1969; Matovinovic 1983). Goitrogens have been detected in the milk from cows grazing on Brassica, but while this may affect the calves there is no evidence that there is sufficient to affect human beings.

As well as these vegetables, goitrogens are present in cassava (a staple of some 250 million people in the tropics), soybean (*Glycine max*), walnut (*Juglans regia*), peanut (*Arachis hypogaea*), pinon (pine nuts, *Pinus* spp.). Rapeseed meal (coleseed, *Brassica napus*), the residue after oil extraction, is a useful animal feed but is rich in glucosinolates which lead to poor growth in pigs and to various disorders in poultry, and hypothyroidism in calves. The Canadian variety of Argentine rape, Canola, was developed by selection from *Brassica napus* Bronowski and contains less than 3 mg glucosinolates /g as well as less than 5 per cent erucic acid—a reduction of about 90 per cent of standard values.

Goitre can also arise from too high an intake of iodine. Amounts of 50 mg /day or serum levels greater than 200 μg /L can disturb thyroid function at stages from synthesis to secretion. Usually there is an adaptation to high levels of intake within a few days, but the problem persists in some 3–4 per cent of people (Wolff 1969). Excessive intakes of iodine can occur from iodine-rich foods such as kelp (seaweed) when eaten in quantity; Suzuki *et al.* (1965) reported a higher incidence of goitre in coastal districts of Japan than in inland towns, apparently due to the consumption of seaweed soups prepared from plants containing 0.8–4.5 g iodine per kg dry weight. Additional sources of iodine arise from iodophors used to disinfect dairy equipment, and the teats and udders of cows, and drinking glasses, the use of the red food colour erythrosine (2.4.5.7–tetra-iodofluoroscein, E-127, FD & C Red No. 3), which contains 580 mg iodine per g, and the use of iodate as a dough-conditioner, although not all of this iodine is available.

27.2.6 Phytate and dietary fibre

At one time, phytates (inositol hexaphosphate as water-soluble sodium and potassium salts and insoluble calcium and magnesium salts) were thought to reduce the availability of calcium (see section 14.1), iron (see section 24.2.3.1), zinc (see section 25.26.1). Enrichment of oatmeal with 1 per cent calcium acid phosphate was instituted as long ago as 1935 in Denmark, to overcome what was believed to be the rachitogenic effect of oatmeal, and an outbreak of rickets in Ireland in the 1940s was attributed to the same cause. However, there is phytase (EC 3.1.3.8 and 3.1.3.26) in the human intestine and also in the yeast used in bread-making, so any effect of phytate appears to be limited. Moreover Walker (1951) reported that the negative calcium balance of subjects fed 900 mg of phytate as wholemeal bread reverted to positive after a few weeks. The same was found by Cullumbine *et al.* (1950) with brown rice.

Contradictory findings reported in the literature may be due to the differing amounts of phytate fed. Some non-starch polysaccharides (NSP, see section 7.3) bind divalent cations such as calcium, iron, copper, and zinc *in vitro*. This may be due to uronic acid residues of NSP or the associated phytate. However, *in vivo* studies in human beings do not show any reduction in mineral availability unless the phytate and NSP levels are high and the minerals only marginally adequate (Department of Health 1991).

27.2.7 Oxalate

There is a relatively high concentration of oxalate in plants such as beetroot, rhubarb, parsley, spinach and tea—and to a small extent in beans. This could theoretically combine with calcium and render it insoluble, so reducing the amount absorbed. The average British diet supplies 70–150 mg of oxalate per day, half of this being provided by five cups of tea. This is sufficient to chelate only 30–70 mg of calcium out of a total intake of 10–20 times this amount, so any deleterious effects of oxalate would appear to be unlikely unless the calcium intake was extremely low.

27.3 Toxins naturally present in foods

Many foods contain alkaloids that are potentially harmful—e.g. myristicin in nutmeg, hallucinogens in many wild mushrooms. Other wild fungi may prove fatal as a result of their toxic alkaloids, and the puffer fish (*Fuga rubripes*) is a prized delicacy in Japan, but must be prepared by chefs skilled in the art of removing the poison gland, which contains the neurotoxin tetrodotoxin.

27.3.1 Glycoalkaloids

The potato, *Solanum tuberosum*, contains toxic alkaloids synthesized from cholesterol, mostly α-solanine and α-chaconine; derivatives of the aglycone solanidine. Total glycoalkaloids range between 2.5 and 15 mg /100 g fresh weight and they are found immediately below the skin. The sprouts of the potato are much richer in glycoalkaloids, the amount being affected by cultivar, growing conditions, and post-harvest treatment. Mechanically and chemically induced stress and exposure to light increase the amount.

Poisoning with solanine results in gastrointestinal and neurological disturbances with haemolytic and haemorrhagic damage. Elevated levels in excess of 11 mg /100 g fresh weight cause a bitter taste and it is generally accepted that levels should not exceed 20 mg /100 g. While outbreaks of solanine poisoning are rare and very few deaths have been reported in the literature, it is suggested that many cases of gastro-intestinal upset may perhaps be due to solanine poisoning but not reported as such.

27.3.2 Cyanogenic glycosides

Cyanides in trace amounts are widely distributed in the plant kingdom as cyanogenic glycosides, e.g. in cassava, sweet potato, yam, maize, millet, sugarcane, butter (Lima) beans, kernels of almond, apple, cherry, apricot, plum. Four of these have been found to be of practical importance, namely amygdalin (bitter almonds), dhurrin (in sorghum and other grasses), and linamarin (phaseolunatin) and methyllinamarin (lotaustralin) in pulses and cassava. Amygdalin yields benzaldehyde on hydrolysis; dhurrin yields *p*-hydroxybenzaldehyde; linamarin yields acetone; lotaustralin yields methylethyl ketone—together with glucose and HCN.

Ingested cyanide is rapidly absorbed in the upper gastrointestinal tract and HCN gas is absorbed in the lungs. It combines with thiosulphate and sulphite catalysed by the enzyme rhodanese (EC 2.8.1.1), which is widespread in tissues, and the resultant thiocyanate is excreted in the urine and saliva. Hydroxocobalamin (vitamin B_{12}, see section 21.5) takes up cyanide to form cyanocobalamin, which is only slowly restored to the metabolically active vitamer.

The minimum lethal dose of cyanide has been estimated at 0.5–3.5 mg /kg body weight. Human poisoning has been reported from various types of *Phaseolus vulgaris*, cassava, and bitter almonds. Cassava is a staple food in some regions and is relatively rich in cyanide. While local methods of processing have been developed to remove most of it, accidents are not uncommon and the chronic intake of small amounts appears to create problems in some areas—tropical ataxic neuropathy and tropical amblyopia, apparently the result of vitamin B_{12} depletion.

27.3.3 Lathyrogens

Lathyrism is an ancient disease caused by the consumption of seeds of many species of *Lathyrus* peas (chickling vetch, flat-podded vetch, Spanish vetchling, Indian vetch). The neurotoxin oxalyl-diamino propionic acid causes muscular weakness and sudden paralysis of the legs as a result of neurological lesions of the spinal cord (neurolathyrism), when the seeds are a high proportion of the diet over a period of some months. Impaired synthesis of connective tissue proteins as a result of inhibition of cross-linkage by β-aminopropionitrile leads to the development of bone abnormalities (osteolathyrism) and in severe cases aortic rupture, in animals fed large amounts of *Lathyrus* spp. (see section 25.11.3).

Growing *Lathyrus* species has been banned in many countries but lathyrism continues to be a public health problem in India, since Kesari dhal (*Lathyrus sativa*) is a hardy crop, with a high yield, that survives adverse conditions, and so is available at times of food shortages

27.3.4 Favism

Favism is an acute haemolytic anaemia caused by eating broad beans (fava beans, *Vicia faba*) or, in severe cases, by inhalation of the pollen of the plant. It is prevalent in insular and littoral regions of the Mediterranean areas and middle East, and is the result of an inborn error of metabolism causing a deficiency in glucose-6–phosphate dehydrogenase in red blood cells (see section 7.7.1). It is one of commonest genetically determined enzyme defects in human beings, affecting some 100 million people world-wide. The toxic agents are vicine and convicine: diamino-dihydroxypyrimidine-glucopyranose and trihydroxy-aminopyrimidine glucopyranoside.

27.3.5 Lectins (phytohaemagglutinins)

Lectins are proteins found in a variety of plants and in some animal species (crustaceans, molluscs, mammalian tissues), which bind to the carbohydrates of cell surface glycoproteins. They are also known as phytohaemagglutinins, since they cause the agglutination of red blood cells; this provides an *in vitro* method of measurement. When ingested they cause growth retardation in animals and sometimes death. They bind to intestinal mucosal cells, causing non-specific interference with absorption.

The main problem in human health arises from beans, most especially *Phaseolus vulgaris* because of the high concentration of lectins. The lectin protein is denatured, and so detoxicated, by heat, but incompletely cooked beans remain toxic and have been the cause of outbreaks of food poisoning. The young *Phaseolus vulgaris* beans (French beans) are often eaten raw but do not cause any problems because the level of lectins is low until the beans reach maturity.

In human beings the phaseolus lectins cause diarrhoea and vomiting 1–3 hours after ingestion, usually with rapid recovery (Noah *et al.* 1980). In the late 1970s there were several hundred outbreaks involving about 900 people in Great Britain, due both to the consumption of raw beans softened by soaking, and to slow cooking at 70–80°C of dishes such as chilli con carne—even when continued for several hours (Bender 1983*a*). The hazard appears to have been overcome after advice that beans should be vigorously boiled for at least 10 min.

27.3.6 Amines and migraine

Amines formed by bacterial and fungal decarboxylation of the aromatic amino acids (phenylethylamine from phenylalanine and tyramine from tyrosine) are present in a number of foods, especially fermented foods and ripe cheeses; chocolate contains a relatively large amount of phenylethylamine. They are also formed to some extent in the large intestine, by bacterial metabolism of free amino acids. Both amines are potent vasoconstrictors, but are normally oxidized to the inactive aldehydes and then acids by the action of monoamine oxidase (EC 1.4.3.4) and aldehyde oxidase (EC 1.2.3.1) in the intestinal mucosa and liver. Nevertheless, amine-rich foods such as cheese and chocolate are common triggers of diet-induced migraine, and there is some evidence that in susceptible individuals a significant amount of dietary amines may enter the peripheral circulation.

27.3.7 Potential carcinogens and cocarcinogens

The development of cancer can be divided into two stages, initiation and promotion. Initiation (in animal experiments) requires only a single treatment with a carcinogen and is regarded as irreversible; such compounds are detected as mutagens in *in vitro* bacterial assays. The dietary compounds recognized as risk factors in cancer are thought to act mainly as promoters of tumour development after the initiation of the tumour.

Doll and Peto (1981) estimated that the likely contributions of various environmental factors to human cancers in the United States were 35 per cent from the diet, 30 per cent from tobacco, 3 per cent from alcohol and less than 1 per cent from food additives, with 15 per cent from non-dietary sources. Ames (1983) listed many mutagens and putative carcinogens in natural foodstuffs including safrole in root beer, piperine and safrole in black pepper, various hydrazides in mushrooms, photocarcinogens in celery and parsnips, various flavonoids and pyrrolizidine alkaloids in many plant foods, mutagenic quinones in rhubarb, caffeic acid in coffee, theobromine in tea and cocoa, allyl isothiocyanate in mustard and horseradish—together with numerous tumour-promoting,

and potentially teratogenic, phenolic compounds in plant foods (see Table 27.9). It is noteworthy, however, that many of these cocarcinogenic phenolic compounds also have potentially protective actions, since they can form stable radicals, and can therefore act as radical-trapping antioxidants (see sections 15.5.1 and 23.3).

27.3.7.1 Phyto-oestrogens
A number of compounds naturally present in plants (as distinct from those produced by mould growth) have oestrogenic activity, including lignans in cereals, berries, and nuts, flavones and isoflavones in chickpeas, cherries, plums, and soybean; isocoumarin derivatives in carrots, oestrone in apple and pomegranate, and oestradiol in French beans. While animal studies, feeding high levels of these phyto-oestrogens, suggest potential adverse effects, evidence from epidemiological studies suggests that at normal levels of intake they may have a protective role against the development of prostate and other hormone-dependent cancers (Adlerkreutz *et al.* 1993; Herman *et al.* 1995; Price and Fenwick 1985).

27.4 Toxic factors resulting from food processing

Because of advanced analytical techniques, many toxic agents, previously unrecognized, have been discovered in processed foods, some being formed during storage and domestic cooking. This does not mean that such foods are unsafe since most toxic materials can be tolerated at levels commonly found in food.

27.4.1 The Maillard reaction (non-enzymic browning)

The reaction between proteins and reducing sugars, the Maillard reaction or non-enzymic browning, has been intensively investigated. The reaction takes place particularly with the ε-amino group of lysine in the intact protein molecule to an extent dependent on temperature, time, and the presence of moisture (see Fig. 10.5).

Maillard complex is formed on the outside of the crust of bread and roasted meat, where it makes a contribution to the flavour. The reaction occurs during storage, where the development of colour and the loss of available lysine are deleterious. The *N*-substituted amino sugars undergo a complex series of reactions, depending on pH, temperature, oxygen and the presence of other substances, to give rise eventually to reductones, furfurals, their oxidation derivatives and other cyclic compounds (Hurrel and Finot 1983; Finot 1983).

In experimental animals, Maillard compounds can give rise to hypertrophy of the liver and caecum, damage to reproduction, and to kidneys, but there is no evidence of harm in human beings.

27.4.2 Pyrolysis products of lipids and amino acids

Considerable changes take place when fats and oils are stored, and especially when subjected to the high temperature of frying, baking and roasting. A large number of compounds are produced and they can form a significant proportion of the lipid in question; many of these are toxic such as hydroperoxides, cyclic derivatives, and oxidized fatty acid dimers. The amount of benzo(a)pyrene, a potent carcinogen, may exceed 50 μg /kg in smoked foods; some of the polycyclic aromatic hydrocarbons are powerful inducers of drug-metabolizing enzymes which may create problems (Yennai 1980).

The more unsaturated the fatty acids, the greater the production of potentially harmful substances. Pyrolysis products of carbohydrates, proteins and nucleic acids, as well as fats, have been shown to be toxic. However, all these findings refer to animal experiments and there is little evidence that heated fats pose a hazard to human beings. Some of the literature shows that fatty foods prepared domestically or commercially are relatively safe compared with lipids heated in the laboratory for experimental purposes. This may partly be due to the higher temperatures employed in the laboratory, and to the volatilization with steam of some compounds when the food is heated under practical conditions, as distinct from model systems.

27.4.3 Ethyl carbamate (urethane)

Ethyl carbamate is formed during fermentation by reaction of carbamyl compounds such as urea and the amino acid citrulline (see Fig. 10.3) with ethanol. It is found especially in distilled alcoholic beverages, but also in wines, beers, bread, yoghurt and cheeses; it is carcinogenic in experimental animals.

27.4.4 Nitrosamines

Nitrite, present in many cured meats, and naturally present in small amounts in saliva, can react with amines under acid conditions as occur in the sto-

mach, to yield *N*-nitroso derivatives. The various nitrosamines are potent carcinogens in experimental animals. However, it is not known to what extent nitrosamines are formed in the stomach, or whether the (small) amounts that may be formed pose a significant hazard. As discussed in section 22.4.2.2, ascorbic acid (vitamin C) inhibits the formation of nitrosamines, and may have some protective action.

27.5   Toxins arising from microbial contamination

In addition to spoilage of food by bacteria and fungi (see Table 26.9), so that it is obviously unfit for consumption, many micro-organisms produce toxins that may accumulate to hazardous levels without any adverse effect on the appearance or flavour of the food.

27.5.1 Mycotoxins

A number of fungi that grow on foods, especially when stored under damp conditions, produce toxins that may be carcinogenic or acutely or chronically toxic. The most important of these are as follows.

1. Aflatoxins, produced by *Aspergillus flavus*, *A. parasiticus*, and *A. nominus*, found especially in nuts, but also cereals, cassava, dried fruit and cheese. In UK the main sources are imported nuts and dried figs; the maximum permissible amount is 4 μg /kg total aflatoxins for foods that are to be sold directly, and 10 μg /kg for foods that are to undergo further processing before sale. Aflatoxins are secreted in milk, and may accumulate in the flesh of animals; the maximum amounts permitted in animal feedingstuffs are between 0.01–0.05 μg /kg.

2. Ochratoxins, formed by *Aspergillus* and *Penicillium* spp. growing on cereals; in both animals and human beings high intakes of ochratoxins have been associated with nephropathy, and there is evidence that they are also carcinogenic and teratogenic. Ochratoxins are cleaved by protozoan enzymes in cattle, but monogastric animals, such as the pig, can accumulate relatively high concentrations in blood and tissues.

3. Moniliformin, formed by *Fusarium moniliforme*, *F. oxysporum*, *F. anthopilum*, and *F. graminearum*, growing especially on maize. Moniliformin is toxic in experimental animals, and has been associated with Keshan disease in

areas of China where selenium intake is extremely low (see section 15.6.3).

4. Patulin is a broad-spectrum antibiotic produced by a variety of *Penicillium* and *Aspergillus* spp., of which *P. expansum* is the most important, since this is a common storage rot of apples, apricots, bananas, cherries, grapes, peaches, pears, and pineapples. It is a mutagen, and potentially carcinogenic and teratogenic. Patulin reacts with sulphur dioxide and sulphydryl groups to yield inactive products, and it is also destroyed during alcoholic fermentation of fruit juice. The main source is apple juice, especially where mouldy apples have been used in manufacture. The Food Advisory Committee of the UK Ministry of Agriculture, Fisheries and Food (MAFF 1993) recommends that the concentration of patulin in apple juice should not exceed 50 μg /kg.

5. The ergot alkaloids are produced by *Claviceps purpurea* growing on rye; ingestion of moderately large amounts leads to ergotism (also known as St Anthony's fire)—dizziness, chest pains, abnormal and variable heart rate, nausea, vomiting, and digital paraesthesia with severe cramping and vasoconstriction, possibly fatal. In small amounts, ergot alkaloids are used in treatment of migraine, and in obstetric practice to stimulate uterine contraction.

27.5.2 Dinoflagellate toxins in shellfish

Various species of dinoflagellate phytoplankton produce toxins; normally the organisms are present in only small numbers, but under environmentally favourable conditions they can grow rapidly to produce toxic algal blooms or 'red tides'; when this occurs shellfish can accumulate dangerous concentrations of the toxins.

27.5.2.1 Paralytic shellfish poisoning
Three related neurotoxic compounds, saxitoxins, neosaxitoxins, and gonyautoxins, are produced by *Protogonylaux* spp., *Alexandrium* spp., and *Prodinium* spp. Consumption of contaminated shellfish leads to paraesthesia of the peri-oral region, tongue and limbs, with lower back pain and a sensation of floating; in severe cases there may be loss of consciousness and respiratory failure. The onset of symptoms is within 2 hours of eating contaminated shellfish, and they persist for 12–24 hours; after high intakes death occurs within 2–12 hours.

The maximum permissible level of these toxins in the EU is 80 μg /100 g of mollusc flesh, and if this threshold is exceeded then commercial fisheries are closed by law until the contamination falls to within the acceptable limit.

27.5.2.2 Diarrhetic shellfish poisoning
Mussels and scallops can accumulate okaidic acid, a polyether carboxylic acid, and a variety of methylated derivatives, collectively known as dinophysis toxins, from dinoflagellates; *Dinophysis* spp. are a common problem in Europe, and *Prorocentrum* spp. in Japan. The toxins cause acute gastrointestinal disorders: diarrhoea, abdominal pain, nausea and vomiting; the onset of symptoms is between 0.5–12 hours after ingestion, persisting for 3–4 days. No fatalities have been reported.

27.6 Bacterial food poisoning

Bacterial contamination of food (and sometimes also water) can lead to gastrointestinal symptoms, including cramps, diarrhoea and vomiting, through two mechanisms.

1. Infection of the gastrointestinal tract. Symptoms may persist for several days, and severe cases may require treatment with broad-spectrum antibiotics that are not absorbed, such as neomycin.

2. Bacterial toxins, which may be present if infected food has been sterilized by heat or irradiation. The onset of symptoms is generally more rapid than when colonization of the gastrointestinal tract by invading micro-organisms occurs, and treatment with antibiotics will have no effect.

Table 6.12 lists the normal intestinal flora, and Table 6.14 the major bacteria associated with food- and water-borne gastrointestinal disease; in addition, rotaviruses and protozoa including *Entamoeba histolytica* and *Giarda lamblia* can cause persistent, antibiotic-resistant gastrointestinal disease.

Further reading

Brostoff, J. and Challacombe, S.J. (1987). *Food Allergy and Intolerance.* Baillière-Tindall, London.

Cliver, D.O. (1990). *Foodborne Diseases.* Academic Press, San Diego, CA.

Liener, I.E. (1980). *Toxic Constituents of Plant Foodstuffs.* Academic Press, New York.

Metcalfe, D. D., Sampson, H. A., and Simon, R.A. (1991). *Food Allergy: Adverse reactions to Foods and Food Additives*. Blackwell Scientific Publications, Oxford.

Miller, K. (1987). *Toxicological Aspects of Food*. Elsevier Applied Science, London.

Watson, D.H. (1987). *Natural Toxicants in Food: Progress and Prospects*. Ellis Horwood.

Table 27.1: Action levels for pesticide residues in foods Levels at or above which FDA will take action to remove products from the market; where a range is shown this represents the range for different crops and foodstuffs.

	action level, ppm
aldrin and dieldrin	0.03-0.1
benzene hexachloride (BHC)	0.05-0.3
chlordane	0.1-0.3
chlordecone	0.3-0.4
dicofol	0.5
DDT, DDE, TDE	0.1-1.0
dimethylnitrosamine	0.0005-0.001
ethylene dibromide	30-150
heptachlor, heptachlor epoxide	0.01-0.3
lindane	0.1-0.5
mercury	1
mirex	0.1
polychlorinated biphenyls	3

Source: FDA/IAS 1994.

Table 27.2: Common symptoms of allergic reactions in children and adults

gastrointestinal tract	frequent possetting regurgitation, vomiting
	frequent loose stools, mucus, diarrhoea
	colic, bloating, excessive flatulence
	constipation
	abdominal pain
	blood in stools
	poor appetite, poor weight gain in infants
skin	dry patches, cracks
	spots, rashes
	eczema
	hives, welts, swelling around eyes
	itchiness (scratching or rubbing in infants)
	sweatiness
	redness around mouth, anus or on cheeks
	easy bruising
respiratory tract	nasal stuffiness, mucus, runny nose
	noisy breathing, sniffing, snorting
	sneezing
	coughing
	hiccups
	bad breath
	dyspnoea
	bronchospasm
	recurrent croup
	frequent ear infections
	angio-oedema (swelling)
genitourinary tract	cystitis
	vulvovaginitis
	haematuria
	nephrosis
circulation	cold hands and feet
	changes in pulse rate and regularity, palpitations
	changes in temperature
	changes in skin colour, especially around lips
	anaemia, haemolysis

Table 27.3: Types of allergic reaction

Type I	Anaphylactic (immediate response)	Antigens react with mast cells sensitized with IgE, leading to release of vasoactive and myoactive substances, including histamine.
Type II	Cytotoxic	Antigen attached to cell membranes reacts with complement-fixing antibodies; the cells then lyse under the influence of complement, or are destroyed by cytotoxic lymphocytes.
Type III	Immune-complex mediated	Antigen and antibody react in varying proportions to form an immune complex which is attacked by macrophages and complement; the lytic enzymes liberated also damage tissues. Rarely associated with food.
Type IV	Cell-mediated (delayed reaction)	Antigen binds to T-lymphocytes and triggers activity of cytotoxic lymphocytes to secrete lymphokines which alter capillary permeability and produce inflammation. Commonly occurs in children

Table 27.4: Hypoallergenic diets

	A	B
meat	lamb or turkey	beef or chicken
starch staple	rice or potato	rye, maize or tapioca
fruit	banana or pineapple	exclude citrus fruits and apples
vegetables	brassicas or carrots	exclude beans and peas
milk substitutes	soya milk, casein hydrolysate	
oil	olive oil	maize, sunflower, cottonseed
bread spread	kosher (vegetable) margarine	

Table 27.5: Frequency with which different foods are claimed to be responsible for allergies

		% of patients
cereals	wheat	60
	maize	44
	oats	34
	rye	30
	barley	24
	rice	15
dairy produce	milk	44
	cheese	39
	eggs	26
	butter	25
	yoghurt	24
fish	white fish	10
	shellfish	10
	smoked fish	7
meat	beef	16
	pork	14
	chicken	13
	lamb	11
	turkey	8
fruit	citrus	24
	rhubarb	12
	apples	12
	bananas	11

Table 27.5: (Cont'd)

		% of patients
	pineapple	8
	pears	8
	strawberries	8
	grapes	7
	melon	5
	avocado	5
	raspberries	4
vegetables	onions	22
	potatoes	20
	cabbage	19
	Brussels sprouts	18
	peas	17
	carrots	15
	lettuce	15
	leeks	15
	broccoli	14
	soya beans	13
	spinach	13
	mushrooms	12
	parsnips	12
	tomatoes	11
	cauliflower	11
	celery	11
	green beans	10
	cucumber	10
	turnip / swede	10
	marrow	8
	beetroot	8
	peppers	6
miscellaneous	coffee	33
	tea	25
	nuts	22
	chocolate	22
	preservatives	20
	yeast	20
	cane sugar	13
	beet sugar	12
	alcohol	12
	saccharin	9

Table 27.6: The scope of the food intolerance databank

Ingredients	includes	interpretation of free from
milk	milk and milk powders, cheese, yoghurt, cream, butter, caseinates, whey, whey syrup sweetener, margarine or shortening containing whey, lactose	no added milk or milk derivative
egg	fresh or dried egg, egg albumin, egg lecithin, egg yolk	no added egg or egg derivative
wheat	wholewheat, wheat flour, wheat starch, breadcrumbs, rusk, wheat bran, wheat binder, wheat thickener, wheat germ, wheat germ oil, raising agent containing wheat starch	no added wheat or wheat derivative
soya	soya protein products, hydrolysed vegetable protein (soya), soya lecithin (E-322), soya flavouring, soya oil or shortening	no added soya or soya derivative
cocoa	cocoa powder, cocoa butter	no added cocoa or cocoa derivative
BHA / BHT	butylated hydroxyanisole (E-320), butylated hydroxytoluene (E-321)	< 1mg /kg
sulphur dioxide	sulphur dioxide, sulphites and metabisulphite (E-220-228)	< 10 mg /kg SO_2
benzoates	benzoic acid, benzoates and hydroxybenzoates (E-210-219)	< 1 mg /kg
glutamates	glutamic acid, monosodium glutamate, potassium and calcium glutamates (E-620-625)	no added glutamate and <0.20% from other ingredients
azo colours	amaranth (E-123), black PN (E-151), brown FK (E-154), brown HT (E-155), carmoisine (E-122), pigment rubine, Ponceau 4R (E-124), rose 2G, sunset yellow (E-110, FD&C yellow no 6), tartrazine (E102, FD&C yellow no 6), yellow 2G	contains no added azo colour

See section 26.2 for discussion of food additives.

Table 27.7: Biochemical families of foods that may contain similar antigens

1	Graminae	barley, maize, millet, oats, rye, sugar cane, wheat
2	Palmae	coconut, dates, sago,
3		asparagus, chives, garlic, onions
4	Polygonaceae	buckwheat, rhubarb
5		avocados, cinnamon
6	Brassicaeae	Brussels sprouts, cabbage, cauliflower, kale, mustard greens, turnips
7	Rosaceae	apples, apricots, blackberries, cherries, loganberries, pears, plums, raspberries, strawberries
8	Leguminosae	kidney beans, lentils, liquorice, peanuts, peas, soya beans
9	citrus	lemons, mandarins, oranges
10		cashews, mangoes, pistachios
11	Umbelliferae	caraway, carrots, celery, fennel, dill, parsnip
12	Solanaceae	aubergines, green peppers, physalis, potatoes, tomatoes
13		basil, lavender, peppermint, rosemary, sage, thyme
14		cucumbers, watermelons
15	Compositae	artichokes, chicory, endive, lettuce, safflower, sunflower
16		hickory, pecan, walnuts
17		filberts, hazelnuts
18	molluscs	clams, cockles, oysters, scallops, snails
19	crustaceans	crab, crayfish, lobster, prawns, shrimps

Table 27.8: Protease inhibitors in plant foods

trypsin inhibitors

alfalfa	*Medicago sativa*
bamboo sprouts	*Bambusa arundinaria*
barley	*Hordeum vulgare*
beetroot	*Beta vulgaris*
buckwheat	*Fagopyrum esculentum*
cashew nut	*Anacardium occidentale*
finger millet	*Eleusine coracana*
garlic	*Allium sativum*
Indian mustard	*Brassica juncea*
jack fruit seed	*Artocarpus integrifolia*
maize	*Zea mays*
oats	*Avena sativa*
onion	*Allium cepa*
rapeseed	*Brassica campestris*
rice	*Oryza sativa*
sorghum	*Sorghum bicolor*
spinach	*Spinacia oleracea*
squash (leaves)	*Cucurbita maxima*
sunflower seed	*Helianthus annuus*
sweet potato	*Ipomea batata*
vine leaves	*Vitis vinifera*

trypsin and chymotrypsin inhibitors

cassava	*Manihot utillisima*
cucumber	*Cucumis sativus*
peanut (groundnut)	*Arachis hypogea*
rye	*Secale cereale*
tamarind	*Tamarindus indica*
taro	*Colocasia esculenta*
triticale	*Triticale*
wheat	*Triticum durum, T. vulgare*

trypsin, chymotrypsin and carboxypeptidase inhibitors

potato	*Solanum tuberosum*

trypsin, chymotrypsin and elastase inhibitors

kidney bean	*Phaseolus vulgaris*

Most legumes contain inhibitors of trypsin and chymotrypsin.
Source: from data reported by Liener, 1980.

Table 27.9: Naturally occurring compounds in plant foods that are carcinogenic in experimental animals

	major sources
bergaptin	celery, parsley, parsnips
benzyl acetate	basil, honey, jasmine tea
caffeic acid	anise, apple, aubergine, basil, caraway, carrot, celery, cherry, coffee beans, dill, endive, grapes, lettuce, marjoram, pear, plum, rosemary sage, savory, tarragon, thyme, tomato
catechol	coffee beans
coumestrol (phyto-oestrogen)	alfalfa, soybean sprouts
cycasin (methyl azoxymethyl glucoside)	cycad nuts
estragole	anise, basil, fennel, tarragon
genistin (phyto-oestrogen)	soybean, clover
p-hydrazinobenzoates	mushrooms
ipomeanol, ipomearone	sweet potatoes
isoflavones	soybean
lubminin	potatoes
lupulonic acid	hops
methyl benzyl alcohol	cocoa
methylpsoralens	celery, parsley, parsnip
mirestrol (phyto-oestrogen)	legumes
oestrone	palm kernels
phaseolin	green beans
pisatin	peas
pyrrazolidone alkaloids	coltsfoot, comfrey, *Crotolaria* spp., *Heliotropum* spp., *Senecio* spp.
rishitin	potatoes
safrole	mace, nutmeg, pepper (black), sassafras oil
sesamol	sesame oil
sinigrin (allylisothiocyanate)	Brussels sprouts, cabbage, cauliflower, collard greens, horserdish, mustard (brown)
xanthotoxin	celery, parsley, parsnips
zearalonone (phyto-oestrogen)	*Fusarium roseum* growing on maize

Source: from data reported by Ames 1993; Ames *et al.* 1990 *a,b;* Tricker & Preusmann 1990.

28

Systematic classification of foodstuffs

Table 28.1: Cereal crops

adlay, Job's tears	*Coix lacryma-jobi*
barley four-row	*Hordeum vulgare*
barley six-row	*Hordeum hexasticum*
barley two-row	*Hordeum disticum*
buckwheat[1]	*Fagopyrum esculentum*
canagua or coaihua	*Chenopodium pallidicaule*
canary seed	*Phalaris canariensis*
feijoa	*Feijoa sellowiana*
fonio, black (hungry rice)	*Digitaria iburua*
fonio,findi	*Digitaria exilis*
guinea corn	*Sorghum guineense*
Inca wheat (quihuicha, quinoa)	*Amaranthus caudatus, Chenopodium quinoa, C. album*
Job's tears (adlay)	*Coix lacryma-jobi*
jowar, durra, kaoliang	*Sorghum dura*
kaffir corn (common sorghum)	*Sorghum vulgare*
maize (corn, Indian corn, mealies)	*Zea mays*
millet, barnyard or Japanese	*Echinocloa frumentacea*
millet, bulrush	*Pennisetum gluacum, P. americanum, P. typhoideum*
millet, common, golden or proso	*Panicum miliaceum*
millet, ditch (koda)	*Paspalum scrobiculatum*
millet, finger or African (ragi)	*Eleusine coracana, E.* spp.
millet, foxtail	*Setaria italica*
millet, haraka, kodo	*Paspalum scobiculatum*
millet, jajeo	*Acroceras amplectens*
millet, pearl or cattail	*Pennisetum glaucum*
oats	*Avena sativa and other* spp.
quihuicha (Inca wheat)	*Amaranthus caudatus*
quinoa	*Chenopodium quinoa, C. album*
rice	*Oryza sativa and other* spp.
rice, glutinous	*Oryza glutinosa*
rice, hungry (black fonio)	*Digitaria iburua*
rice, wild	*Zizania aquatica*
rye	*Secale cereale*
sorghum, common (milo, feterita, kaffir corn)	*Sorghum bicolor, S. vulgare, Andropogon sorghum, Holchus sorghum*
teff	*Eragrostis abyssinica*

Table 28.1: (Cont'd)

teosinte	*Euchlaena mexicana*
triticale	*Triticum x Secale*
wheat, common	*Triticum aestivum*
wheat, durum	*Triticum durum*
wheat, spelt	*Triticum spelta*

(1) Buckwheat is considered a cereal, although it is one of Polygonaceae, not one of the Graminaceae.

Table 28.2 Non-cereal starch crops (mainly roots and tubers)

arracacha	*Arracacoa xanthorrhiza*
arrowroot	*Maranta arundinacea*
artichoke, Jerusalem	*Helianthus tuberosus*
breadfruit	*Artocarpus communis, A. altilis*
burdock root (great burdock)	*Arctium lappa*
cassava (manioc, mandioca, yuca)	*Manihot esculenta (syn. M. utilissima)*
cassava, bitter	*Manihot esculenta*
cassava, sweet	*Manihot palmata*
chufa (tigernut, nutsedge, ground almond)	*Cyperus esculentus, C. aureus*
cocoyam, new (tannia)	*Xanthosoma sagittifolium*
cocoyam, old (dasheen, eddo, taro)	*Colocasia esculenta*
dasheen (taro, old cocoyam)	*Colocasia esculenta*
eddo (taro, old cocoyam)	*Colocasia esculenta*
ensete (false or wild banana)	*Ensete ventricosum*
jak fruit	*Artocarpus integrifolia*
jicama (yam bean)	*Pachyrhizus erosus, P. angulatus*
lotus, Hindu	*Nelumbo nucifera*
malanga (new cocoyam, tannia)	*Xanthosoma sagittifolium*
manioc, mandioca (cassava)	*Manihot esculenta (pp. M. utilissima)*
mashua	*Tropaeolum tuberosum*
oca	*Oxalis tuberosa*
ocumo (new cocoyam, tannia)	*Xanthosoma sagittifolium*
plantain	*Musa paradaisica*
potato, Irish	*Solanum tuberosum*
potato, sweet	*Ipomoea batatas*
sago palm	*Metroxylon spp., M. sago*
tannia (new cocoyam)	*Xanthosoma sagittifolium*
taro (old cocoyam)	*Colocasia esculenta*
taro, giant	*Alocasia spp., Cyrtosperma spp.*
tigernut (chufa)	*Cyperus esculentus*
topinambur (Jerusalem artichoke)	*Helianthus tuberosus*
ullucu	*Ullucus tuberosus*
yam	*Dioscorea spp.*
yam bean (jicama)	*Pachyrhizus erosus, P. angulatus*
yautia (new cocoyam, tannia)	*Xanthosoma sagittifolium*
yuca (cassava)	*Manihot esculenta (syn. M. utilissima)*
yuca dulce	*Manihot palmata (syn. M. dulcis)*

Table 28.3: Legumes and pulses

aduki (adzuki) bean	*Vigna angularis (Phaseolus angularis)*
Angola pea (*pigeon pea*)	*Cajanus cajan (C. indicus)*
asparagus bean	*Vigna unguiculata-subspecies - sesquipedalis (L)*
asparagus pea	*Lotus tetragonolobus*
Bambar(r)a groundnut	*Voandzeia subterranea*
Bengal gram	*Cicer aretinum*
black gram	*Vigna mungo (Phaseolus mungo)*
black-eyed bean or pea	*Vigna unguiculata (or V. sesquipedalis or V. sinensis)*
bonavista bean	*Lablab purpureus (Dolichos lablab*
Boston bean	*Phaseolus vulgaris*
broad bean	*Vicia faba var. major*
Burma bean	*Phaseolus lunatus (P. lumensis P. inamoenus)*
butter bean	*Phaseolus lunatus (P. lumensis P. inamoenus)*
castor oil bean	*Ricinus communis*
catjang	*Vigna unguiculata (or V. sesquipedalis or V. sinensis)*
chick pea	*Cicer aretinum*
chickling pea, vetch	*Lathyrus sativus*
China pea	*Vigna unguiculata (or V. sesquipedalis or V. sinensis)*
cluster bean	*Cyamopsis tetragonoloba*
cow pea	*Vigna unguiculata (or V. sesquipedalis or V. sinensis)*
cowgram	*Vigna unguiculata (or V. sesquipedalis or V. sinensis)*
Dolichos bean	*Lablab purpureus (Dolichos lablab)*
earth pea	*Voandzeia subterranea*
Egyptian kidney bean	*Lablab purpureus (Dolichos lablab)*
faba bean	*Vicia faba*
field bean	*Vicia faba var. minor*
field pea	*Pisum arvense*
flageolet (*yellow variety*)	*Phaseolus vulgaris*
four-cornered bean	*Psophocarpus tetragonolobus*
French bean	*Phaseolus vulgaris*
garden, green pea	*Pisum sativum*
garbanzo	*Cicer aretinum*
Goa bean	*Psophocarpus tetragonolobus*
grass pea	*Lathyrus sativus*
green or golden gram	*Phaseolus radiatus*
ground bean	*Voandzeia subterranea*

Table 28.3: (Cont'd)

guar bean	*Cyamopsis tetragonoloba*
haricot bean	*Phaseolus vulgaris*
horse bean	*Vicia faba* var. *equina*
horse gram, grain	*Macrotyloma uniflorum (Dolichos uniflorus, D. biflorus)*
hyacinth bean	*Lablab purpureus (Dolichos lablab)*
Indian butter bean	*Lablab purpureus (Dolichos lablab)*
Indian vetch	*Lathyrus sativus*
jack bean	*Canavalia ensiformis*
Kaffir pea	*Voandzeia subterranea*
kesari dhal	*Lathyrus sativus*
kidney bean	*Phaseolus vulgaris*
kulthi bean	*Macrotyloma uniflorum (Dolichos uniflorus, D. biflorus)*
lablab bean	*Lablab purpureus (Dolichos lablab)*
lathyrus pea	*Lathyrus sativus*
lentil	*Lens culinaris (L. esculenta), Ervum lens*
Lima bean	*Phaseolus lunatus (P. lumensis, P. inamoenus)*
lupins	*Lupinus* spp.
Madagascar butter bean	*Phaseolus lunatus (P. lumensis, P. inamoenus)*
Madagascar groundnut	*Voandzeia subterranea*
Madras gram	*Macrotyloma uniflorum (Dolichos uniflorus, D. biflorus)*
mange tout	*Pisum sativum* var *macrocarpon*
Manila bean	*Psophocarpus tetragonolobus*
mash bean	*Vigna mungo (Phaseolus mungo)*
masur dhal	*Lens culinaris (L. esculenta)*
mat bean	*Vigna aconitifolia (Phaseolus aconitifolia)*
Mauritius bean	*Psophocarpus tetragonolobus*
moth bean	*Vigna aconitifolia (Phaseolus aconitifolia)*
multiflora bean	*Phaseolus coccineus (P. multiflora)*
mung bean	*Vigna mungo (Phaseolus mungo)*
navy bean	*Phaseolus vulgaris*
non-eye pea, Congo bean or pea	*Cajanus cajan (C. indicus)*
overlook bean	*Canavalia ensiformis*
pea bean	*Vigna unguiculata–subspecies sesquipedalis (L)*
pigeon bean	*Vicia faba*

Table 28.3: (Cont'd)

pigeon pea	*Cajanus cajan (C. indicus)*
pinto bean	*Phaseolus vulgaris*
Rangoon bean	*Phaseolus lunatus (P. lumensis, P. inamoenus)*
red bean	*Vigna umbelfata (Phaseolus calcaratus)*
red dhal	*Lens culinaris (L. esculenta)*
red gram	*Cajanus cajan (C. indicus)*
rice bean	*Vigna umbelfata (Phaseolus calcaratus)*
rice haricot bean	*Phaseolus acutifolius (var. latifolius)*
runner bean, scarlet	*Phaseolus coccineus (P. multiflora)*
Sieva bean	*Phaseolus lunatus (P. lumensis, P. inamoenus)*
snapbean	*Phaseolus vulgaris*
Southern pea	*Vigna unguiculata (or V. sesquipedalis or V. sinensis)*
soya bean	*Glycine max (G. soja)*
split pea	*Lens culinaris (L. esculenta)*
string bean	*Phaseolus vulgaris*
sugar pea	*Pisum sativum* var. *macrocarpon*
sword bean	*Canavalia ensiformis*
tepary bean	*Phaseolus acutifolius (var. latifolius)*
Texan bean	*Phaseolus acutifolius (var. latifolius)*
tillseed	*Lens culinaris*
tonga bean	*Lablab purpureus (Dolichos lablab*
tonka bean	*Dipteryx odorata*
trick bean	*Vicia faba*
Turkish gram	*Vigna radiata (Phaseolus aureus)*
urd bean	*Vigna mungo (Phaseolus mungo)*
velvet bean	*Mucuna pruriens, Stilobium* spp.
vetch, spring, common	*Vicia sativa*
wax bean	*Phaseolus vulgaris*
windsor bean	*Vicia faba*
winged bean, pea	*Psophocarpus tetragonolobus*
yam bean	*Pachyrrhizus erosus*
yard long bean	*Vigna unguiculata-subspecies sesquipedalis (L)*
yellow dhal	*Cajanus cajan (C. indicus)*

Table 28.4: Synonyms for legumes

Cajanus cajan (*C. indicus*)	Angola pea, no-eye pea, Congo bean or pea, pigeon pea, red gram, yellow dhal
Canavalia ensiformis	jack bean, overlook bean, sword bean
Cicer arietinum	Bengal gram, chick pea, garbanzo, yellow gram
Cyamopsis tetragonoloba	cluster bean, guar bean
Dipteryx odorata	tonka bean
Dolichos buchamenii	dolichos flower, wild lupin, bully-beef plant
Glycine max (*G. soja*)	soya bean
Lablab purpureus (*Dolichos lablab*)	Bonavista bean, Dolichos bean, Egyptian kidney bean, hyacinth bean, Indian butter bean, lablab bean, tonga bean
Lathyrus sativus	chickling pea, vetch, grass pea, Indian vetch, kesari dhal, lathyrus pea,
Lens culinaris (*L. esculenta*)	masur dhal, red dhal, split pea, lentil, tillseed
Lotus tetragonolobus	asparagus pea
Lupinus spp.	lupins
Macrotyloma uniflorum (*Dolichos uniflorus*)	horse gram, grain, kulthi bean, Madras gram
Mucuna pruriens, Stilobium spp.	velvet bean
Pachyrrhizus erosus	yam bean
Phaseolus acutifolius (var. *latifolius*)	rice haricot bean, tepary bean, Texan bean
Phaseolus coccineus (*P. multiflora*)	multiflora bean, runner bean
Phaseolus radiatus	green or golden gram, mung bean, Boston bean, flageolet, French bean, kidney bean, navy bean, pinto bean, snapbean, string bean, wax bean
Phaseolus lunatus (*P. lumensis, P. inamoenus*)	Burma bean, butter bean, Lima bean, Madagascar butter bean, Rangoon bean, Sieva bean
Pisum arvense	field pea
Pisum sativum	garden pea, green pea, mange tout, sugar pea
Psophocarpus tetragonolobus	four-cornered bean, Goa bean, Manila bean, Mauritius bean, winged bean, pea
Ricinus communis	castor oil bean
Vicia faba	faba bean, pigeon bean, trick bean, windsor bean, horse bean, broad bean, field bean
Vicia sativa	vetch, spring, common

Table 28.4: (Cont'd)

Vigna aconitifolia (*Phaseolus aconitifolia*)	mat bean, moth bean, aconite-leaved bean, dew bean
Vigna angularis (*Phaseolus angularis*)	aduki (adzuki) bean
Vigna mungo (*Phaseolus mungo*)	black gram, mash bean, urd bean, mung bean
Vigna radiata (*Phaseolus aureus*)	Turkish gram, green or golden gram, mung bean
Vigna umbelfata (*Phaseolus calcaratus*)	red bean, rice bean
Vigna unguiculata (or *V. sesquipedalis* or *V. sinensis*)	black-eyed bean or pea, catjang, China pea, cow pea, cowgram, Southern pea
*Vigna unguiculata-*subspecies *sesquipedalis*	asparagus bean, pea bean, yard long bean
Voandzeia subterranea	Bambar(r)a groundnut, earth pea, ground bean, Kaffir pea, Madagascar groundnut

Table 28.5: Nuts

acorn	*Quercus* spp.
almond	*Prunus amygdalus, P. communis, P. dulcis, Amygdalus communis*
almond, java (pili nut)	*Canarium* spp.
areca nut (betel nut)	*Areca catechu*
Brazil nut	*Bertholletia excelsa*
butter (swarri) nut	*Caryocar nuciferum, Juglans cinerea*
caltrops (water chestnut)	*Trapa natans, T. bicornis*
cashew nut	*Anacardium occidentale*
chestnut (sweet)	*Castanea vesca, C. vulgaris, C. sativa , C. dentata*
chestnut, Japanese	*Castanea crenata*
cob (hazel)	*Corylus avellana, C. colurna*
cola (kola) nut	*Cola nitida, C. vera, C. acuminata*
cream or para (Brazil nut)	*Bertholletia excelsa*
filbert	*Corylus maxima*
groundnut (peanut)	*Arachis hypogea*
groundnut, Hausa	*Kerslingiella geocarpa,*
hazelnut (cob)	*Corylus avellana, C. colurna*
karoka nuts	*Pandanus* spp.
kola (cola) nut	*Cola nitida, C. vera, C. acuminata*
macadamia nut	*Macadamia ternifolia*
matai (Chinese water chestnut)	*Eleocharis tuberosa, E. dulcis*
monkey nut (groundnut, peanut)	*Arachis hypogea*
Moreton bay chestnut	*Castanospermum australe*
olive, Chinese (pili nut)	*Canarium* spp.
para or cream nut (Brazil nut)	*Bertholletia excelsa*
paradise (sapucaia) nut	*Lecythis zabucajo*
peanut (groundnut)	*Arachis hypogea*
pecan nut	*Carya illinoensis*
pili nut (Java almond, Chinese olive)	*Canarium* spp.
pine nuts (pignolia)	*Pinus pinea*
pine nuts (pion)	*Pinus cembroides* var. *edulis*
pistachio	*Pistacia vera*
Queensland (macadamia) nut	*Macadamia ternifolia*
sapucaia (paradise) nut	*Lecythis zabucajo*
sinharanut (water chestnut)	*Trapa natans* and *T. bicornis,*
swarri (butter) nut	*Caryocar nuciferum*
walnut, black	*Juglans nigra*
walnut, English, Persian	*Juglans* spp.: esp. *J. regia*
water chestnut	*Trapa natans, T. bicornis*
water chestnut, Chinese (waternut)	*Eleocharis tuberosa, E. dulcis*

Table 28.6: crops grown as sources of oil

arachis (groundnut)	*Arachis hypogaea*
babassu kernel	*Orbignya speciosa*
beech nut	*Fagus sylvatica*
benniseed (sesame seed)	*Sesamum indicum*
candlenut	*Aleurites moluccana*
carapa seed	*Carapa guineensis*
castor bean	*Ricinus communis*
coconut	*Cocos nucifera*
colza (rapeseed)	*Brassica napus* var. *oleifera*
copra (coconut)	*Cocos nucifera*
corn (maize)	*Zea mais*
cottonseed	*Gossypium* spp.
croton seed	*Croton tiglium*
flaxseed (linseed)	*Linum usitatissimum*
ginkgo seed	*Ginkgo biloba*
grape pip	*Vitis vinifera*
groundnut (arachis)	*Arachis hypogaea*
hempseed	*Cannabis sativa*
illipe seed	*Bassia latifolia*
jojoba	*Simmondsia californica* (syn. *S. chinensis*)
kapok fruit	*Ceiba pentandra*
karite nuts (sheanuts)	*Butyrospermum parkii*
linseed (flaxseed)	*Linum usitatissimum*
maize	*Zea mais*
melonseed	*Cucumis melo* and other Cucurbitaceae
mustard, black	*Brassica nigra, Sinapis nigra*
mustard, white	*Brassica alba, B. hirta, Sinapis alba*
niger seed	*Guizotia abyssinica*
oiticica seed	*Licania rigida*
olive	*Olea europaea*
palm	*Elaeis guineensis*
peanut (arachis)	*Arachis hypogaea*
perilla seed	*Perilla frutescens*
physic nut	*Jatropha curcas*
pongam seed	*Pongamia glabra*
rapeseed (colza)	*Brassica napus* var. *oleifera*
rubberseed	*Hevea brasiliensis*
safflower seed	*Carthamus tinctorius*
sal tree seed	*Shorea robusta*
sesame seed (til)	*Sesamum indicum*
sheanuts (karite nuts)	*Butyrospermum parkii*
soybean	*Glycine max* (*G. soja*)
stillingia (Chinese tallow tree)	*Sapium sebiferum, Stillingia sebifera*
sunflower seed	*Helianthus annuus*
tallow tree, Borneo	*Shorea aptera, S. stenocarpa*
tallow tree, Chinese (stillingia)	*Sapium sebiferum, Stillingia sebifera*
til (sesame seed)	*Sesamum indicum*
tukuma kernel	*Astrocaryum* spp.
tung nut	*Aleurites cordata, A. fordii*

See Table 8.5 for fatty acid composition of major oils and fats.

Table 28.7: Crops grown for sugar

black maple	*Acer nigrum*
palmyra (borassus) palm	*Borassus flabellifer*
sugar beet	*Beta vulgaris* var. *altissima*
sugar cane	*Saccharum officinarum*
sugar maple	*Acer saccharum*
sugar palm	*Arenga saccharifera*
sweet sorghum	*Sorghum saccharatum*
wild date palm	*Phoenix sylvestris*

Table 28.8: Vegetables[1]

accoub	*Goundelia tournefortii*
alfalfa (lucerne)	*Medicago sativa*
amaranth, grain	*Amaranthus cruentus, A. caudatis, A. hypochondriacus*
amaranth, leaves	*Amaranthus sylvestris, A. tricolor, A. dubius, A. lividus*
artichoke, Chinese	*Stachys affinis*
artichoke, globe	*Cynara scolymus*
artichoke, Japanese	*Stachys sieboldi*
artichoke, Jerusalem	*Helianthus tuberosus*
asparagus	*Asparagus officinalis*
aubergine (eggplant)	*Solanum melongena*
avocado	*Persica (Persea) americana*
balsam pear (bitter gourd)	*Manordica charantia*
bamboo shoots	*Bambusa arundinacea, Phyllostachys* spp.
bamya (bamies, okra)	*Hibiscus esculentus.*
bath sponge	*Luffa aegyptica*
beans, green, string	*Phaseolus* spp., *Vigna* spp.
beet, leaf, silver, white leaf	*Beta vulgaris* var. *cicla*
beetroot	*Beta vulgaris*
bhaji	*Amaranthus gangeticus*
bhindi (okra, gumbo)	*Hibiscus esculentus*
brinjal (aubergine, egg plant)	*Solanum melongena*
broccoli, Chinese (Chinese kale)	*Brassica oleracea* var. *alboglabra*
broccoli, sprouting	*Brassica oleracea italica*
Brussels sprouts	*Brassica oleracea gemmiferra.*
butterburr, Japanese	*Petasites japonicus*
cabbage	*Brassica oleracea capitata*
cabbage, Chinese, Pekin, snow (petsai)	*Brassica pekinensis*
cabbage, palm (coyoli palm)	*Acrocomia mexicana*
cabbage, swamp	*Ipomea reptans*
calabash (bottle gourd)	*Lagenaria vulgaris*
calabrese	*Brassica olearacea italica*
callaloo	*Amaranthus gangeticus*
caltrops (water chestnut)	*Trapa natans*
camash	*Camassia quamash*
cardoon	*Cynara cardunculus.*
carrot	*Daucus carota*
cassareep (cassava leaves)	*Manihot esculenta, M. utilissima*

Table 28.8: (Cont'd)

cauliflower	*Brassica olearacea botrytis*
celeriac	*Apium graveolens* var. *rapaceum*
celery	*Apium graveolens* var. *dulce.*
chard	*Beta vulgaris*
chayote	*Sechium edule*
chervil, turniprooted	*Chaerophyllum bulbosum*
chestnut, water (caltrops)	*Trapa natans*
chestnut, Chinese (pi-tsi)	*Eleocharis tuberosa*
chicory (endive, escarole)	*Chicorium endivia* var. *latifolia*
chicory (witloof)	*Cichorium intybus* var. *foliosum*
chikli	*Brassica pekinensis*
chilli (red pepper)	*Capsicum frutescans*
Chinese leaves (pak choi)	*Brassica chinensis*
Chinese spinach	*Amaranthus gangeticus*
chives	*Allium schoenoprasum*
chives, Chinese	*Allium tuberosum*
chufle	*Calathea macrosepala*
coocha (chayote)	*Sechium edule*
corn salad (lamb's lettuce)	*Valerianella locusta, V. olitoria*
coyoli palm (palm cabbage)	*Acrocomia mexicana*
cress, American, land, winter	*Barbarea verna*
cress, garden cress (peppergrass)	*Lepidium sativum*
cress, watercress	*Nasturtium officinale*
cucumber	*Cucumis sativus*
cushaw	*Curcurbita moschata*
daisy crown	*Chrysanthemum coronarium*
dandelion	*Taraxacum officinale (Leontodon taraxacum)*
eggplant (aubergine, brinjal)	*Solanum melongena*
eggplant, gboma	*Solanum macrocarpon*
eggplant, scarlet	*Solanum aethiopicum*
endive (chicory)	*Cichorium endivia* var. *latifolia*
fennel, Florence (finnochio)	*Foeniculum dulce, F. vulgare* var. *azoricum*
fern	*Athyrum esculentum*
garlic	*Allium sativum*
gherkin	*Cucumis anguria*
glasswort (marsh samphire)	*Salicornia spp*
gourd, ash	*Benincasa hispida*
gourd, bitter (balsam pear)	*Momordica charantia*
gourd, bottle (calabash)	*Lagenaria vulgaris*
gourd, common	*Cucurbita pepo, Lagenaria vulgaris, Benincasa* spp.
gourd, snake	*Trichosanthes anguina*
gourd, towel	*Luffa acutangula*
gourd, wax	*Benincasa hispida*
gumbo (okra, bhindi)	*Hibiscus esculentus.*
gundelia	*Gundelia tournefortii*
honeywort, Japanese	*Cryptotaenia japonica*

Table 28.8: (Cont'd)

jew's mallow (potherb jute)	*Corchorus olitorius*
kohlrabi	*Brassica oleracea gongylodes*
ladies' fingers (okra)	*Hibiscus esculentus.*
lamb's lettuce (corn salad)	*Valerianella locusta, V. olitoria*
lambsquarters	*Chenopodium album*
leek	*Allium ampeloprasum*
leek, bulk	*Allium porrum*
lettuce	*Lactuca sativa var. longifolia*
lettuce, prickly, Chinese	*Lactuca scariola, L. serriola*
lotus	*Nelumbium nuciferum, N. nelumbo*
lucerne (alfalfa)	*Medicago sativa*
mallow	*Malva spp.*
mangetout	*Pisum sativum var macrocarpum (macrocarpon)*
mangelwurzel, mangoldwurzel	*Beta vulgaris rapa*
marrow	*Cucurbita pepo*
mooli	*Raphanus sativa*
motate (pinguin)	*Bromelia pinguin*
mountain ebony	*Bauhinia variegata*
mustard, field	*Brassica campestris*
mustard, Indian	*Brassica juncea*
mustard spinach	*Brassica perviridis*
nasturtium, tuberous (ysao)	*Tropaeolum tuberosum*
nettle	*Urtica dioica*
oca	*Oxalis tuberosa*
okra (gumbo, bhindi)	*Hibiscus esculentus*
orache	*Atriplex hortensis*
onion	*Allium cepa*
onion, Egyptian (tree onion)	*Allium cepa (proliform)*
onion, everlasting	*Allium perutile*
onion, Japanese bunching	*Allium fistulosum,*
onion, Welsh,	*Allium cepa perutile*
oxalis	*Oxalis crenata*
oyster plant (salsify)	*Tragopogon porrifolius*
pak choi (Chinese greens, chard)	*Brassica chinensis*
palm, African fan	*Borassus aethiopum*
palm cabbage (coyoli palm)	*Acrocomia mexicana*
parsley, leaves	*Petroselinum crispum, P. hortense*
parsley, Hamburg (turnip-rooted)	*Petroselinum crispum var. tuberosum*
parsnip	*Pastinaca sativa*
pea	*Pisum sativum*
petsai (Chinese cabbage)	*Brassica pekinensis*
pepper grass	*Lepidium sativum.*
pepper, hot (Chilli)	*Capsicum frustescens*
pepper, sweet	*Capsicum annuum*
pimiento	*Capsicum annuum*
pinguin (motate)	*Bromelia pinguin*

Table 28.8: (Cont'd)

pi-tsi (Chinese water chestnut)	*Eleochgaris tuberosa*
pumpkin	*Cucurbita moschata, C. pepo*
purslane (pigweed)	*Portulaca oleracea*
quamash (camash)	*Camassia quamash*
radish	*Raphanus sativus*
rocambole	*Allium sativum, A. scorodoprasum*
rocket	*Eruca sativa*
rutabaga (swede turnip)	*Brassica napus, B. rutabaga, B. napobrassica*
sag cholai	*Amaranthus gangeticus*
sag kulfa	*Portulaca oleracea*
salsify	*Tragopogon porrifolius*
salsify, black (scorzonera)	*Scorzonera hispanica*
samphire, marsh (sea asparagus)	*Salicornia spp*
samphire, rock	*Crithmum maritimum*
samphire, golden	*Inula crithmoides*
scorzonera (black salsify)	*Scorzonera hispanica*
sea kale	*Crambe maritima*
sea kale (beet, chard)	*Beta vulgaris var. cicla*
shallot	*Allium ascalonium*
shungiku	*Chrysanthemum coronarium*
snake gourd	*Trichosanthes cucumerina*
sorrel	*Rumex spp., Hibiscus sabdariffa*
spinach	*Spinacea oleracea.*
spinach beet	*Beta vulgaris var. cicla,*
spinach, Chinese	*Amaranthus gangeticus*
spinach, garden	*Atriplex hortensis*
spinach, Philippine	*Talinum triangulare*
spinach, New Zealand	*Tetragonia espansa, T. tetragonoides*
spinach, vine (Ceylon spinach)	*Basella alba, B. rubra*
sponge gourd	*Luffa cylindrica*
squash	*Cucurbita maxima, Cucurbita spp.*
sweet corn	*Zea mays var. saccharata*
swede (swede turnip, rutabaga)	*Brassica napus, B. rutabaga*
Swiss chard	*Beta vulgaris var. cicla*
thistle, edible	*(Goundelia tournefortii)*
tinda	*Citrulus fistulosus, Lycopersicum esculentum*
tomatillo (purple gooseberry, jamberry)	*Physalis ixocarpa*
tomato	*Lycopersicon esculentum*
tomato, English (tree tomato)	*Cyphomandra betacea*
tomato, ground (tomatillo)	*Physalis ixocarpa*
turnip	*Brassica campestris*
turniprooted chervil	*Chaerophyllum bulbosum*
turnip, Swedish	*Brassica rutabaga*

Table 28.8: (Cont'd)

vegetable oyster (salsify)	*Tragopogon porrifolius.*
vine leaves	*Vitis vinifera*
vine spinach	*Basella* spp.
water convulvulus	*Ipomea aquatica, I. reptanus*
watercress	*Nasturtium officinale, N. microphyllum x officinale*
witloof (chicory)	*Cichorium intybus* var. *foliosum*
wong bok	*Brassica pekinensis*
ysaño (tuberous nasturtium)	*Tropaeolum tuberosum*

(1) Those fruits (by the botanical definition) that are conventionally eaten as savoury items have been included here as vegetables; fruits are listed in Table 28.10.
See Table 28.3 for legumes, and Table 28.9 for mushrooms and edible fungi.

Table 28.9: Mushrooms and edible fungi[1]

amethyst deceiver	*Laccaria amethystea*
beefsteak fungus	*Fistulina hepatica*
black forest mushroom (shiitake)	*Lentinula (Lentinus) edodes*
black fungus (wood ears)	*Auriculia polytricha*
blewits	*Tricholoma (Lepista) saevum, Lepista* spp.
blusher toadstool	*Amanita caesarea*
boletus (cèpe, yellow mushroom)	*Boletus edulis, B. granulatus*
boletus, red	*Leccinum aurantiacum*
boletus, ringer	*Suillus luteus*
boletus, rough-stemmed	*Leccinum scabrum*
cèpe (boletus, yellow mushroom)	*Boletus edulis, B. granulatus*
chanterelle (girolle, egg mushroom)	*Cantharellus cibarius*
chestnut (Paris) mushroom	*Agaricus bisporus*
enokitake	*Flammulina velutipes*
fairy ring mushroom	*Marasmius oreades*
field mushroom	*Agaricus campestris, A. vaporarius*
honey fungus	*Armillaria mellea*
horn of plenty	*Craterellus cornucopioides*
horse mushroom	*Agaricus arvensis*
ink cap	*Coprinus atramentarius*
Jew's ear	*Auricularia auricula-judae*
matsutake (pine mushroom)	*Tricholoma matsutake*
morel (sponge mushroom)	*Morchella esculenta, M. vulgaris*
mu-esh	*Hirneola polytricha*
orange agaric	*Lactarius deliciosus*
orange peel fungus	*Aleuria aurantia*
oyster mushroom	*Pleurotus ostreatus*
parasol mushroom	*Macrolepiota procera*
parasol, shaggy	*Lepiotra rhacodes*
Paris (chestnut) mushroom	*Agaricus bisporus*

Table 28.9: (Cont'd)

pholiotte	*Agrocybe aegerita*
puffball, giant	*Calvatia (Lycoperdon) gigantea*
puffball, mosaic	*Calvatia (Lycoperdon) caelata*
rubber brush (wood hedgehog)	*Hydnum repandum*
shiitake (black forest mushroom, Chinese mushroom)	*Lentinula (Lentinus) edodes*
straw mushroom	*Volvariella volvacea*
truffle, black Périgord	*Tuber melanospermum*
truffle, summer	*Tuber aestivum*
truffle, violet	*Tuber brumale*
truffle, white Piedmontese	*Tuber magnatum*
wood blewits	*Tricholoma (Lepista) nudum*
wood ears (Chinese black fungus, cloud ears)	*Auriculia polytricha*
wood hedgehog (rubber brush)	*Hydnum repandum*
yellow mushroom	*Boletus granulatus*

(1) The common cultivated mushroom is *Agaricus bisporus, A. campestris.*

Table 28.10: Fruits[1]

akee	*Blighia sapida*
alingaro (lingaro)	*Elaeagnus latifolia*
anonang (chachalaca)	*Cordia dentata*
apple	*Malus pumila, M. sylvestris, M. communis, Pyrus malus*
apple, Mexican (white sapote)	*Casimiroa edulis*
apricot	*Prunus armeniaca*
arbute	*Arbutus unedo*
avocado	*Persea americana*
avron (cloudberry)	*Rubus chamaemorus*
azarole	*Crataegus azarolus*
babaco	*Carica pentagona*
bacuri	*Platonia insignis*
baked apple berry (cloudberry)	*Rubus chamaemorus*
balsam apple (balsam pear, bitter melon)	*Momordica charantia*
banana	*Musa sapientum, M. cavendishii, M. nana*
banana, cooking (plantain)	*Musa paradisiaca*
banana, false	*Ensete ventricosum*
bandaria (gandaria)	*Bouea macrophylla*
baobab	*Adansonia digitata*
bergamot	*Citrus bergamia, Pyrus persica*
bilberry	*Vaccinium myrtillus,*
bilimbi	*Averrhoa bilimbi*
blackberry	*Morus nigra, Rubus fruticosus, R. ulmifolius*

Table 28.10: (Cont'd)

blackcurrant	*Ribes nigra*
blackthorn (sloe)	*Prunus spinosa*
blueberry, American	*Vaccinium corymbosum, V. augustifolium*
blueberry, European (bilberry, whortleberry)	*Vaccinium myrtillus*
blueberry, high bush	*Vaccinium corymbosum*
blueberry, low bush	*Vaccinium augustifolium*
bog myrtle	*Myrica gale*
boysenberry	*Rubus ursinus* var. *loganbaccus*
breadfruit	*Artocarpus incisa, A. altilis*
buffalo currant	*Ribes odoratum, R. aureum*
bullace	*Prunus insititia*
bullock's heart (custard apple)	*Anona reticulata*
cacao (pataste)	*Theobroma bicolor*
cainito, star apple	*Chrysophyllum* spp.
camucamu	*Myrciaria paraensis*
canihua	*Chenopodium pallidicaule*
Cape gooseberry (Peruvian cherry)	*Physalis peruviana (P. pubescens, P. edulis)*
capulin montes	*Saurauja pauciserrata*
carambola (star fruit)	*Averrhoa carambola, A. bilimbi*
carisa (Natal plum)	*Carissa grandiflora*
carob	*Ceratonia siliqua*
cashew apple	*Anacardium occidentale*
cerimani	*Monstera deliciosa*
chachalaca (anonang)	*Cordia dentata*
cherimoya (custard apple)	*Annona squamosa, Annona* spp.
cherry, bird	*Prunus padus*
cherry, Central American wild	*Prunus serotina*
cherry, ground (wild Cape gooseberry)	*Physalis pruinosa, P. angulata*
cherry, morello (sour)	*Prunus cerasus, P. acida, Cerasus acida*
cherry plum	*Prunus cerasifera*
cherry, Surinam (pitanga)	*Eugenia uniflora, E. michelii*
cherry, sweet	*Prunus avium, Cerasus avium*
cherry, West Indian	*Malpighia punicifolia*
chinotto	*Citrus myrtifolia,*
Christ's thorn	*Zizyphus spina Christi*
citrange	*Poncirus trifoliata*
citron	*Citrus medica* var. *cedrata,*
clementine, satsuma	*Citrus unshiu, C. nobilis* var. *deliciosa*
cloudberry	*Rubus chamaemorus*
coco plum (icaco)	*Chrysobalus icaco*
cow berry (mountain cranberry)	*Vaccinium vitis-idaea*
cranberry, American	*Vaccinium macrocarpon,*
cranberry, European	*Vaccinium oxycoccus*
cranberry, mountain (cow berry)	*Vaccinium vitis-idaea*

Table 28.10: (Cont'd)

currants, red and white	*Ribes rubrum*
custard apple (cherimoya, bullock s heart)	*Anona squamosa, A.* spp.
damson	*Prunus damascena*
dangleberry	*Gaylussacia baccata*
date	*Phoenix dactylifera*
date plum (kaki)	*Diospyros kaki*
date, desert (soapberry, thorntree)	*Balanites aegyptica*
date, Chinese (jujube)	*Ziziphus jujuba*
date, wild	*Phoenix sylvestris*
dewberry	*Rubus caesius*
duku (langsat)	*Lansium domesticum*
durian	*Durio zibethinus*
elderberry	*Sambucus nigra*
falsa	*Grewia asiatica*
fig	*Ficus carica*
fruit salad fruit	*Monstera deliciosa*
gages	*Prunus italica*
gandaria (bandaria)	*Bouea macrophylla*
gean	*Prunus avium*
golden currant	*Ribes odoratum, R. aureum*
gooseberry	*Ribes grossularia*
gooseberry, American (worcesterberry)	*Ribes diverticatum*
gooseberry, Ceylon	*Aberia garneri*
gooseberry, Indian	*Phyllanthus emblica*
grapefruit, pomelo	*Citrus maxima, C. grandis, C. paradisi*
grape	*Vitis vinifera*
grape, sea (papaturos)	*Coccolaba caracasana*
greengage, plum	*Prunus domestica*
grenadilla (passion fruit)	*Passiflora edulis, P. quadrangularis*
guamachil (kuamochil)	*Pithecolobium dulce*
guava	*Psidium guajava*
guava, strawberry	*Psidium littorale*
haw, hawthorn	*Craetagus* spp.
haw, red (manzanilla)	*Craetagus pubescens*
hog plum, mombin	*Spondias* spp.
huckleberry (dangleberry)	*Gaylussacia baccata*
icaco (coco plum)	*Chrysobalus icaco*
ilama	*Anona diversifolia*
jackfruit	*Artocarpus integrifolia, A. heterophyllus*
jalpai (kalomala)	*Elaeocarpus serratus*
jaman	*Eugenia jambos*
jelly palm	*Butia capitata*
jujube (Chinese date)	*Ziziphus jujuba*
kalomala (jalpai)	*Elaeocarpus serratus*
kaki	*Diospyros kaki*
kanapy	*Melicocca bijuga*
karanda	*Carissa carandas*
kechapi (sandal tree, santol)	*Sandoricum indicum*
kiwi fruit	*Actinidia chinensis*
kuamochil (guamachil)	*Pithecolobium dulce*
kumquat	*Fortunella japonica*

Table 28.10: (Cont'd)

langsat (duku)	*Lansium domesticum*
lemon	*Citrus limon*
lemon, sweet	*Citrus limetta*
lime, sour	*Citrus aurantifolia*
lime, sweet	*Citrus limetta, C. limetioides*
lingaro (alingaro)	*Elaeagnus latifolia*
litchi (lychee)	*Nephelium litchi, Litchi chinensis*
locust bean (carob)	*Ceratonia siliqua*
loganberry	*Rubus ursinus* var. *loganobaccus,*
longan	*Nephelium longan, Euphoria longan*
loquat	*Eriobotrya japonica*
loquat, wild	*Uapaca kirkiana*
lulu (ludde, marula plum)	*Sclerocarya birroea*
madrono	*Rheedia madruno*
mamey colorado, sapote	*Calocarpum mammosum*
mammee (mammy apple)	*Mammea americana*
mandarin (tangerine)	*Citrus reticulata, C. nobilio, C. deliciosa*
mango	*Mangifera indica*
mango, wild or bush	*Cordyla africana*
mangosteen	*Garcinea mangostana*
manzanilla (red haw)	*Craetagus pubescens*
mazzard (sweet cherry)	*Prunus avium, Cerasus avium*
medlar	*Mespilus germanica*
melon	*Cucumis melo*
melon, egusi	*Cucumeropsis edulis, C. manii*
melon, water	*Citrullus vulgaris*
mirabelle, plum	*Prunus domestica*
miracle berry	*Richardella dulcifica* (syn. *Synsepalum dulcificum*)
mombin, hog plum, Spanish plum	*Spondias* spp.
monstera	*Monstera deliciosa*
mulberry, black, common	*Morus nigra*
mulberry, Indian	*Morinda citrifolia*
mulberry, red	*Morus rubra*
mulberry, white	*Morus alba*
myrtle berry	*Myrtus communis*
nance	*Byrsonima crassifolia*
naranjillo	*Solanum quitoense*
nectarines, peaches	*Prunus persica* var. *nectarina, Amygdalus persica*
orange, bitter (Seville)	*Citrus aurantium*
orange, Kaffir (monkey balls)	*Strychnos* spp.
orange, sweet	*Citrus sinensis*
orange, temple	*Citrus sinensis* x *C. reticulata*
palm fruit, palm peach	*Bactris utilis, B. gasipaes*
palm, palmyra, borassus	*Borassus flabellifer*
pandanus	*Pandanus* spp.

Table 28.10: (Cont'd)

papaturos (sea grape)	*Coccolaba caracasana*
papaw	*Asimina triloba*
papaya (pawpaw)	*Carica papaya*
parchita (passion fruit)	*Passiflora edulis*
passion fruit (grenadilla)	*Passiflora edulis, P. quadrangularis*
pataste (cacao)	*Theobroma bicolor*
pawpaw (papaya)	*Carica papaya*
pawpaw, mountain	*Carica condamarcensis*
peach, nectarine	*Prunus persica, Amygdalus persica*
pear	*Pyrus communis*
pear, Japanese	*Pyrus serotina*
pejibaye (palm fruit, palm peach)	*Bactris utilis, B. gasipaes*
pepino angelo	*Sicana odorifera*
persimmon, American	*Diospyros virginiana*
persimmon, Japanese (kaki)	*Diospyros kaki*
pineapple	*Ananas sativus,*
pitanga (Surinam cherry)	*Eugenia uniflora, E. michelii,*
plantain (cooking banana)	*Musa paradisiaca*
plum (greengage, mirabelle, damson)	*Prunus domestica*
plum, cherry	*Prunus cerasifera*
plum, coco (icaco)	*Chrysobalus icaco*
plum, hog (Spanish)	*Spondias* spp.
plum, Japanese	*Prunus trifolora (P. salicina)*
plum, marula (lulu, ludde)	*Sclerocarya birroea*
plum, monkey	*Royena pallens*
plum, Oregon	*Prunus subcordata*
plum, Santa rosa	*Prunus salicina*
plum, sour	*Ximenia caffra*
poke (pokeberry)	*Phytolacca americana*
pomegranate	*Punica granatum*
pomelo, grapefruit	*Citrus maxima, C. grandis, C. paradisi*
prickly pear	*Opuntia ficus-indica*
quince	*Cydonia oblonga, C. vulgaris, C. japonica, C. cathayensis*
quince, Japanese	*Chaenomeles lagenaria*
rambutan	*Nephelium lappaceum*
raspberry	*Rubus idaeus*
red currant	*Ribes sativum*
rhubarb	*Rheum rhaponticum*
rose apple	*Eugenia jambos, E. malaccensis*
rose hips	*Rosa* spp.
rowanberry	*Sorbus aucuparia*
santol (sandal tree, kechapi)	*Sandoricum indicum, S. koetjape*
sapodilla (sapota)	*Achras sapota*
sapote, marmalade plum	*Calocarpum sapota*
sapote, mamey colorado	*Calocarpum mammosum*
sapote, white (Mexican apple)	*Casimiroa edulis*

Table 28.10: (Cont'd)

satsuma, clementine	*Citrus unshiu, C. reticulata*
serendipity berry	*Dioscoreophyllum cumminsii*
service-apple	*Sorbus domestica*
sloe (blackthorn)	*Prunus spinosa*
soap berry (desert date, thorntree)	*Balanites aegyptiaca*
soncoya	*Anona purpurea*
sour sop (custard apple)	*Anona muricata*
St John's bread (carob)	*Ceratonia siliqua*
star apple, cainito	*Chrysophyllum cainito*
star fruit (carambola)	*Averrhoa carambola, A. bilimbi*
strawberry	*Fragaria* spp.
strawberry, alpine	*Fragaria vesca semperflorens*
sweet sop (custard apple, sweet apple)	*Anona squamosa*
tacaco	*Polakowski tacaco*
tamarind	*Tamarindus indica*
tampanja	*Cereus hexagonus*
tangelo	*Citrus paradisi x C. reticulata*
tangerine (mandarin)	*Citrus reticulata*
tree-strawberry	*Arbutus unedo*
thorntree (desert date, soap berry)	*Balanites aegyptiaca*
wampee (uampi)	*Clausena lansium*
water lemon (passion fruit)	*Passiflora edulis*
water melon	*Citrullus vulgaris*
whortleberry	*Vaccinium myrtillus*
wineberry	*Rubus phoenicolasius*
winter berry	*Gaultheria procumbens*
worcesterberry (American gooseberry)	*Ribes diverticatum*

(1) This table includes not only true fruits (as defined botanically) but also those vegetables that are conventionally eaten sweet and are commercially considered as fruits; vegetables are listed in Table 28.8.

Table 28.11: Herbs, spices, beverages and plants used for flavouring

cocoa	*Theobroma cacao*
coffee	*Coffea arabica, C. robusta, C. liberica*
tea	*Camellia sinensis, Thea sinensis, T. assaamica*
cassina	*Ilex cassine*
maté	*Ilex paraguayensis*
rooibos tea	*Aspalathus liniearis*
rosella (sorrel, flor de Jamaica)	*Hibiscus sabdariffa*
alecost (costmary, balsam herb, mace)	*Chrysanthemum balsamita*
allspice, Jamaica pepper	*Pimenta officinalis*
ambli (amba)	*Phyllanthus emblica*
anise (aniseed)	*Pimpinella anisum*
anise, star	*Illicium verum*
areca palm (betel nut)	*Arecha catechu*
asafaetida	*Ferula narthea, F. foetida*
badian (star anise)	*Illicium verum*
balm (lemon balm)	*Melissa officinalis*
basil	*Ocimum basilicum, O. minimum*
bay (laurel)	*Laurus nobilis*
betel leaf	*Piper betel*
betel nut (areca)	*Arecha catechu*
bitters, Angostura	*Galispea officinalis*
borage	*Borago officinalis*
brooklime	*Veronica beccabunga*
burnet (salad burnet)	*Poterium sanguisorba*
caper	*Capparis spinosa, C. inermis*
caraway	*Carum carvi, C. capticum*
cardamon, cluster	*Elettaria cardamomum*
cardamons, other	*Aframomum angustifolium, A. hambury, Amomun aromaticum, A. cardamomum*
cassia (Chinese cinnamon)	*Cinnamomum cassia*
chamomile	*Anthemis nobilis, Matricaria recutica*
chervil	*Anthriscus cerefolium*
chilli pepper	*Capsicum frutescens*
cinnamon, Ceylon	*Cinnamomum zeylanicum*
cinnamon, Chinese (cassia)	*Cinnamomum cassia*
clove	*Eugenia caryophyllus, Caryophyllus aromaticus*
comfrey	*Symphytum officinale*
coriander (dhania)	*Coriandrum sativum*
cumin (cummin)	*Cuminum cyminum*
cumin, black	*Nigella sativa*
cumin, sweet (anise)	*Pimpinella anisum*
curry plant (curry leaves)	*Murraya koenigii*
dhania (coriander)	*Coriandrum sativum*
dill	*Anethum graveolens*
fennel	*Foeniculum vulgare*
fenugreek	*Trigonella foenum-graecum*

Table 28.11: (Cont'd)

ginger	*Zingiber officinale*
hops	*Humulus lupulus*
haldi (turmeric)	*Curcuma longa*
horseradish	*Cochlearia armoriaca, Armorica rusticana*
hyssop	*Hyssopus officinialis*
juniper	*Juniperis communis*
kava	*Piper methysticum*
liquorice	*Glycyrrhiza glabra*
locust beans, African	*Parkia filicoidea*
lovage	*Levisticum officinale*
lovage, Scotch	*Ligusticum scoticum*
mace	*Myristica fragrans*
malaguetta pepper, grains of paradise	*Aframomum melegueta*
marjoram	*Origanum majorana, Majorana hortensis,Thymus mastichina*
marjoram, pot	*Origanum onites*
marjoram, sweet	*Majorana hortensis*
milfoil (yarrow)	*Achillea millefolium*
mint	*Mentha spp*
mustard, black or brown mustard	*Brassica nigra, B. juncea*
mustard, white or yellow	*Sinapsis alba*
nigerseed (nug)	*Guizotia abyssinica*
nutmeg (mace)	*Myristica fragrans*
omum	*Carum copticum*
parsley	*Petroselinum crispum, P. hertense, P. sativum*
pepper, black, white	*Piper nigrum*
pepper, chilli (or chili),	*Capsicum frutescens, C.annuum*
pepper, Japan	*Zanthoxylum piperitum*
pepper, long	*Piper longum*
pepper, melegueta, Guinea	*Amomum melegueta*
pepper dulse	*Laurencia pinnatifida*
peppergrass (pepperwort)	*Lepidium sativum*
peppermint	*Mentha piperita*
poppy seed	*Papaver somniferum*
rosemary	*Rosmarinus officinalis*
saffron	*Crocus sativus*
saffron, Mexican	*Carthamus tinctoria*
sage	*Salvia officinalis*
sarsaparilla	*Smilax officinalis*
sassafras	*Sassafras albidum*
savory, summer	*Satureja hortensis*
savory, winter	*Satureja montana*
smallage	*Apium graveolens*
southernwood (lad s love)	*Artemesia abrotanum*
spearmint	*Mentha spicata*
sweet cecily	*Myrrhis odorata*
tamarind	*Tamarindus indica*
tansy	*Tanacetum vulgare*
tarragon	*Artemisia dracunculus*
tarragon, Russian or false	*Artemisia dracunculoides*

Table 28.11: (Cont'd)

thyme	*Thymus vulgaris, Thymus spp.*
thyme, lemon	*Thymus citridorius*
turmeric (haldi)	*Curcuma longa*
vanilla	*Vanilla planifolia, V. pompona, V. aromaticus*
wormwood	*Artemisia absinthium*
yarrow (milfoil)	*Achillea millefolium*
yerba dulce	*Stevia rebaudiana*
zedoary root	*Curcuma zedoaria*

Table 28.12: Meat, livestock, and game

alpaca	*Glama pacos*
moose	*Alces alces andersonii*
moose, American	*Alces americana*
ass	*Equus asinus*
beaver	*Castor canadensis*
bee	*Apis mellifica, A. dorsata, A. florea, A. indica*
beeffalo	*Bison x Bos*
bison, American	*Bison bison*
bison, European	*Bison bonasus*
boar, wild	*Sus scrofa*
Brahman cattle	*Bos indicus*
buffalo, African	*Syncerus caffer*
buffalo, Asiatic	*Bubalus arnee*
buffalo, Indian	*Bubalus bubalus*
buffalo, water	*Bubalus bubalus, B. arnee, B. depressicornis*
camel, Arabian	*Camelus dromedarius*
camel, bactrian	*Camelus bactrianus*
capercaillie (capercailzie, wood grouse)	*Tetrao urogallus*
chicken	*Gallus domesticus*
deer	*Odocoileus* spp.
dormourse, fat or edible	*Glis glis*
duck	*Anas* spp.
duck, mallard	*Anas platyrhynchos*
duck, muscovy	*Cairina moschata*
duck, North American wood	*Aix sponsa*
fowl, Guinea	*Numida meleagris*
fowl, red jungle	*Gallus gallus*
frog	*Rana esculenta*
goat	*Capra* spp.
goat, North American mountain	*Oreamnos americanus*
goose	*Anser anser domesticus*
goose, barnacle	*Branta leucopsis*
goose, Canada	*Branta canadiensis canadiensis*
grouse	*Lagopus lagopus*
grouse, ruffed	*Bonasa umbellicus*
grouse, spruce	*Canachites canadiensis canadiensis*

Table 28.12: (Cont'd)

grouse, wood (capercaillie)	*Tetrao urogallus*
Guinea fowl	*Numida meleagris*
hare	*Lepus* spp.
hinny	sterile offspring of a female ass and a male horse
hog (domestic pig)	*Sus domestica*
horse	*Equus caballus*
kangaroo	*Macropus giganteus, M. major*
llama	*Glama peruana*
mule	sterile offspring of a male ass and a female horse
muskrat	*Ondatra zibethica*
opossum	*Didelphis virginiana*
ostrich	*Struthio camelus*
ox, Asiatic	subgenus *Bibos*
ox, common	*Bos taurus*
ox, humped (zebu)	*Bos indicus*
partridge	*Alectoris rufa*
peacock	*Pavo cristatus*
pheasant	*Phasianus colchicus, Chrysalophus* spp.
pig, domestic (hog)	*Sus domestica*
pigeon (squab)	*Columba livia*
quail, American	*Bonasa umbellus, Colinuis virginianus*
quail, European	*Coturnix coturnix*
quail, Japanese	*Coturnix coturnix japonica*
quail, mountain	*Oreortyx pictus*
quail, Californian	*Lophortyx californica*
rabbit	*Lepus cuniculus, Oryetolagus cuniculus, O. euniculus*
rabbit, American wild	*Sylvilagus floridanus*
raccoon	*Procyon lotor*
reindeer	*Rangifer tarandus*
sheep	*Ovis* spp.
snail	*Helix pomatia*
snail, white-lipped edible	*Helix vermiculata*
snail, little edible	*Helix pisana*
snail, giant African	*Achatima fulica*
squab (pigeon)	*Columba livia*
turkey	*Meleagris gallopavo*
water buffalo	*Bubalus bubalus, B. arnee, B. depressicornis*
witchetty grubs	*Xylentes* spp.
yak	*Poephagus grunniens*
zebu (humped ox)	*Bos indicus*

Table 28.13: Fish

alewife	*Alosa pseudoharengus*
amberfish	*Serioloa quinqueradiata*
anchovy	*Engraulis* spp.
angler (goosefish, monkfish)	*Lophius piscatorius*
barracuda	*Sphyraena* spp.
bass	*Dicentrarchus labrax*
bass, black	*Micropterus salmoides, M. dolomieu*
bass, calico	*Pomoxis nigromaculatus*
bass, channel	*Sciaenops ocellatus*
bass, kelp	*Palabrax clathratus*
bass, rock	*Ambloplites rupestris*
bass, sea, black	*Centropristes striata*
bass, striped, yellow, white	*Morone saxatilis, M. chrysops, M. mississippiensis, Roccus saxatilis, R. chrysops*
blackfish (tautog)	*Tautoga onitis*
bluefish	*Pomatus saltatrix*
bonito	*Katsuwonus pelamys*
bonito, Atlantic	*Sarda sarda*
bonito, striped	*Sarda orientalis*
bream, bluegill	*Leponis machrochinus*
bream, European	*Abramis brama*
brill	*Scophthalmus rhombus*
brill, rough-scaled	*Pseudorhombus digodon*
brisling (young sprats)	*Sprattus (Clupea) sprattus*
buffalo fish	*Ictiobus cyprinellus, I. bubalus, I. niger*
bullhead	*Ictalurus Ameiurus nebulosus, I. A. melas*
burbot	*Lota lota*
butterfish (harvest fish)	*Peprilus triacanthus, Poronotus triacanthus*
butter fish (spade fish)	*Scatophagus argus*
candle fish (eulachon)	*Thaleichthys pacificus*
carp	*Cyprinus carpio*
cat shark (rock salmon, dog fish)	*Scyliorhinus caniculus*
catfish	Ariidae and Plotosidae families, *Anargichas* spp.
catfish, freshwater	*Clarias batrachus*
chub	*Hybopsis* spp., *Gila* spp., *Coregonus* spp.
cisco (lake herring, whitefish)	*Coregonus artedi*
coalfish (coley, pollock)	*Pollachius virens*
cod	*Gaddus morrhua*
cod, Arctic	*Boreogadus saida*
cod, Pacific	*Gaddus macrocephalus*
codling (hake)	*Urophycis blennoides, U. chuss, U. tenuis*
coley	*Pollachius virens.*
conger eel	*Conger myriaster*
crappie, white	*Pomoxis annularis*
croaker	*Pseudosciaena aneus*
croaker, Atlantic	*Micropodon undulatus*
croaker, Atlantic white	*Genyonemus lineatus*

Table 28.13: (Cont'd)

croaker, Atlantic yellow	*Umbrina roncador*
croaker, freshwater (drumfish)	*Aplodinotus grunniens*
cusk	*Brosme brosme*
cutlass fish (hairtail, ribbon fish)	*Trichiurus* spp.
dab	*Limanda limanda*
dogfish (rock salmon, huss, rigg)	*Scyliorhinus* spp., *Galeorhinus* spp., *Mustelus* spp, *Galeus melastomus*, *Squalus acanthias*
dogfish, Mediterranean spotted	*Scyliorhinus caniculus, S. stellaris*
dogfish, smooth	*Mustelus manazo*
dogfish, spiny	*Squalus acanthus*
dolly vardon	*Slavelinus malma*
dolphin	*Coryphaena hippurus*
dory	*Zeus faber*
drumfish, freshwater (croaker)	*Aplodinotus grunniens*
drumfish, red (redfish)	*Sciaenops ocellatus*
eel, American	*Anguilla rostratus*
eel, conger	*Conger myriaster*
eel, European	*Anguilla anguilla, Anguilla* spp.
eel, silver pike	*Muraenesox cinereus*
eulachon (candle fish)	*Thaleichthys pacificus*
flatfish (flounder, sole, sand dab)	*Pseudopleuronectes americanum, Paralichthys dentatus, P. lethostigma, Platichthys stellata, Limanda ferruginea, Atherestes stomias, Parophrys vetulus, Microstomas pacificus, Eopsetta jordani, Hippoglossoides elassodon, Glyptocephalus zachirus, Lepidopsetta bilineata, Citharichthys sordidus, Psettichthys malanotinctus*
flathead, Indian	*Platycephalus indicus*
flounder (fluke)	*Platichthys stellatus, P. flesus, Hippoglossoides elassodon, Paralichtys olivaceus*
flounder, four-spot	*Platichthys oblongus*
flounder, righteye	*Glyptocephalus* spp.
flounder, slime	*Microstomus stelleri*
flounder, summer	*Paralichthys dentatus*
flounder, winter	*Pseudoplectonectes americanus*
flounder, yellowtail	*Limanda ferruginea*
flying fish	*Cypselurus* spp., *Exocoetus volitans*
forkbeard	*Phycis* spp., *Urophycis* spp., *Raniceps raninus*

Table 28.13: (Cont'd)

fugu (puffer fish)	*Fuga rubripes*
fusilier, golden	*Caesio chrysozonus, C. cunning*
gaper	*Schizothaerus* spp.
garfish	*Belone* spp., *Tylosurus giganteus*
goby	*Gobidae* spp., *Glossobius giurus*
goosefish (angler, monkfish)	*Lophius piscatorius*
gouramy	*Trichogaster pectoralis*
grayling	*Thymallus arcticus, T. thymallus*
grouper	*Epinephelus* spp., *Myctoperca* spp.
grunion	*Leuresthes tenuis*
gurnard	*Peristedion cataphactum, Triglidae* family
haddock	*Melanogrammus aeglefinus*
hairtail (cutlass fish, ribbon fish)	*Trichiurus* spp.
hake (codling)	*Urophycis blennoides, U. chuss, U. tenuis*
hake, Atlantic	*Merluccius hubbsi, M. bilinearis*
hake, Cape	*Merluccius capensis, M. paradoxus*
hake, European	*Merluccius merluccius*
hake, Pacific	*Merluccius productus, M. gayi*
hake, silver	*Merluccius bilinearis*
halibut, Atlantic	*Hippoglossus hippoglossus*
halibut, arrow toothed	*Reinhardtius matsuurae*
halibut, black, Greenland	*Reinhardtius hippoglossoides*
halibut, Californian	*Paralichthys californicus*
halibut, Pacific	*Hippoglossus stenolepsis*
hard tail (torpedo)	*Megalaspis cordyla*
harvest fish	*Peprilus alepidotus, P. simillimus, P. triacanthus*
herring, Atlantic	*Clupea harengus harengus*
herring, fall, blueback, spring	*Alosa mediocxris, A. aestivalis, A. pseudoharengus*
herring, lake (whitefish, cisco)	*Coregonus artedi*
herring, Pacific	*Clupea harengus pallasi*
huss (dogfish, rock salmon, rigg)	*Scyliorhinus* spp., *Galeorhinus* spp., *Mustelus* spp, *Galeus melastomus, Squalus acanthias*
inconnu (sheefish)	*Stenodus leucichthys*
jack mackerel	*Thrachurus symmetricus*
john dory	*Zeus faber*
kingfish (surf whiting)	*Menticirrhinus americanus, M. littoralis, M. saxatilis*
lampern (river lamprey)	*Lampetra fluviatilis, Entosphenus japonicus*

Table 28.13: (Cont'd)

lamprey	*Petromyzon marinus*
lascar	*Pegusa lascaris*
ling	*Molva* spp.
lingcod	*Ophiodon elongatus*
loach	*Misgurnus anguillacaudatus*
lumpfish	*Cylopterus lumpus*
mackerel	*Scomber scombrus, Scomber* spp.
mackerel, atka	*Pleurogrammus azonus*
mackerel, chub mackerel	*Scomber japonicus*
mackeral, horse or jack	*Trachurus japonicus*
mackerel, Spanish	*Scomberomorus maculatus*
marlin, black	*Makaira indica*
marlin, sailfish	*Istiophorus* spp.
marlin, striped, white	*Tetrapuyrus audax, T. albidus*
megrim	*Lepidorhombus* spp.
menhaden	*Brevoortia patronus, B. tyrannus*
monkfish (angler, goosefish)	*Lophius piscatorius*
moonfish	*Mene maculata*
mullet	*Mugil* spp.
mullet, grey	*Liza* spp., *Chelon* spp.
mullet, harder	*Mugil cephalus*
mullet, mountain	*Agonostomus monticola*
mullet, red	*Mullus* spp.
mullet, striped	*Mugil cephalus*
muskellunge	*Esox masquinongy*
parrot fish	*Leptoscatus japonicus*
perch, climbing	*Ctenopoma* spp.
perch, common	*Perca fluviatilis*
perch, Pacific	*Sebastes alutus*
perch, white	*Roccus americanus*
perch, yellow	*Perca flavescens*
pike, blue	*Stizostedion vitreum glaucum*
pike, chain pickerel	*Esox niger*
pike, northern	*Esox lucius*
pike, walleye	*Stizostedion vitreum vitreum*
pilchard	*Clupea pilchardus, Sardina pilchardus*
pilchard, Pacific	*Sardinops sagax*
plaice	*Pleuronectus platessa*
pollock (pollack)	*Pollachius virens*
pollock (pollack), European	*Pollachius pollachius*
pollock (pollack), Pacific, Alaska	*Theregra chalcogramma*
pollock (pollack, coley)	*Pollachius virens.*
pompano, Florida	*Trachinotus carolinus*
porgy, American (scup)	*Stenotomus chrysops, S. caprinus, Calamus* spp.
porgy, European, red	*Pagrus pagrus*
pout (pouting)	*Trisopterus luscus*
puffer fish (fugu)	*Fuga rubripes*
ray	*Raja raja*

Table 28.13: (Cont'd)

redfish (ocean perch)	*Sebastes fasciatus, S. marinus, S. mentella, S. viviparus, S. norvegicus, Helicolenus maculatus, H. dactylopterus*
redfish (red drum)	*Sciaenops ocellatus*
redhorse, silver	*Moxostoma anisurum*
ribbon-finned fish	*Nemipterus taenitrus*
ribbon fish (cutlass fish, hairtail)	*Trichiurus* spp.
rigg (rock fish, dogfish, rock salmon, huss)	*Scyliorhinus* spp., *Galeorhinus* spp., *Mustelus* spp, *Galeus melastomus, Squalus acanthias*
rockfish	*Sebastodes* spp.,
roach	*Rutilis rutilis*
roughback	*Hippoglossoides platessoides*
sable fish	*Anaplopoma finibris, A. fimbria*
sailfish	*Istiophorus platyperus, I. orientalis*
saithe (coley)	*Pollachius virens*
salmon, Atlantic	*Salmo salar*
salmon, cherry	*Oncorhynchus masou*
salmon, chum or keta	*Oncorhynchus keta*
salmon, medium red, Coho, silver	*Oncorhynchus kisutch*
salmon, pink, humpback	*Oncorhynchus gorbuscha*
salmon, red or sockeye	*Oncorhynchus nerka*
salmon, spring or King or Chinook	*Oncorhynchus tschwytscha*
sandfish	*Artoscopus japonica*
sardine (young pilchard)	*Sardina (Clupea) pilchardus*
sardine, Pacific	*Sardinops sadax*
sardinella	*Sardinella* spp.
sauger	*Stizostedion canadense*
saury, Pacific	*Cololabis saira*
scad	*Trachurus* spp., *Decapterus macrocosma*
scad, big-eyed	*Caranx crumenopthalmus*
scup (American porgy)	*Stenotomus chrysops, S. caprinus, Calamus* spp.
sea bass	*Serranus scriba, Lateolabrax japonicus, Cynoscion nobilis*
sea bream	*Sparidae* family, *Nemipterus virugatus, Pagrus major*
shad, American	*Alosa sapidissima*
shad, gizzard	*Clupandon punctatus, Dorosoma cepedianum*
sheefish (inconnu)	*Stenodus leucichthys*
sheepshead	*Archosargus probatocephalus*
siscowet (lake trout)	*Salvelinus namaucush*

Table 28.13: (Cont'd)

skate	*Raja* spp.
smelt	*Osmerus* spp., *Thaleichthys pacificus, Atherinopsis affinis, A. californiensis*
snapper, gray	*Lutjanus griseus*
snapper, red	*Lutjanus campechanus, L. blackfordi*
sole	*Solea* spp.
sole, Canary	*Solea senegalensis*
sole, Dover	*Solea solea*
sole, lemon	*Microstomus kitt*
spade fish (butter fish)	*Scatophagus argus*
spot	*Leiostomus xanthurus*
sprat	*Clupea (Sprattus) sprattus*
St. Peter s fish (john dory)	*Zeus faber*
sturgeon	*Acipenser* spp.
sturgeon, Russian beluga	*Huso huso*
sucker	*Catostomus* spp.
sucker, carp	*Carpiodes forbesi, C. cyprinus*
surgeon fish	*Acanthurus bleekeri*
swordfish	*Xiphias gladius*
tarpon	*Megalops cyprinoides, M. atlanticus*
tautog (blackfish)	*Tautoga onitis*
terrapin	*Malaclemus* spp.
thickback	*Microchirus variegatus*
tigerfish	*Therapon* spp.
tilapia	*Tilapia mossambica*
tilefish	*Lopholatilis chamaeleonticeps*
tomcod	*Microgadus tomcod*
torpedo (hard tail)	*Megalaspis cordyla*
trout, brook	*Savelinas fontinelis*
trout, brown	*Salmo trutta*
trout, cut-throat	*Salmo clarkii*
trout, lake (siscowet)	*Salvelinus namaucush*
trout, mountain, American	*Oncorhyncus clarki*
trout, rainbow (steelhead)	*Salmo gairdneri, S. irideus*
trout, rainbow, American	*Oncorhyncus mykiss*
trout, sea	*Salmo trutta*
tuna, albacore	*Thunnus alalunga*
tuna, Atlantic bonito	*Sarda sarda*
tuna, bluefin	*Thunnus thynnus*
tuna, skipjack	*Euthynnus* spp., *Katsuwonus pelamis*
tuna, yellowfin	*Thunnus albacore, T. albacares*
turbot, diamond	*Hypsopsetta guttualata*
turbot, European	*Scophthalmus maximus*
turbot, spotted, hornyhead	*Pleuronichthys ritteri, P. verticalis*
turtle, green	*Chelonia mydas*
tusk	*Brosme brosme*
weakfish (sold as sea trout)	*Cynoscion regalis*
whale	*Balaenoptera* spp., *Physeter catadon*

Table 28.13: (Cont'd)

whitebait	mixture of young herrings and sprats
whitefish, lake	*Coregonus clupeaformis*
whitefish, lake herring	*Coregnus artedi*
whitefish, mountain	*Prosopium williamsoni*
whiting	*Merlangius merlangus*
whiting, blue	*Micromesistius poutassou*
whiting, common, surf (kingfish)	*Menticirrhinus americanus, M. littoralis, M. saxatilis*
witch	*Glyptocephalus cynoglossus*
wreckfish	*Polyprion americanus*
yellowtail	*Seriola dorsalis*

Table 28.14: Crustaceans

crab	*Cancer* spp., *Carcinus* spp.
crab, blue sea	*Neptunus trituberculatus*
crab, king crab	*Limulus polyphemus,* *Paralilthoides comtschaticus*
crab, soft shell	hermit crabs, sub-order *Anomura*
crawfish (sea water)	*Palinuridae*
crayfish (fresh water)	*Canbarus* spp., *Astacus* spp., *Panulirus* spp.
crayfish, European	*Astacus pallipes*
langouste	*Palinurus vulgaris*
lobster, European	*Homarus gammarus*
lobster, northern (American)	*Homarus americanus*
lobster, Norway (scampi)	*Nephrops norvegicus*
lobster, slipper	*Scyllaridae* spp.
lobster, spiny	*Panulirus* spp.
lobster, squat	*Galatheidae* family
prawn	*Palaemonidae* spp., *Penaeidae* spp., *Pandalidae* spp.
prawn, common European	*Palaemon serratus*
prawn, Pacific northwest (a shrimp)	*Crangon franciscorum*
prawn, Dublin bay (scampi) (a lobster)	*Nephrops norvegicus*
prawn, southern (marketed as a shrimp)	*Panaeus setiferus*
prawn, deepwater	*Pandalus borealis*
scampi	*Nephrops norvegicus*
shrimp brown	*Crangon* spp.
shrimp, opossum	*Neomysis* spp.
shrimp, common pink	*Pandalus montagui*
shrimp, pink grooved	*Penaeus duorarum*
shrimp, white	*Penaeus setiferus*

(1) Zoologically, prawns are distinguished from shrimps by having a long serrated rostrum or beak projecting from the shell. Commercially the distinction is on the basis of size, large shrimps are prawns, small prawns are shrimps. UK labelling regulations define shrimps as having a count of more than 330 /kg of peeled cooked tails of *Palaemonidae* spp., *Peneidae* spp., and *Pandalidae* spp., and prawns as less than 330 /kg of peeled cooked tails of the same species.

Table 28.15: Molluscs

abalone	*Haliotus splendens, H. rufescens, H. cracherodii, H. gigantea, H. japonica*
arkshell	*Cardium* spp., *Anadura* spp.
bêche-de-mer, sea slug	*Stichopus japonicus*
calamary	*Lologo vulgaris*
clam (hard shell clam), quahog	*Mercenaria mercenaria, Venus verrucosa, Meretrix lusoria*
clam, baby	*Tapes japonicum, T. philippinarum*
clam, fingernail	*Musculium lacustre*
clam, freshwater (corb shell)	*Corbicula* spp.
clam, hen	*Mactra sinensis*
clam, razor	*Ensis* spp., *Solen* spp., *Siliqua patula*
clam, short neck	*Venerupis semidecussata*
clam, soft	*Mya arenaria*
clam, tongue (lampshell)	*Linguila uguis*
cockles	*Cardium* spp., *Cerastoderma* spp.
corb shell (freshwater clam)	*Corbicula* spp.
cuttlefish	*Sepia officinalis, Sepia* spp.
horn shell	*Terebrallia aulcatus*
ivory shell	*Babylonica japonica*
lampshell (tongue clam)	*Linguila uguis*
limpet	*Patella vulgata*
mussel	*Mytilus edulis, M. californianus, Corbicula sandai*
mussel, freshwater	*Anodonta cellensis, A. cygnea*
mussel, Mediterranean	*Mytilus galloprovincialis*
octopus	*Octopus* spp., *Polypus* spp.
ormer (abalone)	*Haliotus splendens, H. rufescens, H. cracherodii*
oyster	*Ostrea* spp., *Crassostrea* spp.
oyster, Australian rock	*Saxostrea commercialis*
oyster, native	*Ostrea edulis*
oyster, Pacific	*Crassostrea gigas*
oyster, Portuguese	*Crassostrea angulata*
oyster, Virginia	*Crassostrea virginica*
oyster, western	*Ostrea lurida*
periwinkle (winkle)	*Littorina littorea.*
quahog	*Mya arenaria, Venus mercenaria, Mercenaria mercenaria*
rayed shell	*Solatellina* spp.
scallop, bay	*Pecten* spp., *Plactopectens megellanicus*
scallop, clam	*Pecten* spp, *Tridacna gigas*
scallop, Queen	*Chamys opercularis*
sea ear (abalone)	*Haliotus splendens, H. rufescens, H. cracherodii*
sea slug	*Stichopus japonicus*
sea truffle	*Venus verrucosa.*

Table 28.15: (Cont'd)

sea urchin	*Heliocidaris crassispina*
snail	*Helix pomatia*
snail, white-lipped edible	*Helix vermiculata*
snail, little edible	*Helix pisana*
snail, giant African	*Achatima fulica*
topshell	*Turbo cornutus*
whelk	*Buccinum undatum, Fusus antiquus.*
squid (calamar)	*Loligo* spp., *Illex* spp. *Ommastrephes* spp.
winkle (periwinkle)	*Littorina littorea.*

Table 28.16: Seaweeds

ao nori	*Enteromorpha* spp.
badderlocks	*Alaria esculenta*
bladderwrack	*Fucus vesiculosus*
carrageen	*Chondrus crispus, Gigartina stellata*
dulse	*Rhodymenia palmata, Dilsea carnosa, D. edulis*
fingerware	*Laminaria digitata.*
hijiki	*Hizikia fusiforme*
Iberian, Irish moss	*Chondrus crispus*
kelp	*Laminaria* spp.
knotted wrack	*Ascophyllum nodosum*
konbu breton	*Laminaria digitaria*
laver	*Porphyra* spp.
laver, purple	*Porphyra tenera*
nori	*Porphyra tenera*
oarweed	*Laminaria* spp., *L. digitata*
sea lettuce	*Ulva lactuca*
sea spaghetti	*Himanthalia elongata*
sugarware	*Laminaria saccharina*
tangle	*Laminaria japonica*
wakame	*Undaria pinnatifida*

In addition to the species listed above, for which there are common names, the following species of seaweed are eaten, especially in south-east Asia:
Alaria spp., *Amphiroa* spp., *Cambarns clarkii, Carpopeltis affinis, Caulerpa racemosa, Chaetomorpha crassa, Chamois parvura, Chlorella ellipsoides, Chondrococos japonicus, Chondrus ocellatus, Coccophora langsdorfii, Codium* spp., *Costaria costata, Cystophyllum hakadotense, Dictyopterus prolilfera, Ecklonia cava, Ectocarpus* spp., *Eisenia bicyclis, Endarchne binghamise, Engraulis japonica, Euphasia* spp., *Gelidium* spp., *Gracillaria* spp., *Grateloupia* spp., *Halimeda cuneata, Hujika fusiformis, Hypnea seticulosa, Laurencia okamurai, Metapenaeus* spp., *Monostrima nitidum, Myelophycus caespitosus, Neomycis intermedia, Pandalus* spp., *Paneus* spp., *Sargassum* spp., *Sergestes lucens, Ulva pertusa.*

29

Miscellaneous tables

Table 29.1: Abbreviations

ADI	Acceptable Daily Intake (of an additive, see section 26.2.9)
AIDS	acquired immunodeficiency syndrome
ATP	adenosine triphosphate
ADP	adenosine diphosphate
AMP	adenosine monophosphate
cAMP	$3',5'$-cyclic adenosine monophosphate
A_r	relative atomic mass (also known as atomic weight)
BMI	body mass index (see Table 2.2)
BMR	Basal Metabolic Rate (see Table 5.6)
BV	Biological Value (of a protein, see section 10.7.2)
CAT	computerized axial tomography (see section 2.2.1.6)
CRABP	cellular retinoic acid-binding protein (see section 13.2.5)
CRBP	cellular retinol-binding protein (see section 13.2.5)
DEXA-DPX	dual energy, dual photon X-ray absorption (see section 2.2.1.6)
DNA	deoxyribonucleic acid
e	on food labels, signifying a package size that has been declared to the relevant authorities of the EU
E-	prefix for numbers in the EU list of permitted food additives (see Table 26.4)
EAAI	Essential Amino Acid Index (see section 10.7.2)
EC	Enzyme Commission classification of enzymes (see Tables 29.7 and 29.8)
ELISA	enzyme-linked immunosorbent assay
EU	the European Union
FAD	flavin-adenine dinucleotide (see section 18.2)
FAO	Food and Agriculture Organization of the United Nations
FD&C	Colours permitted in USA for Food, Drug and Cosmetic use
FDA	Food and Drug Adminstration (USA)
FDNB	fluorodinitrobenzene
FMN	flavin mononucleotide (riboflavin phosphate, see section 18.2)
fplc	fast protein liquid chromatography

Table 29.1: (Cont'd)

G-protein	guanine nucleotide-binding regulatory protein
GDP	guanosine diphosphate
glc	gas-liquid chromatography
GMP	Good Manufacturing Practice
GMP	guanosine monophosphate
cGMP	$3',5'$-cyclic guanosine monophosphate
GRAS	generally regarded as safe
GSH	reduced glutathione (γ-glutamyl-cysteinyl-glycine)
GSSG	oxidized glutathione
GTP	guanosine triphosphate
Hb	haemoglobin
HIV	human immunodeficiency virus
hplc	high pressure (performance) liquid chromatography
ICRP	International Commission on Radiological Protection
Ig	immunoglobulin
IEI	Integrated Energy Index (see Table 5.6)
i.u.	international units (of vitamin potency, see sections 13.1.1, 14.3, 15.2)
K_m	the Michaelis constant for an enzyme, effectively the concentration of substrate at which the enzyme achieves 50% of its maximum rate of reaction
LRNI	Lower Reference Nutrient Intake (see section 4.1)
M_r	relative molecular mass (also known as molecular weight)
MAFF	Ministry of Agriculture, Fisheries and Food (UK)
MRI	Magnetic resonance imagining (see section 2.2.1.6)
NAD	nicotinamide adenine dinucleotide (see section 19.2)
NADH	reduced nicotinamide adenine dinucleotide (see section 19.2)
NADP	nicotinamide adenine dinucleotide phosphate (see section 19.2)
NADPH	reduced nicotinamide adenine dinucleotide phosphate (see section 19.2)
NDP	Net Dietary Protein (see section 10.7.2)

Table 29.1: (Cont'd)

NEL	No-Effect Level (of an additive, see section 26.2.9)
NER	Nitrogen Efficiency Ratio (see section 10.7.2)
NMR	nuclear magnetic resonance
NPR	Net Protein Ratio (see section 10.7.2)
NPU	Net Protein Utilization (see section 10.7.2)
nsp	non-starch polysaccharide(s) (see section 7.3)
P_i	inorganic phosphate
PAGE	poly-acrylamide gel electrophoresis
PAL	Physical Activity Level (see Table 5.6)
PAR	Physical Activity Ratio (see Table 5.6)
PCR	polymerase chain reaction
PDCAAS	Protein Digestibility-Corrected Amino Acid Score (see section 10.7.2)
PER	Protein Efficiency Ratio (See section 10.7).
PP_i	inorganic pyrophosphate
PRI	Population Reference Intake (see section 4.1)
RBP	retinol binding protein (see section 13.2.4)
RDA	Recommended Daily (or Dietary) Allowance (see section 4.1)
RDI	Recommended Daily Intake (see section 4.1)
re	retinol equivalents (see section 13.1.1)
RIA	radio-immunoassay
RNA	ribonucleic acid
mRNA	messenger RNA
tRNA	transfer RNA
RNI	Reference Nutrient Intake (see section 4.1)
SAMI	socially acceptable monitoring instrument (see section 5.2.2.2)
SD	standard deviation
SI	Système Internationale d'Unités
tlc	thin-layer chromatography
TOBEC	total body electrical conductivity (see section 2.2.1.8.1)
u	unit (of enzyme activity) = 1 µmol of substrate converted /min at 30°C)
UDP	uridine diphosphate
UNU	United Nations University
UTP	uridine triphosphate
uv	ultraviolet
V_{max}	the maximum rate of reaction achieved by an enzyme with a saturating concentration of substrate
WHO	World Health Organization

Abbreviations for amino acids are shown in Table 10.3, and for fatty acids in Table 8.4.

Table 29.2: Units of physical quantities

physical quantity	unit	symbol	definition
amount of substance	mole	mol	SI base unit
electric charge	coulomb	C	s.A
electric conductance	siemens	S	$A.V^{-1}$
electric current	ampere	A	SI base unit
electric potential difference	volt	V	$J.A^{-1}.s^{-1}$
electric resistance	ohm	Ω	$v.A^{-1}$
electrical capacitance	farad	F	$A.s.V^{-1}$
energy	joule	J	$m^2.kg.s^{-1}$
	calorie	cal	4.186 J
force	newton	N	$J.m^{-1}$
frequency	hertz	Hz	s^{-1}
illuminance	lux	lx	$m^{-2}.cd.sr$
length	metre	m	SI base unit
length	ångstrom	Å	10^{-10} m
luminous flux	lumen	lm	cd.sr
luminous intensity	candela	cd	SI base unit
magnetic flux	weber	Wb	V.s
magnetic flux density	tesla	T	$V.s.m^{-2}$
mass	kilogram	kg	SI base unit
plane angle	radian	rad	SI base unit
power	watt	W	$J.s^{-1}$
pressure	pascal	Pa	$N.m^{-2}$
	bar	bar	10^5 Pa
radiation dose absorbed	gray	Gy	$J.kg^{-1}$
radioactivity	becquerel	Bq	s^{-1}
solid angle	steradian	sr	SI base unit
temperature	degree Celsius	°C	thermodynamic temperature -273.15 K
temperature (thermodynamic)	kelvin	K	SI base unit
time	second	s	SI base unit
volume	litre (cubic decimetre)	L (dm^3)	10^{-3} m^3

Table 29.3: Multiples and submultiples of units

	name	symbol
x 10^{21}	zetta	Z
x 10^{18}	exa	E
x 10^{15}	peta	P
x 10^{12}	tera	T
x 10^9	giga	G
x 10^6	mega	M
x 10^3	kilo	k
x 10^2	centa	ca
x 10	deca	da
x 10^{-1}	deci	d
x 10^{-2}	centi	c
x 10^{-3}	milli	m
x 10^{-6}	micro	μ (or mc)
x 10^{-9}	nano	n
x 10^{-12}	pico	p
x 10^{-15}	femto	f
x 10^{-18}	atto	a
x 10^{-21}	zepto	z

Table 29.4: Periodic Table of the elements

Atomic number is top left of each box, and atomic mass bottom right. Values of atomic mass in parentheses are for the most stable or familiar isotope.

1A 1	IIA 2	IIIB 3	IVB 4	VB 5	VIB 6	VIIB 7	VIIIB 8	VIIIB 9	VIIIB 10	IB 11	IIB 12	IIIA 13	IVA 14	VA 15	VIA 16	VIIA 17	VIIIA 18
1 H 1.01																	2 He 4.00
3 Li 6.94	4 Be 9.01											5 B 10.81	6 C 12.01	7 N 14.01	8 O 16.00	9 F 19.00	10 Ne 20.18
11 Na 22.99	12 Mg 24.30											13 Al 26.98	14 Si 28.09	15 P 30.97	16 S 32.07	17 Cl 35.45	18 Ar 39.95
19 K 39.10	20 Ca 40.08	21 Sc 44.96	22 Ti 47.88	23 V 50.94	24 Cr 52.00	25 Mn 54.94	26 Fe 55.85	27 Co 58.93	28 Ni 58.69	29 Cu 63.55	30 Zn 65.39	31 Ga 69.72	32 Ge 72.59	33 As 74.92	34 Se 78.96	35 Br 79.90	36 Kr 83.80
37 Rb 85.47	38 Sr 87.62	39 Y 88.91	40 Zr 91.22	41 Nb 92.91	42 Mo 95.94	43 Tc (98)	44 Ru 101.07	45 Rh 102.91	46 Pd 106.42	47 Ag 107.87	48 Cd 112.41	49 In 114.82	50 Sn 118.71	51 Sb 121.75	52 Te 127.60	53 I 126.90	54 Xe 131.29
55 Cs 132.90	56 Ba 137.33	57 La* 138.91	72 Hf 178.49	73 Ta 180.85	74 W 183.85	75 Re 186.21	76 Os 190.2	77 Ir 192.22	78 Pt 195.08	79 Au 196.97	80 Hg 200.59	81 Tl 204.38	82 Pb 207.2	83 Bi 208.98	84 Po (209)	85 At (210)	86 Rn (222)
87 Fr (223)	88 Ra 226.02	89 Ac** 227.03	104 Unq (261)	105 Unp (262)	106 Unh (263)	107 Uns (262)											

*the lanthanides

58 Ce 140.12	59 Pr 140.91	60 Nd 144.24	61 Pm (145)	62 Sm 150.36	63 Eu 151.96	64 Gd 157.25	65 Tb 158.92	66 Dy 162.50	67 Ho 164.93	68 Er 167.26	69 Tm 168.94	70 Yb 173.04	71 Lu 174.97

**the actinides

90 Th 232.04	91 Pa 231.04	92 U 238.03	93 Np 237.05	94 Pu (244)	95 Am (243)	96 Cm (247)	97 Bk (247)	98 Cf (251)	99 Es (252)	100 Fm (257)	101 Md (258)	102 No (259)	103 Lr (260)

Table 29.5: The elements, arranged alphabetically

element	symbol	atomic number	atomic weight	periodic series	see section
actinium	Ac	89	227.03	IIIB	-
aluminium	Al	13	26.98	IIIA	25.2
americium	Am	95	(243)	actinide	-
antimony	Sb	51	121.75	VA	25.3
argon	Ar	18	39.95	VIIIA	-
arsenic	As	33	74.92	VA	25.4
astatine	At	85	(210)	VIIA	-
barium	Ba	56	137.33	IIA	-
berkelium	Bk	97	(247)	actinide	-
beryllium	Be	4	9.01	IIA	-
bismuth	Bi	83	208.98	VA	-
boron	B	5	10.81	IIIA	25.5
bromine	Br	35	79.90	VIIA	25.6
cadmium	Cd	48	112.41	IIB	25.7
calcium	Ca	20	40.08	IIA	14.1.1
californium	Cf	98	(251)	actinide	-
carbon	C	6	12.01	IVA	-
cerium	Ce	58	140.12	lanthanide	-
caesium	Cs	55	132.90	IA	25.8
chlorine	Cl	17	35.453	VIIA	25.1
chromium	Cr	24	52.00	VIB	25.9
cobalt	Co	27	58.93	VIIIB	25.10
copper	Cu	29	63.55	IB	25.11
curium	Cm	96	(247)	actinide	-
dysprosium	Dy	66	162.50	lanthanide	-
einsteinium	Es	99	(252)	actinide	-
erbium	Er	68	167.26	lanthanide	-
europium	Eu	63	151.96	lanthanide	-
fermium	Fm	100	(257)	actinide	-
fluorine	F	9	19.00	VIIA	25.12
francium	Fr	87	(223)	IA	-
gadolinium	Gd	64	157.25	lanthanide	-
gallium	Ga	31	69.72	IIIA	-
germanium	Ge	32	72.59	IVA	25.13
gold	Au	79	196.97	IB	-
hafnium	Hf	72	178.49	IVB	-
helium	He	2	4.00	VIIIA	-
holmium	Ho	67	164.93	lanthanide	-
hydrogen	H	1	1.01	IA	-
indium	IN	49	114.82	IIIA	-
iodine	I	53	126.90	VIIA	25.14
iridium	Ir	77	192.22	VIIIB	-
iron	Fe	26	55.85	VIIIB	24
krypton	Kr	36	83.80	VIIIA	-
lanthanum	La	57	138.91	IIIB	-
lawrencium	Lr	103	(260)	actinide	-
lead	Pb	82	207.2	IVA	-
lithium	Li	3	6.94	IA	25.15
lutetium	Lu	71	174.97	lanthanide	-
magnesium	Mg	12	24.30	IIA	25.16
manganese	Mn	25	54.94	VIIB	25.17
mendelevium	Md	101	(258)	actinide	-
mercury	Hg	80	200.59	IIB	25.18
molybdenum	Mo	42	95.94	VIB	25.19
neodymium	Nd	60	144.24	lanthanide	-

Table 29.5: (Cont'd)

element	symbol	atomic number	atomic weight	periodic series	see section
neon	Ne	10	20.18	VIIIA	-
neptunium	Np	93	237.05	actinide	-
nickel	Ni	28	58.69	VIIIB	25.20
niobium	Nb	41	92.91	VB	-
nitrogen	N	7	14.01	VA	10.1
nobelium	No	102	(259)	actinide	-
osmium	Os	76	190.2	VIIIB	-
oxygen	O	8	16.00	VIA	-
palladium	Pd	46	106.42	VIIIB	-
phosphorus	P	15	30.97	VA	14.2
platinum	Pt	78	195.08	VIIIB	-
plutonium	Pu	94	(244)	actinide	-
polonium	Po	84	(209)	VIA	-
potassium	K	19	39.10	IA	25.1
praseodymium	Pr	59	140.91	lanthanide	-
promethemium	Pm	61	(145)	lanthanide	-
protactinium	Pa	91	231.04	actinide	-
radium	Ra	88	226.02	IIA	-
radon	Rn	86	(222)	VIIIA	-
rhenium	Re	75	186.21	VIIB	-
rhodium	Rh	45	102.91	VIIIB	-
rubidium	Rb	37	85.47	IA	-
ruthenium	Ru	44	101.07	VIIIB	-
samarium	Sm	62	150.36	lanthanide	-
scandium	Sc	21	44.96	IIIB	-
selenium	Se	34	78.96	VIA	15.5
silicon	Si	14	28.09	IVA	25.21
silver	Ag	47	107.87	IB	-
sodium	Na	11	22.99	IA	25.1
strontium	Sr	38	87.62	IIA	25.22
sulphur	S	16	32.07	VIA	25.23
tantalum	Ta	73	180.95	VB	-
technetium	Tc	43	(98)	VIIB	-
tellurium	Te	52	127.60	VIA	-
terbium	Tb	65	158.92	lanthanide	-
thallium	Tl	81	204.38	IIIA	-
thorium	Th	90	232.04	actinide	-
thulium	Tm	69	168.93	lanthanide	-
tin	Sn	50	118.71	IVA	25.24
titanium	Ti	22	47.88	IVB	-
tungsten	W	74	183.85	VIB	-
unnihexilium	Unh	106	(263)	VIB	-
unnilpentium	Unp	105	(262)	VB	-
unnilquadium	Unq	104	(261)	IVB	-
unnilseptium	Uns	107	(262)	VIIB	-
uranium	U	92	238.03	actinide	-
vanadium	V	23	50.94	VB	25.25
xenon	Xe	54	131.29	VIIIA	-
ytterbium	Yb	70	173.04	lanthanide	-
yttrium	Y	39	88.91	IIIB	-
zinc	Zn	30	65.39	IIB	25.26
zirconium	Zr	40	91.22	IVB	-

Table 29.6: Isotopes of elements of nutritional importance

element	atomic no		atomic mass	decay	decay energy MeV	half-life	natural abundance, %
hydrogen	1	^{1}H	1.0078	stable	-	-	99.985
(deuterium)		^{2}H	2.0140	stable	-	-	0.015
(tritium)		^{3}H	3.016	beta	0.01861	12.26 y	-
carbon	6	^{12}C	12.000	stable	-	-	98.9
		^{13}C	13.003355	stable	-	-	1.10
		^{14}C	14.003241	beta	0.15648	5730 y	-
nitrogen	7	^{14}N	14.03074	stable	-	-	99.63
		^{13}N	13.005738	positron	2.2205	93.97 min	-
		^{15}N	15.000108	stable	-	-	0.37
oxygen	8	^{16}O	15.994915	stable	-	-	99.762
		^{18}O	17.999160	stable	-	-	0.200
sodium	11	^{23}Na	22.989767	stable	-	-	100
		^{22}Na	21.994434	positron, ec	2.842	2.605 y	-
phosphorus	15	^{31}P	30.973762	stable	-	-	100
		^{32}P	31.973907	beta	1.710	14.28 d	-
sulphur	16	^{32}S	31.972070	stable	-	-	95.02
		^{35}S	34.969031	beta	0.167	87.2 d	-
potassium	19	^{39}K	38.963707	stable	-	-	93.2581
		^{40}K	39.963999	beta	1.32	1.25×10^9 y	0.0117
calcium	20	^{40}Ca	39.962591	stable	-	-	96.941
		^{45}Ca	44.956185	beta	0.257	163.8 d	-
		^{47}Ca	46.954543	beta	1.988	4.536 d	-
chromium	24	^{52}Cr	51.940509	stable	-	-	83.79
		^{53}Cr	52.940651	stable	-	-	9.5
		^{55}Cr	54.940842	beta	2.603	3.5 m	-
		^{56}Cr	55.940643	beta	1.62	5.9 m	-
chlorine	17	^{35}Cl	34.968852	stable	-	-	75.77
		^{36}Cl	35.968306	beta	0.7093	3×10^5 y	-
		^{37}Cl	36.965903	stable	-	-	24.23
iron	26	^{55}Fe	54.938296	ec	0.2314	2.7 y	-
		^{56}Fe	55.934939	stable	-	-	91.72
		^{59}Fe	58.934877	beta	1.565	44.51 d	-
cobalt	27	^{57}Co	56.936294	ec	0.836	271 d	-
		^{58}Co	57.935755	ec, positron	2.30	70.91 d	-
		^{59}Co	58.933198	stable	-	-	100
		^{60}Co	59.933819	beta	2.824	5.272 y	-
nickel	28	^{58}Ni	57.935346	stable	-	-	68.27
		^{60}Ni	59.930788	stable	-	-	26.1
		^{63}Ni	62.929669	beta	0.65	100 y	-
copper	29	^{63}Cu	62.939598	stable	-	-	69.17
		^{65}Cu	64.927793	stable	-	-	30.83
zinc	30	^{64}Zn	63.929145	stable	-	-	48.6
		^{65}Zn	64.929243	ec, positron	1.352	243.8 d	-
		^{66}Zn	65.926034	stable	-	-	27.9
		^{68}Zn	67.924846	stable	-	-	18.8
selenium	34	^{75}Se	74.922521	ec	0.864	118.5 d	-
		^{76}Se	75.919212	stable	-	-	9.0
		^{77}Se	76.919912	stable	-	-	7.6

Table 29.6: (Cont'd)

element	atomic no		atomic mass	decay	decay energy MeV	half-life	natural abundance, %
		^{78}Se	77.919912	stable	-	-	23.5
		^{80}Se	79.916520	stable	-	-	49.6
		^{82}Se	81.916698	stable	-	-	9.4
iodine[1]	53	^{127}I	126.9	stable	-	-	-
		^{125}I	124.904620	ec	0.178	59.9 d	-
		^{131}I	130.906114	beta	0.971	8.04 d	-

(1) Naturally occurring iodine is a complex mixture of stable isotopes.
ec=electron capture

Table 29.7: Classification of enzymes by reaction catalysed : classes and subclasses

All enzymes have systematic (Enzyme Commission) numbers, shown as EC N1.N2.N3.N4, where N1 is the class, N2 the sub-class, N3 the sub-sub-class and N4 the unique number for that enzyme within the class, sub-class and sub-sub-class.

1	oxidoreductases	1.1	acting on CH-OH group of donor
		1.2	acting on aldehyde or oxo group of donor
		1.3	acting on CH-CH of donor
		1.4	acting on CH_2-NH_2 group of donor
		1.5	acting on CH-NH group of acceptor
		1.6	acting on NAD(P)H
		1.7	acting on other nitrogenous compounds as donor
		1.8	acting on sulphur group of donor
		1.9	acting on haem group of donor
		1.10	acting on diphenols as donors
		1.11	acting on peroxide as acceptor
		1.12	acting on hydrogen as donor
		1.13	oxygenases acting on single donor with incorporation of molecular oxygen
		1.14	oxygenases acting on paired donors with incorporation of molecular oxygen
		1.15	acting on superoxide radical as acceptor
		1.16	oxidizing metal ions
		1.17	acting on CH_2 groups
		1.18	acting on reduced ferredoxin as donor
		1.19	acting on reduced flavodoxin as donor
		1.97	other oxidoreductases
2	transferases	2.1	transferring one-carbon groups
		2.2	transferring aldehyde or ketone groups
		2.3	transferring acyl groups
		2.4	transferring sugars
		2.5	transferring alkyl or aryl groups other than methyl
		2.6	transferring nitrogenous groups
		2.7	transferring phosphorus-containing groups
		2.8	transferring sulphur-containing groups
3	hydrolases	3.1	acting on ester bonds
		3.3	acting on ether bonds
		3.2	glycosidases
		3.4	acting on peptide bonds
		3.5	acting on carbon-nitrogen bonds other than peptide bonds
		3.6	acting on acid anhydrides
		3.7	acting on carbon-carbon bonds
		3.8	acting on carbon-halide bonds

Table 29.7: (Cont'd)

		3.9	acting on phosphorus-nitrogen bonds
		3.10	actng on sulphur-nitrogen bonds
		3.11	acting on carbon-phosphorus bonds
		3.12	acting on sulphur-sulphur bonds
4	lyases	4.1	carbon-carbon lyases
		4.2	carbon-oxygen lyases
		4.3	carbon-nitrogen lyases
		4.4	carbon-sulphur lyases
		4.5	carbon-halide lyases
		4.6	phosphorus-oxygen lyases
		4.99	other lyases
5	isomerases	5.1	racemases and epimerases
		5.2	*cis-trans-* isomerases
		5.3	intramolecular oxidoreductases
		5.4	intramolecular transferases (mutases)
		5.5	intramolecular lyases
		5.99	other isomerases
6	ligases	6.1	forming carbon-oxygen bonds
		6.2	forming carbon-sulphur bonds
		6.3	forming carbon-nitrogen bonds
		6.4	forming carbon-carbon bonds
		6.5	forming phosphoric ester bonds

Source: Enzyme Nomenclature: *Recommendations (1992) of the Nomenclaturee Committee of the International Union of Biochemistry and Molecular Biology*, Academic Press, San Diego, CA. The enzyme nomenclature database, searchable by EC number, enzyme class, official or alternative names or searching in comments line is available on the World-wide Web from the ExPASy molecular biology server at http://expasy.hcuge.ch/sprot/enzyme.html.

Table 29.8: Classification of enzyme reactions by the reaction catalysed: clasees, subclasses and sub-subclasses

All enzymes have systematic (Enzyme Commission) numbers, shown as EC N1.N2.N3.N4, where N1 is the class, N2 the sub-class, N3 the sub-sub-class and N4 the unique number for that enzyme within the class, sub-class and sub-sub-class.

class		sub-class		sub-sub-class	
1	oxidoreductases	1.1	acting on CH-OH group of donor	1.1.1	NAD(P)$^+$ as acceptor
				1.1.2	cytochrome as acceptor
				1.1.3	oxygen as acceptor
				1.1.4	disulphide as acceptor
				1.1.5	quinone as acceptor
				1.1.99	other acceptor
		1.2	acting on aldehyde or oxo group of donor	1.2.1	NAD(P)$^+$ as acceptor
				1.2.2	cytochrome as acceptor
				1.2.3	oxygen as acceptor
				1.2.5	quinone as acceptor
				1.2.7	iron-sulphur protein as acceptor
				1.2.99	other acceptor
		1.3	acting on CH-CH of donor	1.3.1	NAD(P)$^+$ as acceptor
				1.3.2	cytochrome as acceptor
				1.3.3	oxygen as acceptor
				1.3.4	disulphide as acceptor
				1.3.5	quinone as acceptor
				1.3.7	iron-sulphur protein as acceptor
				1.3.99	other acceptor
		1.4	acting on CH$_2$-NH$_2$ group of donor	1.4.1	NAD(P)$^+$ as acceptor
				1.4.2	cytochrome as acceptor
				1.4.3	oxygen as acceptor
				1.4.4	disulphide as acceptor
				1.4.7	iron-sulphur protein as acceptor
				1.4.99	other acceptor
		1.5	acting on CH-NH group of acceptor	1.5.1	NAD(P)$^+$ as acceptor
				1.5.3	oxygen as acceptor
				1.5.4	disulphide as acceptor
				1.5.5	quinone as acceptor
				1.5.99	other acceptor
		1.6	acting on NAD(P)H	1.6.1	NAD(P)$^+$ as acceptor
				1.6.2	cytochrome as acceptor
				1.6.4	disulphide as acceptor
				1.6.5	quinone as receptor
				1.6.6	nitrogenous group as acceptor
				1.6.8	flavin as acceptor
				1.6.99	other acceptor
		1.7	acting on other nitrogenous compounds as donor	1.7.2	cytochrome as acceptor
				1.7.3	oxygen as acceptor
				1.7.7	iron-sulphur protein as acceptor
				1.7.99	other acceptor
		1.8	acting on sulphur group of donor	1.8.1	NAD(P)$^+$ as acceptor
				1.8.2	cytochrome as acceptor
				1.8.3	oxygen as acceptor
				1.8.4	disulphide as acceptor

Table 29.8: (Cont'd)

class	sub-class		sub-sub-class	
		1.8.5	quinone as receptor	
		1.8.7	iron-sulphur protein as acceptor	
		1.8.99	other acceptor	
	1.9	acting on haem group of donor	1.9.3	oxygen as acceptor
			1.9.6	nitrogenous group as acceptor
			1.9.99	other acceptor
	1.10	acting on diphenols as donors	1.10.1	$NAD(P)^+$ as acceptor
			1.10.2	cytochrome as acceptor
			1.10.3	oxygen as acceptor
			1.10.99	other acceptor
	1.11	acting on peroxide as acceptor	1.11.1	-
	1.12	acting on hydrogen as donor	1.12.1	$NAD(P)^+$ as acceptor
			1.12.2	cytochrome as acceptor
			1.12.99	other acceptor
	1.13	oxygenases acting on single donor with incorporation of molecular oxygen	1.13.11	incorporation of 2 atoms of oxygen
			1.13.12	incorporation of 1 atom of oxygen
			1.13.99	miscellaneous
	1.14	oxygenases acting on paired donors with incorporation of molecular oxygen	1.14.11	2-oxo-glutarate as one donor, incorporation of 1 oxygen atom into each donor
			1.14.12	NAD(P)H as one donor, and incorporation of 2 oxygen atoms into other donor
			1.14.13	NAD(P)H as one donor, and incorporation of 1 oxygen atom
			1.14.14	reduced flavin as one donor, and incorporation of 1 oxygen atom
			1.14.15	reduced iron-sulphur protein as one donor, and incorporation of 1 oxygen atom
			1.14.16	reduced pteridine as one donor, and incorporation of 1 oxygen atom
			1.14.17	ascorbate as one donor, and incorporation of 1 oxygen atom
			1.14.18	another compound as as one donor, and incorporation of 1 oxygen atom
			1.14.99	miscellaneous
	1.15	acting on superoxide radical as acceptor		
	1.16	oxidizing metal ions	1.16.1	$NAD(P)^+$ as acceptor
			1.16.3	oxgen as acceptor
	1.17	acting on CH_2 groups	1.17.1	$NAD(P)^+$ as acceptor
			1.17.3	oxygen as acceptor
			1.17.4	disulphide as acceptor
			1.17.99	other acceptors
	1.18	acting on reduced ferredoxin as donor	1.18.1	$NAD(P)^+$ as acceptor
			1.18.6	dinitrogen as acceptor
			1.18.99	H^+ as acceptor
	1.19	acting on reduced flavodoxin as donor	1.19.6	dinitrogen as acceptor
	1.97	other oxidoreductases		

Table 29.8: (Cont'd)

class		sub-class		sub-sub-class	
2	transferases	2.1	transferring one-carbon groups	2.1.1	methyl groups
				2.1.2	hydroxymethyl, formyl groups
				2.1.3	carboxyl, carbamoyl groups
				2.1.4	amidino groups
		2.2	transferring aldehyde or ketone groups		
		2.3	transferring acyl groups	2.3.1	acyl groups
				2.3.2	amino acids
		2.4	transferring sugars	2.4.1	hexoses
				2.4.2	pentoses
				2.4.99	other glycosyl groups
		2.5	transferring alkyl or aryl groups other than methyl		
		2.6	transferring nitrogenous groups	2.6.1	amino groups
				2.6.2	oximino groups
				2.6.99	other nitrogenous groups
		2.7	transferring phosphorus-containing groups	2.7.1	phosphotransferase to alcohol group
				2.7.2	phosphotransferase to carboxyl group
				2.7.3	phosphotransferase to nitrogenous group
				2.7.4	phosphotransferase to phosphate group
				2.7.6	diphosphotransferases
				2.7.7	nucleotidyltransferases
				2.7.8	transferases for other substituted phosphate groups
				2.7.9	phosphotransferases with paired acceptors
		2.8	transferring sulphur-containing groups	2.8.1	sulphurtransferases
				2.8.2	sulphotransferases
				2.8.3	CoA transferases
3	hydrolases	3.1	acting on ester bonds	3.1.1	hydrolysing carboxylic esters
				3.1.2	hydrolysing thiol esters
				3.1.3	hydrolysing phosphoric monoesters
				3.1.4	hydrolysing phosphoric diesters
				3.1.5	hydrolysing triphosphoric monoesters
				3.1.6	hydrolysing sulphuric esters
				3.1.7	hydrolysing diphosphoric monoesters
				3.1.8	hydrolysing phosphoric triesters
				3.1.11	exo-deoxyribonucleases yielding 5'-phosphomonoesters
				3.1.13	exo-ribonucleases yielding 5'-phosphomonoesters
				3.1.14	other exo-ribonucleases
				3.1.15	exonucleases yielding 5'-phosphomonoesters
				3.1.16	other exonucleases
				3.1.21	endo-deoxyribonucleases yielding 5'-phosphomonoesters
				3.1.22	other endo-deoxyribonucleases
				3.1.25	site-specific endo-deoxyribonucleases specific for altered bases

Table 29.8: (Cont'd)

class		sub-class		sub-sub-class	
				3.1.26	endo-ribonucleases yielding 5′-phosphomonoesters
				3.1.27	other endo-ribonucleases
				3.1.30	yielding 5 -phosphomonoesters
				3.1.31	other endonucleases
		3.2	glycosidases	3.2.1	hydrolysing *O*-glycosyl compounds
				3.2.2	hydrolysing *N*-glycosyl compounds
				3.2.3	hydrolysing *S*-glycosyl compounds
		3.3	acting on ether bonds	3.3.1	hydrolysing thio-ethers
				3.3.2	hydrolysing ethers
		3.4	acting on peptide bonds	3.4.11	aminopeptidases
				3.4.13	dipeptidases
				3.4.14	dipeptidyl-peptidases and tripeptidyl-peptidases
				3.4.15	peptidyl-dipeptidases
				3.4.16	serine-type caarboxypeptidases
				3.4.17	metallo-carboxypeptidases
				3.4.18	cysteine-type carboxypeptidases
				3.4.19	omega peptidases
				3.4.21	serine endopeptidases
				3.4.22	cysteine endopeptidases
				3.4.23	aspartic endopeptidases
				3.4.24	metallo-endopeptidases
				3.4.99	endopeptidases, unknown catalytic mechanism
		3.5	acting on carbon-nitrogen bonds other than peptide bonds	3.5.1	in linear amides
				3.5.2	in cyclic amides
				3.5.3	in linear amidines
				3.5.4	in cyclic amidines
				3.5.5	in nitriles
				3.5.99	in other compounds
		3.6	acting on acid anhydrides	3.6.1	phosphorus containing anhydrides
				3.6.2	sulphonyl-containing anhydrides
		3.7	acting on carbon-carbon bonds	3.7.1	in ketonic substances
		3.8	acting on carbon-halide bonds	3.8.1	in C-halide compounds
		3.9	acting on phosphorus-nitrogen bonds		
		3.10	acting on sulphur-nitrogen bonds		
		3.11	acting on carbon-phosphorus bonds		
		3.12	acting on sulphur-sulphur bonds		
4	lyases	4.1	carbon-carbon lyases		
		4.1.1	carboxy-lyases (decarboxylases)		
		4.1.2	aldehyde-lyases		
		4.1.3	oxo-acid lyases		
		4.1.99	other carbon-carbon lyases		
		4.2	carbon-oxygen lyases		
				4.2.1	hydro-lyases
				4.2.2	acting on polysaccharides
				4.2.99	other carbon-oxygen lyases
		4.3	carbon-nitrogen lyases		
				4.3.1	ammonia lyases

Table 29.8: (Cont'd)

class		sub-class		sub-sub-class	
				4.3.2	amidine lyases
				4.3.3	amine lyases
				4.3.99	other carbon-nitrogen lyases
		4.4	carbon-sulphur lyases		
		4.5	carbon-halide lyases		
		4.6	phosphorus-oxygen lyases		
		4.99	other lyases		
5	isomerases	5.1	racemases and epimerases	5.1.1	acting on amino acids and derivatives
				5.1.2	acting on hydroxy-acids and derivatives
				5.1.3	acting on carbohydrates and derivatives
				5.1.99	acting on other compounds
		5.2	*cis-trans-* isomerases		
		5.3	intramolecular oxidoreductases	5.3.1	interconverting aldoses and ketoses
				5.3.2	interconverting keto and enol groups
				5.3.3	transposing C=C bonds
				5.3.4	transposing S-S bonds
				5.3.99	other intramolecular oxidoreductases
		5.4	intramolecular transferases (mutases)	5.4.1	transferring acyl groups
				5.4.2	transferring phosphate groups (phosphomutases)
				5.4.3	transferring amino groups
				5.4.99	transferring other groups
		5.5	intramolecular lyases		
				5.99	other isomerases
6	ligases	6.1	forming carbon-oxygen bonds	6.1.1	forming aminoacyl-tRNA
		6.2	forming carbon-sulphur bonds	6.2.1	acid-thiol ligases
		6.3	forming carbon-nitrogen bonds	6.3.1	amide synthetases
				6.3.2	peptide synthases
				6.3.3	cyclo-ligases
				6.3.4	other carbon-nitrogen ligases
				6.3.5	carbon-nitrogen ligases with glutamine as amido-N-donor
		6.4	forming carbon-carbon bonds		
		6.5	forming phosphoric ester bonds		

Source: *Enzyme Nomenclature: Recommendations (1992) of the Nomenclaturee Committee of the International Union of Biochemistry and Molecular Biology*, Academic Press, San Diego, CA. The enzyme nomenclature database, searchable by EC number, enzyme class, official or alternative names or searching in comments line is available on the World-wide Web from the ExPASy molecular biology server at http://expasy.hcuge.ch/sprot/enzyme.html.

Table 29.9: Bibliography of systematic nomenclature of compounds of nutritional importance

Systematic rules for naming compounds of nutritional importance have been published by the Nomenclature Comittee of the International Union of Biochemistry and Molecular Biology as shown below. In addition, all the recommendations have been reprinted in *Biochemical Nomenclature and Related Documents, A Compendium* (2nd edn, 1992), published for the International Union of Biochemistry and Molecular Biology by Portland Press, London.

Amino acids and peptides

Nomenclature and symbolism for amino acids and peptides. *European Journal of Biochemistry*, **138**, 9–37 (1984).
Nomenclature of glycoproteins, glycopeptides and peptidoglycans. *European Journal of Biochemistry*, **159**, 1–6 (1986).
The nomenclature of peptide hormones. *European Journal of Biochemistry*, **55**, 485–6 (1975).
Abbreviated nomenclature of synthetic polypeptides (polymerized amino acids). *European Journal of Biochemistry*, **26**, 301–4 (1972).
Abbreviations and symbols for the description of the conformation of polypeptide chains. *European Journal of Biochemistry*, **17**, 193–201 (1970).

Carbohydrates

Tentative rules for carbohydrate nomenclature. *European Journal of Biochemistry*, **21**, 455–77 (1969).
Nomenclarure of cyclitols. *European Journal of Biochemistry*, **57**, 1–7 (1975).
Numbering of atoms in myo-inositol. *European Journal of Biochemistry*, **180**, 485–6 (1989).
Conformational nomenclature for five- and six-membered ring forms of monosaccharides and their derivateves. *European Journal of Biochemistry*, **111**, 295–8 (1980).
Nomenclature of unsaturated monosaccharides. *European Journal of Biochemistry*, **119** 103 (1981).
Nomenclature of branched-chain monosaccharides. *European Journal of Biochemistry*, **119**, 5–8 (1981).
Abbreviated terminology of oligosaccharide chains. *European Journal of Biochemistry*, **126**, 433–7 (1982).
Polysaccharide nomenclature. *European Journal of Biochemistry*, **126**, 439–41 (1982).
Symbols for specifying the conformation of polysaccharide chains. *European Journal of Biochemistry*, **131**, 5–7 (1983).

Lipids and fat-soluble vitamins

The nomenclature of lipids. *European Journal of Biochemistry*, **79**, 11–21 (1976).
The nomenclature of steroids. *European Journal of Biochemistry*, **186**, 429–58 (1989).
Nomenclature of quinones with isoprenoid side chains. *European Journal of Biochemistry*, **53**, 15–18 (1975).
Tentative rules for the nomenclature of carotenoids. *European Journal of Biochemistry*, **25**, 397–408 (1972).
Nomenclature of carotenoids, amendments 1974. *European Journal of Biochemistry*, **57**, 317–8 (1975).
Nomenclature of tocopherols and related compounds. *European Journal of Biochemistry*, **123**, 473–5 (1982).
Nomenclature of vitamin D. *European Journal of Biochemistry*, **124**, 223–7 (1982).
Nomenclature of retinoids. *European Journal of Biochemistry*, **129**, 1–5 (1982).

Water-soluble vitamins

Nomenclature and symbols for folic acid and related compounds. *European Journal of Biochemistry*, **168**, 251–3 (1987).
Nomenclature for vitamins B-6 and related compounds. *European Journal of Biochemistry*, **40**, 325–7 (1973).
The nomenclature of corrinoids. *European Journal of Biochemistry*, **45**, 7–12 (1974).

References

Abboud, M.R., Alexander, D., and Najjar, S.S. (1985). Diabetes mellitus, thiamin-dependent megaloblastic anaemia and sensorineural deafness associated with deficient α-ketoglutarate dehydrogenase activity. *Journal of Pediatrics*, **107**, 537–41.

Abrams, C.K., Hamosh, M., Dutta, S.K., Hubbard, V.S., and Hamosh, P. (1987). Role of nonpancreatic lipolytic activity in exocrine pancreatic insufficiency. *Gastroenterology*, **92**, 125–9.

Adams, P.W., Folkard, J., Wynn, V., and Seed, M. (1976). Influence of oral contraceptives, pyridoxine and tryptophan on carbohydrate metabolism. *Lancet*,(i), 759–64.

Adelakan, D.A., and Thurnham, D.I. (1986). The influence of riboflavin deficiency on absorption and liver storage of iron in the growing rat. *British Journal of Nutrition*, **56**, 171–9.

Adlerkreutz, H., Markannen, H., and Watanabe, S. (1993). Plasma concentrations of phyto-oestrogens in Japanese man. *Lancet*, **342**, 1209–10.

Aggett, P.J. (1991). The assessment of zinc status: a personal view. *Proceedings of the Nutrition Society*, **50**, 9–17.

Aggett, P.J., and Favier, A. (1993). Flair concerted action No 10 status papers: Zinc. *International Journal of Vitamin and Nutrition Research*, **63**, 301–7.

Ainsworth, B.E., Haskell, W.L., Leon, A.S., Jacobs, D.R., Montoye, H.J., Sallis, J.F., and Paffenberger, R.S. (1992). Compendium of physical activities: classification of energy costs of human physical activities. *Medicine and Science in Sports and Exercise*, **25**, 71–80.

Allgood, V.A., and Cidlowski, J.A. (1992). Vitamin B_6 modulates transcriptional activation by multiple members of the steroid hormone receptor superfamily. *Journal of Biological Chemistry*, **267**, 3819–24.

Allgood, V.E., Powell-Oliver, F.E., and Cidlowski, J.A. (1990). Vitamin B_6 influences glucocorticoid receptor-dependent gene expression. *Journal of Biological Chemistry*, **265**, 12424–33.

Allison, J.B. (1959). In *Protein and Amino Acid Nutrition* (ed. A.A. Albanese) Chapter 5. Academic Press, London.

Allison, P.M., Mummah-Schendel, L.L., Kindberg, C.G., Harms, C.S., Bang, N.U., and Suttie, J.W. (1987). Effects of a vitamin K deficient diet and antibiotics in normal human volunteers. *Journal of Laboratory and Clinical Medicine*, **110**, 180–8.

Allison, R.M., Laird, W.M., and Synge, R.L.M. (1973). Notes on a deamination method proposed for determining 'chemically available lysine' of proteins. *British Journal of Nutrition*, **29**, 51–5.

alpha-Tocopherol, beta-Carotene Cancer Prevention Study Group (1994). The effect of vitamin E and beta-carotene on the incidence of lung cancer and other cancers in male smokers. *New England Journal of Medicine*, **330**, 1029–35.

Altar, C.A., Bennett, B.L., Wallace, R., and Yuwiler, A. (1983). Glucocorticoid induction of tryptophan oxygenase: attenuation by intragastrically administered carbohydrate and metabolites. *Biochemical Pharmacology*, **32**, 979–84.

Altman, K., and Greengard, O. (1966). Correlation of kynurenine excretion with liver tryptophan pyrrolase levels in disease and after hydrocortisone induction. *Journal of Clinical Investigation*, **45**, 1527–34.

Ames, B.N. (1983). Dietary carcinogens and anti-carcinogens; oxygen radicals and degenerative diseases. *Science*, **221**, 1256–4.

Ames, B.N., Profet, M., and Gold, L.S. (1990a). Dietary pesticides (99.99% all natural). *Proceedings of the National Academy of Sciences*, **87**, 7777–81.

Ames, B.N., Profet, M., and Gold, L.S. (1990b). Nature's chemicals and synthetic chemicals: comparative toxicity. *Proceedings of the National Academy of Sciences*, **87**, 7782–6

Andersen, T., Juhl, E., and Quaade, F. (1980). Jejunoileal bypass for obesity: what can we learn from a literature study? *American Journal of Clinical Nutrition*, **33**, 440–5.

Andres, R., Elahi, D., Tobin, J.D., Muller, D.C., and Brant, L. (1985). Impact of age on weight goals. *Annals of Internal Medicine*, **103**, 1030–3.

Anon (1989). Zinc fingers and vitamin D resistance. *Lancet* (i), 478.

Appling, D.R., and Chytil, F. (1981). Evidence for a role of retinoic acid (vitamin A acid) in the maintenance of testosterone production in male rats. *Endocrinology*, **108**, 2120–3.

Arinze, J.C., and Mistry, S.P. (1971). Activities of some biotin enzymes and certain aspects of gluconeogenesis during biotin deficiency. *Comparative Biochemistry and Physiology*, **38B**, 285–294.

Arky, R.A., Veverbrants, E., and Abramson, E.A. (1968). Irreversible hypoglycaemia: a complication of alcohol and insulin. *Journal of the American Medical Association*, **206**, 575–8.

Arnaud, J. (1993). Flair concerted action No 10 status papers: Copper. *International Journal of Vitamin and Nutrition Research*, **63**, 308–11.

Aw, T.Y., Jones, D.P., and McCormick, D.B. (1983). Uptake of riboflavin by isolated rat liver cells. *Journal of Nutrition*, **113**, 1249–54.

Aynsley-Green, A., Lucas, A., Lawson, G.R., and Bloom, S.R. (1990). Gut hormones and regulatory peptides in relation to enteral feeding, gastroenteritis, and necrotizing enterocolitis in infancy. *Journal of Pediatrics*, **117**, S24–32.

Baggenstoss, A.H., Christensen, N.A., Berge, K.G., Baldus, W.P., Spieckerman, R.E., and Ellefson, R.D. (1967). Fine structural changes in the liver in hypercholesteremic patients receiving long-term nicotinic acid therapy. *Mayo Clinic Proceedings*, **42**, 385–99.

Bahna, S.L. (1978). Control of milk allergy: a challenge for physicians, mothers and industry. *Annals of Allergy*, **41**, 1–12.

Bailey, L.B. (1990). Folate status assessment. *Journal of Nutrition*, **120**, 1508–11.

Baker, G.L. (1969). Human adipose tissue composition and age. *American Journal of Clinical Nutrition*, **22**, 829–35.

Baker, E.M., Hodges, R.E., Hood, J., Sauberlich, H.E., and March, S. (1969). Metabolism of ascorbic acid-1-^{14}C in experimental human scurvy. *American Journal of Clinical Nutrition*, **22**, 549–58.

Baker, E.M., Hodges, R.E., Hood, J., Sauberlich, H.E., March, S., and Canham, J.E. (1971). Metabolism of ^{14}C and ^{3}H labelled L-ascorbic acid in human scurvy. *American Journal of Clinical Nutrition*, **24**, 444–54.

Baker, H., Frank, O., Rusoff, I.I., Morch, K.R.A., and Huntner, S.H. (1978). Protein quality of foodstuffs determined with *Tetrahymena thermophila* and rat. *Nutrition Reports International*, **17**, 525.

Balfour, J.A., and McTavish, D. (1993). Acarbose: an update of its pharmacology and therapeutic use in diabetes mellitus. *Drugs*, **46**, 1025–54.

Baram, J., Chabner, B.A., Drake, J.C., Fitzhugh, A.L., Sholar, P.W., and Allegra, C.J. (1988). Identification and biochemical properties of 10–formyldihydrofolate, a novel folate found in methotrexate-treated cells. *Journal of Biological Chemistry*, **263**, 7105–11.

Barker, T.C., Oddy, D.J., and Yudkin, J. (1970). *The Dietary Surveys of Dr Edward Smith*, 1862–3. Staples Press, London.

Barker, D.J.P., Osmond, C., Golding, J., Kuh, D., and Wadsworth, M.E.J. (1989*a*). Growth in utero, blood pressure in childhood and adult life, and mortality from cardiovascular disease. *British Medical Journal*, **298**, 564–7.

Barker, D.J.P., Osmond, C., and Law, C.M. (1989*b*). The intrauterine and early post-natal origins of cardiovascular disease and chronic bronchitis. *Journal of Epidemiology and Public Health*, **43**, 237–40.

Barker, D.J.P., Winter, P.D., Osmond, C., Margetts, B., and Simmonds, S.J. (1989*c*). Weight in infancy and death from ischaemic heart disease. *Lancet*, **(ii)**, 577–80.

Barman, T.E. (1968). *Enzyme Handbook*, Vol. 1, 1968, Vol. 2, 1969, Supplement 1, 1974. Springer Verlag, Berlin.

Barnard, H.C., de Kock, J.J., Vermaak, W.J.H., and Potgieter, G.M. (1986). A new perspective in the assessment of vitamin B-6 nutritional status during pregnancy in humans. *Journal of Nutrition*, **117**, 1303–6.

Baron, D.N., Dent, C.E., Harris, H., Hart, E.W., and Jepson, J.B. (1956). Hereditary pellagra-like skin rash with temporary cerebellar ataxia, constant renal aminoaciduria and other bizarre biochemical features. *Lancet* **(ii)**, 421–8.

Bates, C.J. (1989). Metabolism of [^{14}C]adipic acid in riboflavin deficient rats, a test *in vivo* for fatty acid oxidation. *Journal of Nutrition*, **119**, 887–91.

Bates, C.J. (1990). Liberation of $^{14}CO_2$ from [^{14}C]adipic acid and [^{14}C]octanoic acid by adult rats during riboflavin deficiency and its reversal. *British Journal of Nutrition*, **63**, 553–62.

Bates, C.J. (1993). Flair Concerted action no 10 status papers: riboflavin. *International Journal of Vitamin and Nutrition Research*, **63**, 274–7.

Bates, C.J., and Heseker, H. (1994). Human bioavailability of vitamins. *Nutrition Research Reviews*, **7**, 93–128.

Bayoumi, R.A.L., Kirwan, J.R., and Smith, W.R.D. (1972). Some effects of dietary vitamin B_6 deficiency and 4–deoxypyridoxine on GABA metabolism in rat brain. *Journal of Neurochemistry*, **19**, 569–76.

Belavady, B., and Rao, P.U. (1979). Leucine and isoleucine content of jowar and its pellagragenicity. *Indian Journal of Experimental Biology*, **17**, 659–61.

Bell, E. (1980). The excretion of a vitamin B_6 metabolite and the probability of recurrence of early breast cancer. *European Journal of Cancer*, **16**, 297–8.

Bell, G., Higgins, C.F., Payne, G.M., and Payne, J.W. (1977). In *Nutritional Evaluation of Cereal Mutants*. International Atomic Energy Agency, Vienna.

Bender, A.E. (1957). Biological methods of evaluating protein quality. *Proceedings of the Nutrition Society*, **17**, 85–91.

Bender, A.E. (1958). The stability of vitamin C in a commercial fruit squash. *Journal of the Science of Food and Agriculture*, **11**, 754–60.

Bender, A.E. (1961). Protein Values by chemical analysis. *Progress in Meeting Protein Needs of Infants and Preschool Children*. National Academy of Science / National Research Council, Washington, DC.

Bender, A.E. (1982). Evaluation of protein quality. *Proceedings of the Nutrition Society*, **41**, 267–76.

Bender, A.E. (1983*a*). Haemagglutinins (lectins) in beans. *Food Chemistry*, **11**, 309–20.

Bender, D.A. (1983*b*). Effects of a dietary excess of leucine on the metabolism of tryptophan in the rat: a mechanism for the pellagragenic action of leucine. *British Journal of Nutrition*, **50**, 25–32.

Bender, D.A. (1983c). Effects of oestradiol and vitamin B$_6$ on tryptophan metabolism in the rat: implications for the interpretation of the tryptophan load test for vitamin B$_6$ nutritional status. *British Journal of Nutrition*, 50, 33–42.

Bender, D.A. (1984). B vitamins in the nervous system. *Neurochemistry International*, 6, 297–321.

Bender, D.A. (1985). *Amino Acid Metabolism*. Wiley, Chichester.

Bender, D.A. (1987). Oestrogens and vitamin B$_6$ — actions and interactions. *World Review of Nutrition and Dietetics*, 51, 140–88.

Bender, D.A. (1989). Effects of dietary excess leucine and of the addition of leucine and 2–oxo-isocaproate on the metabolism of tryptophan in isolated rat liver cells. *British Journal of Nutrition*, 61, 629–40.

Bender, D.A. (1993). Lack of concordance between two biochemical indices of vitamin B$_6$ nutritional status. *Proceedings of the Nutrition Society*, 52, 315A.

Bender, D.A. (1994). Novel functions of vitamin B$_6$. *Proceedings of the Nutrition Society*, 53, 625–30.

Bender, A.E., and Doell, B.H. (1957). Biological evaluation of proteins: a new aspect. *British Journal of Nutrition*, 11, 140–8.

Bender, D.A., and McCreanor, G.M. (1985). Kynurenine hydroxylase: a potential rate-limiting enzyme in tryptophan metabolism. *Biochemical Society Transactions*, 13, 441–3.

Bender, A.E., and Miller, D.S. (1953). A new brief method of estimating net protein value. *Biochemical Journal*, 53, vii.

Bender, D.A., and Olufunwa, R. (1988). Utilization of tryptophan, nicotinamide and nicotinic acid as precursors for nicotinamide nucleotide synthesis in isolated rat liver cells. *British Journal of Nutrition*, 59, 279–87.

Bender, D.A., and Totoe, L. (1984a). High doses of vitamin B$_6$ in the rat are associated with inhibition of hepatic tryptophan metabolism and increased uptake of tryptophan into the brain. *Journal of Neurochemistry*, 43, 733–6.

Bender, D.A., and Totoe, L. (1984b). Inhibition of tryptophan metabolism by oestrogens in the rat, a factor in the aetiology of pellagra. *British Journal of Nutrition*, 51, 219–25.

Bender, D.A., and Wynick, D. (1981). Inhibition of kynureninase by oestrone sulphate, an alternative explanation for abnormal results of tryptophan load tests in women receiving oestrogenic steroids. *British Journal of Nutrition*, 45, 269–75.

Bender, D.A., Earl, C.J., and Lees, A.J. (1979). Niacin depletion in Parkinsonian patients treated with L-dopa, Benserazide or Carbidopa. *Clinical Science and Molecular Medicine*, 56, 89–93.

Bender, D.A., Magboul, B.I., and Wynick, D. (1982). Probable mechanisms of regulation of the utilization of dietary tryptophan nicotinamide and nicotinic acid as precursors of nicotinamide nucleotides in the rat. *British Journal of Nutrition*, 48, 119–27.

Benesch, R.E., Kwong, S., Benesch, R., and Baugh, C.M. (1985). The binding of folyl- and antifolylpolyglutamates to hemoglobin. *Journal of Biological Chemistry*, 260, 14653–8 .

Benn, R.T. (1971). Some mathematical properties of weight-for-height indices used as measures of adiposity. *British Journal of Preventive and Social Medicine*, 25, 42–50.

Bennett, N., Dodd, T., Flatley, J., Freeth, S., and Bolling, K. (1995). *Health Survey for England, 1993*. OPCS, London.

Benninck, H.J.T.C., and Schreurs, W.H.P. (1975). Improvement of oral glucose tolerance in gestational diabetes by pyridoxine. *British Medical Journal*, (iii), 13–5.

Bennion, L.J., and Grundy, S.M. (1975). Effects of obesity and caloric intake on biliary lipid metabolism in man. *Journal of Clinical Investigation*, 56, 996–1011.

Bergner H (1977). *Proceedings of the Federation of European Biochemical Societies, Copenhagen*, 44, 149.

Bernback, S., and Blackberg, L. (1989). Human gastric lipase. The N terminal tetrapeptide is essential for lipid binding and lipase activity. *European Journal of Biochemistry*, 182, 495–9.

Bernback, S., Blackberg, L., and Hernell, O. (1989). Fatty acids generated by gastric lipase promote human milk triacylglycerol digestion by pancreatic colipase-dependent lipase. *Biochimica et Biophysica Acta*, 1001, 286–93.

Berndt, T.J., Knox, F.G., Kempson, S.A., and Dousa, T.P. (1981). Nicotinamide adenine dinucleotide and renal response to parathyroid hormone. *Endocrinology*, 108, 2005–7.

Bessey, O.A., Adam, D.J.D., and Hansen, A.E. (1957). Intake of vitamin B$_6$ and infantile convulsions, a first approximation of the requirements of pyridoxine in infants. *Pediatrics*, 20, 33–44.

Bettger, W.J., and O'Dell, B.L. (1993). Physiological roles of zinc in the plasma membrane of mammalian cells. *Journal of Nutritional Biochemistry*, 4, 194–207.

Bierman, E.L., Bagdade, J.D., and Porte, D. (1968). Obesity and diabetes: the odd couple. *American Journal of Clinical Nutrition*, 21, 1434–7.

Billings, R.E. (1984). Decreased hepatic 5,10–methylenetetrahydrofolate reductase activity in mice after chronic phenytoin treatment. *Molecular Pharmacology*, 25, 459–66.

Birch, G.G., Bointon, B.M., Rolfe, E.J., and Selman, J.D. (1974). Quality changes related to vitamin C in fruit juice and vegetable processing. In *Vitamin C: Recent Aspects of its Physiological and Technological importance* (ed. G.G. Birch and K.J. Parker), Chapter 4, pp. 40–67. Applied Science Publishers, London.

Birkhed, D., and Bär, A. (1991). Sorbitol and dental caries. *World Review of Nutrition and Dietetics*, 65, 1–37.

Bitsch, R. (1993). Flair Concerted Action no 10 Status Papers: Vitamin B$_6$. *International Journal of Vitamin and Nutrition Resarch*, 63, 278–82.

Bitsch, R. (1993). Vitamin B$_6$. *International Journal of Vitamin and Nutrition Research*, 63, 278–82.

Björntorp, P. (1988). The associations between obesity, adipose tissue distribution and disease. *Acta Medica Scandinavica suppl*, **723**, 121–34.

Björntorp, P. (1990). Classification of obese patients and complications related to the distribution of surplus fat. *Nutrition*, **6**, 131–7.

Black, A.L., Guirard, B.M., and Snell, E.E. (1975). Increased muscle glycogen phosphorylase in rats fed high levels of vitamin B_6. *Journal of Nutrition*, **107**, 1962–8.

Black, A.L., Guirard, B.M., and Snell, E.E. (1978). The behaviour of muscle phosphorylase as a reservoir for vitamin B_6 in the rat. *Journal of Nutrition*, **108**, 670–7.

Blanchard, R.A., Furie, B.C., Jorgensen, M., Kruger, S.F., and Furie, B. (1981). Acquired vitamin K-dependent carboxylation deficiency in liver disease. *New England Journal of Medicine*, **305**, 242–8.

Blass, J.P., Gibson, G.E., and Kark, R.A.P. (1976). Pyruvate decarboxylase deficiency. In *Thiamine* (ed. G.C. Gubler, M. Fujiwara, and P.M. Dreyfus), pp. 321–32. Wiley, New York.

Blaxter, K. (1989). *Energy Metabolism in Animals and Man*. Cambridge University Press.

Block, R.J., and Mitchell, H.H. (1946). The correlation of amino acid composition of proteins with their nutritive value. *Nutrition Abstracts and Reviews*, **16**, 249–78.

Blundell, J. (1991). Pharmacological approaches to appetite suppression. *Trends in Pharmacological Sciences*, **12**, 147–57.

Boffetta, P., and Garfinkel, L. (1990). Alcohol drinking and mortality among men enrolled in an American Cancer Society prospective study. *Epidemiology*, **1**, 342–8.

Bollag, W., and Matter, A. (1981). From vitamin A to retinoids in experimental and clinical oncology: achievements, failures, and outlook. *Annals of the New York Academy of Sciences*, **359**, 9–23.

Booth, R.A.D., Goddard, B.A., and Paton, A. (1966). Measurement of fat thickness in man: a comparison of ultrasound, Harpenden calipers and electrical conductivity. *British Journal of Nutrition*, **20**, 719–25.

Borkan, G.A., Gerzof, S.G., Robbins, A.H., Hults, D.E., Silbert, C.K., and Silbert, J.E. (1982a). Assessment of abdominal fat content by computed tomography. *American Journal of Clinical Nutrition*, **36**, 172–6.

Borkan, G.A., Hults, D.E., Cardarelli, J., and Burrows, B.A. (1982b). Comparison of ultrasound and skinfold measurements in assessment of subcutaneous and total fatness. *American Journal of Physical Anthropology* **58**, 307–13.

Borkan, G.A., Hults, D.E., Gerzof, S.G., Burrows, B.A., and Robbins, A.H. (1983). Relationships between computed tomography tissue areas, thicknesses and total body composition. *Annals of Human Biology*, **10**, 537–46.

Borschel, M., Kirksey, A., and Hannemann, R.E. (1986). Effects of vitamin B_6 intake on nurture and growth of young infants. *American Journal of Clinical Nutrition*, **43**, 7–15.

Bothwell, T.H., Bayner, R.D., MacFarlane, B.J., and MacPhail, A.P. (1989). Nutritional iron requirements and food iron absorption. *Journal of Internal Medicine*, **226**, 357–65.

Bouchard, C., Bray, G.A., and Hubbard, V.S. (1990). Basic and clinical aspects of regional fat distribution. *American Journal of Clinical Nutrition*, **52**, 946–50.

Bouchier, I.A.D. (1983). Biochemistry of gallstone formation. *Clinics in Gastroenterology*, **12**, 25–43.

Bowden, J.-F., Bender, D.A., Symes, E.K., and Coulson, W.F. (1986). Increased uterine uptake and nuclear retention of [^{3}H]oestradiol through the oestrous cycle and enhanced end-organ sensitivity to oestrogen stimulation in vitamin B_6 deficient rats. *Journal of Steroid Biochemistry*, **25**, 359–65.

Boyages, S.C. (1993). Iodine deficiency disorders. *Journal of Clinical Endocrinology and Metabolism*, **77**, 587–91.

Bray, G.A.. (1985). Complications of obesity. *Annals of Internal Medicine*, **103**, 1052–62.

Bray, G.A. (1993). Use and abuse of appetite-suppressant drugs in the treatment of obesity. *Annals of Internal Medicine*, **119**, 707–13.

Bray, T.M., and Bettger, W.J. (1990). The physiological role of zinc as an antioxidant. *Free Radical Biology and Medicine*, **8**, 281–91.

Bredenkamp, B.L.F., and Luck, D.N. (1969). Effect of raw soy beans on levels of protein and nucleic acid in the rat pancreas. *Proceedings of the Society for Experimental Biology and Medicine*, **132**, 537–9.

Brent, G.A. (1994). The molecular basis of thyroid hormone action. *New England Journal of Medicine*, **331**, 847–53.

Bressani, R., and Elias, L.G. (1972). *Nutritional Improvement of Legumes*. Proceedings of a Symposium of the Protein Advisory Group. FAO, Rome.

Briend, A. (1990). Is diarrhoea a major cause of malnutrition among the under-fives in developing countries? *European Journal of Clinical Nutrition*, **44**, 611–28.

Brin, M. (1964). Erythrocyte as a biopsy tissue for functional evaluation of thiamine adequacy. *Journal of the American Medical Association*, **187**, 762–6.

Brise, H., and Hallberg, L. (1962). Effect of ascorbic acid on iron absorption. *Acta Medica Scandinavica (suppl. 376)*, **171** 51–8.

British Nutrition Foundation (1995). *Trans fatty acids*: Report of the British Nutrition Foundation Task Force. British Nutrition Foundation, London.

Brouwer, A., and van den Berg, K.J. (1986). Binding of a metabolite of 3,4,3′,4′-tetrachlorbiphenyl to transthyretin reduces serum vitamin A transport by inhibiting the formation of the protein complex carrying both retinol and thyroxin. *Toxicology and Applied Pharmacology*, **85**, 301–12.

Brown, M.S., and Goldstein, J.L. (1986). A receptor-mediated pathway for cholesterol homeostasis. *Science*, **232**, 34–47.

Brozek, J., and Keys, A. (1951). The evaluation of leanness-fatness in man: norms and interrelationships. *British Journal of Nutrition*, **5**, 194–206.

Brozek, J., Grande, F., Anderson, J.T., and Keys, A. (1963). Densitometric analysis of body composition: revision of some quantitative assumptions. *Annals of the New York Academy of Sciences*, 110, 113–40.

Brummer, R.J., Karibe, M., and Stockbrugger, R.W. (1993). Lactose malabsorption: optimalization of investigational methods. *Scandinavian Journal of Gastroenterology suppl.* 200, 65–9.

Brune, M., Magnusson, B., Persson, H., and Hallberg, L. (1986). Iron losses in sweat. *American Journal of Clinical Nutrition*, 43, 438–43.

Bukowiecki, L.J. (1984). Mechanisms of stimulus-calorigenesis coupling in brown adipose tissue. *Canadian Journal of Biochemistry and Cell Biology*, 62, 623–30.

Bunce, G.E., and Vessal, M. (1987). Effect of zinc and / or pyridoxine deficiency upon oestrogen retention and oestrogen receptor distribution in the rat uterus. *Journal of Steroid Biochemistry*, 26, 303–8.

Burger, M., Hein, L.W., Tepley, L.J. (1956). Vitamin, mineral and proximate composition of frozen fruits, juices and vegetables. *Journal of Agricultural and Food Chemistry*, 4, 418–25.

Burk, R.F., and Hill, K.E. (1994). Selenoprotein P: a selenium-rich extracellular glycoprotein. *Journal of Nutrition*, 124, 1891–7.

Burkinshaw, L., Morgan, D.B., Silverton, N.P., and Thomas, R.D. (1981). Total body nitrogen and its relationship to body potassium and fat-free mass in healthy subjects. *Clinical Science*, 61, 457–62.

Burri, B.J, Sweetman, L., and Nyhan, W.L. (1981). Mutant holocarboxylase synthetase: evidence for the enzyme defect in early infantile biotin-responsive multiple carboxylase deficiency. *Journal of Clinical Investigation*, 68, 1491–5.

Burtis, C.A., and Ashwood, E.R. (1994). *Tietz Textbook of Clinical Chemistry*, 2nd edn. W. B. Saunders, Philadelphia, PA.

Burton, G.W., and Ingold, K.U. (1981). Autoxidation of biological molecules: (i) the antioxidant activity of vitamin E and related chain breaking phenolic antioxidants *in vitro*. *Journal of the American Chemical Society*, 103, 6472–7.

Burton, G.W., and Ingold, K.U. (1984). β-Carotene, an unusual type of lipid antioxidant. *Science*, 224, 569–73.

Burton, G.W., Ingold, K.U., Foster, D.O., Cheng, S.C., Webb, A., Hughes, L., and Lusztyk, E. (1988). Comparison of free α-tocopherol and α-tocopheryl acetate as sources of vitamin E in rats and humans. *Lipids*, 23, 834–40.

Burton, G.W., Wronska, U., Stone, L., Foster, D.O., and Ingold, K.U. (1990). Biokinetics of dietary RRR-α-tocopherol in the male guinea pig at three dietary levels of vitamin C and two levels of vitamin E: evidence that vitamin C does not 'spare' vitamin E *in vivo*. *Lipids*, 25, 199–210.

Butterworth, R.F. (1982). Neurotransmitter function in thiamine deficiency. *Neurochemistry International*, 4, 449–65.

Butterworth, R.F., Giguère, J-F, and Bessnard, A-M (1985). Activities of thiamine-dependent enzymes in two experimental models of thiamine-deficiency encephalopathy: (i) the pyruvate dehydrogenase complex. *Neurochemical Research*, 10, 1417–28.

Butterworth, R.F., Giguère, J-F, and Bessnard, A-M (1986). Activities of thiamine-dependent enzymes in two experimental models of thiamine-deficiency encephalopathy: (ii) α-ketoglutarate dehydrogenase. *Neurochemical Research*, 11, 567–77 .

Cai, L., Chu, Y., Wilson, S.E., and Schlender, K.K. (1995). A metal-dependent form of protein phosphatase 2A. *Biochemical and Biophysical Research Communications*, 208, 274–9.

Calvo, M.S. (1993). Dietary phosphorus, calcium metabolism and bone. *Journal of Nutrition*, 12, 1627–33.

Cameron, E., and Pauling, L. (1974a). The orthomolecular treatment of cancer: (i) the role of ascorbic acid in host resistance. *Chemical-Biological Interactions*, 9, 273–83.

Cameron, E., and Pauling, L. (1974b). The orthomolecular treatment of cancer: (ii) clinical trial of high dose ascorbic acid supplements in advanced human cancer. *Chemical-Biological Interactions*, 9, 285–315.

Campbell, C.H. (1984). The severe lacticacidosis of thiamine deficiency: acute pernicious or fulminating beriberi. *Lancet* (ii), 446–9.

Campbell, R.M., and Kosterlitz, H.W. (1948).. The assay of the nutritive value of a protein by its effect on liver cytoplasm. *Journal of Physiology*, 107, 383–98.

Canham, J.E., Baker, E.M., Harding, R.S., Sauberlich, H.E., and Plough, I.C. (1969). Dietary protein, its relationship to vitamin B_6 requirements and function. *Annals of the New York Academy of Sciences*, 166, 16–29.

Cannon, P.R. (1945). The relationship of protein metabolism to antibody production and resistance to infection. In *Advances in Protein Chemistry*, Vol 2, pp. 135–54. Academic Press, New York.

Canton, M., and Cremin, F.L. (1990). The effect of dietary zinc depletion and repletion in rats: zinc concentration in various tissues and activity of pancreatic γ-glutamyl hydrolase (EC 3.4.22.12) as indices of zinc status. *British Journal of Nutrition*, 64, 201–9.

Cardinale, G.J., Carty, T.J., and Abeles, R.H. (1970). Effect of methylmalonyl coenzyme A, a metabolite which accumulates in vitamin B_{12} deficiency, on fatty acid synthesis. *Journal of Biological Chemistry*, 245, 3771–5.

Carl, G.F., Eto, I., and Krumdieck, C.L. (1987). Chronic treatment of rats with primidone causes depletion of pteroylpentaglutamates in liver. *Journal of Nutrition*, 117, 970–5.

Carlisle, E.M. (1970). Silicon, a possible factor in bone calcification. *Science*, 167, 279–80.

Carpenter, K.J. (1960). The estimation of available lysine on animal-protein foods. *Biochemical Journal*, 77, 604–10.

Carpenter, K.J. (1973). Damage to lysine in food processing: its measurement and its significance. *Nutrition Abstracts and Reviews*, 43, 423–51.

Carpenter, K.J., and Levin, W.J. (1985). A re-examination of the composition of diets associated with pellagra. *Journal of Nutrition*, 115, 543–52.

Carter, E.G.A., and Carpenter, K.J. (1982). The bioavailability for humans of bound niacin from wheat bran. *American Journal of Clinical Nutrition*, 36, 855–61.

Castiello, R.J., and Lynch, P.S. (1972). Pellagra and the carcinoid syndrome. *Archives of Dermatology*, 105, 574–77.

Catignani, G.L. (1980). Hepatic α-tocopherol-binding protein. *Methods in Enzymology*, 67, 117–22.

Chalmers, A.H., Cowley, D.M., and Brown, J.M. (1986). A possible etiological role for ascorbate in calculi formation. *Clinical Chemistry*, 32, 333–6.

Chalmers, T.C. (1975). Effects of ascorbic acid on the common cold: an evaluation of the evidence. *American Journal of Medicine*, 58, 532–6.

Chambers, I., Frampton, J., Goldfarb, P., Affara, N., McBain, W., and Harrison, P.R. (1986). The structure of the mouse glutathione peroxidase gene: the selenocysteine in the active site is encoded by the 'termination' codon TGA. *EMBO Journal*, 5, 1221–7.

Chanarin, I., England, J.M. Mollin, C., and Perry, J. (1973). Methylmalonic acid excretion studies. *British Journal of Haematology*, 25, 45–53.

Chanarin, I., Deacon, R., Lumb, M., Muir, M., and Perry, J. (1985). Cobalamin-folate interrelations: a critical review. *Blood*, 66, 479–89.

Charlton, R.W., Fatti, L.P., Lynch, S.R., Torrance, J.D., and Bothwell, T.H. (1980). Equilibration of tracer radio-iron with body iron. *Clinical Science*, 58, 90–100.

Chastain, J.L., and McCormick, D.B. (1987). Clarification and quantitation of primary (tissue) and secondary (microbial) catabolites of riboflavin that are excreted in mammalian (rat) urine. *Journal of Nutrition*, 117, 468–75.

Chatterjee, I.B. (1978). Ascorbic acid metabolism. *World Review of Nutrition and Dietetics*, 30, 69–87.

Chen, C-C, Heller, J., Ding, L-L, and Horwitz, J. (1981). Retinol transfer from rat liver cytosol retinyl ester lipoprotein complex to serum retinol binding protein. *Archives of Biochemistry and Biophysics*, 207, 392–8.

Chen, Q., Blackberg, L., Nilsson, A., Sternby, B., and Hernell, O. (1994). Digestion of triacylglycerols containing long chain polyenoic fatty acids *in vitro* by colipase dependent pancreatic lipase and human milk bile salt stimulated lipase. *Biochimica et Biophysica Acta*, 1210, 239–43.

Chesney, R.W. (1990). Requirements and upper limits of vitamin D Intake in the term neonate, infant and older child. *Journal of Pediatrics*, 116, 159–66.

Chia, C.P., Addison, R., and McCormick, D.B. (1978). Absorption metabolism and excretion of 8–(amino acid) riboflavins in the rat. *Journal of Nutrition*, 108, 373–81.

Chiang, A-N., and Huang, P-C. (1988). Excess energy and nitrogen balance at protein intakes above the requirement level in young men. *American Journal of Clinical Nutrition*, 48, 1015–22.

Cho-Chung, Y.S., and Pitot, H.C. (1967). Feedback control of rat liver tryptophan pyrrolase. *Journal of Biological Chemistry*, 242, 1192–8.

Chu, B.C.F., and Lawley, P.D. (1975). Increased urinary excretion of nucleic acid and nicotinamide derivatives by rats after treatment with alkylating agents. *Chemical-Biological Interactions*, 10, 333–8.

Cidlowski, J.A., and Thanassi, J.W. (1981). Pyridoxal phosphate, a possible cofactor in steroid hormone action. *Journal of Steroid Biochemistry*, 15, 11–6.

Cimino, J.A., Jhangiani, S., Schwartz, E., and Cooperman, J.M. (1987). Riboflavin metabolism in the hypothyroid human adult. *Proceedings of the Society for Experimental Biology and Medicine*, 184, 151–3.

Clark, W.G., and MacKay, E.M. (1950). The absorption and excretion of rutin and related flavonoid substances. *Journal of the American Medical Association*, 143, 1411–15.

Clarys, J.P., Martin, A.D., and Drinkwater, D.T. (1984). Gross tissue weights in the human body by cadaver dissection. *Human Biology*, 56, 459–73.

Clements, J.E., and Anderson, B.B. (1980). Glutathione reductase activity and pyridoxine (pyridoxamine) phosphate oxidase activity in the red cell. *Biochimica et Biophysica Acta*, 632, 159–63.

Clugston, G.A., and Garlick, P.J. (1982). The response of protein and energy metabolism to food intake in lean and obese man. *Human Nutrition : Clinical Nutrition*, 36C, 57–70.

Coburn, S.P. (1990). Location and turnover of vitamin B_6 pools and vitamin B_6 requirements of humans. *Annals of the New York Academy of Sciences*, 585, 76–85.

Cohn, S.H. (1991). Neutron activation analysis in assessment of body composition. *New Techniques in Nutritional Research*, (ed. R.G. Whitehead and A. Prentice), Chapter 12, pp. 261–79 Academic Press, San Diego, CA.

Cohn, S.H. (1992). *In vivo* neutron activation analysis; a new technique in nutritional research. *Journal of Nutritional Biochemistry*, 3, 378–86.

Cohn, R., Merrell, R.C., and Koslow, A. (1981). Gastric stapling for morbid obesity. *American Journal of Surgery*, 142, 67–72.

Colditz, G.A., Giovannucci, E., Rimm, E.B., Stampfer, M.J., Rosner, B. Speizer, F.E., Gordis, E., and Willett, W.C. (1991). Alcohol intake in relation to diet and obesity in women and men. *American Journal of Clinical Nutrition*, 54, 49–55.

Coles, T.J. (1986). Weight/height^p compared to weight/height^2 for assessing adiposity in childhood: influence of age and bone age on p during puberty. *Annals of Human Biology*, 13, 433–51.

Comstock, G.W., Kendrick, M.A., and Livesay, V.T. (1966). Subcutaneous fatness and mortality. *American Journal of Epidemiology*, 83, 548–63.

Cook, J.D., and Skikne, B.S. (1989). Iron deficiency: definition and diagnosis. *Journal of Internal Medicine*, 226, 349–55.

Coon, W.W., and Nagler, E. (1969). The tryptophan load as a test for pyridoxine deficiency in hospitalized patients. *Annals of the New York Academy of Sciences*, 166, 30–43.

Coppoletta, J.M., and Wolbach, S.B. (1933). Body length and organ weights of infants and children. *American Journal of Pathology*, 9, 55–70.

Cornish, E.J., and Tesoriero, W. (1975). Pyridoxine and oestrogen-induced glucose intolerance. *British Medical Journal*, (iii), 649–50.

Coward, W.A. (1988). The doubly-labelled water ($^2H_2^{18}O$) method: principles and practice. *Proceedings of the Nutrition Society*, 47, 209–18.

Creagan, E.T., Moertel, C.G., O'Fallon, J.R., Schutt, A.J., O'Connell, M.J., Rubin, J., and Frytack, S. (1979). Failure of high dose vitamin C (ascorbic acid) therapy to benefit patients with advanced cancer. *New England Journal of Medicine*, 301, 687–90.

Cronk, C.E., and Roche, A.F. (1982). Race- and sex-specific reference data for triceps and subscapular skinfolds and weight/stature. *American Journal of Clinical Nutrition*, 35, 347–54.

Cronk, C.E. (1983). Fetal growth as measured by ultrasound. *Yearbook of Physical Anthropology*, 26, 65–89.

Culebras, J.M., and Moore, F.D. (1977). Total body water and the exchangeable hydrogen: (i) theoretical calculation of non-aqueous exchangeable hydrogen in man. *American Journal of Physiology*, 232, R54–9.

Culebras, J.M., Fitzpatrick, G.F., Brennan, M.F., Boyden, C.M., and Moore, F.D. (1977). Total body water and the exchangeable hydrogen: (ii) a review of comparative data from animals based on isotope dilution and desiccation, with a report on new data from the rat. *American Journal of Physiology*, 232, R60–5.

Cullumbine, H., Basnayake, J.T., Lemottee, J., and Wickamanayake, T.W. (1950). Mineral metabolism on rice diets. *British Journal of Nutrition*, 4, 101–11.

Cummings, J.H., and Englyst, H.N. (1995). Gastrointestinal effects of food carbohydrates. *American Journal of Clinical Nutrition (Suppl.)*, 61, 938–45s.

Cuthbertson, D.P. (1964). Physical injury and its effects on protein metabolism. In *Human Protein Metabolism*, Vol. II, (ed. H.N. Munro and J.B. Allison), Chapter 19, pp. 373–414 Academic Press, New York.

Czeizel, A.E. (1993). Prevention of congenital abnormalities by periconceptual multivitamin supplement. *British Medical Journal*, 306, 1645–8.

Dakshinamurti, K., and Chauhan, J. (1994). Biotin-binding proteins. In *Vitamin Receptors: Vitamins as Ligands in Cell Communication*, (ed. K. Dakshinamurti), Chapter 8, pp. 200–49 Cambridge University Press.

Dakshinamurti, K., Tarrago-Litvak, L., and Hong, H.C. (1970). Biotin and glucose metabolism. *Canadian Journal of Biochemistry*, 48, 4993–5000.

Dallman, P.R. (1977). New approaches to screening for iron deficiency. *Journal of Pediatrics*, 90, 678–81.

Dallman, P.R. (1989). Iron deficiency: does it matter? *Journal of Internal Medicine*, 226, 367–72.

Danks, D.M. (1995). Disorders of copper transport, Ch 68, pp 2211–35 in *The Metabolic and Molecular Basis of Inherited Disease*, Vol II, Scriver CR, Beaudet AL, Sly WS and Valle D (Eds). McGraw-Hill, New York.

Davies, L., and Holdsworth, M.D. (1985). Nutrition and health at retirement age in the United Kingdom. *Human Nutrition: Applied Nutrition*, 39, 315–32.

Davis, E.A. (1995). Functionality of sugars: physicochemical interactions in foods. *American Journal of Clinical Nutrition, (suppl.)*, 62, (suppl) 170–7s.

Davis, G.R.F., and Sosalki, F.W. (1974). Nutritional quality of oilseed protein isolates as determined with larvae of the yellow mealworm, *Tenebrio molitor*. *Journal of Nutrition*, 104, 1172–7.

Davison, J.S. (1989). *Gastrointestinal Secretion*. Wright, London.

de Lange, P.J., and Joubert, C.P. (1964). Assessment of nicotinic acid status of population groups. *American Journal of Clinical Nutrition*, 15, 169–74.

de Muelenaere, H.J.R. (1964). Studies on the digestion of soy beans. *Journal of Nutrition*, 82, 197–205.

de Pee, S., West, C.E., Muhilal, Kayadi, D., and Hautvast, J.G.A.J. (1995). Lack of improvement in vitamin A status with increased consumption of dark-green leafy vegetables. *Lancet*, 346, 75–81.

Delmas, P.D. (1993). Biochemical markers of bone turnover: theoretical considerations and clinical use in osteoporosis. *American Journal of Medicine, (suppl. 5a)*, 95, 11–6s.

DeLuca, H.M. (1977). The direct involvement of vitamin A in glycosyl transfer reactions of mammalian membranes. *Vitamins and Hormones*, 35, 1–57.

Delves, H.T. (1985). Assessment of trace element status. *Clinics in Endocrinology and Metabolism*, 14, 725–60.

Department of Health (1991). *Dietary Reference Values for Food Energy and Nutrients for the United Kingdom*. HMSO, London.

Department of Health (1994a). *Nutritional Aspects of Cardiovascular Disease*. Report on Health and Social Subjects no 46, HMSO, London.

Department of Health (1994b). *On the state of the public health, Annual report of the Chief Medical Officer of the Department of Health for the year 1993*. HMSO, London.

Department of Health (1994c). Report on Health and Social Subjects no 45: *Weaning and the weaning diet*. HMSO, London.

Department of Health and Social Security (1977). Report on Health and Social Subjects no 12. *The composition of mature human milk*. HMSO, London.

Department of Health and Social Security (1987). Report on Health and Social Subjects no 31: *The use of very low calorie diets in obesity*. HMSO, London.

Deutsch, M.J., and Weeks, C.E. (1965). Microfluorimetric assay for vitamin C. *Journal of the Association of Official Analytical Chemists*, 48, 1248–56.

Dibley, M.J., Goldsby, J.B., Staehling, N.W., and Trowbridge, F.L. (1987a). Development of normalized curves for the international growth reference: historical and technical considerations. *American Journal of Clinical Nutrition*, 46, 36–48.

Dibley, M.J., Staehling, N., Nieburg, P., and Trowbridge, F.L. (1987b). Interpretation of the Z-score anthropometric indicators derived from the international growth reference. *American Journal of Clinical Nutrition*, 46, 749–62.

Dickson, R.C., and Tomlinson, R.N. (1967). Selenium in blood and human tissues. *Clinica Chimica Acta*, 16, 311–21.

Dickson, I.R., Walls, J., and Webb, S. (1989). Vitamin A and bone formation: different responses to retinol and retinoic acid of chick bone cells in organ culture. *Biochimica et Biophysica Acta*, 1013, 254–8.

Diliberto, E.J., Dean, G., Carter, C., and Allen, P.L. (1982). Tissue subcellular and submitochondrial distributions of semidehydroascorbate reductase: possible role of semidehydroascorbate reductase in cofactor regeneration. *Journal of Neurochemistry*, 39, 563–8.

Diplock, A.T. (1993). Indexes of selenium status in human populations. *American Journal of Clinical Nutrition*, 57, 256s-8s.

Diplock, A.T., and Lucy, J.A. (1973). The biochemical modes of action of vitamin E and selenium, a hypothesis. *FEBS Letters*, 29, 205–10.

Doll, R., and Peto, R. (1981). *The Causes of Cancer*. Oxford University Press, New York.

Donahue, R.P., Abbott, R.D., Bloom, E., Reed, D.M., and Yano, K. (1987). Central obesity and coronary heart disease in men. *Lancet*, (i),821–4.

Donald, E.A., and Bosse, T.R. (1979). The vitamin B_6 requirement in oral contraceptive users: (ii) assessment by tryptophan metabolites, vitamin B_6 and pyridoxic acid levels in urine. *American Journal of Clinical Nutrition*, 32, 1024–32.

Donaldson, R.M. (1985). How does cobalamin (vitamin B_{12}) enter and traverse the ileal cell? *Gastroenterology*, 89, 1069–71.

Downs, D.E., and Meckel, R.B. (1943). *Cereal Chemistry*, 20, 352–5.

Drasar, B.S., and Barrow, P.A. (1985). *Intestinal Microbiology*. Van Nostrand Reinhold, London.

Duckworth, W.C., Solomon, S.S., Liepnieks, J., Hamel, F.G., Hand, S., and Peavy, D.E. (1988). Insulin-like effects of vanadate in isolated rat hepatocytes. *Endocrinology*, 122, 2285–9.

Dumont, J.E., Corvilain, B., and Contempre, B. (1994). The biochemistry of endemic cretinism: roles of iodine and selenium deficiency and goitrogens. *Molecular and Cellular Endocrinology*, 100, 163–66.

Dupre, S., Rosei, M.A., Bellusi, L., del Grosso, E., and Cavallini, D. (1973). The substrate specificity of pantetheinase. *European Journal of Biochemistry*, 40, 103–7.

Durkacz, B.W., Omidiji, O., Gray, D.A., and Shall, S. (1980). (ADP-ribose)$_n$ participates in DNA excision repair. *Nature*, 283, 593–6.

Durnin, J.V.G.A., and Rahaman, M.M. (1967). The assessment of the amount of fat in the human body from measurements of skinfold thickness. *British Journal of Nutrition*, 21, 681–9.

Durnin, J.V.G.A., and Womersley, J. (1974). Body fat assessed from total body density and its estimation from skinfold thickness: measurements on 481 men and women aged from 16 to 72 years. *British Journal of Nutrition*, 23, 77–97.

Dutta, P., Pinto, J., and Rivlin, R.S. (1985). Antimalarial effects of riboflavin deficiency. *Lancet*, (ii), 1040–2.

Dykes, M.H.M., and Meier, P. (1975). Ascorbic acid and the common cold: evaluation of its efficacy and toxicity. *Journal of the American Medical Association*, 231: 1073–9.

Eastham, R.D., and Slade, R.R. (1992). *Clinical Haematology*, 7th edn. Butterworth-Heinemann, London.

Eberle, E.D., and Eiduson, S. (1968). Effect of pyridoxine deficiency on aromatic amino acid decarboxylase in developing rat liver and brain. *Journal of Neurochemistry*, 15, 1071–83.

Edwin, E.E., and Jackman, R. (1970). Thiaminase I in the development of cerebrocortical necrosis in sheep and cattle. *Nature*, 228, 772–4.

Egger, J., Carter, C.M., Graham, P.J., Gumley, D., and Soothill, J.F. (1985). A controlled trial of oligo-antigenic diet treatment in the hyperkinetic syndrome. *Lancet*, (i), 540–5.

Eichenbaum, J.W., and Cooper, J.R. (1971). Restoration by thiamin of the action potential in ultra-violet irradiated nerves. *Brain Research*, 32, 258–60.

Einarsson, K., Nilsell, K., Leijd, B., and Angelin, B. (1985). Influence of age on secretion of cholesterol and synthesis of bile acids by the liver. *New England Journal of Medicine*, 313, 277–82.

Ellis, J.M., Folkers, K., Watanabe, T., Kaji, M., Saji, S., Caldwell, J., Temple, C., and Wood, F. (1979). Clinical results of a cross-over treatment with pyridoxine and placebo of the carpal tunnel syndrome. *American Journal of Clinical Nutrition*, 32 2040–6.

Englyst, H.N., Quigley, M.E., Hudson, G.J., and Cummings, H.J. (1992). Determination of dietary fibre as non-starch polysaccharides by gas-liquid chromatography. *Analyst*, 117 1707–14.

Euronut SENECA Investigators (1991). Intake of vitamins and minerals. *European Journal of Clinical Nutrition (suppl. 3)*, 45, 121–38.

European Commission (1990). Council Directive 90/496/EEC on nutrition labelling for foodstuffs. *Official Journal of the European Communities*, L 276, 40–4.

European Commission (1991). Commission Directive 91/321/EEC on infant formulae and follow-on formulae. *Official Journal of the European Communities*, L 175, 35–49.

Evans, G.W., and Johnson, P.E. (1980). Characterization and quantitation of a zinc-binding ligand in human milk. *Pediatric Research*, 14, 876–80.

Evans, E., and Witty, R. (1978). An assessment of methods used to determine protein quality. *World Review of Nutrition and Dietetics*, 32, 1–26.

Evans, G.W., Roginski, E.E., and Mertz, W. (1973). Interactions of the glucose tolerance factor with insulin.

Biochemical and Biophysical Research Communications, 50, 718–22.

Evans, R.M., Currie, L., and Campbell, A. (1982). The distribution of ascorbic acid between various cellular components of blood in normal individuals and its relation to the plasma concentration. *British Journal of Nutrition*, 47, 473–82.

Evans, D.J., Hoffmann, R.G., Kalkhoff, R.K., and Kissebah, A.H. (1984). Relationship of body fat topography to insulin sensitivity and metabolic profiles in premenopausal women. *Metabolism*, 33, 68–75.

Eyton, A. (1982). *The F-Plan Diet*. Penguin Books, Harmondsworth.

Fafunso, M., and Bassir, O. (1976). The effect of cooking on the vitamin C content of fresh leaves and wilted leaves. *Journal of Agricultural and Food Chemistry*, 24, 354–55.

FAO (1955). *Protein requirements*. Food and Agriculture Organization publication no 16. FAO, Rome.

FAO (1995). Data from the United Nations Food and Agriculture Organization Internet pages at http://www.fao.org/.

FAO/WHO (1988). Requirements of vitamin A, iron, folate, and vitamin B_{12}. *FAO Food and Nutrition Series* no 23. FAO, Rome.

FAO/WHO (1991). *Protein quality evaluation*. Report of a joint FAO/WHO expert consultation. FAO Food and \int_{}^{}{}{}Nutrition Paper no 51. FAO, Rome.

FAO/WHO/UNU (1985). *Energy and protein requirements*. Report of a Joint FAO/WHO/UNU Expert Consultation. *WHO Technical Report Series* 724. WHO, Geneva.

Farrer KTH (1955). *Advances in Food Research* 6: 257–311.

FDA (1993). Food Labelling: serving sizes. *Federal Register* 58: 2229–91.

FDA/IAS (1994). Action levels for poisonous or deleterious substances in human food and animal feed. File fdaact at http:\\www.fda.gov.

Feingold, B.F. (1975). Hyperkinesis and learning disabilities linked to artificial food flavours and colours. *American Journal of Nursing*, 75, 797–803.

Felber, J-P (1992). From obesity to diabetes: pathophysiological considerations. *International Journal of Obesity*, 16, 937–52.

Fenton, D.A., Wilkinson, J.D., and Toseland, P.A. (1983). Family exhibiting cerebellar-like ataxia, photosensitivity and shortness of stature—a new inborn error of tryptophan metabolism. *Journal of the Royal Society of Medicine*, 76, 736–9.

Fenwick, G.R., and Heaney, R.K. (1983). Glucosinolates and their breakdown products in cruciferous crops, foods and feedingstuffs. *Food Chemistry*, 11, 249–71.

Finglas, P.M. (1993). Flair concerted action no 10 status papers: thiamin. *International Journal of Vitamin and Nutrition Research*, 63, 270–4.

Finot, P.A. (1983). Lysinoalanine in food proteins. *Nutrition Abstracts and Reviews, Clinical Nutrition*, 53, 67–80.

Fiorotto, M.L. (1991). Measurements of total body electrical conductivity for the estimation of fat and fat-free mass. Chapter 13, pp 281–301 in Whitehead RG and Prentice A (Eds) *New Techniques in Nutritional Research*, Academic Press, San Diego, CA.

Firkin, F., Chesterman, C., Penington, D., and Rush, B. (1989). *de Gruchy's Clinical Haematology in Medical Practice*. Blackwell Scientific, Oxford.

Fisher, A., Waterhouse, T.D., and Adams, A.P. (1975). Obesity: its relation to anaesthesia. *Anaesthesia*, 30, 633–47.

Fleck, A., Colley, C.A., and Myers, M.A. (1985). Liver export proteins and trauma. *British Medical Bulletin*, 41, 265–73.

Folsom, A.R., Kaye, S.A., Sellers, T.A., Hong, C.P., Cerhan, J.R., Potter, J.D., and Prineas, R.J. (1993). Body fat distribution and 5–year risk of death in older women. *Journal of the American Medical Association*, 269, 483–7.

Fomon, S.J. (1967). Body composition of the reference male infant during the first year of life. *Pediatrics*, 40, 863–70.

Fomon, S.J., Hasche, F., Ziegler, E.E., and Nelson, S.E. (1982). Body composition of reference children from birth to age 10 years. *American Journal of Clinical Nutrition*, 35, 1169–75.

Forbes, J.M. (1988). Metabolic aspects of the regulation of voluntary food intake and appetite. *Nutrition Research Reviews*, 1, 145–68.

Forbes, G.B., and Bruining, G.J. (1976). Urinary creatinine excretion and lean body mass. *American Journal of Clinical Nutrition*, 29, 1359–66.

Forbes, R.M., Cooper, A.R., and Mitchell, H.H. (1953). Unpublished data cited by Keys and Brozek (1953).

Freeman, J.B., Meyer, P.D., Printen, K.J., Mason, E.E., and DenBesten, L. (1975). Analysis of gallbladder bile in morbid obesity. *American Journal of Surgery*, 129, 163–6.

Freundlich, E., Statter, M., and Yatziv, S. (1981). Familial pellagra-like skin rash with neurological manifestations. *Archives of Diseases of Childhood*, 56, 146–8.

Friedman, G.D., Kannel, W.B., and Dawber, T.R. (1966). The epidemiology of gall bladder disease: observations from the Framingham study. *Journal of Chronic Diseases*, 19, 273–92.

Fries, M.E., Chrisley, B.M., and Driskell, J.A. (1981). Vitamin B_6 status of a group of preschool children. *American Journal of Clinical Nutrition*, 32, 706–10.

Frimpter, G.W., Andelman, R.J., and George, W.F. (1969). Vitamin B_6 dependency syndromes. *American Journal of Clinical Nutrition*, 22, 794–805.

Frisancho, A.R. (1974). Triceps skin fold and upper arm muscle size norms for assessment of nutritional status. *American Journal of Clinical Nutrition*, 27, 1052–8.

Frisancho, A.R. (1981). New norms of upper limb fat and muscle areas for assessment of nutritional status. *American Journal of Clinical Nutrition*, 34, 2540–5.

Frisancho, A.R. (1984). New standards of weights and body composition by frame size and height for assessment of nutritional status of adults and the elderly. *American Journal of Clinical Nutrition*, 40, 808–19.

Frot-Coutaz, J., Letoublon, R., Degiuli, A., Fayet, Y., Audigier-Petit, C., and Got, R. (1985). Spatial aspects of mannosyl phosphoryl retinol formation. *Biochimica et Biophysica Acta*, **841**, 299–305.

Fry, P.C., Fox, H.M., and Tao, H.G. (1976). Metabolic response to a pantothenic acid deficient diet in humans. *Journal of Nutritional Science and Vitaminology*, **22**, 39–46.

Fu, C.S., Swendseid, M.E., Jacob, R.A., and McKee, R.W. (1989). Biochemical markers for assessment of niacin nutritional status in young men: levels of erythrocyte niacin coenzymes and plasma tryptophan. *Journal of Nutrition*, **119**, 1945–9.

Fuchs, C.S., Stampfer, C.H., Colditz, G.A., Giovannucci, E.L., Manson, J.E., Kawachi, I., Hunter, D.J., Hankinson-Fuchs, S.E., Hennekens, C.H., and Rosner, B. (1995). Alcohol consumption and mortality among women. *New England Journal of Medicine*, **332**, 1245–50.

Fujioka, S., Matsuzawa, Y., Tokunaga, K., and Tarui, S. (1987). Contribution of intra-abdominal fat accumulation to the impairment of glucose and lipid metabolism in human obesity. *Metabolism*, **36**, 54–9.

Gardemann, A., and Domagk, G.F. (1983). The occurence of γ-carboxyglutamate in a protein isolated from ox liver mitochondria. *Archives of Biochemistry and Biophysics*, **220**, 347–53.

Gardner, M.L.G. (1988). Gastrointestinal absorption of intact proteins. *Annual Review of Nutrition*, **8**, 329–50.

Garfinkel, L. (1986). Overweight and mortality. *Cancer*, **58**, 1826–9.

Garn, S.M., Pesick, S.D., and Hawthorne, V.M. (1983). The bony chest breadth as a frame size standard in nutritional assessment. *American Journal of Clinical Nutritiuon*, **37**, 315–8.

Garrow, J.S. (1982). New approaches to body composition. *American Journal of Clinical Nutrition*, **35**, 1152–8.

Garrow, J.S. (1983). Indices of adiposity. *Nutrition Abstracts and Reviews*, **8**, 697–708.

Garrow, J.S. (1988). *Obesity and Related Disorders*, Second Edition. Churchill-Livingstone, Edinburgh.

Garrow, J.S., Fletcher, K., and Halliday, D. (1965). Body composition in severe infantile malnutrition. *Journal of Clinical Investigation*, **44**, 417–25.

Garrow, J.S., Stalley, S., Diethelm, R., Pittet, P.H., Hesp, R., and Halliday, D. (1979). A new method for measuring body density of obese adults. *British Journal of Nutrition*, **42**, 173–83.

Garza, C., Scrimshaw, N.S., and Young, V.R. (1977). Human protein requirements: evaluation of the 1973 FAO/WHO safe level of protein intake for young men at high energy intakes. *British Journal of Nutrition*, **37**, 403–20.

Ge, X., and Yang, G. (1993). The epidemiology of selenium deficiency in the etiologic study of endemic diseases in China. *American Journal of Clinical Nutrition*, **57**, 259s–63s.

Gerber, G.B., and Deroo, J. (1970). Metabolism of labelled nicotinamide coenzymes in different organs of rats and mice. *Proceedings of the Society for Experimental Biology and Medicine*, **134**, 689–93.

Gey, K.F. (1989). Inverse correlation of vitamin E and ischaemic heart disease, pp. 224–31 in *Elevated Dosages of Vitamins* (eds P. Walter, H. Stahelin and G. Brubacher) Hans Huber Publishers, Toronto.

Gibson, R.S. (1990). *Principles of Nutritional Assessment*. Oxford University Press, New York.

Giguère, J-F, and Butterworth, R.F. (1987). Activities of thiamine-dependent enzymes in two experimental models of thiamine-deficiency encephalopathy: (iii) transketolase. *Neurochemical Research*, **12**, 305–10.

Gilbert, J.A., and Gregory, J.F. (1992). Pyridoxine-5–β-D-glucoside affects the metabolic utilization of pyridoxine in rats. *Journal of Nutrition*, **122**, 1029–35.

Glinsmann, W.H., and Mertz, W. (1966). Effect of trivalent chromium on glucose tolerance. *Metabolism*, **15**, 510–20.

Goldberg, A. (1963). The anaemia of scurvy. *Quarterly Journal of Medicine*, **32**, 51–64.

Golden, M.H.N. (1982). Protein deficiency, energy deficiency and the oedema of malnutrition. *Lancet*, (i), 1259–65.

Golden, M.H.N., and Golden, B.E. (1981). Trace elements: potential importance in human nutrition, with particular reference to zinc and vanadium. *British Medical Bulletin*, **37**, 31–66.

Golden, M.H.N., and Ramdath, D. (1987). Free radicals in the pathogenesis of kwashiorkor. *Proceedings of the Nutrition Society*, **46**, 53–68.

Gontzea, I., Rujinski, A., and Sutzesco, P. (1976). Rapide évaluation de l'état de nutrition niacinique. *Bibliotheca Nutritio et Dieta*, **23**, 95–104.

Goode, H.F., Kelleher, J., and Walker, B.E. (1989). Zinc concentrations in pure populations of peripheral blood neutrophils, lymphocytes and monocytes. *Annals of Clinical Biochemistry*, **26**, 89–95.

Goodman, S.I. (1981). Organic aciduria in the riboflavin deficient rat. *American Journal of Clinical Nutrition*, **34**, 2434–7.

Gopalan, C., and Rao, K.S.J. (1975). Pellagra and amino acid imbalance. *Vitamins and Hormones*, **33**, 505–28.

Gopalan, C., and Srikantia, S.G. (1960). Leucine and pellagra. *Lancet*, (i), 954–7.

Gorbak, G., and Regula, E. (1964). *Fette: Seifen: Anstrichmittel*, **66**, 920–5.

Gray, D.S., Bray, G.A., Bauer, M., Kaplan, K., Gemayel, N., Wood, R., Greenaway, F., and Kirk, S. (1990). Skinfold thickness measurements in obese subjects. *American Journal of Clinical Nutrition*, **51**, 571–7.

Greb, A., Bitsch, R., Leinert, J., and Simon-Schnaß, I. (1993). Interaktionen zwischen vitamin B_2 und B_6: einfluss des vitamin-B_2-status auf die vitamin B_6-versorgungslage. *Vitaminspur*, **8**, 79–80.

Gregory, J.F. (1980a). Effects of ε-pyridoxyl-lysine and related compounds on liver and brain pyridoxal kinase and liver pyridoxamine (pyridoxine) 5′-phosphate oxidase. *Journal of Biological Chemistry*, **255**, 2355–9.

Gregory, J.F. (1980b). Effects of ε-pyridoxyl-lysine bound to dietary protein on the vitamin B_6 status of rats. *Journal of Nutrition*, **110**, 995–1005.

Gregory, J.F., and Kirk, J.R. (1981). The bioavailability of vitamin B$_6$ in foods. *Nutrition Reviews*, **39**, 1–8.

Gregory, J., Foster, K., Tyler, H., and Wiseman, M. (1990). *The Dietary and Nutritional Survey of British Adults.* HMSO, London.

Gregory, J.F., Trumbo, P.R., Bailey, L.B., Toth, J.P., Baumgartner, T.G. and Cerda, J.J. (1991). Bioavailability of pyridoxine-5–β-D-glucoside determined in human by stable-isotope methods. *Journal of Nutrition*, **121**, 177–86.

Gregory, J.R., Collins, D.L., Davies, P.S.W., Hughes, J.M., and Clarke, P.C. (1995). *National Diet and Nutrition Survey: Children aged 1 to 4 years.* HMSO, London.

Gries, F.A. (1987). Problems with unusual methods of obesity control. In *Body Weight Control: The Physiology, Clinical Treatment and Prevention of Obesity* (ed. A.E. Bender and L.J. Brooks), Chapter 14, pp. 147–59. Churchill-Livingstone, Edinburgh.

Griffen, W.O. (1979). Gastric bypass for morbid obesity. *Surgical Clinics of North America*, **59**, 1103–12.

Griffen, W.O., Bivins, B.A., and Bell, R.M. (1983). The decline and fall of the jejunoileal bypass. *Surgery*, **157**, 301–8.

Griffin, J.E., and Zerwekh, J.E. (1983). Impaired stimulation of 25-hydroxyvitamin D 24–hydroxylase in fibroblasts from a patient with vitamin D dependent rickets, type II, a form of receptor-positive resistance to 1,25–dihydroxyvitamin D. *Journal of Clinical Investigation*, **72**, 1190–9.

Grøbbæk, M., Deis, A., Sørensen, T.I.A., Becker, U., Schnohr, P., and Jensen, G. (1995). Mortality associated with moderate intake of wine, beer, or spirits. *British Medical Journal*, **310**, 1165–9.

Gromisch, D.S,. Lopez, R., Cole, H.S., and Cooperman, J.M. (1977). Light (phototherapy)-induced riboflavin deficiency in the neonate. *Journal of Pediatrics*, **90**, 118–22.

Gruber, H.E., and Baylink, D.J. (1991). The effects of fluoride on bone. *Clinics in Orthopaedics*, **267**, 264–77.

Guggenheim, K.Y. (1981). *Nutritional Diseases, the Evolution of Concepts.* Collamore Press, Lexington, MA.

Guilarte, T.R., and Wagner, H.N. (1987). Increased concentrations of 3–hydroxykynurenine in vitamin B$_6$ deficient neonatal rat brain. *Journal of Neurochemistry*, **49**, 1918–26.

Gundlach, B.L., Nijkrake, H.G.M., and Hautvast, J.G.A.J. (1980). A rapid and simplified plethysmographic method for measuring body volume. *Human Biology*, **52**, 23–33.

Gunn, A.D.G. (1985). Vitamin B$_6$ and the premenstrual syndrome. *International Journal of Vitamin and Nutrition Research*, **27**, 213–24.

Gurdill, S.L., and Suttie, J.W. (1990). Vitamin K epoxide and quinone reductase activities: evidence for reduction by a common enzyme. *Biochemical Pharmacology*, **40**, 1055–61.

Habicht, J-P, Martorell, R., Yarbrough, C., Malina, R., and Klein, R.E. (1974). Height and weight standards for preschool children: how relevant are ethnic differences in growth potential. *Lancet*, **1**, 611–615.

Hahn, C.J., and Evans, G.W. (1973). Identification of a low molecular weight ^{65}Zn complex in rat intestine. *Proceedings of the Society for Experimental Biology and Medicine*, **144**, 793–5.

Halevy, S., and Grosswicz, N. (1953). A microbiological approach to nutritional evaluation of proteins. *Proceedings of the Society of Experimental Biology*, **82**, 567–71.

Hall, R., and Malia, R.G. (1991). *Medical Laboratory Haematology*, 2nd edn. Butterworth-Heinemann, London.

Hallberg, L. (1982). Iron absorption and iron deficiency. *Human Nutrition : Clinical Nutrition*, **36C**, 259–78.

Hallberg, L., and Rossander-Hultén, L. (1991). Iron requirements in menstruating women. *American Journal of Clinical Nutrition*, **54**, 1047–58.

Hallberg, L., Brune, M., Erlandsson, M., Sandberg, A-S, and Rossander-Hultén, L. (1991). Calcium: effect of different amounts on nonheme- and heme-iron absorption in humans. *American Journal of Clinical Nutrition*, **53**, 112–9.

Hallberg, L., Rossander-Hultén, L., Brune, M., and Gleerup, A. (1992). Inhibition of haem iron.absorption in man by calcium. *British Journal of Nutrition*, **69**, 533–40.

Haller, R.G., Dempsey, W.B., Feit, H., Cook, J.D., and Knochel, J.P. (1983). Low muscle levels of pyridoxine in McArdle's syndrome. *American Journal of Medicine*, **74**, 217–20.

Hamill, P.V., Drizd, T.A., Johnson, C.L., Reed, R.B., Roche, A.F., and Moore, W.M. (1979). Physical growth: National Center for Health Statistics percentiles. *American Journal of Clinical Nutrition*, **32**, 607–29.

Hamilton, E.I., Minski, M.J., and Cleary, J.J. (1992). Problems concerning multi-element assay in biological materials. *Science of the Total Environment*, **1**, 1–14.

Hamosh, M. (1990). Lingual and gastric lipases. *Nutrition*, **6**, 421–8.

Handler, C.E., and Perkin, G.D. (1982). Anorexia nervosa and Wernicke's encephalopathy: an under-diagnosed association. *Lancet*, (ii), 771–2.

Hannah, S.S., and Norman, A.W. (1994). 1α-25(OH)$_2$ Vitamin D$_3$-regulated expression of the eukaryotic genome. *Nutrition Reviews*, **52**, 376–82.

Hansen, A.E., Knott, E.M., Wiese, F., Shaperman, E., and McQuarrie, I. (1947). Eczema and essential fatty acids. *American Journal of Diseases of Childhood*, **73**, 1–18.

Harper, C. (1979). Wernicke's encephalopathy: a more common disease than realized. A neuropathological study of 51 cases. *Journal of Neurology, Neurosurgery and Psychiatry*, **42**, 226–31.

Harrison, H.C., and Long, C.N.H. (1945). Regeneration of liver protein in the rat. *Journal of Biological Chemistry*, **161**, 545–57.

Hartz, A.J., Rupley, D.C., Klakhoff, R.D., and Rimm, A.A. (1983). Relationship of obesity to diabetes: influence of obesity level and body fat distribution. *Preventive Medicine*, **12**, 351–7.

Hayes, K.C. (1988). Taurine nutrition. *Nutrition Research Reviews*, 1, 99–113

Heitman, B.L. (1990). Evaluation of body fat estimated from body mass index, skinfolds and impedance: a comparative study. *European Journal of Clinical Nutrition*, 44, 831–7.

Hellendoorn, E.W., de Groot, A.P., van der Dekker, L.P., Slump, P., and Willems, J.J. (1971). Nutritive value of canned meals. *Journal of the American Dietetic Association*, 58, 434–41.

Heller, S., Salkeld, R.M., and Korner, W.F. (1973). Vitamin B_6 status in pregnancy. *American Journal of Clinical Nutrition*, 26, 1339–48.

Henry, C.J.K., and Rees, D.G. (1991). New predictive equations for the estimation of basal metabolic rate in tropical peoples. *European Journal of Clinical Nutrition*, 45, 177–85.

Henry, H.L., and Norman, A.W. (1978). Vitamin D, two dihydroxylated metabolites are required for normal egg hatchability. *Science*, 201, 835–7.

Henry, H.L., Taylor, A.N., and Norman, A.W. (1977). Response of chick parathyroid glands to the vitamin D metabolites, 1,25–dihydroxycholecalciferol and 24,25–dihydroxy cholecalciferol. *Journal of Nutrition*, 107, 1918–26.

Herbert, V. (1962). Experimental nutritional folate deficiency in man. *Transactions of the Association of American Physicians*, 75, 307–20.

Herbert, V. (1987*a*). Recommended dietary intakes (RDI) of folate in humans. *American Journal of Clinical Nutrition*, 45, 661–70.

Herbert, V. (1987*b*). Recommended dietary intakes (RDI) of vitamin B_{12} in humans. *American Journal of Clinical Nutrition*, 45, 671–8.

Herbert, V. (1987*c*). The 1986 Herman Award Lecture, Nutrition Science as a continually unfolding story: the folate and vitamin B_{12} paradigm. *American Journal of Clinical Nutrition*, 46, 387–402.

Herbert, V. (1988). Vitamin B_{12}: plant sources, requirements, and assay. *American Journal of Clinical Nutrition*, 48, 852–8.

Herman, C., Adlerkreutz, T., Goldin, B.R., Gorbach, S.L., Hockerstedt, K.A., Watanabe, S., Hamalainen, E.K., Markkanen, M.H., Makela, T.H., and Wahala, K.T. (1995). Soybean phytoestrogen intake and cancer risk. *Journal of Nutrition*, 125, 757s-70s.

Hernell, O., and Blackberg, L. (1994). Human milk bile salt stimulated lipase: functional and molecular aspects. *Journal of Pediatrics*, 125, S56–61.

Hers, H.G. (1976). The usefulness of 'futile cycles'. *Biochemical Society Transactions*, 4, 985–8.

Hertog, M.G., Kromhout, D., Aravanis, C., Blackburn, H., Buzina, R., Fidanza, F., Giampaoli, S., Jansen, A., Menotti, A., and Nedelijkovic, S. (1995). Flavonoid intake and long-term risk of coronary heart disease and cancer in the seven countries study. *Archives of Internal Medicine*, 155, 381–6.

Heymsfield, S.B., McManus, C., Smith, J., Stevens, V., and Nixon, D.W. (1982). Anthropometric measurement of muscle mass: revised equations for calculating bone-free arm muscle area. *American Journal of Clinical Nutrition*, 36, 680–90.

Hicks, R.M. (1983). The scientific basis for regarding vitamin A and its analogues as anti-carcinogenic agents. *Proceedings of the Nutrition Society*, 42, 83–93.

Hicks, R.M., and Turton, J. (1986). Retinoids and cancer. *Biochemical Society Transactions*, 14, 939–42.

Hodges, R.E., Baker, E.M., Hood, J., Sauberlich, H.E., and March, S.C. (1969). Experimental scurvy in man. *American Journal of Clinical Nutrition*, 22, 535–48.

Hodges, R.E., Hood, J., Canham, J.E., Sauberlich, H.E., and Baker, E.M. (1971). Clinical manifestations of ascorbic acid deficiency in man. *American Journal of Clinical Nutrition*, 24, 432–43.

Hodges, R.E., Sauberlich, H.E., Canham, J.E., Wallace, D.L., Rucker, R.B., Mejia, L.A., and Mohanram, M. (1978). Hematopoietic studies in vitamin A deficiency. *American Journal of Clinical Nutrition*, 31, 876–85.

Hohenauer, L. (1980). Intrauterine growth curves for German-speaking countries. *Zeitschrift für Geburtshilfe und Perinatalogie*, 184, 167–79.

Holick, M.F. (1990). The use and interpretation of assays for vitamin D and its metabolites. *Journal of Nutrition*, 120, 1464–9.

Holliday, M.A. (1986). Body composition and energy needs during growth. In *Human Growth: A Comprehensive Treatise*, (eds F. Falkner F and J.M. Tanner), Chapter 5, pp. 101–17. Plenum Press, New York.

Holman, R.T. (1971). Biological activities of, and requirements for, polyunsaturated fatty acids. In *Progress in Chemistry of Fats vol 9* (ed. R.T. Holman), pp. 607–82. Pergamon Press, Oxford.

Holroyd, C.P., Gabudza, T.G., Putnam, R.C., Paul, P., and Reichard, G.A. (1975). Altered glucose metabolism in metastatic carcinoma. *Cancer Research*, 35, 3710–4.

Holst, J.J., and Schmidt, P. (1994). Gut hormones and intestinal function. *Ballière's Clinical Endocrinology and Metabolism*, 81, 137–64.

Holst, J.J. (1994). Glucagonlike peptide 1: a newly discovered gastrointestinal hormone. *Gastroenterology*, 107, 1848–55.

Hoorn, R.F.H., Flickweert, J.P., and Westrink, D. (1975). Vitamin B_1, B_2 and B_6 deficiencies in geriatric patients measured by coenzyme stimulation of enzyme activities. *Clinica Chimica Acta*, 61, 151–62.

Horn, M.J., Blum, A.E., Womack, M., and Gersdorff, C.E.F. (1952). Nutritional evaluation of food proteins by measuring availability of amino acids to micro-organisms: (i) cottonseed protein. *Journal of Nutrition*, 48, 231–41.

Horne, D.W., Patterson, D., and Cook, R.J. (1989). Effect of nitrous oxide inactivation of vitamin B_{12}-dependent methionine synthetase on the subcellular distribution of folate coenzymes in rat liver. *Archives of Biochemistry and Biophysics*, 270, 729–33.

Hornig, D. (1975). Distribution of ascorbic acid metabolites and analogues in man and animals. *Annals of the New York Academy of Sciences*, 258, 103–18.

Horwitt, M.K., and Kreisler, O. (1949). The determination of early thiamine deficient states by estimation of blood lactic and pyruvic acids after glucose administration and exercise. *Journal of Nutrition*, 37, 411–27.

Horwitt, M.K. (1965). Role of vitamin E selenium and polyunsaturated fatty acids in clinical and experimental muscle disease. *Federation Proceedings*, 24, 68–72.

Horwitt, M.K., Harvey, C.C., Dahm, C.H., and Searcy, M.T. (1972). Relationship between tocopherol and serum lipid levels for determination of nutritional adequacy. *Annals of the New York Academy of Sciences*, 203, 223–36.

Horwitt, M.K., Harvey, C.C., Rothwell, W.S., Cutler, J.L., and Haffron, D. (1956). Tryptophan-niacin relationships in man. *Journal of Nutrition*, 60, suppl 1: 1–43.

Hoyumpa, A.M., Nichols, S.G., Wilson, F.A., and Schenker, S. (1977). Effect of ethanol on intestinal (Na, K) ATPase and intestinal thiamine transport in rats. *Journal of Laboratory and Clinical Medicine*, 90, 1086–95.

Hume, E.M., and Krebs, H.A. (1949). Vitamin A requirement of human adults. *Report of the Vitamin A Subcommittee of the Accessory Food Factors Committee.* Medical Research Council, HMSO London.

Hume, R., Vallance, B., and Weyers, E. (1977). Ascorbic acid and stress. *International Journal of Vitamin and Nutrition Research*, 47, (suppl 16) 89–98.

Huque, T.A. (1982). A survey of human liver reserves of retinol in London. *British Journal of Nutrition*, 47, 165–72.

Hurley, L.S., Duncan, J.R., Sloan, M.V., and Eckhertt, C.D. (1977). Zinc binding ligands in milk and intestine: a role in neonatal nutrition. *Proceedings of the National Academy of Sciences*, 74, 3547–9.

Hurrel, R.F., and Finot, P.A. (1983). Food processing and storage as a determinant of protein and amino acid availability. pp 135– 56 in *Nutritional Adequacy, Nutrient Availability and Needs*. J. Mauron, Ed. Birkhauser Verlag, Basel. *Experimentia Supplementum* Vol. 44.

Hytten, F.E., Taylor, K., and Taggart, N. (1966). Measurement of total body fat in man by absorption of [85]Kr. *Clinical Science*, 31, 111–9.

IARC (1977). International Agency for Research on Cancer, Intestinal Microecology Group: Dietary fibre, transit time, faecal bacteria, steroids and colon cancer in two Scandinavian populations. *Lancet*, (ii), 207–11.

Ikeda, M., Tsuji, H., Nakamura, S., Ichiyama, A., Nishizuka, Y., and Hayaishi, O. (1965). Studies on the biosynthesis of nicotinamide adenine dinucleotide (ii) a role of picolinic carboxylase in the biosynthesis of nicotinamide adenine dinucleotide from tryptophan in mammals. *Journal of Biological Chemistry*, 240, 1395–401.

Ingold, K.U., Burton, G.W., Foster, D.O., Hughes, L., Lindsy, D.A., and Webb, W. (1987). Biokinetics of, and discrimination between, dietary *RRR*- and *SRR*-α-tocopherols in the male rat. *Lipids*, 22, 163–72.

International Vitamin A Consultative Group (1983). *Biochemical Methodology for the Assessment of Vitamin A Status*. The Nutrition Foundation, Washington, DC.

Intersalt Cooperative Research Group (1988). Intersalt: an international study of electrolyte excretion and blood pressure. Results for 24 hour urinary sodium and potassium excretion. *British Medical Journal*, 297, 319–28.

Irwin, M.I., and Hegsted, D.M. (1971). A conspectus of research on amino acid requirements of man. *Journal of Nutrition*, 101, 541–66.

Itokawa, Y., and Cooper, J.R. (1970a). Ion movements and thiamine in nervous tissue: (i) intact preparations. *Biochemical Pharmacology*, 19, 985–92.

Itokawa, Y., and Cooper, J.R. (1970b). Ion movements and thiamine: (ii) the release of the vitamin from membrane fragments. *Biochimica et Biophysica Acta*, 196, 274–84.

Jackson, A.A. (1983). Amino acids, essential and non-essential. *Lancet*, (i), 1034–7.

Jackson, A.A. (1991) The glycine story. *European Journal of Clinical Nutrition*, 45, 59–65.

Jackson, A.A. (1993). Chronic malnutrition: protein metabolism. *Proceedings of the Nutrition Society*, 52, 1–10.

Jackson, A.S., and Pollock, M.L. (1978). Generalized equations for predicting body density of men. *British Journal of Nutrition*, 40, 497–507.

Jacob, R.A., Kelley, D.S., Pianalto, F.S., Swendseid, M.E., Henning, S.M., Zhang, J.Z., Ames, B.N., Fraga, C.G., and Peters, J.H. (1991). Immunocompetence and oxidant defense during ascorbate depletion of healthy men. *American Journal of Clinical Nutrition*, 54, 1302–9s.

Jaksic, T., Wagner, D.A., Burke, J.F., and Young, V.R. (1991). Proline metabolism in adult male burned patients and healthy control subjects. *American Journal of Clinical Nutrition*, 54, 408–13.

James, W.P.T., and Schofield, E.C.. (1980) *Human Energy Requirements: a Manual for Planners and Nutritionists.* Oxford University Press for the Food and Agriculture Organization of the UN.

James, W.P.T., Ferro-Luzzi, A., Isaksson, B., and Szostak, W.B. (1988). *Healthy nutrition: preventing nutrition-related diseases in Europe.* WHO Regional Publications, European Series no 24. WHO, Copenhagen.

Janero, D.A., Hreniuk, D., Sharif, H.M., and Prout, K.C. (1993). Hydroperoxide-induced oxidative stress alters pyridine nucleotide metabolism in neonatal heart muscle cells. *American Journal of Physiology*, 264, C1401–10.

JECFI (1970). *Joint Expert Committee on the Wholesomeness of Irradiated Foods. WHO Technical Report Series 451.* WHO, Geneva.

JECFI (1977). *Joint Expert Committee on the Wholesomeness of Irradiated Foods. WHO Technical Report Series 604.* WHO, Geneva.

JECFI (1981). *Joint Expert Committee on the Wholesomeness of Irradiated Foods. WHO Technical Report Series 659.* WHO, Geneva.

Jelliffe, D.B., and Jelliffe, E.F.P. (1989). *Community Nutritional Assessment*, Oxford University Press.

Jelliffe, D.B. (1966). *Assessment of the Nutritional Status of the Community*. WHO, Geneva.

Jennens, M.L., and Lowe, M.E. (1994). A surface loop covering the active site of human pancreatic lipase influences interfacial activation and lipid binding. *Journal of Biological Chemistry*, 269, 25470–4.

Jolly, D.W., Craig, C., and Nelson, T.E. (1977). Estrogen and prothrombin synthesis: effect of estrogen on absorption of vitamin K_1. *American Journal of Physiology*, 232, H12–7.

Joshi, J.G. (1990). Aluminium, a neurotoxin which affects diverse metabolic reactions. *Biofactors*, 2, 163–9.

Juan, D., and DeLuca, H.F. (1977). The regulation of 24,25–dihydroxy-vitamin D_3 production in cultures of monkey kidney cells. *Endocrinology*, 101, 1184–93.

Kabir, H., Leklem, J.E., and Miller, L.T. (1983). Comparative vitamin B_6 availability from tuna, whole wheat bread and peanut butter in humans. *Journal of Nutrition*, 113, 2412–20.

Kakade, M.L., Thompson, R.D., Engelstad, W.E., Behrens, G.C., Yoder, R.D., and Crane, M.F. (1976). Failure of soy bean trypsin inhibitor to exert deleterious effect in calves. *Journal of Dairy Science*, 59, 1484–9.

Kakade, M.L., Hoffa, D.E., and Liener, I.E. (1973). Contribution of trypsin inhibitors to the deleterious effect of unheated soybeans fed to rats. *Journal of Nutrition*, 103, 1772–8.

Kallner, A., Hartmann, D., and Hornig, D. (1979). Steady-state turnover and body pool of ascorbic acid in man. *American Journal of Clinical Nutrition*, 32, 530–9.

Kallner, A., Hartmann, D., and Hornig, D. (1981). On the requirements of ascorbic acid in man: steady state turnover and body pool in smokers. *American Journal of Clinical Nutrition*, 34, 1347–55.

Kallner, A., Hornig, D., and Pellikka, R. (1985). Formation of carbon dioxide from ascorbate in man. *American Journal of Clinical Nutrition*, 41, 609–13.

Kanis, J.A., and Passmore, R. (1989). Calcium supplementation in the diet: not justified by present evidence. *British Medical Journal*, 298, 205–8.

Kappus, H., and Diplock, A.T. (1992). Tolerance and safety of vitamin E: a toxicological position report. *Free Radicals in Biology and Medicine*, 13, 55–74.

Karlson, B., Leijd, B., and Hellström, K. (1986). On the influence of vitamin K rich vegetables and wine on the effectiveness of warfarin treatment. *Acta Medica Scandinavica*, 220, 347–50.

Kawai, C., Wakabayashi, A., Matsumura, T., and Yui, Y. (1980). Reappearance of beriberi heart disease in Japan: a study of 23 cases. *American Journal of Medicine*, 69, 383–6.

Kelly, D., Weir, D., Reed, B., and Scott, J. (1979). Effect of anticonvulsant drugs on the rate of folate catabolism in mice. *Journal of Clinical Investigation*, 64, 1989–96.

Kelsay, J., Miller, L.T., and Linkswiler, H. (1968a). Effect of protein intake on the excretion of quinolinic acid and niacin metabolites by men during vitamin B_6 depletion. *Journal of Nutrition*, 94, 27–31.

Kelsay, J., Baysal, A., and Linkswiler, H. (1968b). Effects of vitamin B_6 depletion on the pyridoxal, pyridoxamine and pyridoxine content of the blood and urine of man. *Journal of Nutrition*, 94, 490–4.

Kelsay, J.L. (1969). A compendium of nutritional status studies and dietary evaluation studies in the USA, 1957–1967. *Journal of Nutrition*, 99, suppl 1, 119–66.

Kesteloot, H., Roelandt, J., Willems, J., Claes, J.H., and Joossens, J.V. (1968). An enquiry into the role of cobalt in the heart disease of chronic beer drinkers. *Circulation*, 37, 854–64.

Keutsch, G.T., and Farthing, M.J.G. (1990). Nutritional aspects of AIDS. *Annual Review of Nutrition*, 10, 475–501.

Keys, A. and Brozek, J. (1953). Body fat in adult man. *Physiological Reviews*, 33, 245–325.

Killberg, M.S., Stevens, B.R., and Novak, D.A. (1993). Recent advances in mammalian amino acid transport. *Annual Review of Nutrition*, 13, 137–65.

Killmann, S-A (1964). Effect of deoxyuridine on incorporation of tritiated thymidine: difference between normoblasts and megaloblasts. *Acta Medica Scandinavica*, 175, 483–8.

King, C.E., and Toskes, P.P. (1983). The use of breath tests in the study of malabsorption. *Clinics in Gastroenterology*, 12, 591–610.

Kirchgessner, M., Krziwanek, S., and Grassman, E. (1977). The influence of dietary protein quality on the activities of several metallo-enzymes. *Zeitschrift für Tierenphysiologie, Tierernährung und Futtermittelkunde*, 38, 273–82.

Kirksey, A., Keaton, K., Abernathy, R.P., and Greger, J.L. (1978). Vitamin B_6 nutritional status of a group of female adolescents. *American Journal of Clinical Nutrition*, 31, 946–54.

Klein, G.L. (1995). Aluminium in parenteral solutions revisited—again. *American Journal of Clinical Nutrition*, 61, 449–56.

Kley, H.K., Edelman, P., and Krüskemper, H.L. (1980). Relationship of plasma sex hormones to different parameters of obesity in male subjects. *Metabolism*, 29, 1041–5.

Knapp, A. (1960). Uber eine neue hereditäre, von Vitamin-B_6 abhängige Störung im Tryptophan-Stoffwechsel. *Clinica Chimica Acta*, 5, 6–13.

Komrower, G.M., Wilson, V., Clamp, J.R., and Westall, R.G. (1964). Hydroxykynureninuria: a case of abnormal tryptophan metabolism probably due to a deficiency of kynureninase. *Archives of Diseases of Childhood*, 39, 250–6.

König, K.G., and Navia, J.M. (1995). Nutritional role of sugars in oral health. *American Journal of Clinical Nutrition*, 62, (supplement) 275–83s.

Kopple, J.D., and Swendseid, M.E. (1975). Evidence that histidine is an essential amino acid in normal and chronically uremic man. *Journal of Clinical Investigation*, 55, 881–91.

Kotake, Y., Ueda, T., Mori, T., Murakami, E., and Hattori, M. (1975). The physiological significance of the xanthurenic acid-insulin complex. *Journal of Biochemistry (Tokyo)*, 77, 685–7.

Krebs, H.A. (1968). The effects of ethanol on the metabolic activities of the liver. *Advances in Enzyme Regulation*, 6, 467–80.

Krebs, H.A., Hems, R., and Tyler, B. (1976). The regulation of folate and methionine metabolism. *Biochemical Journal*, 158, 341–53.

Krinke, G., Schaumburg, H.H., Spencer, P.S., Suter, J., Thomann, O., and Hess, R. (1980). Pyridoxine megavitaminosis produces degeneration of peripheral sensory neurons (sensory neuronopathy) in the dog. *Neurotoxicology*, 2, 13–24.

Krinsky, N.I., and Deneke, S.M. (1982). Interaction of oxygen and oxy-radicals with carotenoids. *Journal of the National Cancer Institute*, 69, 205–10.

Krishnamurthy, K., Suriola, N., and Adiga, P.R. (1984). Mechanism of foetal wastage following immunoneutralization of riboflavin carrier protein in the pregnant rat: disturbances in flavin coenzyme levels. *FEBS Letters*, 178, 87–91.

Kushner, R.F. (1993). Body weight and mortality. *Nutrition Reviews*, 51, 127–36.

Kushner, R.F., Schoeller, D.A., Fjeld, C.R., and Danford, L. (1992). Is the impedance index (ht^2/R) significant in predicting total body water? *American Journal of Clinical Nutrition*, 56, 835–9.

Laburthe, M., Couvineau, A., Amiranoff, B., and Voisin, T. (1994). Receptors for gut regulatory peptides. *Ballière's Clinical Endocrinology and Metabolism*, 8:1, 77–110.

Laidlaw, S.A., and Kopple, J.D. (1987). Newer concepts of the indispensable amino acids. *American Journal of Clinical Nutrition*, 46, 593–605.

Lakshmi, A.V., and Bamji, M.S. (1974). Tissue pyridoxal phosphate concentration and pyridoxamine phosphate oxidase activity in riboflavin deficiency in rats and man. *British Journal of Nutrition*, 32, 249–55.

Lands, W.E.M., and Zakhari, S. (1991). The case of the missing calories. *American Journal of Clinical Nutrition*, 54, 47–8.

Lane, P.A., and Hathaway, W.E. (1985). Vitamin K in infancy. *Journal of Pediatrics*, 106, 351–9.

Langstein, H.N., and Norton, J.A. (1991). Mechanisms of cancer cachexia. *Haematology and Oncology Clinics of North America*, 5, 103–23.

Larsson, A., and Erlanson-Albertsson, C. (1991). The effect of pancreatic procolipase and colipase on pancreatic lipase activation. *Biochimica et Biophysica Acta*, 1083, 283–8.

Larsson, B., Bengtsson, C., Björntorp, P., Lapidus, L., Sjöström, L., Svärdsudd, K., Tibblin, G., Weidel, H., Welin, L., and Wilhelmsen, L. (1992). Is abdominal body fat distribution a major explanation for the sex difference in the incidence of myocardial infarction? *American Journal of Epidemiology*, 135, 266–73.

Lavis, G.J., Ofei, V., and Bender, D.A. (1986). Differences in the zinc content of different regions of the toe-nail. *Proceedings of the Nutrition Society*, 46, 59A.

Lee, S-S, and McCormick, D.B. (1985). Thyroid hormone regulation of flavocoenzyme biosynthesis. *Archives of Biochemistry and Biophysics*, 237, 197–201.

Lehman, J. (1972). Mental and neuromuscular symptoms in tryptophan deficiency. *Acta Psychiatrica Scandinavica suppl*, 237, 5–28.

Leklem, J.E. (1990). Vitamin B-6: a status report. *Journal of Nutrition*, 120, 1503–7.

Leklem, J.E., and Schultz, T.D. (1983). Increased plasma pyridoxal 5'-phosphate and vitamin B_6 after a 4500 meter run. *American Journal of Clinical Nutrition*, 38, 541–8.

Lemoine, A., le Devehat, C., Codaccioni, J.L., Monges, A., Bermond, P., and Salkeld, R.M. (1980). Vitamin B_1, B_2, B_6 and C status in hospital inpatients. *American Journal of Clinical Nutrition*, 33, 2595–600.

Lentze, M.J. (1995). Molecular and cellular aspects of hydrolysis and absorption. *American Journal of Clinical Nutrition*, 61, (suppl) 946–61s.

Leo, M.A., and Lieber, C.S. (1985). New pathway for retinol metabolism in liver microsomes. *Journal of Biological Chemistry*, 260, 5228–31.

Leo, M.A., Kim, C-I, and Lieber, C.S, (1989). Role of vitamin degradation in the control of hepatic levels in the rat. *Journal of Nutrition*, 119, 993–1000.

Levenson, D.I., and Bockman, R.S. (1994). A review of calcium preparations. *Nutrition Reviews*, 52, 221–32.

Levine, R.A,, Streeten, D.H.P., and Doisy, R.J. (1968). Effects of oral chromium supplementation on the glucose tolerance of elderly human subjects. *Metabolism*, 17, 114–25.

Lew, E.A. (1985). Mortality and weight: insured lives and American Cancer Society studies. *Annals of Internal Medicine*, 103, 1024–9.

Lew, E.A., and Garfinkel, L. (1979). Variation in mortality by weight among 750,000 men and women. *Journal of Chronic Diseases*, 12, 563–76.

Lieber, C.S. (1985). Alcohol and liver: metabolism of ethanol, metabolic effects and pathogenesis of injury. *Acta Medica Scandinavica suppl.*, 703, 11–55.

Liener, I.E. (1980). *Toxic Constituents of Plant Foodstuffs*. Academic Press, New York.

Lind, C., Hochstein, P., and Ernster, L. (1982). DT-diaphorase as a quinone reductase: a cellular control device against semiquinone and superoxide radical formation. *Archives of Biochemistry and Biophysics*, 216, 178–85.

Linkswiler, H.M. (1981). Methionine metabolite excretion as affected by a vitamin B_6 deficiency. In *Methods in Vitamin B-6 Nutrition, Analysis and Status Assessment* (ed. J.E. Leklem and R.D. Reynolds), pp. 373–382. Plenum Press, New York.

Litwack, G., Williams, J.N., Chen, L., and Elvehjem, C.A. (1952). A study of the relationship of liver xanthine oxidase to quality of dietary protein. *Journal of Nutrition*, 47, 299–306.

Livesey, G. (1984). The energy equivalents of ATP and the energy values of food proteins and fats. *British Journal of Nutrition*, 51, 15–28.

Livesey, G. (1992). The energy values of dietary fibre and sugar alcohols for man. *Nutrition Research Reviews*, 5, 61–84.

Livesey, G., and Elia, M. (1988). Estimation of energy expenditure, net carbohydrate utilization, and net fat oxidation and synthesis by indirect calorimetry: evaluation of errors with special reference to the detailed composition of fuels. *American Journal of Clinical Nutrition*, 47, 608–28.

Llovera, M., López-Soriano, F.J.,, and Argilés, J.P. (1993). Effects of tumor necrosis factor-α on muscle protein turnover in female Wistar rats. *Journal of the National Cancer Institute*, 85, 1334–9.

Lloyd, K.C. (1994) Gut hormones in gastric function. *Ballière's Clinical Endocrinology and Metabolism*, 8:1, 111–6.

Loerch, J.D., Underwood, B.A., and Lewis, K.C. (1979). Response of plasma levels of vitamin A to a dose of vitamin A as an indicator of hepatic vitamin A reserves in rats. *Journal of Nutrition*, 109, 778–86.

Lohman, T.G. (1971). Skinfolds and body density and their relation to body fatness: a review. *Human Biology*, 53, 181–225.

Lonergan, M.E., Milne, J.S., Maule, M.M., and Williamson, J. (1975). A dietary study of older people in Edinburgh. *British Journal of Nutrition*, 34, 517–27.

Loschiavo, S.R. (1960). *Journal of Science of Food and Agriculture*, 31, 351.

Lubchenko, L.O., Hansmann, C., Dressler, M., and Boyd, E. (1963). Intrauterine growth as estimated from liveborn birthweight at 24–42 weeks of gestation. *Pediatrics*, 32, 793–800.

Lubchenko, L.O., Hansman, C., and Boyd, E. (1966): Intrauterine growth in length and head circumference as estimated from live births at gestational ages from 26 to 42 weeks. *Pediatrics*, 37, 403–8.

Luhby, A.L., Brin, M., Gordon, M., David, P., Murphy, M., and Spiegel, H. (1971). Vitamin B_6 metabolism in users of oral contraceptive agents (i) abnormal urinary excretion of xanthurenic acid and its correction by pyridoxine. *American Journal of Clinical Nutrition*, 24, 684–93.

Lukaski, H.C. (1987). Methods for the assessment of human body composition: traditional and new. *American Journal of Clinical Nutrition*, 46, 537–56.

Lukaski, H.C., Johnson, P.E., Bolonchuk, W.W., and Lykken, G.I. (1985). Assessment of fat-free mass using bio-electrical impedance measurements of the human body. *American Journal of Clinical Nutrition*, 41, 810–7.

Lumb, M., Perry, J., Deacon, R., and Chanarin, I. (1982). Urinary folate loss following inactivation of vitamin B_{12} by nitrous oxide in rats. *British Journal of Haematology*, 51, 235–42.

Lumeng, L., Brashear, R.E., and Li, T-K (1974). Pyridoxal 5'-phosphate in plasma: source, protein binding and cellular transport. *Journal of Laboratory and Clinical Medicine*, 84, 334–43.

Lunn, P.G., Northrop-Clewes, C.A., and Downes, R.M. (1991). Intestinal permeability, mucosal injury, and growth faltering in Gambian infants. *Lancet*, 338, 907–10.

Mabee, T.M., Meyer, P., DenBesten, L., and Mason, E.E. (1976). The mechanism of increased gallstone formation in obese human subjects. *Surgery*, 79, 460–8.

MacFarlane, T.W., and Samaranayake, L.P. (1989). *Clinical Oral Microbiology*. Wright, London.

MacKenzie, R.E., and Baugh, C.M. (1980). Tetrahydropteroylpolyglutamate derivatives as substrates of two multifunctional proteins with folate-dependent enzyme activities. *Biochimica et Biophysica Acta*, 611, 187–95.

MacLaughlin, J., and Holick, M.F. (1985). Aging decreases the capacity of human skin to produce vitamin D_3. *Journal of Clinical Investigation*, 76, 1536–8.

Maclure, K.M., Hayes, K.C., Colditz, G.A., Stampfer, M.J., Speizer, F.E., and Willett, W.C. (1989). Weight, diet and the risk of symptomatic gallstones in middle-aged women. *New England Journal of Medicine*, 321, 563–9.

MAFF (1993). Ministry of Agriculture, Fisheries and Food. *Food Surveillance Paper no 36: Mycotoxins, 3rd report*. HMSO, London.

Magboul, B.I., and Bender, D.A. (1983). The effects of a dietary excess of leucine on the synthesis of nicotinamide nucleotides in the rat. *British Journal of Nutrition*, 49, 321–4.

Maiorino, M., Coassin, M., Roveri. A., and Ursini, F. (1989). Microsomal lipid peroxidation: effect of vitamin E and its functional interaction with phospholipid hydroperoxide glutathione peroxidase. *Lipids*, 24, 721–6.

Man, E.H., and Bada, J.L. (1987). Dietary D-amino acids. *Annual Review of Nutrition*, 7, 209–25.

Manson, J.A., and Carpenter, K.J. (1978a). The effects of a high level of dietary leucine on the niacin status of chicks and rats. *Journal of Nutrition*, 108, 1883–8.

Manson, J.A., and Carpenter, K.J. (1978b). The effect of a high level of dietary leucine on the niacin status of dogs. *Journal of Nutrition*, 108, 1889–98.

Manson, J.E., Colditz, G.A., Stampfer, M.J., Willett, W.C., Rosner, B., Monson, R.R., Speizer, F.E., and Hennekens, C.H. (1990). A prospective study of obesity and risk of coronary heart disease in women. *New England Journal of Medicine*, 322, 882–889.

Manwaring, J.D., and Csallany, A.S. (1988). Malondialdehyde-containing proteins and their relationship to vitamin E. *Lipids*, 23, 651–5.

Mapson, L.W. (1956). Effect of processing on the vitamin content of foods. *British Medical Bulletin*, 12, 73–7.

March, B.E., Wong, E., Seier, L., Sim, J., and Biely, J. (1973). Hypervitaminosis E in the chick. *Journal of Nutrition*, 103, 371–7.

Marchesini, A., Majorino, G., Montuori, F., and Gagna, D. (1975). Changes in the ascorbic acid and dehydroascorbic acid content of fresh and canned beans. *Journal of Food Science*, 40, 665–8.

Marletta, M.A., Tayeh, M.A., and Hevel, J.M. (1990). Unravelling the biological significance of nitric oxide. *Biofactors*, 2, 219–25.

Marmot, M., and Brunner, E. (1991). Alcohol and cardio-vascular disease: the status of the U-shaped curve. *British Medical Journal*, **303**, 565–8.

Martin, A.D., Drinkwater, D.T., and Clarys, J.P. (1984). Human body surface area: validation of formulae based on a cadaver study. *Human Biology*, **56**, 475–88.

Martner-Hawes, P.M., Hunt, I.F., Murphy, N.J., Swendseid, M.E., and Settlage, R.H. (1986). Vitamin B_6 nutriture and plasma diamine oxidase in pregnant Hispanic teenagers. *American Journal of Clinical Nutrition*, **44**, 907–13.

Mason, J.B., and Kodicek, E. (1970). The metabolism of niacytin in the rat, trigonelline as a major metabolite of niacytin in the urine. *Biochemical Journal*, **120**, 515–21.

Mason, J.B., and Selhub, J. (1988). Folate-binding protein and the absorption of folic acid in the small intestine of the suckling rat. *American Journal of Clinical Nutrition*, **48**, 620–5.

Mason, J.B., Gibson, N., and Kodicek, E. (1973). The chemical nature of the bound nicotinic acid of wheat bran, studies of nicotinic acid containing macromolecules. *British Journal of Nutrition*, **30**, 297–311.

Massachussetts General Hospital (1986). Normal Reference Laboratory Values. *New England Journal of Medicine*, **314**, 39–49.

Matovinovic, J. (1983). Endemic goitre and cretinism at the dawn of the third millenium. *Annual Review of Nutrition*, **3**, 341–412.

Matsubara, T., Touchi, A., Harauchi, T., Takno, K., and Yoshizaki, T. (1989). Depression of liver microsomal vitamin K epoxide reductase activity associated with antibiotic-induced coagulopathy. *Biochemical Pharmacology*, **38**, 2693–701.

Matsuoka, L.Y., Wortsman, J., Haddad, J.G., and Hollis, B.W. (1989). *In vivo* threshold for cutaneous synthesis of vitamin D_3. *Journal of Laboratory and Clinical Medicine*, **114**, 301–5.

Matsusaka, T., Fujii, M., Nakano, T., Terai, T., Kurata, A., Imaizumi, M., and Abe, H. (1988). Germanium-induced nephropathy: report of two cases and review of the literature. *Clinical Nephrology*, **30**, 342–5.

Matthews, R.G. (1982). Are the redox properties of tetrahydrofolate cofactors utilized in folate-dependent reactions? *Federation Proceedings*, **41**, 2600–4.

Mavrelis, P.G., Ammon, H.V., Gleysteen, J.J., Komorowski, R.A., and Charaf, U.K. (1983). Hepatic free fatty acids in alcoholic liver disease and morbid obesity. *Hepatology*, **3**, 226–31.

Mawer, E.B., Backhouse, J., Taylor, C.M., Lumb, G.A., and Stanbury, S.W. (1973). Failure of formation of 1,25–dihdroxycholecalciferol in chronic renal insufficiency. *Lancet*, (i), 626–8.

May, M.E., and Hill, J.O. (1990). Energy content of diets of variable amino acid composition. *American Journal of Clinical Nutrition*, **52**, 770–6.

Mazur, A., Green, S., and Carleton, A. (1960). Mechanism of plasma iron incorporation into hepatic ferritin. *Journal of Biological Chemistry*, **235**, 599–603.

McCandless, D.W., Hanson, C., Speeg, K.V., and Schenker, S. (1970). Cardiac metabolism in thiamin deficiency in rats. *Journal of Nutrition*, **100**, 991–1002.

McCandless, D.W., Carley, A.D., and Cassidy, C.E. (1976). Thiamine deficiency and the pentose phosphate pathway in rats: intracerebral mechanisms. *Journal of Nutrition*, **106**: 1144–51.

McChrisley, B., and Thye, F.W. (1988). Plasma B_6 vitamer and 4–pyridoxic acid concentrations of men fed controlled diets. *Journal of Chromatography*, **428**, 35–42.

McConalogue, K., and Furness, J.B. (1994). Gastrointestinal neurotransmitters. *Ballière's Clinical Endocrinology and Metabolism*, **8**, 1–6.

McCreanor, G.M., and Bender, D.A. (1983). The role of catabolism in controlling tissue concentrations of nicotinamide nucleotide coenzymes. *Biochimica et Biophysica Acta*, **759**, 222–8.

McDowell, I., and Savage-King, F. (1982). Interpretation of arm circumference as an indicator of nutritional status, *Archives of Disease in Childhood*, **57**, 292–6.

McLaren, D.S., Pellett, P.L., and Read, W.W.C. (1967). A simple scoring system for classifying the severe forms of protein-calorie malnutrition of early childhood. *Lancet*, (i), 533–5.

McLaughlan, J.M. (1976). The relative nitrogen method for evaluating protein quality. *Journal of the Association of Official Analytical Chemists*, **59**, 42–5.

McLaughlan, J.M., Anderson, G.H., Heckler, L.R., Hill, D.C., Jansen, G.R., Keith, M.O., Sarwar, G., and Sosulski, F.W. (1980). Assessment of rat growth methods for estimating protein quality: interlaboratory study. *Journal of the Association of Official Analytical Chemists*, **63**, 462–7.

McPartlin, J., Courtney, G., McNulty, H., Weir, D., and Scott, J. (1992). The quantitative analysis of endogenous folate catabolites in human urine. *Analytical Biochemistry*, **206**, 256–61.

McPartlin, J., Halligan, A., Scott, J.M., Darling, M., and Weir, D.G. (1993). Accelerated folate breakdown in pregnancy. *Lancet*, **341**, 148–9.

McTigue, J.J., and Suttie, J.W. (1983). Vitamin K-dependent carboxylase: demonstration of a vitamin K and O_2-dependent exchange of ^3H from ^3H_2O into glutamic acid residues. *Journal of Biological Chemistry*, **258**, 12129–31.

Means, A.L., and Gudas, L.J. (1995). The roles of retinoids in vertebrate development. *Annual Review of Biochemistry*, **64**, 201–33.

Medical Research Council Vitamin C Sub-committee of the Accessory Food Factor Committee (1948). Vitamin C requirement of human adults. *Lancet*, (i), 835–58.

Medrano, J.F., and Bressani, R. (1977). Evaluation of nutritional quality of food with the red flour beetle (*Tribolium castaneum*): effects of protein concentration in the diet on larval growth and development time. *Nutrition Reports International*, **16**, 255–66.

Medsger, T.A. (1990). Tryptophan-induced eosinophilia-myalgia syndrome. *New England Journal of Medicine*, **322**, 926–8.

Meeks, R.G., Zaharevitz, D., and Chen, R.F. (1981). Membrane effects of retinoids: possible correlation with toxicity. *Archives of Biochemistry and Biophysics*, **207**, 141–7.

Mehler, A.H., Yano, K., and May, E.L. (1964). Nicotinic acid biosynthesis control by an enzyme that competes with a spontaneous reaction. *Science*, **145**, 817–9.

Mennita, F.S., Knoth, J., and Diliberto, E.J. (1986). The role of ascorbic acid in dopamine-beta-hydroxylation: the endogenous enzyme cofactor and putative electron donor for cofactor regeneration. *Journal of Biological Chemistry*, **261**, 16901–8.

Mertz, W. (1974). Biological function of nicotinic acid-chromium complexes. *Federation Proceedings*, **33**, 659.

Mertz, W. (1995). Risk assessment of essential trace elements: new approaches to setting Recommended Dietary Allowances and safety limits. *Nutrition Reviews*, **53**, 179–85.

Metropolitan Life Assurance Society (1983). *Metropolitan Life Assurance Statistical Bulletin*, **64**, part 2.

Metzger, A.L., Heymsfield, S., and Grundy, S.M. (1972). The lithogenic index, a numerical expression for the relative lithogenicity of bile. *Gastroenterology*, **62**, 499–501.

Michajlovskij, N., and Langer, P.. (1959). The occurrence of preformed thiocyanate in some vegetables with regard to seasonal and regional differences. *Hoppe-Seyler's Zeitschrift für Physiologische Chemie*, **317**, 30–3.

Michajlovskij, N., Sedlak, J., Jusic, M., and Buzina, R. (1969). Goitrogenic substances of kale and their possible relation to the endemic goitre of the island of Krk (Jugoslavia). *Endocrinologica Experimentalis (Bratislava)*, **3**, 65–73.

Mickell. J.J. (1982). Urea nitrogen excretion in critically ill children. *Pediatrics*, **70**, 949–55.

Mifflin, M.D., St Jeor, S.T., Hill, L.A., Scott, B.J., Daugherty, S.A., and Koh, Y.O. (1990). A new predictive equation for resting energy exendture in healthy individuals. *American Journal of Clinical Nutrition*, **51**, 241–7.

Mikkelson, K., Rasmussen, E.L., and Zinck, O. (1984). Retention of vitamin B_1, B_2 and B_6 in frozen meats, pp 777–81 in *Thermal Processing and Quality of Foods* (Zeuthen P, Ed), Elsevier Applied Science Publishers, London.

Miller, D.F. (1978). Pellagra deaths in the United States. *American Journal of Clinical Nutrition*, **31**, 558.

Miller, D.S., and Bender, A.E. (1955). The determination of net utilization of proteins by a shortened method. *British Journal of Nutrition*, **9**, 382–8.

Miller, L.T., and Linkswiler, H. (1967). Effect of protein intake on the development of abnormal tryptophan metabolism by men during vitamin B_6 depletion. *Journal of Nutrition*, **93**, 53–9.

Millward, D.J. (1993). Stable isotope tracer studies of amino acid balance and human indispensable amino acid requirements. *American Journal of Clinical Nutrition*, **57**, 81–91.

Millward, D.J. (1994). Can we define indispensable amino acid requirements and assess protein quality in adults? *Journal of Nutrition*, **124**, 1509–16S.

Millward, D.J., and Bates, P.C. (1983). 3–Methylhistidine turnover in the whole body and the contribution of skeletal muscle and intestine to urinary 3–methylhistidine excretion in the adult rat. *Biochemical Journal*, **214**, 607–15.

Millward, D.J., and Rivers, J.P.W. (1988). The nutritional role for indispensable amino acids and the metabolic basis for their requirements. *European Journal of Clinical Nutrition*, **42**, 367–93.

Millward, D.J., Jackson, A.A., Price, G., and Rivers, J.P.W. (1989). Human amino acid and protein requirements: current dilemmas and uncertainties. *Nutrition Research Reviews*, **2**, 109–32.

Millward, D.J., Price, G.M., Pacy, P.J.H., and Halliday, D. (1991). Whole body protein and amino acid turnover in man: what can we measure with confidence? *Proceedings of the Nutrition Society*, **50**, 197–216.

Milne, D.B. (1994). Assessment of copper nutritional status. *Clinical Chemistry*, **40**, 1479–84.

Milne, D.B., and Johnson, P.E. (1993). Assessment of copper status: effect of age and gender on reference ranges in healthy adults. *Clinical Chemistry*, **39**, 883–7.

Minister of National Health and Welfare (1988). *Canadian Guidelines for Healthy Weights: Report of an expert group*. Ottawa.

Ministry of Agriculture, Fisheries and Food / Department of Health (1991). *Dietary Supplements and Health Foods*; report of the working party. MAFF Publications, London.

Mirabelli, F., Salis, A., Marinoni, V., Finardi, G., Bellomo, G., Thor, H., and Orrenius, S. (1988). Menadione-induced bleb formation in hepatocytes is associated with the oxidation of thiol groups in actin. *Archives of Biochemistry and Biophysics*, **264**, 261–9.

Mitchell, H.H. (1924). A method of determining the biological value of protein. *Journal of Biological Chemistry*, **58**, 873–903.

Mitchell, H.H., Hamilton, T.S., Steggerda, F.R., and Bean, H.W. (1945). Chemical composition of the human body and its bearing on the biochemistry of growth. *Journal of Biological Chemistry*, **158**, 625–37.

Mizutani, T., Kurata, H. and Yamada, K. (1991). Study of mammalian selenocysteine-tRNA synthesis with $[^{75}Se]H_2Se$. *FEBS Letters*, **289**, 59–63.

Mock, D.M., Baswell, D.L., Baker, H., Holman, R.T., and Sweetman, L. (1985). Biotin deficiency complicating parenteral alimentation: diagnosis, metabolic repercussions, and treatment. *Journal of Pediatrics*, **106**, 762–9.

Mock, D.M., Mock, N.I., Johnson, S.B., and Holman, R.T. (1988). Effects of biotin deficiency on plasma and tissue fatty acid composition: evidence for abnormalities in rats. *Pediatric Research*, **24**, 396–402.

Mohyuddin, M., Sharma, T.R., Dhar, P., and Niemann, E.G. (1977). Nutritive values of some wheat varieties assessed with *Aspergillus flavus* in comparison to rat feeding experiments. *Qualitas Plantarum*, **27**, 249–54.

Mokady, S., Viola, S., and Zimmermann, G. (1969). A new biological method for estimating protein nutritive value. *British Journal of Nutrition*, **23**, 491–5.

Momoi, T., Hanoaka, K., and Momoi, M. (1990). Spatial and temporal expression of cellular retinoic acid binding protein (CRABP) along the antero-posterior axis in the central nervous system of mouse embryos. *Biochemical and Biophysical Research Communications*, **169**, 991–6.

Moorjani, M.N., and Subrahmanyan, V. (1950). Comparative values of vegetable-milk proteins and casein for the formation of blood proteins. *Indian Journal of Medical Research*, **38**, 145–50.

Morgan, D.B., and Burkinshaw, L. (1983). Estimation of non-fat body tissue from measurements of skinfold thickness, total body potassium and total body nitrogen. *Clinical Science*, **65**, 407–14.

Morrison, M.H. (1974). *Journal of Food Technology*, **9**, 491–500.

Morrison, A.B., and Campbell, J.A. (1960). Vitamin absorption studies: (i) factors influencing the excretion of oral test doses of thiamine and riboflavin by human subjects. *Journal of Nutrition*, **72**, 435–40.

Morrison, A.N., Qi, C.J., and Tokita, A. (1994). Prediction of bone density from vitamin D receptor alleles. *Nature*, **67**, 284–7.

Motil, K.J., Matthews, D.E., Bier, D.M., Burke, J.F., Munro, H.N., and Young, V.R. (1981). Whole body leucine and lysine metabolism: response to dietary protein intake in young men. *American Journal of Physiology*, **240**, E712–21.

MRC Research Group (1991). Prevention of neural tube defects: the results of the Medical Research Council study. *Lancet*, **338**, 131–7.

Mudd, S.H. (1971). Pyridoxine-responsive genetic disease. *Federation Proceedings*, **30**, 970–6.

Muller, D.P.R. (1986). Vitamin E—its role in neurological function. *Postgraduate Medical Journal*, **62**, 107–12.

Muller, D.P.R., Lloyd, J.K., and Wolff, O.H. (1983). Vitamin E and neurological function. *Lancet*, (i), 225–8.

Münchow, H., and Bergner, J. (1968). Empfehlung zur Proteinbewertung von Eiweissfuttermitteln anhand der Bestimmung der Harstoffkonzentration im Blut von Ratte und Schwein. *Archives Tierernährung*, **18**, 222–8

Muniyappa, K., and Adiga, P.R. (1980). Occurrence and functional importance of a riboflavin carrier protein in the pregnant rat. *FEBS Letters*, **110**, 209–12.

Munnich, A., Saudubray, J.M., Coude, F.X., Charpentier, C., Saurat, J.H., and Frezal, J. (1980). Fatty acid responsive alopecia in multiple carboxylase deficiency. *Lancet*, (i), 1080–1.

Munro, H.N., Lazarus, S., and Bell, G.H. (1947). The value of capillary strength tests in the diagnosis of vitamin C and vitamin P deficiency in man. *Nutrition Abstracts and Reviews*, **17**, 291.

Muraoka, S., Sugiyama, M., and Yamasaki, H. (1962). Histamine metabolism via the nucleotide pathway. *Nature*, **196**, 441–3.

Murray, C.J.L., and Lopez, A.D. (1994). Global and regional causes-of-death patterns in 1990. *Bulletin of the World Health Organization*, **72**, 447–80.

Muto, Y., Smith, J.E., Milch, P.O., and Goodman, D.S. (1972). Regulation of retinol-binding protein metabolism by vitamin A status in the rat. *Journal of Biological Chemistry*, **247**, 2542–50.

Myllylä, R., Kuutki-Savolainen, E-R, and Kivirrikko, K.I. (1978). The role of ascorbate in the prolyl hydroxylase reaction. *Biochemical and Biophysical Research Communications*, **83**, 441–8.

Naimark, A., and Cherniak, R.M. (1960). Compliance of the respiratory system and its components in health and obesity. *Journal of Applied Physiology*, **15**, 377–82.

Najjar, M.F., and Rowland, M. (1987). *Anthropometric reference data and prevalence of overweight*. Vital Health Statistics, Series 11, No 238, DHHS Publication no (PHS). 87–1688. National Center for Health Statistics, Hyattsville, MD.

Nakagawa, T., Takahashi, T., Suzuki, T., and Masana, Y. (1969). Effect in man of the addition of tryptophan or niacin to the diet on the excretion of their metabolites. *Journal of Nutrition*, **99**, 325–30.

Nakagawa, T., Ohguri, S., Sasaki, A., Kujimoto, M., Sasaki, M., and Takahashi, T. (1975). Effects of excess intake of leucine and valine deficiency on tryptophan metabolism in humans. *Journal of Nutrition*, **105**, 1241–52.

Nakahiro, M., Fujita, N., Fukuchi, I., Saito, K., Nishimura, T., and Yoshida, H. (1985). Pantoyl-γ-aminobutyric acid facilitates cholinergic function in the central nervous system. *Journal of Pharmacology and Experimental Therapeutics*, **232**, 501–6.

Nakamura, T., Shinno, H., and Ichihara, A. (1980). Insulin and glucagon as a new regulator system for tryptophan oxygenase activity demonstrated in primary cultured rat hepatocytes. *Journal of Biological Chemistry*, **255**, 7533–5.

National Advisory Committee on Hyperkinesis and Food Additives (1980). Final Report to the Nutrition Foundation, New York.

National Research Council (1989). *Recommended Dietary Allowances*, 10th edn. National Academy Press, Washington, DC.

National Research Council Committee on Diet and Health (1989). *Diet and Health: Implications for Reducing Chronic Disease Risk*. National Academy Press, Washington, DC.

Nellhaus, G. (1968). Head circumference from birth to eighteen years: practical composite international and interracial graphs. *Pediatrics*, **41**, 106–14.

Nève, J., Vertongen, F., and Molle, L. (1985). Selenium deficiency. *Clinics in Endocrinology and Metabolism*, **14**, (3) 629–56.

Nielsen, F.H., Hunt, C.D., Mullen, L.M., and Hunt, J.R. (1987). Effect of boron on mineral, estrogen, and testosterone metabolism in postmenopausal women. *FASEB Journal*, **1**, 394–7.

Nielsen, F.H. (1991). Nutritional requirements for boron, silicon, vanadium, nickel, and arsenic: current knowledge and speculation. *FASEB Journal*, **5**, 2661–7.

NIH consensus conference on osteoporosis (1993). *American Journal of Medicine 95*: supplement 5a.

Noah, D.N., Bender, A.E., Reaidi, G.B., and Gilbert, R.J. (1980). Food poisoning from raw kidney beans. *British Medical Journal*, **281**, 236–7.

Norgan, N.G., and Ferro-Luzzi, A. (1985). The estimation of body density in men: are general equations general? *Annals of Human Biology*, **12**, 1–15.

Norum, K.R., Blomhoff, R., Green, M.H., Green, J.B., Wathne, K-O, Gjoen, T., Botilsrud, M., and Berg, T. (1986). Metabolism of retinol and other retinoids. *Biochemical Society Transactions*, **14**, 923–5.

Noto, Y., and Okamoto, H. (1978). Inhibition by kynurenine metabolites of pro-insulin synthesis in isolated pancreatic islets. *Acta Diabetologica Latina*, **15**, 273–82.

Nugon-Baudon, L., and Rabot, S. (1994). Glucosinolates and glucosinolate derivatives: implications for protection against chemical carcinogenesis. *Nutrition Research Reviews*, **7**, 205–31.

O'Keefe, S.J.D., and Marks, V. (1977). Lunchtime gin and tonic a cause of reactive hypoglycaemia. *Lancet*, **(i)**, 1286–8.

O'Keefe, S.J.D., Sender, P.M., and James, W.P.T. (1974). 'Catabolic' loss of body nitrogen in response to surgery. *Lancet*, **(ii)**, 1035–8.

Oduho, G.W., Han, Y., and Baker, D.H. (1994). Iron deficiency reduces efficacy of tryptophan as a niacin precursor. *Journal of Nutrition*, **124**, 444–60.

Oguntoga, T.H.E., and Bender, A.E. (1976). *Journal of Food Technology*, **11**, 347–52.

Ohkawa, H., Ohishi, N., and Yagi, K. (1983a). New metabolites of riboflavin appear in human urine. *Journal of Biological Chemistry*, **258**, 5623–8.

Ohkawa, H., Ohishi, N., and Yagi, K. (1983b). Hydroxylation of the 7- and 8-methyl groups of riboflavin by the microsomal electron transfer system of rat liver. *Journal of Biological Chemistry*, **258**, 5629–33.

Ohkawa, H., Ohishi, N., and Yagi, K. (1986). Distribution of 8-hydroxyriboflavin in rat organs. *Journal of Biochemistry*, **99**, 945–50.

Olson, J.A. (1986). Metabolism of vitamin A. *Biochemical Society Transactions*, **14**, 928–30.

Olson, J.A. (1987a). Recommended Daily Intakes (RDI) of vitamin K in humans. *American Journal of Clinical Nutrition*, **45**, 687–92.

Olson, J.A. (1987b). Recommended dietary intakes (RDI) of vitamin A in humans. *American Journal of Clinical Nutrition*, **45**, 704–16.

Olson, J.A., and Hodges, R.E. (1987). Recommended Dietary Intakes (RDI) of vitamin C in humans. *American Journal of Clinical Nutrition*, **45**, 693–703.

Omdhal, J.L., and DeLuca, H.F. (1971). Strontium-induced rickets—a metabolic basis. *Science*, **174**, 949–51.

Osborne, T.B., Mendel, L.B., and Ferry, E.L. (1919). A method of expressing numerically the growth-promoting value of proteins. *Journal of Biological Chemistry*, **37**, 223–9.

Oser, B.L. (1951). Method for integrating essential amino acid content in the nutritional evaluation of foods. *Journal of the American Dietetic Association*, **27**, 396–402.

Ott, S.M., and Chesnut, C.H. (1989). Calcitriol treatment is not effective in post-menopausal osteoporosis. *Annals of Internal Medicine*, **110**, 267–74.

Page, M.G., Ankoma-Sey, V., Coulson, W.F., and Bender, D.A. (1989). Brain glutamate and γ-aminobutyrate (GABA) metabolism in thiamin deficient rats. *British Journal of Nutrition*, **62**, 245–53.

Paine, A.J., Allen, C.M., Durkacz, B.W., and Shall, S. (1982). Evidence that poly(ADP-ribose) polymerase is involved in the loss of NAD from cultured rat liver cells. *Biochemical Journal*, **202**, 551–3.

Palm, D., Klein, H.W., Schinzel, R., Buehner, M., and Helmreich, E.J.M. (1990). The role of pyridoxal 5'-phosphate in glycogen phosphorylase catalysis. *Biochemistry*, **29**, 1099–107.

Paquin, J., Baugh, C.M., and MacKenzie, R.E. (1985). Channeling between the active sites of formiminotransferase-cyclodeaminase: binding and kinetic studies. *Journal of Biological Chemistry*, **260**, 14925–31.

Parfitt, A.M. (1988). Use of calciferol and its metabolites and analogues in osteoporosis: current status. *Drugs*, **36**, 513–20.

Parsons, W.B. (1961). Treatment of hypercholesterolemia by nicotinic acid: progress report with review of studies regarding mode of action. *Archives of Internal Medicine*, **107**, 639–52.

Passmore, R., and Durnin, J.V.G.A. (1955) Human energy expenditure. *Physiological Reviews*, **35**, 801–40.

Paukert, J.L., Straus, L.D.A., and Rabinowitz, J.C, (1976). Formylmethenyl-methylenetetrahydrofolate synthetase (combined), an ovine protein with multiple catalytic activities. *Journal of Biological Chemistry*, **251**, 5104–11.

Paul, A.A., and Southgate, D.A.T. (1978). *McCance and Widdowson's 'The Composition of Foods'*, HMSO, London.

Pauling, L. (1970). Evolution and the need for vitamin C. *Proceedings of the National Academy of Sciences*, **67**, 1643–8.

Paumgartner, G., and Sauerbruch, T. (1991). Gallstones: pathogenesis. *Lancet*, **338**, 1117–21.

Pawlik, F., Bischoff, A., and Bitsch, I. (1977). Peripheral nerve changes in thiamine deficiency and starvation, an electron microscopic study. *Acta Neuropathologica (Berlin)*, **39**, 211–8.

Pelliniemi, T-T, and Beck, W.S. (1980). Biochemical mechanisms in the Killmann experiment, critique of the deoxyuridine suppression test. *Journal of Clinical Investigation*, **65**, 449–60.

Pendrys, D.G., and Stamm, J.W. (1990). Relationship of total fluoride intake to beneficial effects and enamel fluorosis. *Journal of Dental Research*, **69**, 529–38.

Peppler, W.W., and Mazess, R.B. (1981). Total body bone mineral and lean body mass by dual photon absorptiometry: (i) theory and measurement procedure. *Calcified Tissue International*, 33, 353–9.

Perry, T.L., Yong, V.W., Kish, S.J., Ito, M., Foulks, J.G., Godolphin, W.J., and Sweeney, V.P. (1985). Neurochemical abnormalities in brains of renal failure patients treated by repeated haemodialysis. *Journal of Neurochemistry*, 45, 1043–8.

Peters, R.A. (1963). *Biochemical Lesions and Lethal Synthesis*. Pergamon, Oxford.

Peterson, P.A., Nilsson, S.F., Ostberg, L., Rask, L., and Vahlquist, A. (1974). Aspects of the metabolism of retinol-binding protein and retinol. *Vitamins and Hormones*, 32, 181–214.

Peto, R., Doll, R., Buckley, J.D., and Sporn, M.B. (1981). Can dietary β-carotene materially reduce human cancer risk? *Nature*, 290, 201–8.

Phelps, D.L. (1987). Current perspectives on vitamin E in infant nutrition. *American Journal of Clinical Nutrition*, 46, 187–91.

Phillips, W.E.J., Mills, J.H.L., Charbonneau, S.M., Tryphonas, L., Hatina, G.V., Zawidzka, Z., Bryce, F.R., and Munro, I.C. (1978). Sub-acute toxicity of pyridoxine hydrochloride in the beagle dog. *Toxicology and Applied Pharmacology*, 44, 323–33.

Pi-Sunyer, F.X. (1991). Health implications of obesity. *American Journal of Clinical Nutrition*, 53, 1595–603s.

Picou, D., and Taylor-Roberts, T. (1969). The measurement of total protein synthesis and catabolism and nitrogen turnover in infants in different nutritional states and receiving different amounts of dietary protein. *Clinical Science*, 36, 283–96.

Pinto, J., Huang, Y.P., and Rivlin, R.S. (1981). Inhibition of riboflavin metabolism in rat tissues by chlorpromazine, imipramime, and amitriptyline. *Journal of Clinical Investigation*, 67, 1500–6.

Pirie, A., Werb, Z., and Burleigh, M.C. (1975). Collagenase and other proteinases in the cornea of the retinol deficient rat. *British Journal of Nutrition*, 34, 297–309.

Pisters, P.W.T., and Brennan, M.F. (1990). Amino acid metabolism in human cancer cachexia. *Annual Review of Nutrition*, 10, 100–32.

Portale, A.A., Halloran, B.P., and Morris, R.C. (1989). Physiological regulation of the serum concentration of 1,25–dihydroxyvitamin D by phosphorus in normal men. *Journal of Clinical Investigation*, 83, 1494–9.

Porter, J.W.G., and Thompson, S.Y. (1976). *Proceedings of the 4th International Congress of Food Science and Technology*, Madrid.

Postlethwait, R.W., and Johnson, W.D. (1972). Complications following surgery for duodenal ulcer in obese patients. *Archives of Surgery*, 105, 438–40.

Powell, J.J., and Thompson, R.P.H. (1993). The chemistry of aluminium in the gastrointestinal lumen, and its uptake and absorption. *Proceedings of the Nutrition Society*, 52, 241–53.

Prasad, A.S., Halsted, J.A., and Nadimi, M. (1961). Syndrome of iron deficiency anemia, hepatosplenomegaly, hypogonadism, dwarfism and geophagia. *American Journal of Medicine*, 31, 532–46.

Prasad, A.S., Miale, A., Farid, A., Schulert, A., and Sandstead, H.H. (1963). Zinc metabolism in patients with the syndrome of iron deficiency anemia, hypogonadism and dwarfism. *Journal of Laboratory and Clinmical Medicine*, 61, 537–49.

Prasad, A.S., Schoomaker, E.B., Ortega, J., Brewer, G.J., Oberleas, D., and Oelshlegel, F. (1975). Zinc deficiency in sickle cell disease. *Clinical Chemistry*, 21, 582–7.

Prasad, A.S., Meftah, S., Abdallah, J., Kaplan, J., Brewer, G.J., Bach, J.F., and Dardenne, M. (1988). Serum thymulin in human zinc deficiency. *Journal of Clinical Investigation*, 82, 1202–10.

Prentice, A.M., and Bates, C.J. (1981). A biochemical evaluation of the erythrocyte glutathione reductase (EC 1.6.4.2) test for riboflavin status: (i) rate and specificity of response in acute deficiency. *British Journal of Nutrition*, 45, 37–52.

Preusch, P.C., and Suttie, J.W. (1981). Vitamin K-dependent reactions in rat liver: role of flavoproteins. *Journal of Nutrition*, 111, 2087–97.

Preusch, P.C., and Suttie, J.W. (1984). Relationship of dithiothreitol-dependent microsomal vitamin K epoxide reductases inhibition of epoxide reduction by vitamin K quinone. *Biochimica et Biophysica Acta*, 798, 141–3.

Price, K.R., and Fenwick, G.R. (1985). Naturally occurring oestrogens in foods; a review. *Food Additives and Contaminants*, 2, 73–106.

Price, G., Millward, D.J., Pacy, P.J.H., and Halliday, D. (1990). Whole body protein homeostasis and protein requirement in man: validation studies of a new metabolic model. *Proceedings of the Nutrition Society*, 49, 194A.

Price, J.M., Yess, N., Brown, R.R., and Johnson, A.M. (1967). Tryptophan metabolism: hitherto unreported abnormality occurring in a family. *Archives of Dermatology*, 95, 462–72.

Priest, N.D. (1993). The bioavailability and metabolism of aluminium compounds in man. *Proceedings of the Nutrition Society*, 52, 2312–40.

Prosky, L., Asp, N-G, Furda, I., DeVries, J.W., Schweizer, T.F., and Harland, B.F. (1985). Determination of total dietary fiber in foods and food products: collaborative study. *Journal of the Association of Official Analytical Chemists*, 68, 677–9.

Prosky, L., Asp, N-G, Schweizer, T.F., DeVries, J.W., and Furda, I. (1988). Determination of insoluble, soluble and total dietary fiber in foods and food products: interlaboratory study. *Journal of the Association of Official Analytical Chemists*, 71, 1017–23.

Quigley, M.E., and Englyst, H.N. (1992). Determination of neutral sugars and hexosamines by high-performance liquid chromatography with pulsed amperometric detection. *Analyst*, 117, 1715–8.

Raffin, S.B., Woo, C.K., Roost, K.T., Price, D.C., and Schmid, R. (1974). Intestinal absorption of heme iron—heme cleavage by mucosal heme oxygenase. *Journal of Clinical Investigation*, 54, 1344–52.

Raisz, L.G., and Smith, J-A (1989). Pathogenesis, prevention and treatment of osteoporosis. *Annual Review of Medicine*, **40**, 251–67.

Ramotar, K., Conly, J.M., Chubb, H., and Louie, J. (1984). Production of menaquinones by intestinal anaerobes. *Journal of Inherited Diseases*, **150**, 213–22.

Rao, G.H., and Mason, K.E. (1975). Antisterility and anti-vitamin K activity of D-α-tocopheryl hydroquinone in the vitamin E deficient female rat. *Journal of Nutrition*, **105**, 495–8.

Rasmussen, K.N., Barsa, P.M., and McCormick, D.B. (1979). Pyridoxamine (pyridoxine) 5′-phosphate oxidase activity in rat tissues during development of riboflavin or pyridoxine deficiency. *Proceedings of the Society for Experimental Biology and Medicine*, **161**, 527–30.

Ray, C.S., Sue, D.Y., Bray, G., Hansen, J.E., and Wasserman, K. (1983). Effects of obesity on respiratory function. *American Review of Respiratory Diseases*, **128**, 501–6.

Rebuffé-Scrive, M. (1988). Steroid hormones and distribution of adipose tissue. *Acta Medica Scandinavica suppl.*, **723**, 143–6.

Reddy, V., and Sivakumar, B. (1972). Studies on vitamin A absorption. *Indian Paediatrics*, **9**, 307–10.

Redegeld, F.A.M., Moison, R.M.W., Koster, A.S.J., and Noordhoek, J. (1989). Alterations in energy status by menadione metabolism in hepatocytes isolated from fasted and fed rats. *Archives of Biochemistry and Biophysics*, **273**, 215–22.

Reichel, H., Koeffler, H.P., and Norman, A.W. (1989). The role of vitamin D endocrine system in health and disease. *New England Journal of Medicine*, **320**, 980–91.

Rennie, M.J., Tadros, L., Khogali, S., Ahmed, A., and Taylor, P.M. (1994). Glutamine transport and its metabolic effects. *Journal of Nutrition*, **124**, 1503–8S.

Reynolds, E.H. (1967). Effects of folic acid on the mental state and fit frequency of drug-treated epileptic patients. *Lancet*, **(i)**, 1986–9.

Reynolds, R.D. (1988). Bioavailability of vitamin B₆ from plant foods. *American Journal of Clinical Nutrition*, **48**, 863–7.

Riis, B.J. (1993). Biochemical markers of bone turnover (ii) diagnosis, prophylaxis and treatment of osteoporosis. *American Journal of Medicine*, **95**, (suppl 5a) 17–21s.

Rindi, G., and Ventura, U. (1972). Thiamine intestinal transport. *Physiological Reviews*, **52**, 821–827

Rink, T.J. (1994). In search of a satiety factor. *Nature*, **372**, 406–7.

Rivers, J.M. (1987). Safety of high-level vitamin C ingestion. *Annals of the New York Academy of Sciences*, **498**, 445–51.

Rivlin, R.S. (1970). Regulation of flavoprotein enzymes in hypothyroidism and in riboflavin deficiency. *Advances in Enzyme Regulation*, **8**, 239–50.

Rivlin, R.S., and Langdon, R.G. (1966). Regulation of hepatic FAD levels by thyroid hormone. *Advances in Enzyme Regulation*, **4**, 45–58.

Robertson, J., and Sissons, D.J. (1966). *Nutrition*, **20**, 21–7.

Robertson, J.A., and Gallagher, N.D. (1985). *In vivo* evidence that cobalamin is absorbed by receptor-mediated endocytosis in the mouse. *Gastroenterology*, **88**, 908–12.

Robinson, S.M., Jacquard, C., Peraud. C., Jackson, A.A., Jequier, E., and Schultz, Y. (1990). Protein turnover and thermogenesis in response to high-protein and high-carbohydrate feeding in men. *American Journal of Clinical Nutrition*, **52**, 72–80.

Robishaw, J.D., Berkich, D., and Neely, J.R. (1982). Rate-limiting step and control of coenzyme A synthesis in cardiac muscle. *Journal of Biological Chemistry*, **257**, 10967–72.

Robscheitt-Robbins, F.S., and Whipple, G.H. (1949a). Dietary effects on anaemia plus hypoproteinaemia in dogs: some protein further production of hemoglobin and others plasma plasma protein production. *Journal of Experimental Medicine*, **89**, 339–351.

Robscheitt-Robbins, F.S., and Whipple, G.H. (1949b). Dietary effects on anaemia plus hypoproteinaemia in dogs: findings with milk products, wheat and peanut flour as compared with liver. *Journal of Experimental Medicine*, **89**, 359–68.

Rockland, L.B., and Dunn, M.S. (1940). *Food Technology*, **3**, 289.

Roe, A., and Brickell, P.M. (1993). The nuclear retinoid receptors. *International Journal of Experimental Pathology*, **74**, 117–28.

Romessen, J.J. (1992). Fructose and related food carbohydrates. *Scandinavian Journal of Gastroenterology*, **27**, 819–28.

Rose, W.C. (1957). The amino acid requirements of adult man. *Nutrition Abstracts and Reviews*, **27**, 631–47.

Rose, D.P. (1966a). Excretion of xanthurenic acid in the urine of women taking progesterone-oestrogen preparations. *Nature*, **210**, 196–7.

Rose, D.P. (1966b). The influence of oestrogens on tryptophan metabolism in man. *Clinical Science*, **31**, 265–72.

Rose, C.S., Gyorgy, P., Butler, M., Andres, R., Norris, A.H., Shock, N.W., Tobin, J., Brin, M., and Spiegel, H. (1976). Age difference in vitamin B₆ status of 617 men. *American Journal of Clinical Nutrition*, **29**, 847–53.

Rosen, G.D., and Fernell, W.R. (1956). Microbiological evaluation of protein quality with *Tetrahymena pyriformis* W. *British Journal of Nutrition*, **10**, 156–69.

Ross, C.R., Diezi-Chomety, F., and Roch-Rachel, F. (1975). Renal excretion of N-methyl nicotinamide in the rat. *American Journal of Physiology*, **228**, 1641–5.

Rowan, M.J. (1993). Recent research on the causes of Alzheimer's disease. *Proceedings of the Nutrition Society*, **52**, 255–62.

Royal College of Physicians (1987). *A Great and Growing Evil: the Medical Consequences of Alcohol Abuse*. Tavistock, London.

Royal College of Physicians and the British Nutrition Foundation. (1984). Food Intolerance and Food Aversion. *Journal of the Royal College of Physicians*, **18**, 83–122.

Rumessen, J.J. (1992). Fructose and related food carbohydrates: sources, intakes, absorption and clinical implications. *Scandinavian Journal of Gastroenterology*, **27**, 819–28.

Ruz, M., Cavan, K.R., Bettger, W.J., and Gibson, R.S.. (1992) Erythrocytes, erythrocyte membranes, neutrophils and platelets as biopsy materials for the assessment of zinc status in humans. *British Journal of Nutrition*, **68**, 515–27.

Ryberg, D., and Alexander, J. (1990). Mechanisms of chromium toxicity in mitochondria. *Chemical-Biological Interactions*, **75**, 141–51.

Ryzen, E., Elbaum, N., Singer, F., and Rue, R.K. (1985). Parenteral magnesium tolerance testing in the evaluation of magnesium deficiency. *Magnesium*, **4**, 137–47.

Sadowski, J.A., Hood, S.J., Dallal, G.E., and Garry, P.J. (1989). Phylloquinone in plasma from elderly and young adults: factors influencing its concentration. *American Journal of Clinical Nutrition*, **50**, 100–8.

Saleh, A.M., Pheasant, A.E., Blair, J.A., Allan, R.N., and Walters, J. (1982). Folate metabolism in man: the effect of malignant disease. *British Journal of Cancer*, **46**, 346–53.

Salih, M.M., Bender, D.A., and McCreanor, G.M. (1985). Lethal familial pellagra-like skin lesion associated with neurologic and developmental impairment and the development of cataracts. *Pediatrics*, **76**, 787–93.

Salter, M., Bender, D.A., and Pogson, C.I. (1985). Leucine and tryptophan metabolism in rats. *Biochemical Journal*, **225**, 277–81.

Samonds, K.W., and Hegsted, D.M. (1977). Animal bioassays: a critical evaluation with special reference to assessing nutritive value for the human. In *Evaluation of Proteins for Humans* (ed. C.E. Bodwell) pp. 68–80. Avi Publishing, Westport.

Sanchez-Castillo, P., Warrender, S., Whitehead, T.P., and James, W.P.T. (1987). An assessment of the sources of dietary salt in a British population. *Clinical Science*, **72**, 95–102.

Sandström, B. (1992). Dose-dependence of zinc and manganese absorption in man. *Proceedings of the Nutrition Society*, **51**, 211–8.

Sankey, K. (1984). The practical effect of obesity on the insured life-relative risks associated with obesity and various disease states — 'the impaired life'. *Postgraduate Medical Journal*, **60**, suppl. 3, 5–12.

Sarwar, G., and McDonough, F.E. (1990). Evaluation of protein digestibility corrected amino acid score method for assessing protein quality of foods. *Journal of the Association of Official Analytical Chemists*, **73**, 347–56.

Sauberlich, H.E. (1975). Vitamin C status: methods and findings. *Annals of the New York Academy of Sciences*, **258**, 438–450.

Sauberlich, H.E., Canham, J.E., Baker, E.M., Raica, N., and Herman, Y.F. (1972). Biochemical assessment of the nutritional status of vitamin B6 in the human. *American Journal of Clinical Nutrition*, **25**, 629–642.

Sauberlich, H.E., Dowdy, R.P., and Skala, J.H. (1974a). *Laboratory Tests for the Assessment of Nutritional Status*. CRC Press, Cleveland, OH.

Sauberlich, H.E., Hodges, R.E., Wallace, D.L., Kolder, H., Canham, J.E., Hood, J., Raica, N., and Lowry, L.K. (1974b). Vitamin A metabolism and requirements in the human studied with the use of labelled retinol. *Vitamins and Hormones*, **32**, 251–75.

Schaeppi, U., and Krinke, G. (1982). Pyridoxine neuropathy: correlation of functional tests and neuropathology in beagle dogs treated with large doses of vitamin B6. *Agents and Actions*, **12**, 575–82.

Schaumburg, H., Kaplan, J., Windeland, A., Vick, N., Rasmus, S., Pleasure, D., and Brown, N.J. (1983). Sensory neuropathy from pyridoxine abuse, a new megavitamin syndrome. *New England Journal of Medicine*, **309**, 445–8.

Schiffman, S.S., and Gatlin, C.A. (1993). Clinical physiology of taste and smell. *Annual Review of Nutrition*, **13**, 405–36.

Schimke, R.T., Sweeney, E.W., and Berlin, C.M. (1965a). The roles of synthesis and degradation in the control of rat liver tryptophan pyrrolase. *Journal of Biological Chemistry*, **240**, 322–31.

Schimke, R.T., Sweeney, E.W., and Berlin, C.M. (1965b). Studies on the stability *in vivo* and *in vitro* of rat liver tryptophan pyrrolase. *Journal of Biological Chemistry*, **240**, 4609–20.

Schoeller, D.A., and Van Santen, E. (1982). Measurement of energy expenditure in humans by doubly-labelled water method. *Journal of Applied Physiology*, **53**, 955–9.

Schoental, R. (1983). Mycotoxins and nutritional deficiencies. *Nutrition and Health*, **2**, 147–52.

Schoffeniels, E., Dandrifose, G., and Bettendorf, L. (1984). Phosphate derivatives of thiamine and Na+ channel in conducting membrane. *Journal of Neurochemistry*, **43**, 269–71.

Schofield, W.N., Schofield, C., and James, W.P.T. (1985). Basal metabolic rate—review and prediction, together with an annotated bibliography of source material. *Human Nutrition : Clinical Nutrition*, **39C**, suppl. 1, 5–41.

Schorah, C.J., Habibzadeh, N., Hancock, M., and King, R.F.G.J. (1986). Changes in plasma and buffy layer vitamin C concentrations following major surgery: what do they reflect? *Annals of Clinical Biochemistry*, **23**, 5660–70.

Scott, J.M., Dinn, J.J., Wilson, P., and Weir, D.G. (1981). Pathogenesis of subacute combined degeneration, a result of methyl group deficiency. *Lancet*, **(ii)**, 334–7.

Schramm, W., and Bitsch, R. (1993). Selective measurement of vitamin B-6 derivatives in plant foods. *Bioavailability '93*, FECS event no 181, ISSN 0933–5463.

Schrijver, J., van Veelen, B.W., and Schreurs, W.H. (1985). Biochemical evaluation of the vitamin and iron status of an apparently healthy Dutch free-living elderly population: comparison with younger adults. *International Journal of Vitamin and Nutrition Research*, **55**, 337–49.

Schuster, K., Bailey, L.B., and Mahan, C.S. (1981). Vitamin B6 status of low income adolescent and adult pregnant women and the condition of their infants at birth. *American Journal of Clinical Nutrition*, **34**, 1731–5.

Schuster, K., Bailey, L.B., Dimperio, D., and Mahan, C.S. (1985). Morning sickness and vitamin B₆ status of pregnant women. *Human Nutrition Clinical Nutrition*, **39C**, 75–9.

Schwarz, K. (1974). Recent dietary trace element research, exemplified by tin, fluorine and silicon. *Federation Proceedings*, **33**, 1748–57.

Scientific Committee for Food (1993). *Nutrient and energy intakes for the European Community*. Commission of the European Communities, Luxembourg.

Scriver, C.R., Gregory, D.M., Sovetts, D., and Tissenbaum, G. (1985). Normal plasma free amino acids in adults: the influence of some common physiological variables. *Metabolism*, **34**, 868–73.

Scrutton, M.C., Griminger, P., and Wallace, (1972). Pyruvate carboxylase. *Journal of Biological Chemistry*, **247**, 3305–13.

Segal, K.R., Gutin, B., Presta, E., Wang, J., and Van Itallie, T.B. (1985). Estimation of human body composition by electrical impedance methods: a comparative study. *Journal of Applied Physiology*, **58**, 1565–71.

Seidell, J.C., Bakx, J.C., de Boer, E., Deurenberg, P., and Hautvast, J.G.A.J. (1985). Fat distribution of overweight persons in relation to morbidity and subjective health. *International Journal of Obesity*, **9**, 363–74.

Serdula, M.K., Koong, S.L., Williamson, D.F., Anda, R.F., Madans, J.H., Kleinman, J.C., and Byers, T. (1995). Alcohol intake and subsequent mortality: findings from the NHANES I follow-up study. *Journal of Studies on Alcohol*, **56**, 233–9.

Sethi, S., Gibney, M.J., and Williams, C.M. (1993). Postprandial lipoprotein metabolism. *Nutrition Research Reviews*, **6**, 161–83.

Sharma, R.V., Mathur, S.N., and Ganguly, J. (1976). Studies on the relative biopotencies and intestinal absorption of different apo-β-carotenoids in rats and chickens. *Biochemical Journal*, **158**, 377–83.

Sharma, R.V., Mathur, S.N., Dmitrovskii, A.A., Das, R.C., and Ganguly, J. (1977a). Studies on the metabolism of β-carotene and apo-β-carotenoids in rats and chickens. *Biochimica et Biophysica Acta*, **486**, 183–94.

Sharma, T.R., Kaul, A.K., and Niemann, G.G. (1977b). Evaluation of nutritional quality in plant cultivars using confused flour beetle, *Tribolium confusum*. *Qualitas Plantarum*, **27**, 303–12.

Shearer, M.J. (1990). Vitamin K and vitamin K-dependent proteins. *British Journal of Haematology*, **75**, 156–62.

Shearer, M.J., McBurney, A., and Barkhan, P. (1974). Studies on the absorption and metabolism of phylloquinone (vitamin K₁) in man. *Vitamins and Hormones*, **32**, 513–42.

Shen, Q., Chu, F.F., and Newburger, P.E. (1993). Sequences in the 3′-untranslated region of the human glutathione peroxidase gene are necessary and sufficient for selenocysteine incorporation at the UGA codon. *Journal of Biological Chemistry*, **268**, 11463–9.

Sherlock, S. (1995). Alcoholic liver disease. *Lancet*, **345**, 227–8.

Sherwood, L.M., and Russell, J. (1989). The role of 1,25–(OH)₂D₃ in regulating parathyroid gland function. *Proceedings of the Society for Experimental Biology and Medicine*, **191**, 233–7.

Shibata, K., Gross, C.J., and Henderson, L.M. (1983). Hydrolysis and absorption of pantothenate and its coenzymes in the rat small intestine. *Journal of Nutrition*, **113**, 2207–15.

Shiratori, T. (1974). Uptake storage and excretion of chylomicra-bound ³H-α-tocopherol by the skin of the rat. *Life Sciences*, **14**, 929–35.

Shulkes, A. (1994). Somatostatin: physiology and clinical applications. *Ballière's Clinical Endocrinology and Metabolism*, **8**, 215–36.

Shulman, G.I., Ladenson, P.W., Wolfe, M.H., Ridgway, E.C., and Wolfe, R.R. (1985). Substrate cycling between gluconeogenesis and glycolysis in euthyroid, hypothyroid, and hyperthyroid man. *Journal of Clinical Investigation*, **76**, 757–64.

Sies, H., Stahl, W., and Sundquist, (1992). Antioxidant functions of vitamins C and E, beta-carotene and other carotenoids. *Annals of the New York Academy of Sciences*, **669**, 7–20.

Silber, R.H., and Porter, C.C. (1950). In *Protein and Amino Acid Requirements of Mammals* (ed. A.A. Albanese). Academic Press, New York.

Sinclair, H.M. (1982). Essential fatty acids (vitamin F), In *Vitamins in Medicine*, 4th Ed, Vol II, (ed. B.M. Barker and D.A. Bender), Chapter 5, pp. 168–98. Heinemann Medical, London.

Sinden, S.L., and Deahl, K.L. (1976). Effect of glycoalkaloids and phenolics on potato flavour. *Journal of Food Science*, **41**, 520–3.

Siri, W.E. (1956). The gross composition of the body. In *Advances in Biological and Medical Physics*, Vol 4, (ed. C.A. Tobias and J.H. Laurence). Academic Press, New York.

Siri, W.E. (1961). Body composition from fluid spaces and density: analysis of methods. In *Techniques for measuring body composition*, (ed. J. Brozek and A. Henschel) National Academy of Sciences / National Research Council, Washington, DC.

Skulachev, V.P. (1991). Fatty acid circuit as a physiological mechanism of uncoupling of oxidative phosphorylation. *FEBS Letters*, **294**, 158–62.

Slaughter, M.H., Lohman, T.G., Boileau, R.A., Horswill, C.A., Stillman, R.J., van Loan, M.D., and Bemben, D.A. (1988). Skinfold equations for estimation of body fatness in children and youth. *Human Biology*, **60**, 709–23.

Smith, G.P., and Gibbs, J. (1992). Are gut peptides a new class of anorectic agents? *American Journal of Clinical Nutrition*, **55**, 283–5s.

Smith, J. (1991). *Food Additive User's Handbook*. Blackie Academic and Professional, London.

Smith, J.C., McDaniel, E.G., Fan, F.F., and Halsted, J.A. (1973). Zinc: a trace element essential in vitamin A metabolism. *Science*, **181**, 945–55.

Snedden, W., Mellor, C.S., and Martin, J.R. (1983). Familial hypertryptophanaemia, tryptophanuria and indoleketonuria. *Clinica Chimica Acta*, **131**, 247–56.

Snell, K. (1984). Enzymes of serine metabolism in normal developing and neoplastic rat tissues. *Advances in Enzyme Regulation*, **22**, 325–400.

Snyder, W.S., Cook, M.J., Nassett, E.S., Karkhausen, L.R., Parry-Howells, G., and Tipton, I.H. (1975). International Commission on Radiological Protection, *Report of the Task Group on Reference Man*. Pergamon, Oxford.

Sokol, R.J. (1988). Vitamin E deficiency and neurologic disease. *Annual Review of Nutrition*, **8**, 351–73.

Soll, A.H. (1990). Pathogenesis of peptic ulcer and implications for treatment. *New England Journal of Medicine*, **322**, 909–16.

Solomons, N.W., and Russell, R.M. (1980). The interaction of vitamin A and zinc: implications for human nutrition. *American Journal of Clinical Nutrition*, **33**, 2031–40.

Sommer, A. (1982). *Field Guide to the Detection and Control of Xerophthalmia*, 2nd edn. WHO, Geneva.

Somogyi, J.C. (1980). Naturally occurring toxicants in food. *Bibliotheca Nutritio et Dieta*, **29**, 110–27.

Somogyi, J.C., and Nageli, U. (1976). Antithiamin effect of coffee. *International Journal of Vitamin and Nutrition Research*, **46**, 149–53.

Sones, K., Heaney, R.K., and Fenwick, G.R. (1984). An estimate of the mean daily intake of glucosinolates from cruciferous vegetables in the UK. *Journal of the Science of Food and Agriculture*, **35**, 712–20.

Soprano, D.R., Smith, J.E., and Goodman, D.S. (1982). Effect of retinol status on retinol-binding protein biosynthesis rate and translatable messenger RNA level in rat liver. *Journal of Biological Chemistry*, **257**, 7693–7.

Souba, W.W. (1993). Intestinal glutamine metabolism and nutrition. *Journal of Nutritional Biochemistry*, **4**, 2–9

Souba, W.W. (1994). Cytokine control of nutrition and metabolism in critical illness. *Current Problems in Surgery*, **31**, 577–643.

Southgate, D.A.T. (1969). Determination of carbohydrates in foods: (ii) unavailable carbohydrates. *Journal of the Science of Food and Agriculture*, **20**, 331–5.

Spallholz, J.E. (1994). On the nature of selenium toxicity and carcinostatic action. *Free Radicals in Biology and Medicine*, **17**, 45–64.

Speck, W.T., Chen, C.C., and Rosenkranz, H.S. (1975). *In vitro* studies of effects of light and riboflavin on DNA and HeLa cells. *Pediatric Research*, **9**, 150–3.

Spector, R. (1986). Development and characterization of pantothenic acid transport in brain. *Journal of Neurochemistry*, **47**, 563–8.

Spellacy, W.N., Buki, W.B., and Birch, S.A. (1977). Vitamin B$_6$ treatment of gestational diabetes mellitus: studies of blood glucose and plasma insulin. *American Journal of Obstetrics and Gynecology*, **127**, 599–602.

Spencer, H., and Kramer, L. (1986). The calcium requirement and factors causing calcium loss. *Federation Proceedings*, **45**. 2758–62.

Srikantia, S.G., Narasinga-Rao, B.S., Raghuramulu, N., and Gopalan, C. (1968). Pattern of nicotinamide nucleo-tides in the erythrocytes of pellagrins. *American Journal of Clinical Nutrition*, **21**, 1306–9.

Stahl, W., Schwarz, W., Sundquist, A.R., and Sies, H. (1992). *Cis-trans* isomers of lycopene and beta-carotene in human serum and tissues. *Archives of Biochemistry and Biophysics*, **29**, 173–7.

Stamler, R., Stamler, J., Riedinger, W.F., Algera, G., and Roberts, R.H. (1978). Weight and blood pressure: findings in hypertension screening of 1 million Americans. *Journal of the American Medical Association*, **240**, 1607–12.

Stampfer, M.J., Maclure, K.M., Colditz, G.A., Manson, J.E., and Willett, W.C. (1992). Risk of symptomatic gallstones in women with severe obesity. *American Journal of Clinical Nutrition*, **55**, 652–8.

Steinberg, S., Campbell. C.L., and Hillman, R.S. (1979). Kinetics of the normal folate enterohepatic cycle. *Journal of Clinical Investigation*, **64**, 83–8.

Stenflo, J., Fernlund, P., Egan, W., and Roepstorff, P. (1974). Vitamin K-dependent modifications of glutamic acid residues in prothrombin. *Proceedings of the National Academy of Sciences*, **71**, 2730–5.

Stewart, R.A., Hensley, G.W., and Peters, F.N. (1943). Nutritive value of protein: effect of processing on oat protein. *Journal of Nutrition*, **26**, 519–26.

Strain, J.J.. (1994). Aspects of micronutrients in chronic disease: copper. *Proceedings of the Nutrition Society*, **53**, 583–98.

Sturman, J.A. (1988). Taurine in development. *Journal of Nutrition*, **118**, 1169–76.

Sutcliffe, J.F., Knight, G.S., Pinilla, J.C., and Hill, G.L. (1993). New and simple equations to estimate the energy and fat contents and energy density of humans in sickness and health. *British Journal of Nutrition*, **69**, 631–44.

Suttie, J.W., Mummah-Schendel, L.L., Shah, D.V., Lyle, B.J., and Greger, J.L. (1988). Vitamin K deficiency from dietary vitamin K restriction in humans. *American Journal of Clinical Nutrition*, **47**, 475–80.

Suzuki, H., Higuchi, T., Sawa, K., Ohtaki, S., and Horiuchi, Y. (1965). 'Endemic coast goitre' in Hokkaido, Japan. *Acta Endocrinologica* (Copenhagen), **50**, 161–76.

Swiatlow, N., O'Connor, D.L., Andrews, J., and Picciano, M.F. (1990). Relative folate bioavailability from diets containing human, bovine and goat milk. *Journal of Nutrition*, **120**, 172–7.

Symes, E.K., Bender, D.A., Bowden, J-F, and Coulson, W.F. (1984). Increased target tissue uptake of and sensitivity to testosterone in the vitamin B$_6$ deficient rat. *Journal of Steroid Biochemistry*, **20**, 1089–93.

Taché, Y., Garrick, T., and Raybould, H. (1990). Central nervous system action of peptides to influence gastrointestinal motor function. *Gastroenterology*, **98**, 517–28 .

Tada, K., Ito, H., and Wada, Y. (1963). Congenital tryptophanuria with dwarfism ('H' disease-like clinical features without indicanuria and generalized aminoaciduria): a probably new inborn error of tryptophan metabolism. *Tokohu Journal of Experimental Medicine*, **80**, 118–34.

Tajima, M., Iida, T., Yoshida, S., Komatsu, K., Namba, R., Yanagi, M., Noguchi, M., and Okamoto, H. (1990). The reaction product of peptidylglycine α-amidating enzyme is a hydroxyl derivative at α-carbon of the carboxyl-terminal glycine. *Journal of Biological Chemistry*, **265**, 9602–5.

Takai, S., and Shimaguchi, S. (1986). Are height and weight sufficient for the estimation of human body surface area? *Human Biology*, **58**, 625–38.

Tannenbaum, S.R., and Wishnok, J.S. (1987). Inhibition of nitrosamine formation by ascorbic acid. *Annals of the New York Academy of Sciences*, **258**, 354–61.

Tanner, J.M., and Whitehouse, R.H. (1973): Height and weight charts from birth to 5 years allowing for length of gestation: for use in infant welfare clinics. *Archives of Disease in Childhood*, **48**, 786–9.

Tanner, J.M., Whitehouse, R.H., and Takaishi, M. (1966a). Standards from birth to maturity for height, weight, height velocity and weight velocity: British children, 1965. Part i. *Archives of Disease in Childhood*, **41**, 454–71.

Tanner, J.M., Whitehouse, R.H., and Takaishi, M. (1966b). Standards from birth to maturity for height, weight, height velocity and weight velocity: British children, 1965. Part ii. *Archives of Disease in Childhood*, **41**, 613–35.

Tanumihardjo, S.A., Barua, A.B., and Olson, J.A. (1987). Use of 3,4–didehydroretinol to assess vitamin A status in rats. *International Journal of Vitamin and Nutrition Research*, **57**, 127–32.

Tappel, A.L., and Dillard, C.J. (1981). *In vivo* lipid peroxidation measurement via exhaled pentane and protection by vitamin E. *Federation Proceedings*, **40**, 174–78.

Tarr, J.B., Tamura, T., and Stokstad, E.L.R. (1981). Avalability of vitamin B_6 and pantothenate in average American diet. *American Journal of Clinical Nutrition*, **34**, 1328–37.

Taruvinga, M., Jackson, A.A., and Golden, M.H. (1979). Comparison of ^{15}N labelled glycine, aspartate, valine and leucine for measurement of whole body protein turnover. *Clinical Science*, **57**, 281–3.

Tayeh, M.A., and Marletta, M.A. (1989). Macrophage oxidation of L-arginine to nitric oxide, nitrite and nitrate: tetrahydrobiopterin is required as a cofactor. *Journal of Biological Chemistry*, **264**, 19654–8.

Tenenhouse, H.S., and Chu, Y.L. (1982). Hydrolysis of nicotinamide adenine dinucleotide by purified renal brush border membranes, mechanism of NAD^+ inhibition of brush border membrane phosphate transport activity. *Biochemical Journal*, **204**, 635–8.

Teratology Society (1987). Recommendations for vitamin A use during pregnancy. *Teratology*, **35**, 269–75.

Thaller, C., and Eichele, G. (1987). Identification and spatial distribution of retinoids in the developing chick limb bud. *Nature*, **327**, 625–8.

Thilly, C-H, Swennen, B., Bourdoux, P., Ntambue, K., Moreno-Reyes, R., Gillies, J., and Vanderpas, J.B. (1993). The epidemiology of iodine-deficiency disorders in relation to goitrogenic factors and thyroid-stimulating-hormone regulation. *American Journal of Clinical Nutrition*, **57**, 267s-70s.

Thomas, K. (1909). Uber die biologische Wertigkeit der Stickstoff-Substanzen in verschiedenen Nährungsmitteln. *Archive Anatomie und Physiologie*, 219–302, cited in Evans and Witty, 1978.

Thomas, P.J., and Hofmann, A.F. (1973). A simple calculation of the lithogenic index of bile: expressing biliary lipid composition on rectangular coordinates. *Gastroenterology*, **65**, 698–700.

Thompson, J.N., and Scott, M.L. (1970). Impaired lipid and vitamin E absorption related to atrophy of the pancreas in selenium-deficient chicks. *Journal of Nutrition*, **100**, 797–809.

Thompson, R.P.H. (1991). Assessment of zinc status. *Proceedings of the Nutrition Society*, **50**, 19–28.

Thornber, E.J., Dunlop, R.H., and Gawthorne, J.M. (1980). Thiamin deficiency in the lamb: changes in thiamin phosphate esters in the brain. *Journal of Neurochemistry*, **35**, 713–7.

Thornton, J.R., Emmett, P.M., and Heaton, K.W. (1983). Diet and gallstones: effects of refined and unrefined carbohydrate diets on bile cholesterol saturation and bile acid metabolism. *Gut*, **24**, 2–6.

Tomarelli, R.M., and Barnhart, F.W. (1947). Bioassay for proteins and protein digests. *Journal of Nutrition*, **34**, 263–72.

Tomkins, A., Behrnes, R., and Roy, S. (1993). The role of zinc and vitamin A deficiency in diarrhoeal syndromes in developing countries. *Proceedings of the Nutrition Society*, **52**, 131–42.

Traber, M.G., Ingold, K.U., Burton, G.W., and Kayden, H.J. (1988). Absorption and transport of deuterium substituted $2R4'R8'R$-α-tocopherol in human lipoproteins. *Lipids*, **23**, 791–7.

Tracey, K.J., and Cerami, A. (1990). Metabolic responses to cachectin/TNF: a brief review. *Annals of the New York Academy of Sciences*, **587**, 325–31.

Transport and Road Research Laboratory (1983). *The Facts About Drinking and Driving*. Crowthorne, Berks.

Trichopolou, A., and Vassilakou, T. (1990). Recommended dietary intakes in the European community member states: an overview. *European Journal of Clinical Nutrition*, **44**, (suppl 2) 51–125.

Tricker, A.R., and Preussmann, R. (1990). Chemical food contaminants in the initiation of cancer. *Proceedings of the Nutrition Society*, **49**, 133–44.

Trowell, H.C., Southgate, D.A.T., Wolever, T.M.S., Leeds, A.R., Gassull, M.A., and Jenkins, D.J.A. (1976). Dietary fibre redefined. *Lancet*, (i), 967.

Truswell, A.S., Irwin, T., Beaton, G.H., Suzue, R., Haenel, H., Hejda, S., Hou, X-C, Leveille, G., Morava, E., Pederson, J., and Stephen, J.M.L. (1983). Recommended Dietary Intakes around the world. *Nutrition Abstracts and Reviews, Reviews in Clinical Nutrition*, **53**, 939–1015 and 1075–19.

Tsuzaki, S., Matsuo, N., Saito, M., and Osano, M. (1990). The head circumference growth curve for Japanese children between 0–4 years of age: comparison with Caucasian children and correlation with stature. *Annals of Human Biology*, **17**, 297–303.

Uchida, K., Mitsui, M., and Kawakishi, S. (1989). Mono-oxygenation of N-acetylhistamine mediated by L-ascorbate. *Biochimica et Biophysica Acta*, **991**, 377–9.

Ul-Haq, R., and Chytil, F. (1988). Early effects of retinol and retinoic acid on protein synthesis in retinol deficient rat testes. *Biochemical and Biophysical Research Communications*, **151**, 53–60.

Underwood, E.J. (1977). *Trace Elements in Human and Animal Nutrition*. Academic Press, New York.

Underwood, B.A. (1990). Methods for assessment of vitamin A status. *Journal of Nutrition*, **120**, 1459–63.

Underwood, B.A. (1989). Teratogenicity of vitamin A. In *Elevated Dosages of Vitamins* (eds. P. Walter, H. Stahelin and G. Brubacher), pp. 42–55. Hans Huber Publishers, Toronto.

United Nations (1995a). Population Division, Department for Economic and Social Information, and Policy Analysis of the United Nations Secretariat. *World Population Prospects: the 1994 Revision*, Population Information Gopher of the United Nations Population Division, world-wide web http://www:undcp.org/unlinks.html.

United Nations (1995b) *Population Issues Briefing Kit*, United Nations Population Fund, Information and External Relations Division, world-wide web http://www:undcp.org/unlinks.html.

US Department of Agriculture and US Department of Health and Human Services (1990). *Dietary Guidelines for Americans, 3rd edn*. US Government Printing Office, Washington, DC.

van Deel, P., and Deelstra, H. (1993). Flair concerted action no 10 status papers: selenium. *International Journal of Vitamin and Nutrition Research*, **63**, 312–6.

van den Berg, H. (1993). Flair concerted action no 10 status papers: vitamin B_{12}. *International Journal of Vitamin and Nutrition Research*, **63**, 282–9.

van den Berg, H., Louwerse, E.S., Bruinse, H.W., Thissen, J.T.N.M., and Schrijver, J. (1986). Vitamin B_6 status of women suffering from premenstrual syndrome. *Human Nutrition Clinical: Nutrition*, **40C**, 441–50.

van der Meer, R.A., Groen, B.W., Jongejan, J.A., and Duine, J.A. (1990). The redox cycling assay is not suited for the detection of pyrroloquinoline quinone in biological samples. *FEBS Letters*, **26**, 131–4.

van der Westhuyzen, J., Fernandes-Costa, F., and Metz, J. (1982). Cobalamin inactivation by nitrous oxide produces severe neurological impairment in fruit bats: protection by methionine and aggravation by folates. *Life Sciences*, **31**, 2001–10.

van Gossum, A., Shariff, R., Lemoyne, M., Kurian, R., and Jeejeebhoy, K. (1988). Increased lipid peroxidation after lipid infusion as measured by breath pentane output. *American Journal of Clinical Nutrition*, **48**, 1394–9.

van Loan, M., and Mayclin, P. (1987). A new TOBEC instrument and procedure for the assessment of body composition: use of Fourier coefficients to predict lean body mass and total body water. *American Journal of Clinical Nutrition*, **45**, 131–7.

van Tilbeurgh, H., Sarda, L., Verger, R., and Cambillau, C. (1992). Structure of the pancreatic lipase-procolipase complex. *Nature*, **359**, 159–62.

Vanderslice, J.T., and Higgs, D.J. (1993). Quantitative determination of ascorbic, dehydroascorbic, isoascorbic, and dehydroisoascorbic acids by hplc in foods and other matrices. *Journal of Nutritional Biochemistry*, **4**, 184–90.

Vannuchi, H., and Moreno, F.S. (1989). Interaction of niacin and zinc metabolism in patients with alcoholic pellagra. *American Journal of Clinical Nutrition*, **50**, 364–9.

Vardi, P., and Tatar, I. (1955). *Nutrition Abstracts and Reviews*, **25**, 432.

Veenstra, J. (1991). Moderate alcohol use and coronary heart disease: a U-shaped curve? *World Review of Nutrition and Dietetics*, **65**, 38–71.

Veitch, K., Draye, J-P, van Hoof, F., and Sherratt, H.S.A. (1988). Effects of riboflavin deficiency and clofibrate treatment on the five acyl CoA dehydrogenases in rat liver mitochondria. *Biochemical Journal*, **254**, 477–81.

Vernet, O., Christin, L., Schutz, Y., Danforth, E., and Jequier, E. (1986). Enteral versus parenteral nutrition: comparison of energy metabolism in healthy subjects. *American Journal of Physiology*, **250**, E47–54.

Vesely, D.L., Kemp, S.F., and Elders, M.J. (1987). Isolation of a biotin receptor from hepatic membranes. *Biochemical and Biophysical Research Communications*, **143**, 913–6.

Vidal-Cros, A., Gaudrey, M., and Marquet, A. (1990). Vitamin K-dependent carboxylation: mechanistic studies with 3–fluoroglutamate-containing substrates. *Biochemical Journal*, **266**, 749–55.

Vimokesant, S.L., Nakornchai, S., Dhanamittas, S., and Hilker, D.M. (1974). Effect of tea consumption on thiamin status in man. *Nutrition Reports International*, **9**, 371–6.

Vir, S., and Love, A.H.G. (1878). Vitamin B_6 status of the hospitalized aged. *American Journal of Clinical Nutrition*, **31**, 1383–91.

Visek, W.J. (1984). An update of concepts of essential amino acids. *Annual Review of Nutrition*, **4**, 137–55.

von der Decken, A. (1983). Experimental studies on the quality of food proteins. *Comparative Biochemistry and Physiology* (B), **74**, 213–20.

Wadden, T.A., Stunkard, A.J., and Brownell, K.D. (1983). Very low calorie diets: their efficacy, safety and future. *Annals of Internal Medicine*, **99**, 675–84.

Wagner, C. (1964). Regulation of the tryptophan-nicotinic acid-DPN pathway in the rat. *Biochemical and Biophysical Research Communications*, **28**, 289–93.

Walker, A.R.P. (1951). Cereals, phytic acid and calcification. *Lancet*, **(ii)**, 244–8.

Wallin, R., Rossi, F., Loeser, R., and Key, L.L. (1990). The vitamin K-dependent carboxylation system in human osteosarcoma U2–OS cells: antidotal effect of vitamin K_1 and a novel mechanism for the action of warfarin. *Biochemical Journal*, **269**, 459–64.

Walters, M.R. (1992). Newly identified actions of the vitamin D endocrine system. *Endocrine Reviews*, **13**, 719–64.

Watanabe, I., Tomita, T., Hung, K-S, and Iwasaki, Y. (1981). Edematous necrosis in thiamine deficient encephalopathy of the mouse. *Journal of Neuropathology and Experimental Neurology*, **40**, 454–71.

Waterlow, J.C. (1972). Classification and definition of protein-calorie malnutrition. *British Medical Journal*, **(iii)**, 566–9.

Waterlow, J.C. (1973). Note on the assessment and classification of protein-energy malnutrition in children. *Lancet*, **(ii)**, 87–9.

Waterlow, J.C. (1984). Protein turnover with special reference to man. *Quarterly Journal of Experimental Physiology*, **69**, 409–38.

Waterlow, J.C.. (1992) *Protein-Energy Malnutrition*. Edward Arnold, London.

Waterlow, J.C., and Stephen, J.M.L. (1967). The measurement of total lysine turnover in the rat by intravenous infusion of L[U-^{14}C]lysine. *Clinical Science*, **33**, 489–506.

Waterlow, J.C., Buzina, R., Keller, W., Lane, J.M., Nichaman, M.Z., and Tanner, J.M. (1977). The presentation and use of height and weight data for comparing the nutritional status of groups of children under the age of 10 years. *Bulletin of the World Health Organization*, **55**, 489–98.

Waterlow, J.C., Garlick, P.J., and Millward, D.J. (1978). *Protein turnover in mammalian tissues and the whole body*. North-Holland, Amsterdam.

Wayner, D.D.M., Burton, G.W., and Ingold, K.U. (1986). The antioxidant efficiency of vitamin C is concentration dependent. *Biochimica et Biophysica Acta*, **884**, 119–23.

Webb, A. R., and Holick, M. F. (1988). The role of sunlight in the cutaneous production of vitamin D$_3$. *Annual Review of Nutrition*, **8**, 375–99.

Weir, J.B.deV (1949). New methods for calculating metabolic rate, with special reference to protein metabolism. *Journal of Physiology*, **109**, 1–9.

Wellcome Trust Working Party (1970). Classification of infantile malnutrition. *Lancet*, (ii), 302–3.

Wertz, A.W., Lojkin, M.I., Bouchard, B.S., and Derby, M.B. (1958). Tryptophan-niacin relationships in pregnancy. *Journal of Nutrition*, **64**, 339–53.

Westfall, R.J., Bosshardt, D.K., and Barnes, R.H. (1948). Influence of crude trypsin inhibitor on utilisation of hydrolysed protein. *Proceedings of the Society for Experimental Biology and Medicine*, **68**, 498–500.

Wetterhahn, K.E., and Hamilton, J.W. (1989). Molecular basis of hexavalent chromium carcinogenicity: effect on gene expression. *Science of the Total Environment*, **86**, 113–29.

Whitaker, T.R., and Patrick, H. (1971). A plasma amino acid method for determining protein quality. *Bulletin of Agriculture Experimental Station No 605 T*. West Virginia University, Virginia.

Whitehead, R.G. (1965). Hydroxyproline creatinine ratio as an index of nutritional status and rate of growth. *Lancet*, **(ii)**, 567–70.

Whitehead, R.G., and Dean, R.F.A. (1964). Serum amino acids in kwashiorkor: (i) relationship to clinical conditions. *American Journal of Clinical Nutrition*, **14**, 313–9.

Whiting, SJ. (1995). The inhibitory effect of dietary calcium on iron bioavailability: a cause for concern? *Nutrition Reviews*, **53**, 77–80.

WHO (1990). *Diet, Nutrition and the Prevention of Chronic Diseases*. WHO Technical Reports Series 797. WHO, Geneva.

WHO (1995). Global Health Situation and Projections Unit, world-wide web http://www/who

WHO/FAO (1973). *Energy and protein requirements: Report of a joint FAO/WHO ad hoc expert committee*. WHO Technical Reports Series 522, WHO, Geneva.

Widdowson, E.M., McCance, R.A., and Spray, C.M. (1951). The chemical composition of the human body. *Clinical Science*, **10**, 113–25.

Williams, D.L., and Marks, V. (1983). *Biochemistry in Clinical Practice*. Heinemann Medical, London.

Wilson, R.G., and Davis, R.E. (1984). Vitamin B$_6$ intake and plasma pyridoxal phosphate concentrations in the first two weeks of life. *Acta Paediatrica Scandinavica*, **73**, 218–24.

Wilson, S.D., and Horne, D.W. (1984). High performance liquid chromatographic determination of the distribution of naturally occurring folic acid derivatives in rat liver. *Analytical Biochemistry*, **142**, 529–35.

Wilson, A.T., and Reilly, C.S. (1993). Anaesthesia and the obese patient. *International Journal of Obesity*, **17**, 427–35.

Wittwer, C.T., Burkhard, D., Ririe, K., Rasmussen, R., Brown, J., Wyse, B.W., and Hansen, R.G. (1983). Purification and properties of a pantetheine-hydrolysing enzyme from pig kidney. *Journal of Biological Chemistry*, **258**, 9733–8.

Wojtczak, L., and Schonfeld, P. (1993). Effect of fatty acids on energy coupling processes in mitochondria. *Biochimica et Biophysica Acta*, **1183**, 41–57.

Wolf, B., and Feldman, G.L. (1982). The biotin-dependent carboxylase deficiencies. *American Journal of Human Genetics*, **34**, 699–716.

Wolff, J. (1969). Iodine goiter and the pharmacological effects of excess iodine. *American Journal of Medicine*, **47**, 101–24.

Wong, P.W.K., Forman, P., Tabahoff, B., and Justice, P. (1976). A defect in tryptophan metabolism. *Pediatric Research*, **10**, 725–30.

Woodward, B., and March, B.E. (1974). Effects of vitamin A on blood coagulation and clot lysis times. *Canadian Journal of Physiology and Pharmacology*, **52**, 984–90.

Woolley, D.W. (1946). The occurence of a pellagragenic agent in corn. *Journal of Biological Chemistry*, **163**, 773–4.

Wrong, O. (1978). Nitrogen metabolism in the gut. *American Journal of Clinical Nutrition*, **31**, 1587–93.

Wynn, V., and Doar, J.W.H. (1966). Some effects of oral contraceptives on carbohydrate metabolism. *Lancet*, **(i)**, 715–9.

Xerophthalmia Club (1990). Bulletin no 45. International Centre for Eye Health, 27 Cayton Street, London EC1V 9EJ, UK.

Yamada, O., Shin, M., Sano, K., and Umezawa, C. (1979). Effects of dietary excess leucine on nicotinamide nucleotide level in rat liver. *International Journal of Vitamin and Nutrition Research*, **49**, 376–85.

Yamamoto, H., Matsumoto, T., Fukumoto, S., Ikeda, K., Ishizuka, S., and Ogata, E. (1989). Effect of 24,25–dihydroxyvitamin D_3 on 1,25– dihydroxyvitamin D_3 metabolism in vitamin D deficient rats infused with 1,25–$(OH)_2D_3$. *Endocrinology*, **124**, 511–7.

Yang, G.Q., Wang, S.Z., Zhou, R.H., and Sun, S.Z. (1983). Endemic selenium intoxication of humans in China. *American Journal of Clinical Nutrition*, **37**, 872–81.

Yang, G., Zhou, L. Yin, S., Gu, L., Yan, B., Liu, Y., and Li, X. (1989a). Studies of safe maximal dietary Se intake in a seleniferous area in China (i) selenium intake and tissue selenium levels of the inhabitants. *Journal of Trace Elements and Electrolytes in Health and Disease*, **3**, 77–87.

Yang, G., Yin, S., Zhou, L. Gu, L., Yan, B., Liu, Y., and Liu, Y. (1989b). Studies of safe maximal dietary Se intake in a seleniferous area in China (ii) Relation between Se intake and the manifestation of clinical signs and certain biochemical alterations in blood and urine. *Journal of Trace Elements and Electrolytes in Health and Disease*, **3**, 123–30.

Yennai, S. (1980). Toxic factors induced by processing. In *Toxic Constituents of Plant Foodstuffs*. (ed I.E. Liener), pp. 371–427. Academic Press New York, London.

Young, V.R. (1994). Adult amino acid requirements: the case for a major revision in current recommendations. *Journal of Nutrition*, **124**, 1517–23s.

Young, V.R., and Marchini, J.S. (1990). Mechanisms and nutritional significance of metabolic responses to altered intakes of protein and amino acids with reference to nutritional adaptation in humans. *American Journal of Clinical Nutrition*, **51**, 270–89.

Young, V.R., and Munro, H.N. (1978). N^τ-methylhistidine (3–methylhistidine) and muscle protein turnover: an overview. *Federation Proceedings*, **37**, 2291–300.

Young, V.R., and Pellet, P.L. (1987). Protein intake and requirements with reference to diet and health. *American Journal of Clinical Nutrition*, **45**, 1323–43.

Young, V.R., Taylor, Y.S.M., Rand, W.R., and Scrimshaw, N.S. (1973). Protein requirements of man: efficiency of egg protein utilization at maintenance and submaintenance levels in young men. *Journal of Nutrition*, **103**, 1164–74.

Young, E., Patel, S., Stoneham, M.D., Rona, R.J., and Wilkinson, J.D. (1987). The prevalence of reaction to food additives in a survey population. *Journal of the Royal College of Physicians*, **21**, 241–7.

Young, V.R., Bier, D.M., and Pellett, P.L. (1989). A theoretical basis for increasing current estimates of the amino acid requirements in adult men, with experimental support. *American Journal of Clinical Nutrition*, **50**, 80–92.

Young, E., Stoneham, M.D., Petruckevitch, A., Barton, J., and Rona, R. (1994). A population study of food intolerance. *Lancet*, **343**, 1127–30.

Yudkin, J. (1971). *This Slimming Business*. MacGibbon and Kee, London

Zaman, Z., and Verwilghen, R.L. (1977). Effects of riboflavin deficiency on the activity of NADH-FMN oxidoreductase (ferriductase) and iron content of rat liver. *Biochemical Society Transactions*, **5**, 306–8.

Zerez, C.R., Wong, M.D., and Tanaka, K.R. (1990). Synthetase from human erythrocytes: evidence that enzyme activity is a sensitive indicator of lead exposure. *Blood*, **75**, 1576–82.

Zhang, Y., Proenca, R., Maffei, M., Barone, M., Leopold, L., and Friedman, J.M. (1994). Positional cloning of the mouse *obese* gene and its human homologue. *Nature*, **372**, 425–32.

Zitnak, A., and Filadefi, M.A. (1985). Estimation of taste thresholds of three potato glycoalkaloids. *Canadian Institute of Food Science and Technology Journal*, **18**, 337–9.

Zumoff, B. (1988). Hormonal abnormalities in obesity. *Acta Medica Scandinavica suppl.*, **723**, 153–60.

Index